Step By Step

HAIR TRANSPLANTATION

A special thanks to Dr Priyadarshini Das and Dr Alok Sahoo for doing all corrections in a short span of time

Step By Step
HAIR TRANSPLANTATION

Expand the Dermatologist's knowledge on concepts and techniques of FUE hair transplantation

Editors

Pradeep Sethi
MBBS MD (AIIMS, New Delhi)
Honorary Professor Dermatology—Hair Transplant
DY Patil University, Mumbai
Hair Transplant Surgeon
Eugenix Hair Sciences
Mumbai, Maharashtra, India

Arika Bansal
MD (AIIMS, New Delhi) Gold Medalist
Diplomate ABHRS (American Board of Hair Restoration Surgery)
Hair Transplant Surgeon
Eugenix Hair Sciences
Gurugram, Delhi NCR, India

Abhinav Kumar
MBBS (MAMC) MD (LHMC)
Hair Transplant Surgeon
Eugenix Hair Sciences
Gurugram, Delhi NCR, India

Sarita Sanke
MBBS (BMCRI) MD DNB (LHMC)
Senior Resident
Lady Hardinge Medical College
New Delhi, India

Foreword

Robert H True

JAYPEE BROTHERS MEDICAL PUBLISHERS
The Health Sciences Publisher
New Delhi | London | Panama

JAYPEE Jaypee Brothers Medical Publishers (P) Ltd.

Headquarters
Jaypee Brothers Medical Publishers (P) Ltd
4838/24, Ansari Road, Daryaganj
New Delhi 110 002, India
Phone: +91-11-43574357
Fax: +91-11-43574314
Email: jaypee@jaypeebrothers.com

Overseas Offices

J.P. Medical Ltd
83 Victoria Street, London
SW1H 0HW (UK)
Phone: +44 20 3170 8910
Fax: +44 (0)20 3008 6180
Email: info@jpmedpub.com

Jaypee-Highlights Medical Publishers Inc
City of Knowledge, Bld. 235, 2nd Floor
Clayton, Panama City, Panama
Phone: +1 507-301-0496
Fax: +1 507-301-0499
Email: cservice@jphmedical.com

Jaypee Brothers Medical Publishers (P) Ltd
Bhotahity, Kathmandu, Nepal
Phone: +977-9741283608
Email: kathmandu@jaypeebrothers.com

Website: www.jaypeebrothers.com
Website: www.jaypeedigital.com

Step by Step Hair Transplantation

First Edition: **2019**

ISBN: 978-93-5270-537-5

Printed at: Samrat Offset Pvt. Ltd.

CONTRIBUTORS

Abhinav Kumar
MBBS (MAMC) MD (LHMC)
Hair Transplant Surgeon
Eugenix Hair Sciences
Gurugram, Delhi NCR, India

Alok Sahoo
MBBS MD (AIIMS, New Delhi)
Hair Transplant Surgeon
Eugenix Hair Sciences
Gurugram, Delhi NCR, India

Anil Kumar Garg
MS MCh ABHRS FISHRS
Plastic Surgeon
Rejuvenate Hair Transplant Center
Indore, Madhya Pradesh, India

Arika Bansal
MD (AIIMS, New Delhi) Gold Medalist
Diplomate ABHRS (American Board of Hair Restoration Surgery)
Hair Transplant Surgeon
Eugenix Hair Sciences
Gurugram, Delhi NCR, India

Arvind Poswal (Ex-Capt)
MBBS (AFMC)
Hair Transplant Surgeon
Dr A's Clinic
New Delhi, India

Bessam Farjo
MB ChB ABHRS
Hair Transplant Surgeon
Farjo Hair Institute
Quay Street
Manchester, UK

Chiara Insalaco MD PhD
Plastic and Reconstructive Surgeon
Via Flaminia, Rome, Italy

Hyun-Wook Baik MD
Nobline Clinic
Seoul, South Korea

Manas Chatterjee MD DNB
Associate Professor
Department of Dermatology
Institute of Naval Medicine
INHS Asvini
Mumbai, Maharashtra, India

Nicole Rogers MD FAAD FISHRS
Hair Restoration of the South
Galleria Drive Ste.
Metairie, Louisiana, USA

Piero Tesauro MCh (Plastic Surgery)
Hair Transplant Surgeon
Via Melchiorre Gioia
Milan, Italy

Pradeep Sethi
MBBS MD (AIIMS, New Delhi)
Honorary Professor Dermatology—Hair Transplant
DY Patil University, Mumbai
Hair Transplant Surgeon
Eugenix Hair Sciences
Mumbai, Maharashtra, India

Priyadarshini Das MBBS
Hair Transplant Surgeon
Eugenix Hair Sciences
Mumbai, Maharashtra, India

Raghunatha Reddy
MD DNB FRGUHS
Dermatologists and Dermatologic Surgeon
Dr Raghu's Mathapitha Skin Clinic
Bengaluru, Karnataka, India

Rajesh Kumar MD
Associate professor
Grant Medical College
Mumbai, Maharashtra, India

Robert Haber MD
Clinical Associate Professor
Department of Dermatology and Pediatrics
Case Western Reserve University
School of Medicine
Beachwood, Ohio, USA

Sarita Sanke
MBBS (BMCRI) MD DNB (LHMC)
Senior Resident
Lady Hardinge Medical College
New Delhi, India

FOREWORD

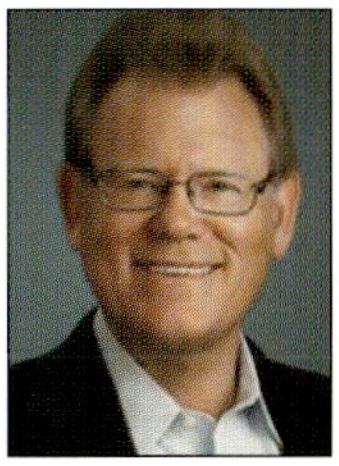

Drs Pradeep Sethi, Arika Bansal, Abhinav Kumar, and Sarita Sanke have teamed up to write an important practical guide to modern hair transplantation. All of the authors have entered the field of hair restoration surgery (HRS) within the past ten years and so what they present is truly a 21st century view of the field.

The book is comprehensive in discussion of all aspects of HRS. They begin with the all-important topics of patient evaluation, preoperative planning, and pre-, intra-, and postoperative care. The authors outline underlying principles and practical tips in design elements for the hairline, temples, and crown.

The authors have focused their surgical approach on follicular unit excision (FUE), which has emerged as a dominant, if not preferred, technique of harvesting grafts for transplantation. They present a thorough discussion of details in the techniques required to excise high quality grafts, to extract the grafts and handle them while out of the body and during placement to achieve optimal outcomes.

There is a special emphasis in this book on the importance of minimizing time out of the body for the grafts. The authors' approach is to perform graft removal and placement simultaneously, which they call "direct hair transplantation (DHT)." This is an excellent approach. HRS surgeons who remove the grafts in-toto before they start to place are faced with special challenges in survival of grafts held out of body over extended time. These doctors have to resort to expensive designed cold storage solutions and systems in order to optimize graft survival. The DHT approach side-steps this necessity. The DHT technique is similar in concept to the approach of the direct hair implantation (DHI) from Greece. However, to the best of my knowledge the DHI technique has not been described in such academic detail as in this book.

As a bonus, the authors have added chapters on beard harvesting and transplantation, eyebrow transplantation, eyelash reconstruction, as well as the unique aspects of treating women with hair loss. In addition, they present a well-conceived and executed approach to the difficult cases of those requiring corrective surgery and to the causes, prevention, and management of surgical complications.

In the final chapter, they give well thought through practical advice on how to start and manage a hair transplant practice.

I have been a hair restoration surgeon for over 25 years and as a clinician I know how hard it is to work on professional papers and textbooks in the midst of keeping up with a busy practice. But Drs Pradeep Sethi, Arika Bansal, Abhinav Kumar, and Sarita Sanke deserve high praise for their accomplishment in writing this guide. Who better than clinical practitioners to create a step-by-step guide that is indeed practical and useful to other doctors including beginners and experienced surgeons. My congratulations to the authors and my welcome to you fortunate readers.

Robert H True MD MPH
Fellow and Past Scientific Chair
International Society of Hair Restoration Surgery
Diplomate and Past President
American Board of Hair Restoration Surgery
Editor Emeritus *Hair Transplant Forum International*

PREFACE

In last one decade, the science of hair transplantation has evolved to a great extent and moreover it has been accepted by patients widely. The incidence, detection and overall androgenetic alopecia cases have also increased including the female patients. While this was happening, baring few books and annual meets, there were not much teaching materials available for systematic training. When we started in 2010 we hardly had much materials to read and not much training in Asia. Over the years of working upon more than 4000 odd patients, we were very particular about scientific documentation of the pictures of all the cases in right angles, background. Who has ever entered into the field of aesthetics including hair restoration would agree that the artistry of the work is as important or more important than the science alone. One has to evolve daily as an artist with each procedure.

In the meantime, the teacher in me found junior doctors who wanted to learn from us the way we do the procedure. Teaching helps in learning more. We thought it is important to put the well-documented self-explanatory pictures in a book format with systematic step-by-step explanations. (This book is primarily pictures, but having enough explanations). We have tried to compile chapters relevant to the practical procedure that is done in the theater. There is more focus upon hairline design as we believe that hairline is the gateway into the face of the person and it has to be a designer's job. Also, there is a focus upon DHT (direct hair transplantation)—a modified FUE (follicular unit excision) technique where grafts are planted simultaneously with extraction which enhances the survival chances of the grafts by reducing the time outside body for the grafts, thus reduces the chances of damage by mechanical trauma, desiccation and infection. Another highlight of the book would be the graft implantation in the pre-made slits by implanters. The implanters ensure that the grafts are not damaged during plantation. It is very important in the hands of the not very experienced technicians who do placement of the grafts. The precision and control required by the small muscles of the hand is high, lest a little bit of extra pressure while handling the grafts and placing them can damage the grafts. Here the loaded grafts in the implanters are to be unloaded in the pre-made slits, which are made in right depth, density and angle by the primary surgeon, who controls the whole procedure. Also, we have added the chapter of evaluation of cases of hair transplantation as it is a very important aspect of hair transplantation. With the rise of female hair transplantation cases, it was also important to highlight the important practical points. Advanced grades of baldness needed special mention because it is usually difficult for neophyte as well as veteran surgeons to provide the adequate density required to cover grade 6–7 baldness cases. Due to inadequate training and whatsoever many patients get botched up jobs and we are encountering a lot of patients with a demand for "re do". So, there is a chapter upon corrective hair transplantation.

Pradeep Sethi

ACKNOWLEDGMENTS

अपूर्वः कोपि कोशोयं विद्यते तव भारती
व्ययतो वृद्धिम् आयाति क्षयम् आयाति संचयात्

Apoorvah kopi koshoyam vidyate tav Bharati
Vyayato vruddhim aayaati kshyam aayaati sanchayaat.

The meaning of the above shloka is "O Goddess Saraswati, your treasure is unique in nature. It increases when it is freely spent and gets destroyed if it is hoarded (and not shared with others)".

The underlying idea in this message is that more the knowledge is shared, the more it tends to broaden and improve the basis of the concept of this knowledge as and when shared, leading to opening of new vistas of knowledge. If knowledge is kept by a person to himself, it perishes and is wasted and lost forever. This has been and observed many a times over time. (I had first read this Sanskrit verse on a plaque that was hanging on the entrance wall of our library of my MBBS medical college. I always remember this verse when I intend to write, speak or publish any important paper on any subject).

One of my latest work is this book I have co-authored *Step by Step Hair transplantation*. It is about my wondrous journey for me as an individual, my delights, my pains and struggle all have been a massive learning and to be honest I loved every bit of it. I have learnt and unlearnt a lot over this time. As the saying goes 'One who thinks that he has devoured all the knowledge there is in this universe, he brings death unto himself' and so I believe learning is an everyday affair.

These past two years of my life that I have dedicated to completion of this book and it would not have been possible without the help of many people. My heartfelt gratitude to each and everyone involved in the book no matter how minuscule their role has been.

I would like to specially mention my whole surgical team Drs Arika Bansal, Shishir, Abhinav Kumar and Priyadarshini Das who have consistently worked hard along with me and absorbed my "perfectionist" episodes. My ever reliable OT technicians Ravi Kumar, Manoranjan Sethi, Giridhari Sethi, Adarsha Sahoo, Kharabela Samal, Rakshyakar Behera to name a few. To my zealous and conscientious group of counsellors; Nelson, Shikha, Vrushali, and Alkesh who play a key role regarding patient associations.

To my efficient technical staff, Debashish and Rajesh who made sure I had every picture or video that I needed which have been collected over the years. Thanks to all my fellow doctors and colleagues; Robert True, Robert Haber, Nicole Rogers, Anil Kumar Garg, Bessam Farjo, Chiara Insalaco, Michael Baik, Arvind Poswal, Piero Tesauro, Manas Chatterjee, Raghunath Reddy and Rajesh Kumar who have provided critical inputs to me whenever they were required.

I am deeply indebted to my patients without whom not only would this book, but I myself as a surgeon would be incomplete. I would like to mention the names of Ashish Joneja and Rahul Raichand who as patients helped me to know more about the psychology of hair loss patients and the expectations of them from the doctor. Mrs (Dr) Dalmiya helped me a lot understanding the details of the female hairline aesthetics.

A loud mention of two senior doctors; Dr Kiran Godse and Dr Kabeer Sardana, they both pressed me hard with affection to write down my experiences of the subject that I am so passionate about. Without their constant pressure this book would not have seen the daylight! The name *Step by Step Hair Transplantation* was suggested by Dr Kabeer Sardana in one flight from Delhi to Dehradun.

Special gratitude to the team at M/s Jaypee Brothers Medical Publishers (P) Ltd, New Delhi, India; Shri Jitendar P Vij (Group Chairman), Mr Ankit Vij (Managing Director), Ms Chetna Malhotra Vohra (Associate Director—Content Strategy), Ms Prerna Bajaj (Development Editor) and Subrato Adhikari (Commissioning Editor) who were wonderful supports to me and a pleasure to work with.

No credit is enough for my co-authors Dr Arika Bansal, Dr Abhinav Kumar, Dr Sarita Sanke who have also given their sweat and blood in this book and made it happen. There is a special mention needed for the hard work and sacrifices of Abhinav Kumar who shaped the dream of this book into reality. Dr Priyadarshini Das, who just joined us recently helped us in fine tuning the copy and many miscellaneous aspects. She is an amazing creative writer with scientific approach.

Lastly I am forever grateful to my loving family for their undying support; my late father (I inherited the passion for work from him), my mother Sashi Sethi, my wife Arika Bansal, and my high spirited sons Arkin and Aryaveer. With a heavy heart I also take this opportunity to state that I have not always been there for my family when consumed by this journey. I hope they have it in them to forgive me.

I have attempted to bring out to the readers, my unbiased knowledge and observations in this book to help and introspect the ever evolving field of Hair Transplant Science.

CONTENTS

Norwood-Hamilton scale/Classification of hair loss in men

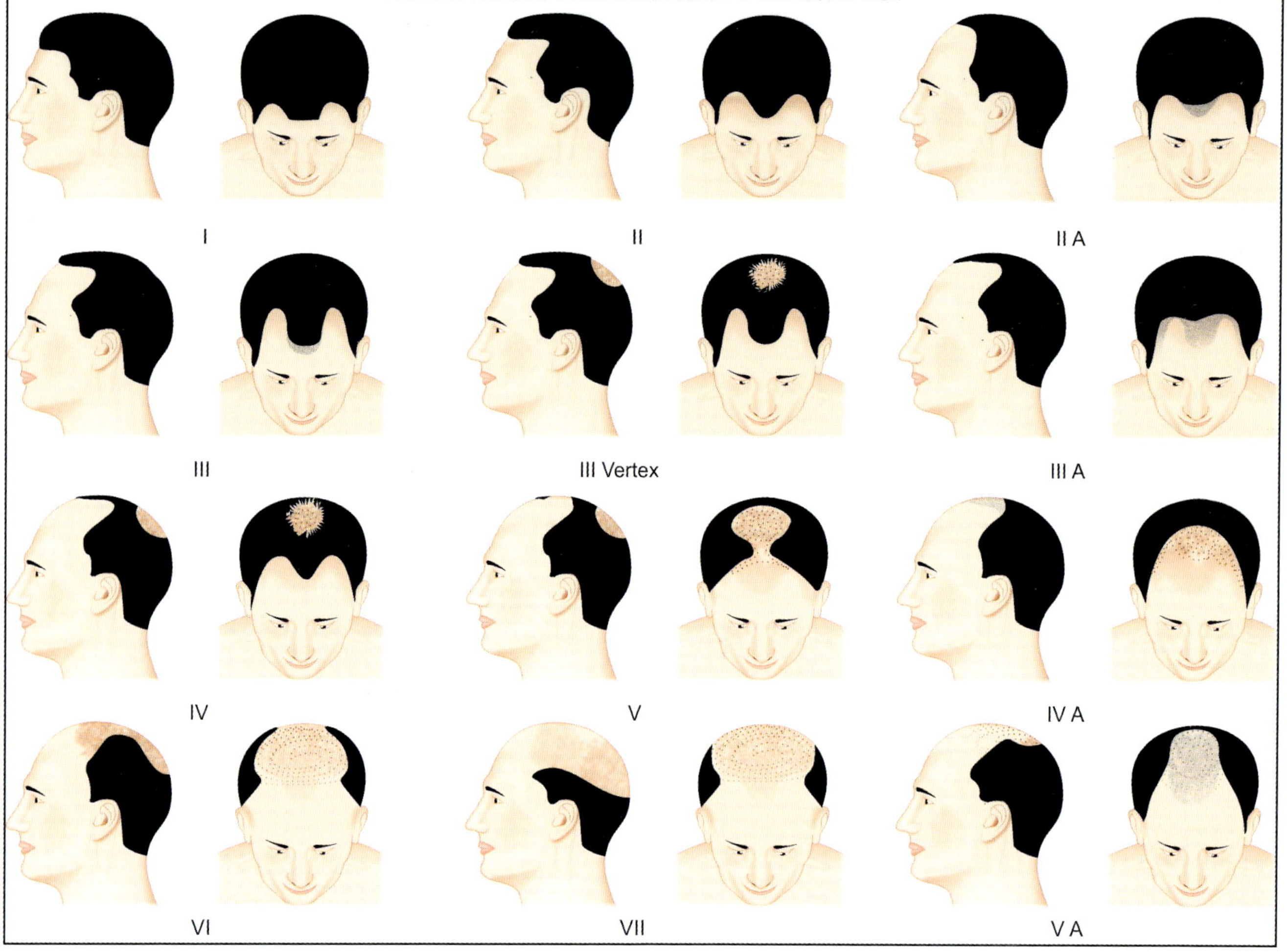

The Norwood or Norwood-Hamilton Scale

The progression of male pattern baldness is generally classified on the *Hamilton-Norwood scale*, which ranges from stages I to VII. This measurement scale was first introduced by James Hamilton in the 1950s and later revised and updated by O'Tar Norwood in the 1970s. It is sometimes referred to as the *Norwood-Hamilton scale* or simply the *Norwood scale.*

Type I: Minimal to no hair loss along the frontotemporal region.

Type II: The anterior border of the hairline exhibits frontotemporal recession that does not extend farther than a line drawn through the coronal plane 2 cm anterior to the external auditory meatus.

Type III: Frontotemporal recession extends beyond the coronal plane drawn 2 cm anterior to the external auditory meatus.

Type IV: It has greater frontotemporal recession than type III along with significant hair loss in crown area. The two areas are connected by a bridge which is relatively dense compared to other areas.

Type V: There is extensive alopecia in frontotemporal and vertex region. There is only small bridge of dense hair between two areas.

Type VI: There is complete absence of hair in the bridge joining the vertex and frontotemporal region. Hair loss extends posteriorly and laterally. The hump is not lost.

Type VII: It is the most severe variant with horse-shoe shaped hairy zone that remains on the posterior and lateral border of hairline.

Variant of Norwood scale

In this variant, the frontotemporal recession marches posteriorly along with the posterior march of central or anterior peninsula of hair.

Type IIA: It refers to a condition in which the entire hairline is receded uniformly across the forehead, but does not extend posterior to the coronal plane drawn 2 cm anterior to the external auditory meatus.

Type IIIA: In this, the entire hairline extends to the mid-coronal plane drawn 2 cm anterior to the external auditory meatus.

Type IVA: The hair loss extends past the mid-coronal line drawn 2 cm anterior to the external auditory meatus.

Type VA: The hair loss extends to the vertex and severe form of this variant becomes indistinguishable from Type V and Type VI.

CHAPTER 1

Evaluation, Workup and Postoperative Care in Hair Transplant

Rajesh Kumar, Pradeep Sethi, Abhinav Kumar, Sarita Sanke

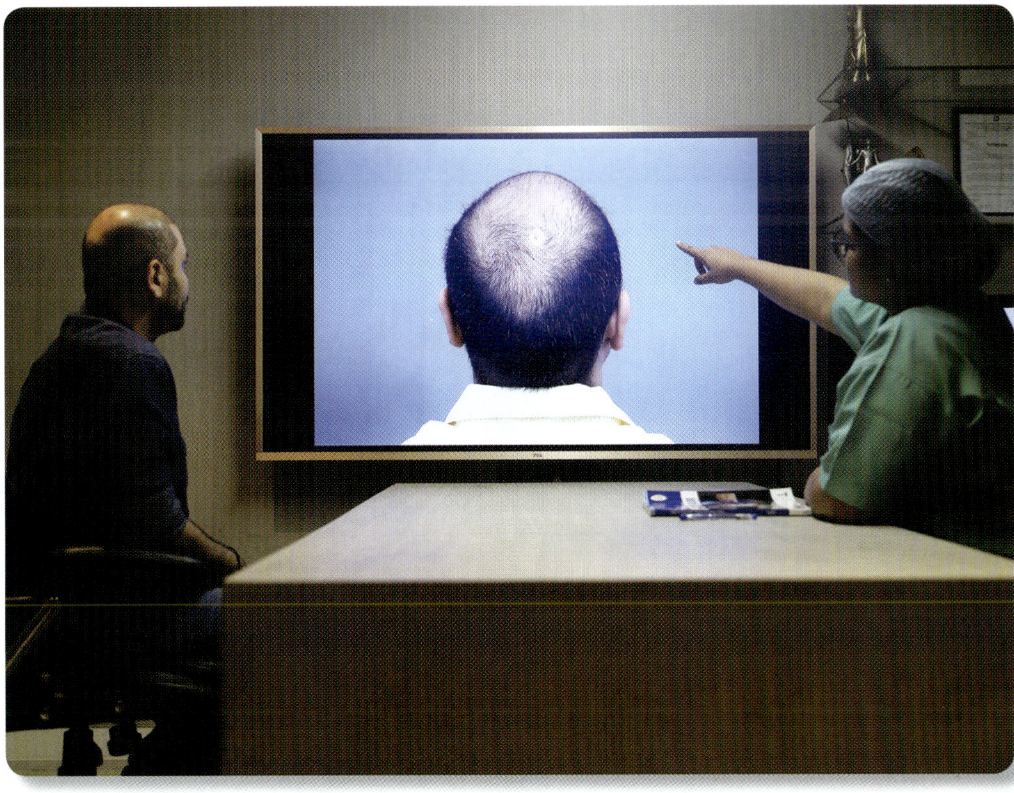

"What the mind doesn't know, the eyes cannot see."

A complete knowledge of the possibilities of each and every individual case depending upon the assessment of the donor area, recipient zone, expectations of the patient and the futuristic approach would end up having a great outcome in terms of a happy patient for ever.

INTRODUCTION

A good patient selection is of utmost importance in order to get a good result. An important thing to keep in mind is that androgenetic alopecia is an ongoing process with no specific boundaries. The age of the patient, the donor area, expectations of the patient are all important things to consider.

Before hair transplantation (HT), thorough examination of the scalp should be done to evaluate any type of lesions.

Any kind of scalp pathology should be dealt with first. Scalp folliculitis should be dealt with antibiotics, seborrhea with an antidandruff shampoo and mild steroid if necessary.

The number of grafts to be offered in any patient is always an approximate calculation based on the patient's age, family history of hair loss and the present extent of hair loss and the donor quality. A young patient or a candidate with grade III or grade IV baldness should initially be prescribed the medical treatment and reassessed after a year to assess the response and need of surgery.

CONSULTATION

It is important for an HT surgeon to understand the patient's needs and demands and to make it very clear to the patient about the expected results. A simple question like "what do you expect?" makes many things clear. The HT surgeon must be able to make him understand that hair loss is an ongoing process and more than one session will eventually be needed. The patient must understand that facial framing is far more important than the density of hair and also that the transplanted hairline is permanent. Disadvantages of keeping a low hairline must be clearly explained especially in a young patient. Satisfying a young patient may lead to problems in their older age.

HISTORY

A history regarding any bleeding problems, hypertension, diabetes mellitus, any medications, drug allergies, vitamin supplementation or heart surgery should be taken. Medicines like aspirin should be stopped 2 weeks prior to surgery, clopidogrel should be stopped 5 days prior and heparin and warfarin 24 hours prior. Alcohol intake should be stopped 3–4 days before surgery.

COUNSELING

A counselor plays the role of a mediator between the physician and the patient. He should be available to answer any type of silly questions pertaining to surgery by the patient. He should be able to win the patient's confidence and make him comfortable. He should be able to provide factual information rather than just persuading the patient. An honest and clear opinion must be given to the patient. The counselor should educate the patient about the nature of the medical aspects of hair loss problems and the various etiological factors involved. He should explain about the concept of visual density which will be achieved after HT. The salient points about step-by-step procedure of HT should be explained in detail. The patient should also be counseled regarding the use of the Food and Drug Administration (FDA) approved topical minoxidil and oral finasteride (in males and postmenopausal women) both pre- and post-HT surgery and the progressive nature of hair loss. The care of hair, post-transplant should also be explained in detail. It is always better to under promise and over deliver.

PATIENT SELECTION

According to the authors, surgery should be postponed in young patients under the age of 25 years due to their unreasonable expectations and demands. Also they are likely to have further hair loss in their coming years and would need further sessions of hair restoration. If at all a young patient demands for hair restoration surgery, care should be taken to set a higher hairline and avoiding grafting in the vertex area. However, in cases where patient achieved Norwood grade VI we can go ahead with full coverage with a higher hairline by mixing scalp and beard hair. It is advisable to not do temple reconstruction in such cases.

Candidates with thin and fine hair should be chosen with care as poor outcome with less density is common in such patients. Even if the growth of transplanted hair in these patients is good, they will not appreciate significant difference in their pre- and post-transplant look. Those with large caliber hair shaft (>80 μm) obtain a denser coverage than those with silky hair. Patients with a good density of donor area [>80 follicular units (FUs)/cm^2] are excellent candidates. Those with less than 40 FUs/cm^2 are considered poor candidates.

Most patients with advanced Norwood type VI and type VII are poor candidates for surgery unless they have a donor area of at least 6,500 grafts to donate. However, coverage in such candidates is now possible with the use of beard grafts. If the donor area is sparse, it is a sensible option to just make a frontal forelock connecting the temporal zones rather than trying to give a full coverage. The vertex transplantation is the most problematic area as it consumes considerable donor grafts. In later years, the patient often becomes dissatisfied due to progressive peripheral loss of nontransplanted hair. In patients with scarring alopecia, the graft uptake and survival will be affected and should be counseled regarding the same before taking up for the surgery.

CALCULATING THE NUMBER OF GRAFTS

A surgeon must always estimate the number of grafts required to give a satisfying result to the patient. There is no hard and fast rule of estimating the number of grafts that can be obtained from a particular donor area. However, a cosmetically acceptable extraction ratio should not exceed one of every four follicles (25% extraction). To estimate the total number of follicles that can be extracted, we have to divide the total number of FUs by 4 for obtaining a 25% yield.[1] In practice, we extract much more than what guidelines say but do not see any impact on donor aesthetics even with slightly more aggressive extraction.

PREPARING THE DONOR AREA

Another challenge for a hair surgeon is to identify the safe donor area (SDA) (Fig. 1.1).

The safe donor area differs in each patient and is usually concentrated around the occipital protuberance arching upward laterally in a crescentic manner up to around 2 cm above the superior helix of the ear.[2] Thus, it covers parts of temporal, parietal and occipital areas. Precaution must be taken to avoid extraction of follicles from beyond the SDA (Figs. 1.2A and B).

The margins of the SDA should be drawn and the entire area divided into six to eight zones. These zones will help the surgeon to extract approximately equal

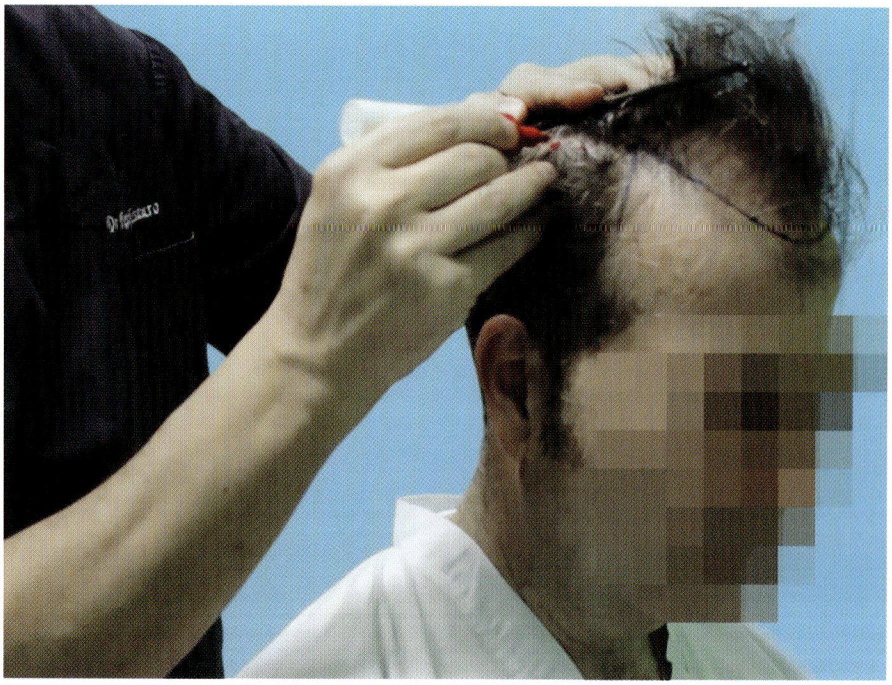

Figure 1.1

Outlining of safe donor region from unsafe donor region.
Courtesy: Dr Piero Tesauro.

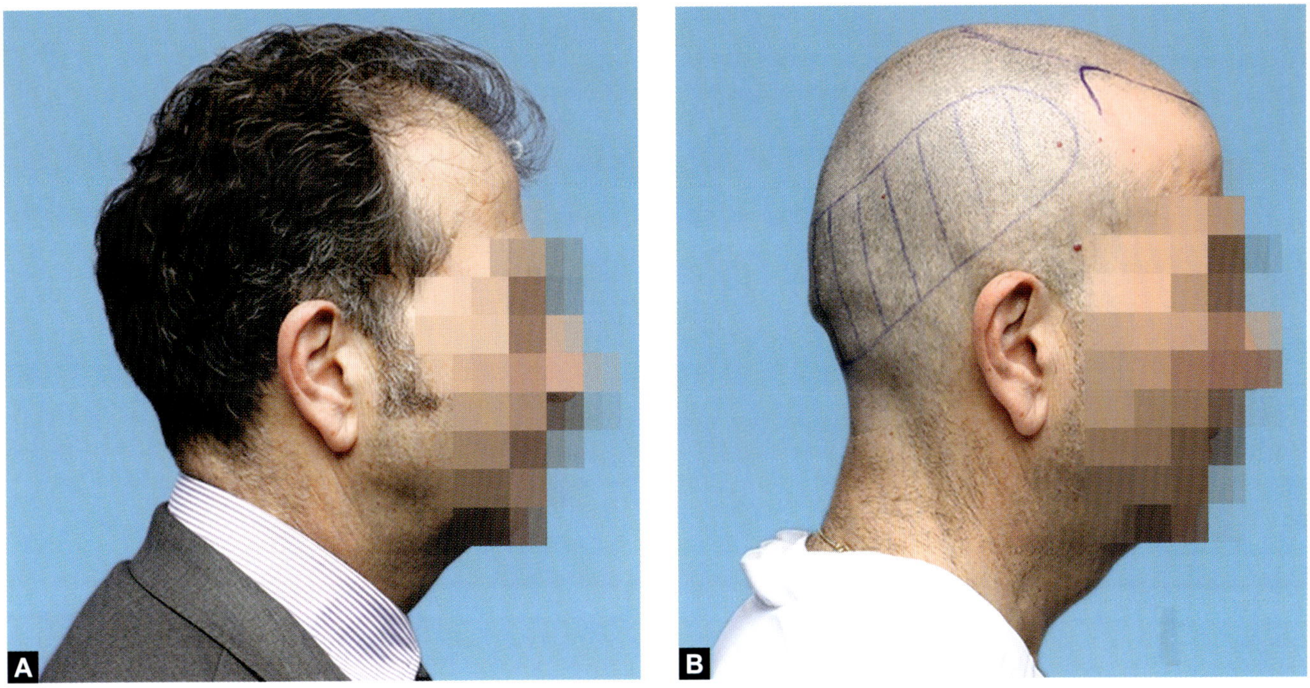

Figures 1.2A and B

Demarcation of safe donor region.
Courtesy: Dr Piero Tesauro.

number of grafts from each zone, thus ensuring equal distribution over the extracted areas (Fig. 1.3).

However, one should remember that extraction numbers in two grids of same surface area may vary as there may be huge variation in density and graft quality in occipital region and temporal region. This may be because of presence of miniaturization in the donor region, retrograde thinning which has not become apparent yet (Fig. 1.4).

Concentrating the extraction of grafts in a particular area will later give a cosmetically unacceptable look, thus it is important to extract uniformly from wider zone of safe donor area even if the surgery is of smaller session size of 500–1,500 grafts.

Once the SDA is identified, it is trimmed closely to a length of 1–1.5 mm. Window stripping can also be done in cases where the hair length is longer (Figs. 1.5A and B).

INFORMED CONSENT

An informed consent should always be taken from the patients prior to surgery. While taking the consent the physician should know about the nature of

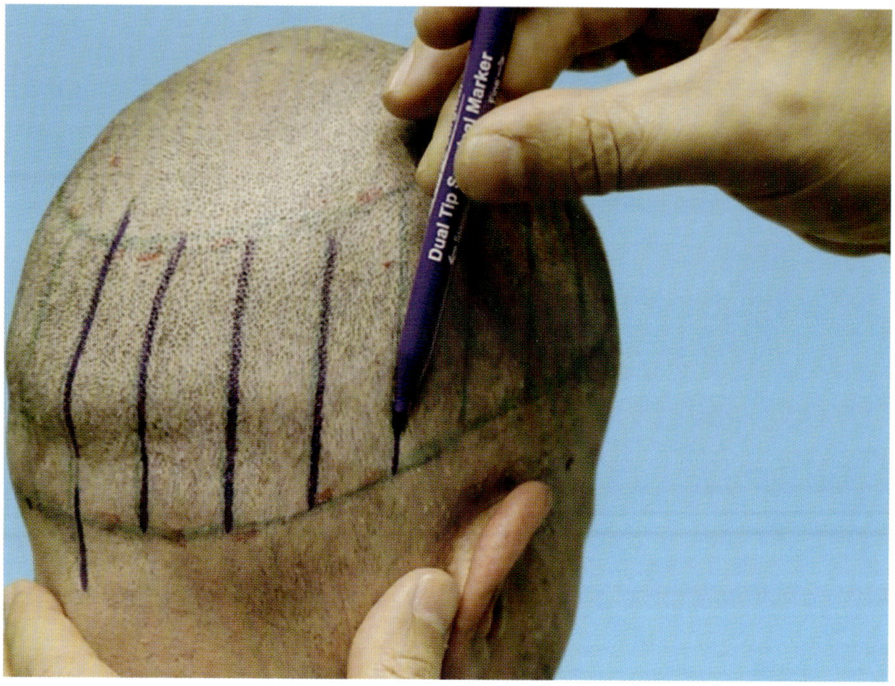

Figure 1.3

Making of grids in safe donor region to ensure that extraction from these grids can be calculated.
Courtesy: Dr Piero Tesauro.

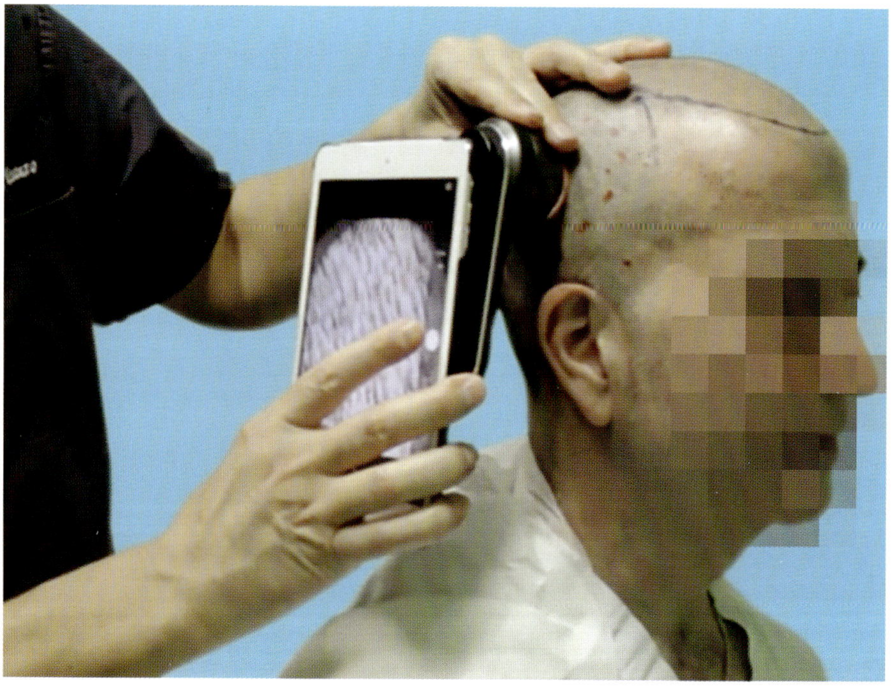

Figure 1.4

Density check of the donor region by dermatoscope.
Courtesy: Dr Piero Tesauro.

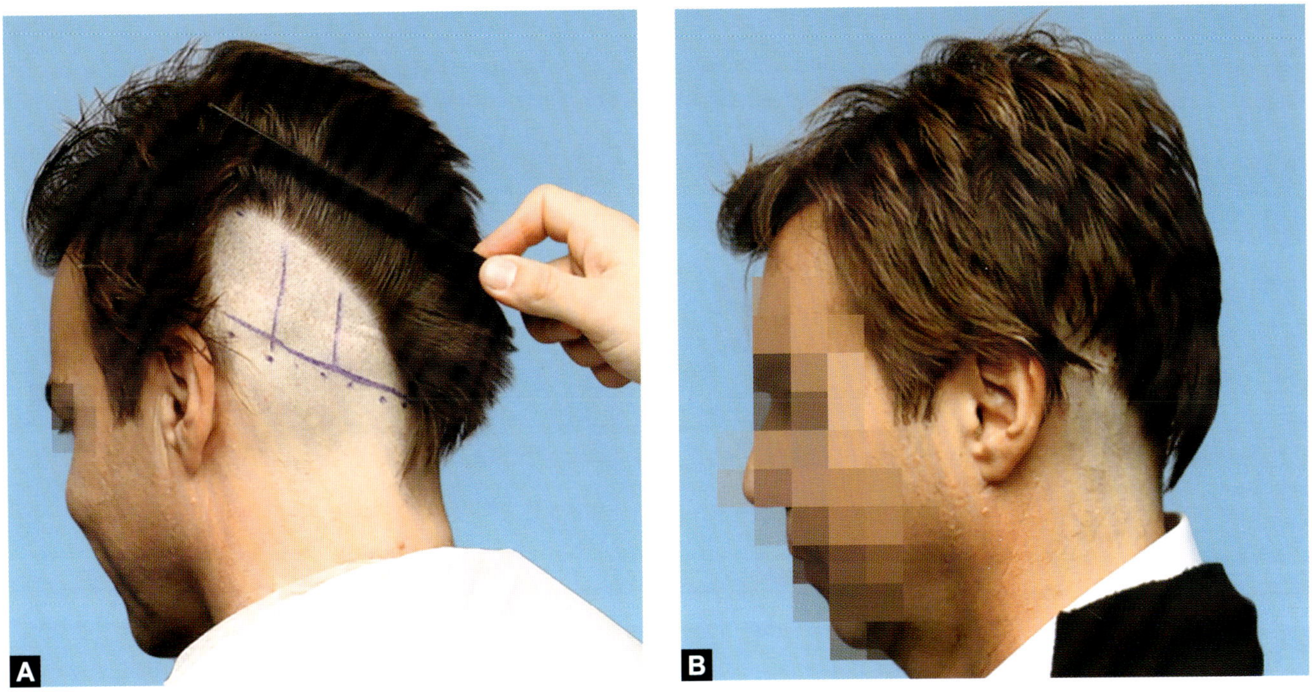

Figures 1.5A and B

(A) Window stripping with hair raised; (B) The same patient postoperatively of window stripping with hair down. *Courtesy:* Dr Piero Tesauro.

patient's condition, the prognosis, the risks, adverse effects, complications and associated benefits of the procedure. Consent regarding complications during harvesting from non-conventional sites like beard and chest should be taken. Patient should be clear that he has given consent for the procedure. He should be given realistic expectation according to his donor quality and grade of baldness. The physician should also discuss other treatment alternatives available to restore hair loss. Need for concomitant medical therapy should be emphasized. Patients should understand that proper hair growth with good density will take 6–9 months after transplantation.

POSTOPERATIVE CARE

The most important aspect of postoperative care is to keep the graft hydrated by spraying normal saline on the recipient site. We recommend the patients to spray every 2 hourly for next 7 days with 5–7 hours of sleep at night. Normal saline spray is also recommended to soften the crust formed around the grafts. It also helps in rapid re-epithelization due to moisture around the grafts.

It is important that there is no trauma in any form to the recipient sites. Trauma can happen in any form, for example patient can rub the graft against the pillow during sleep or he can bang his head while entering his car. The sleeping posture is determined by the area which is transplanted. He cannot sleep prone if hairline restoration has been done. He cannot sleep supine if crown restoration has been done. He can sleep only on the sides if there is complete restoration from hairline to crown. There should be no bandaging around the donor scalp if temple has been restored as there is a risk of dislodgment of grafts. He should take prophylactic oral antibiotic. He should be on anti-inflammatory drug. Regular massaging of forehead should be done to minimize periorbital swelling.

CONCLUDING THOUGHTS

Selecting the right patient for hair transplant surgery will help in ensuring success. Right counseling, developing a rapport and gaining the confidence of the patient are the key steps in making the patient happy.

Comments by Dr Piero Tesauro

Every line of this chapter starting from the first: *"a good patient selection is of utmost importance"* is a pearl of wisdom! Even though many of the concepts outlined in the paragraphs may seem a repetition of all the warnings I have heard in the last 20 years, here they are divided into clear steps and written down to outline all of the "red flags".

But what is selection in reality?

Selection is essentially the collection of subjective parameters that we can put together by looking, touching and listening to our patients.

In fact, we can often immediately understand our patients' expectations and how they live their hair loss situation. When we first examine our patients, moving our fingers from the base of the neck throughout their scalps, we can frequently be quite confident that our evaluation will coincide with the objective data we can retrieve with a dermoscope or any other instrument.

All the objective parameters are a formidable confirmation of our good instincts. They are necessary, especially to avoid being overconfident, but human understanding in this phase is unique and irreplaceable.

Listening is the most difficult part of our job, it presumes that we gain the confidence and the trust of our patients. To do so we must show them we care and understand their problem.

For example to be realistically useful, and not to simply clear our conscience, the therapeutical assignment must be based on three fundamental pillars:

(1) results, (2) irrelevant side effects, and (3) most of all, long-term compliance. So far, our clinics can play, during this first consultations, a wonderful and ethical work in patients education.

SUMMARY

- A detailed consultation, history and counseling are essential for correct patient selection which ultimately provides good result.
- Calculating the number of grafts is required as it decides coverage.
- Safe donor area is to be marked out before hand as extraction from permanent zone can only give desired result.
- Informed consent is prerequisite.
- Postoperative care is crucial as it takes time for the body to take up the grafts. One should be careful and follow all the instructions strictly during this time period.

REFERENCES

1. Boden AS. FUE donor evaluation and surgical planning. In: Lam SM, Jr Williams KL (Eds). Hair Transplant 360, 1st edn. New Delhi: Jaypee Brothers Medical Publishers (P) Ltd. 2010;4:116-7.
2. Lam SM. Hair Transplant operative 360. In: Lam SM (Ed). Hair Transplant 360 for Physicians, 1st edn. New Delhi: Jaypee Brothers Medical Publishers (P) Ltd. 2010;1:63.

CHAPTER 2

Direct Hair Transplantation

Pradeep Sethi, Arika Bansal

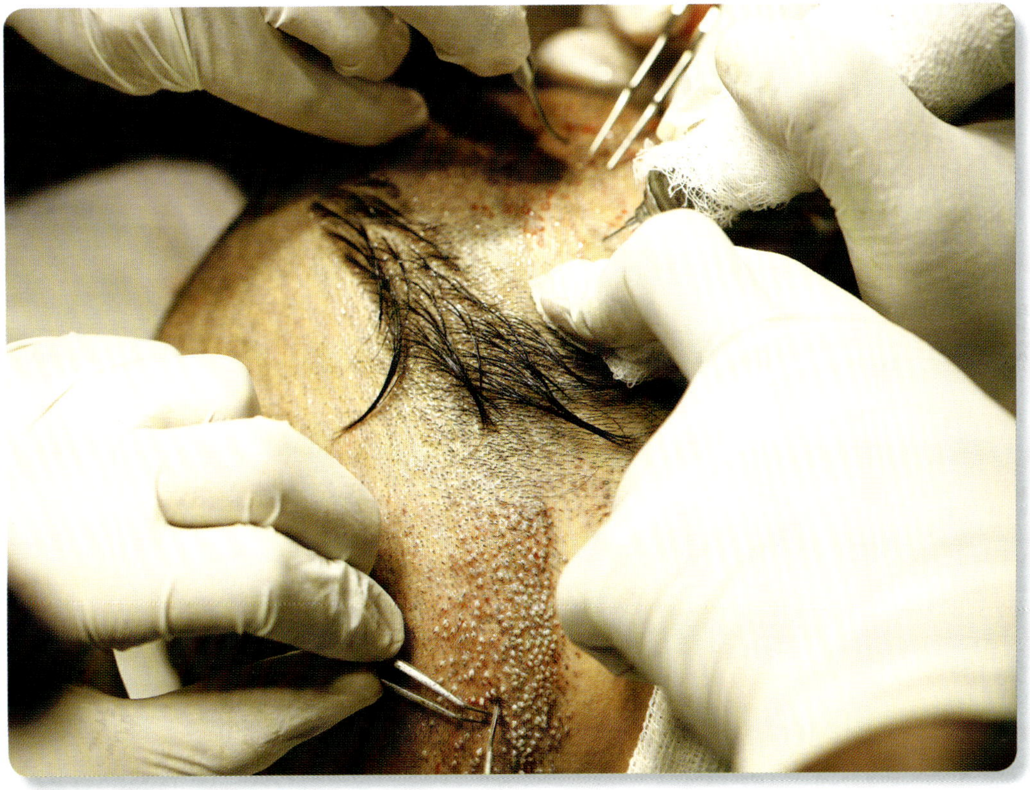

A living tissue should not be challenged enough by keeping outside the mother tissue for long, which is supposed to grow back as a happy bunny!

INTRODUCTION

During the last decade, hair transplant surgery has become a very popular means for hair restoration especially in patients with androgenetic alopecia. A good hair transplant is assessed by the naturalness of the end result in terms of hair growth, hairline and density.[1] These parameters depend on the total number of grafts extracted, implanted and grown.[2] The follicular unit excision, earlier called follicular unit extraction (FUE) technique of hair transplantation has been gaining increased acceptance among patients and physicians. One of the main drawbacks of this procedure is that the grafts are "skinny" and can be easily damaged by handling during the process of transplantation.[3] The use of implanters has circumvented this problem by decreasing the handling of the graft to the minimum.[4]

We have previously reported modification of the conventional FUE technique in which slits at the recipient site are premade and simultaneous extraction and implantation of the grafts is being done using the implanters.[2] We have been following this technique in our patients and have found this technique yielding faster results and also enabled us to implant up to 7,410 grafts in a single visit to the surgeon.

METHOD

The direct hair transplantation (DHT) surgery technique is a modification of FUE and comprises three key steps: (1) premade slits; (2) simultaneous scoring, graft extraction and graft placement; and (3) graft placement.

Premade Slits

The recipient area is prepared by giving a ring block, followed by extraction of test grafts to know the depth of slits needed for the placement of grafts at recipient sites. Slits are made in the hairline zone which consisted of 3–4 rows using 20G needles in males and 21G needles in females. The slits in the area posterior to this are made using 19G needles. The average number of slits is 40–50/cm^2 (Figs. 2.1A and B).

Simultaneous Scoring, Graft Extraction and Graft Placement

After the desired number of slits are made, the patient is made to lie to on the left lateral or right lateral side. Ring block is given in donor area followed by scoring of grafts with sharp, serrounded or trumpet punches of 0.85–1.0 mm. The grafts are harvested using a forester forcep without teasing the dermal part of the graft. Once the desired number of maximum grafts are scored and harvested from one side, patient is shifted to the other lateral side and then finally patient is shifted to the prone position for scoring and harvesting grafts from the occipital area.

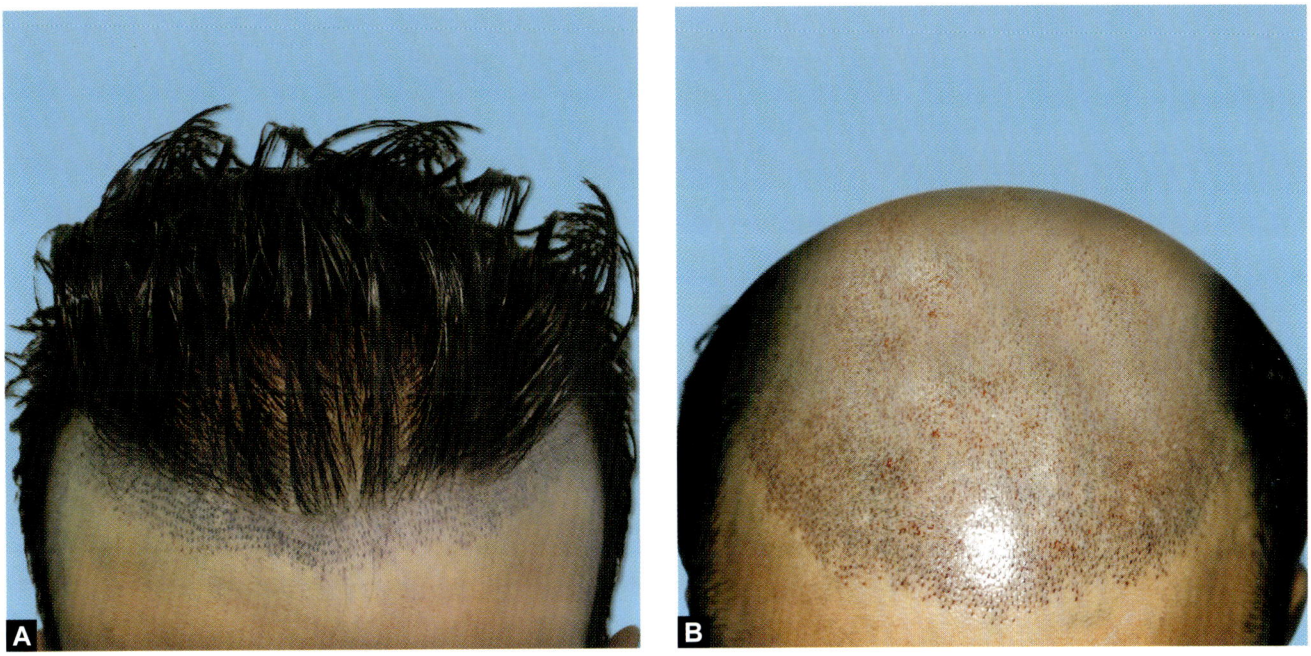

Figures 2.1A and B

The slits are made before the extraction process.

In prone position, graft placement is done on the crown following segregation of grafts into singles, doubles and triplets followed by loading into dull needle implanters (Figs. 2.2 and 2.3).[2]

Meticulous attempts are made to plant some 20–50% of the grafts into the premade slits by the end of the scoring.

Graft Implantation

The rest of the grafts are planted in supine position by two surgical assistants simultaneously so as to reduce the 'out of the body' time. The implanters are inserted into the slits up to the bevel of the needle in the sagittal plane and then rotated by 90°. The graft is pushed in from above using a jeweller's forcep and the implanter is gently withdrawn from the slit while pressing the epidermis from above. A little epidermis of the graft is left slightly protruding over the epidermis of the recipient area (Fig. 2.4).

POSTOPERATIVE CARE

Postoperatively, patients are advised to use a povidone-iodine scrub and mupirocin 2% ointment on the donor area and a normal saline spray 2–3 hourly on the recipient area along with oral antibiotic and painkiller for 7 days. Patients are followed up on day 7 and then at monthly intervals.

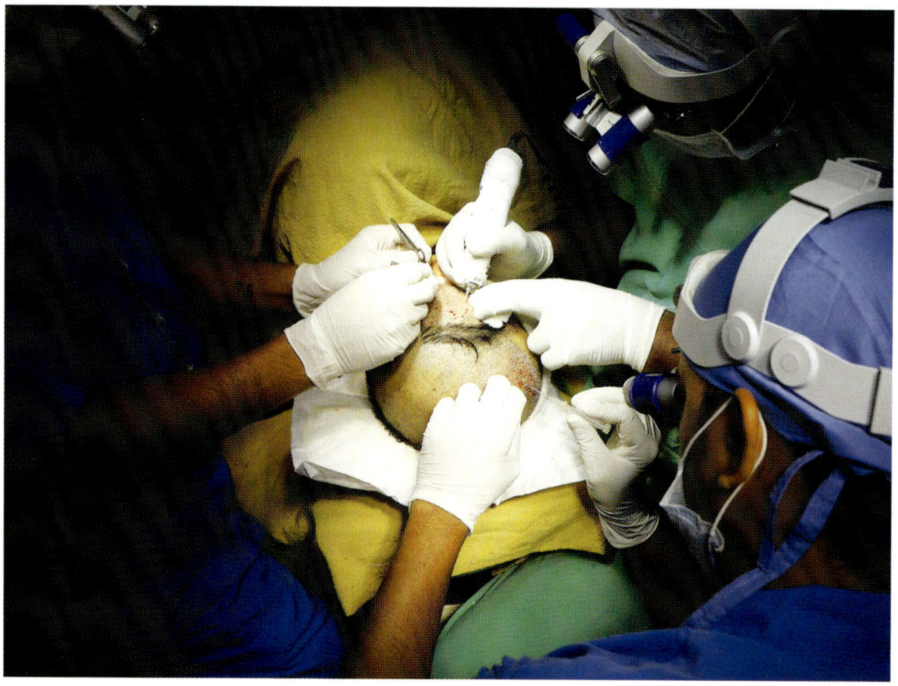

Figure 2.2A

Graft scoring, extraction and placement (DHT) being done in the patient.

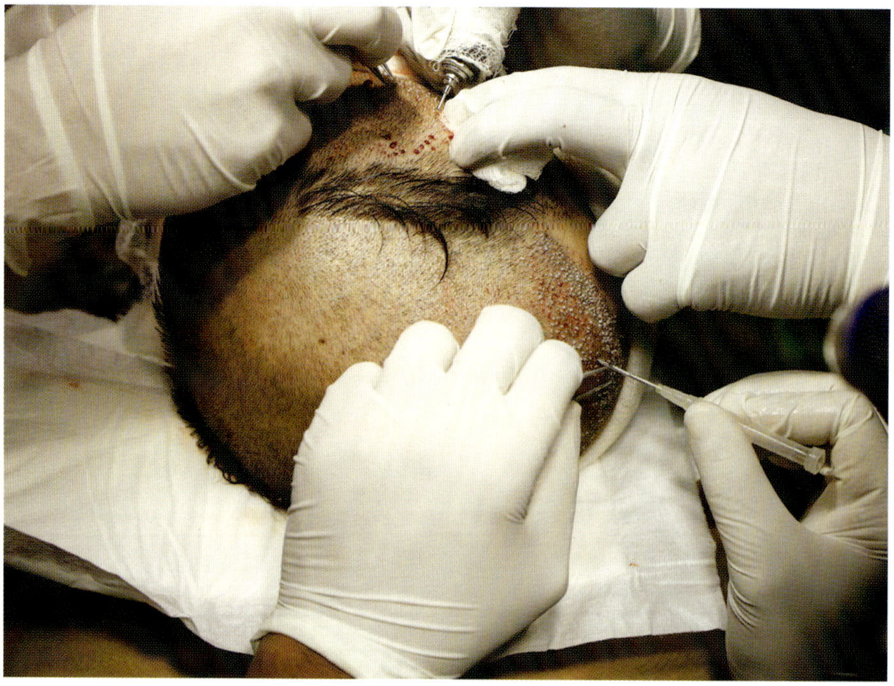

Figure 2.2B

Close-up view of the direct hair transplantation with placement being done by dull needle implanter.

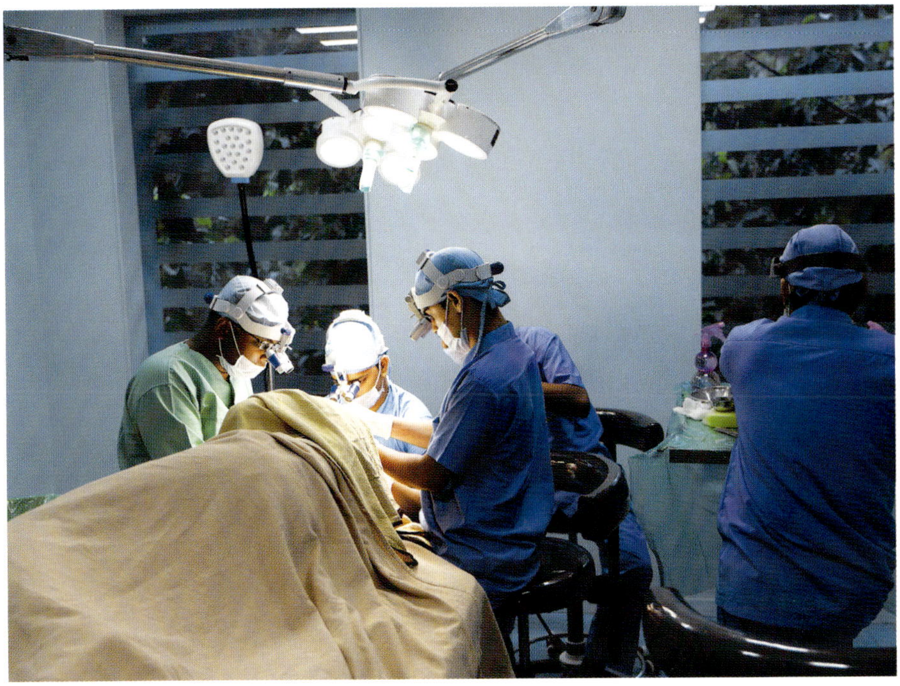

Figure 2.2C

Scene of operation theater: One surgical assistant is loading the graft in the implanter on the table. Another surgical assistant is passing the implanter to the assistant sitting below and behind the head of the patient for simultaneous graft plantation.

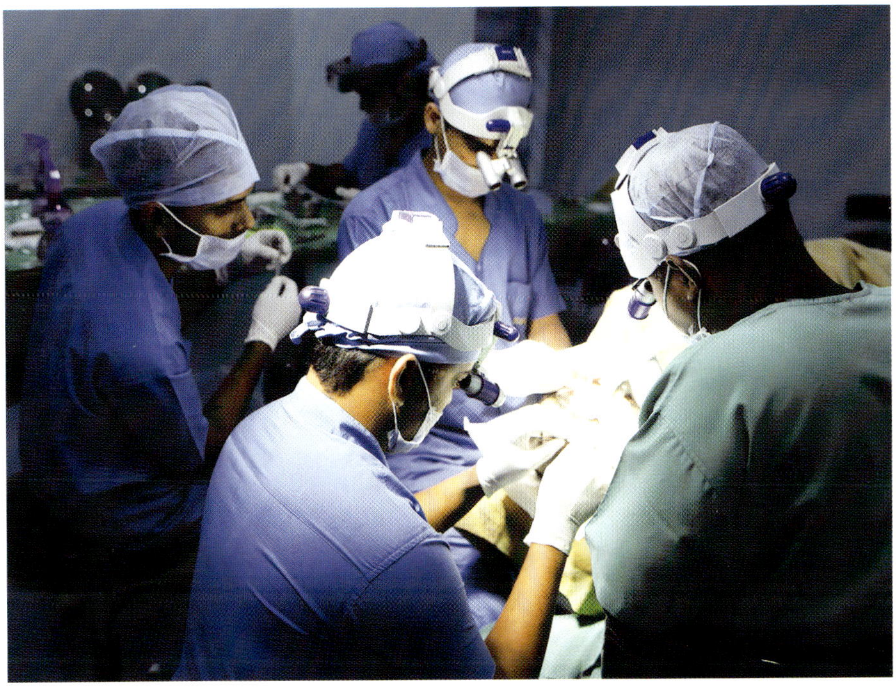

Figure 2.2D

Scene of the operation theater from a different angle.

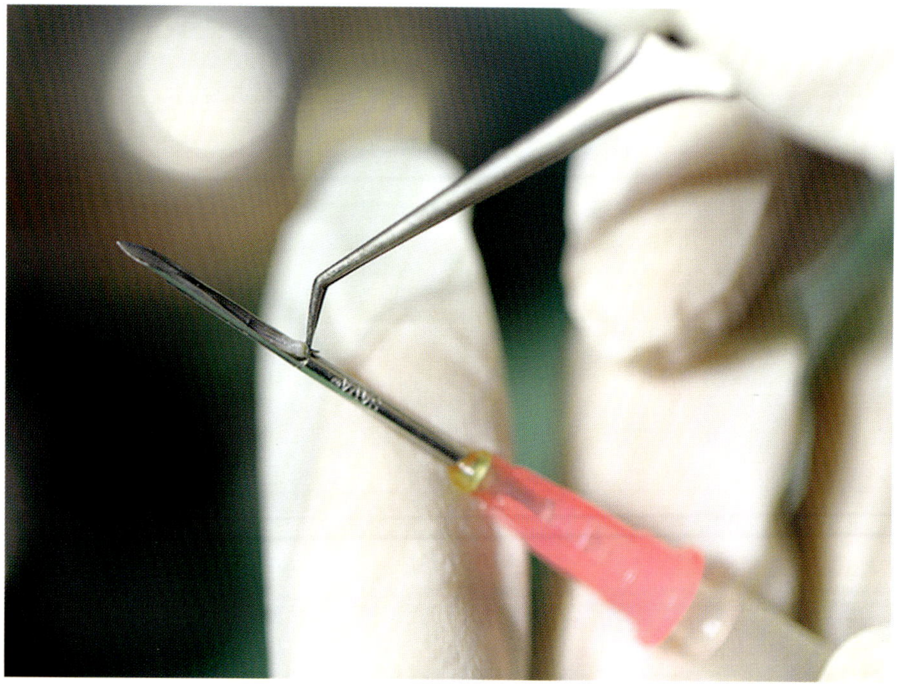

Figure 2.3

Loading of graft into SAVA™ implanter (dull needle implanter) ensuring near to zero mechanical handling of graft during implantation.

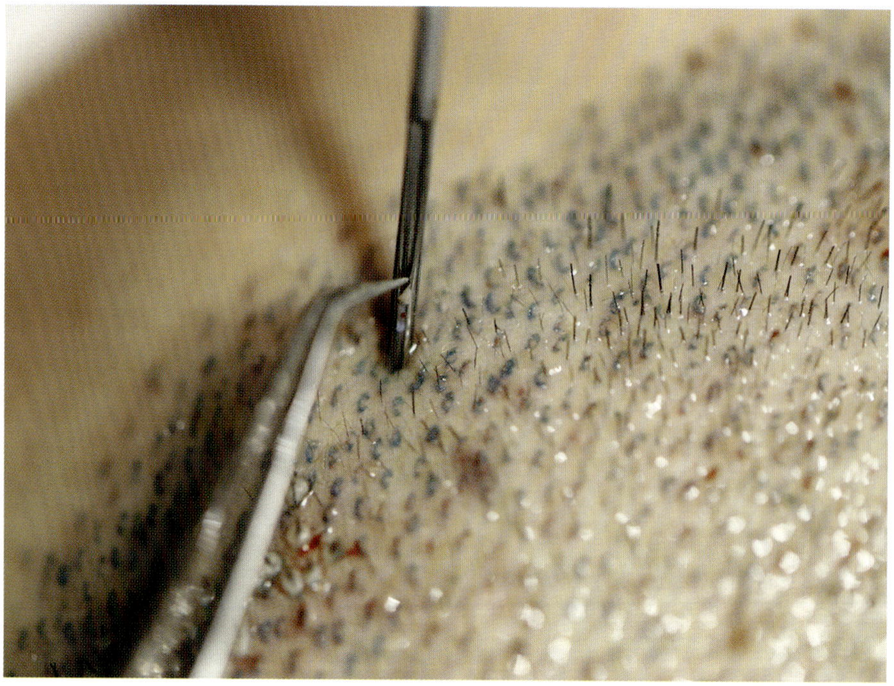

Figure 2.4

Pushing of the graft from the epidermal end while unloading the graft from the implanter.

ADVANTAGES OVER CONVENTIONAL FUE SURGERY

Direct hair transplantation technique is a modification of FUE which entails combining premade recipient sites, simultaneous extraction and plantation of grafts using implanters for the maximum possible number of grafts followed by placement of the rest of the extracted grafts by two assistants after completion of scoring of grafts. The word "direct" is added to the name because grafts are planted into premade slits immediately without splitting them into individual follicles and the process is done as rapidly as possible to minimize out of body time of the grafts.

The advantages of our method include:

- Decreased force is required to insert the graft due to the premade sites[5] and graft enter the slits without being touched below the epidermal portion, hence preserving the viability of graft.
- Minimal mechanical handling of grafts due to use of implanters and no dissection of grafts into follicles.
- Little risk of popping due to decreased resistance encountered in premade slits.[6]
- Reduction in number of sharp implanters needed for plantation due to premade slits.
- Saving surgeon's time as the design of hairline, density and angulations are decided in premade sites along with possibility to implant in any head position with implanters which is not possible when we implant with forceps.[7]
- Little out of body graft time due to use of implanters and simultaneous extraction-plantation in major part of surgery.[6]

Our ability to implant grafts in premade slits with implanters, made even on the previous day of surgery, reduces bleeding from slit sites, increases stickiness of grafts thus reducing popping of grafts.[7] It has been observed that the recipient sites become more hospitable bed for grafts over time and risk of reperfusion injury is almost nil as diffusion rather than neovascularization is the predominant method of graft survival on second day of surgery.[7]

Our DHT technique has enabled us to conduct hair transplantation up to 8,000 grafts in a single visit and up to 10,410 grafts in two visits to the hair transplant surgeon, thus it has greatly increased the speed of surgery and enabled us to give full coverage in patients with highest grade of baldness in two sittings. Patients who get surgery done in single visit often opt for complete coverage as it has the benefit of complete change in look within a year. It should be kept in mind that large number of grafts are needed to be negotiated in such cases and every possible way to increase the survival should be adopted and surgery should be done on 2 consecutive days. The number of assistants needed in DHT are six or

Table 2.1: Parameters of follicular unit extraction (FUE) and direct hair transplant (DHT).

Parameters	*Follicular unit extraction*	*Direct hair transplant®*
Points of difference	• *Step 1*: Graft extraction • *Step 2*: Making slits • *Step 3*: Graft placement	• *Step 1*: Slit creation • *Step 2*: Graft extraction and placement (minimizes outside body time)
Transit time: Time for which grafts remain outside the body	3–5 hours	Up to 30 minutes
Chance of graft damage	• Present if forceps are used • Minimal if implanters are used	Minimal due to use of implanters
Root handling	Slight to more	Nil
Storage solution	Required	Not required (normal saline)
Surveillance by doctors	Less	All important steps like premade slits and scoring of grafts are done by doctors

more along with the hair transplant surgeon. There is no limitation in access, angulations and direction while transplanting the grafts as body is shifted into various positions as mentioned in the procedure along with sitting position which is used for transplantation by two assistants simultaneously.

Parameters of FUE and DHT have been shown in Table 2.1.

SUMMARY

- Direct hair transplant is modified version of conventional FUE technique. It comprises of prior making of recipient area slits followed by simultaneous scoring, extraction and implantation followed by implantation of remaining grafts.
- The Zen factor being decreased 'out of the body time' of grafts which ensures graft survivability.
- Implantation of grafts in premade slits decreases bleeding and increases stickiness of grafts thus reducing popping of grafts.

REFERENCES

1. Rose PT. Hair restoration surgery: challenges and solutions. Clin Cosmet Investig Dermatol. 2015;8:361-70.
2. Sethi P, Bansal A. Direct hair transplantation: a modified follicular unit extraction technique. J Cutan Aesthet Surg. 2013;6(2):100-5.
3. Harris JA. Follicular unit extraction. Facial Plast Surg Clin North Am. 2013;21(3):375-84.
4. Lee SJ, Lee HJ, Hwang SJ, et al. Evaluation of survival rate after follicular unit transplantation using the KNU implanter. Dermatol Surg. 2001;27(8):716-20.
5. Lee DY, Choi YL, Kim MG, et al. The combined use of needle with hair transplanter for hair recipient sites. Dermatol Surg. 2007;33(1):128-9.
6. Bicknell LM, Kash N, Kavouspour C, et al. Follicular unit extraction hair transplant harvest: a review of current recommendations and future considerations. Dermatol Online J. 2014;20(3).
7. Bernstein RM, Rassman WR. Pre-making recipient sites to increase graft survival in manual and robotic FUE procedures. Hair Transplant Forum Intl. 2012;22(4):128-30.

CHAPTER 3

Anesthesia, Pain Management and Hemostasis in Hair Transplant

Abhinav Kumar, Arika Bansal, Raghunatha Reddy

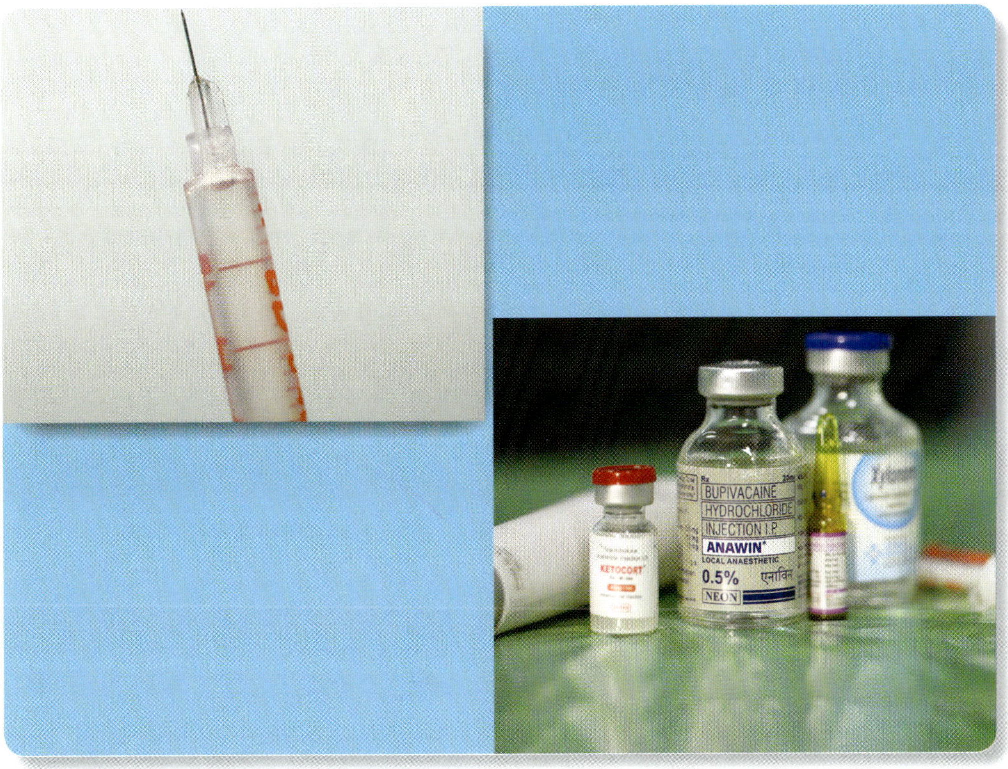

Though patients are aware that they have to negotiate with some pain at the beginning of the procedure, the aim should be at providing least substance for the long-term memory of this. And it is doable!

INTRODUCTION

Pain is the first thing that comes in mind of any patient who hears the word "surgery". Promising a surgery with minimal pain not only helps in reducing the patient's anxiety but also helps in building the confidence of the patient. Patients who have had a bad experience in the first surgery are unlikely to return to you for subsequent procedures and are also likely to spread a bad word about you among family and friends. In order to master a surgery with minimal pain, a thorough knowledge about anesthetic agents is a must. The goal of the surgeon should be to minimize discomfort and toxicity.

Many choices for anesthesia are available these days either in the type of anesthesia or route of administration. For local nerve blocks, injection or infiltration is preferred, while for systemic action, anesthesia can be given either orally, intravenously or by inhalation.

PREOPERATIVE SEDATION[1]

Before giving any form of injections over scalp, an oral benzodiazepine is given to relax the patient while maintaining consciousness. It also causes profound retrograde and anterograde amnesia and hence patients are unable to remember the pricks, thus have higher chance of coming for second sitting, if required.

Midazolam has sedative, anxiolytic and amnesic actions which is 2–4 times more potent than diazepam. It is highly selective for amnesia, with its amnesic dose being 1/10th of its hypnotic dosage. Intravenous (2–5 mg) or subcutaneously 2.5 mg to 5 mg midazolam is given by many surgeons, 10–20 minutes before starting the procedure. Lorazepam 1 mg sublingually 1 hour before the procedure is given and can be repeated in 4–5 hours as per the need. Maximum dose should not exceed 0.05 mg/kg. Oral alprazolam 0.25 mg or diazepam 10–20 mg also helps a person to calm his nerves. All these measures reduce the risk of vasovagal syncope. A test dose of lignocaine and bupivacaine should always be given over left forearm (0.1 ml) and right forearm respectively to test the sensitivity.

LOCAL AND TUMESCENT ANESTHESIA

Local anesthetic solution: Its composition is variable depending on doctor. We use 20 ml normal saline, 0.5 ml adrenaline and 20 ml bupivacaine (0.5% at 5 mg/ml). Total dosage of bupivacaine given to patient is 100 mg in 24 hours. We avoid giving sodium bicarbonate because of its edema propensity. The rationale behind giving bupivacaine as local anesthetic is due to its prolonged action.

Tumescent solution: We use 30 ml of 2% lignocaine which has 21.3 mg of lignocaine hydrochloride per ml. Thus we use a total dosage of 639 mg of lignocaine in 24 hours. We mix 0.5 ml of adrenaline with lignocaine, 40 mg of triamcinolone acetonide (40 mg/ml) and 60 ml of normal saline in the final cocktail of tumescent solution.

LOCAL ANESTHESIA

The basic techniques to achieve adequate anesthesia include nerve blocks, ring blocks and field infiltration. In nerve block, we inject a small amount of lidocaine around a sensory nerve root which will anesthetize the area supplied by that nerve. In hair restoration, this is usually performed for the supraorbital nerve (Fig. 3.1). We usually resort to nerve blocks only if complete anesthesia is not achieved in the central scalp after the ring block.

For anesthetizing, usually lignocaine or bupivacaine with adrenaline is preferred. Adrenaline increases the efficacy of local anesthetic due to its vasoconstrictive properties and gives us a bloodless field during the procedure. Since hair transplantation is a long process requiring at least 4–6 hours, we need to add an anesthetic agent whose duration of action is long. Bupivacaine fulfills this

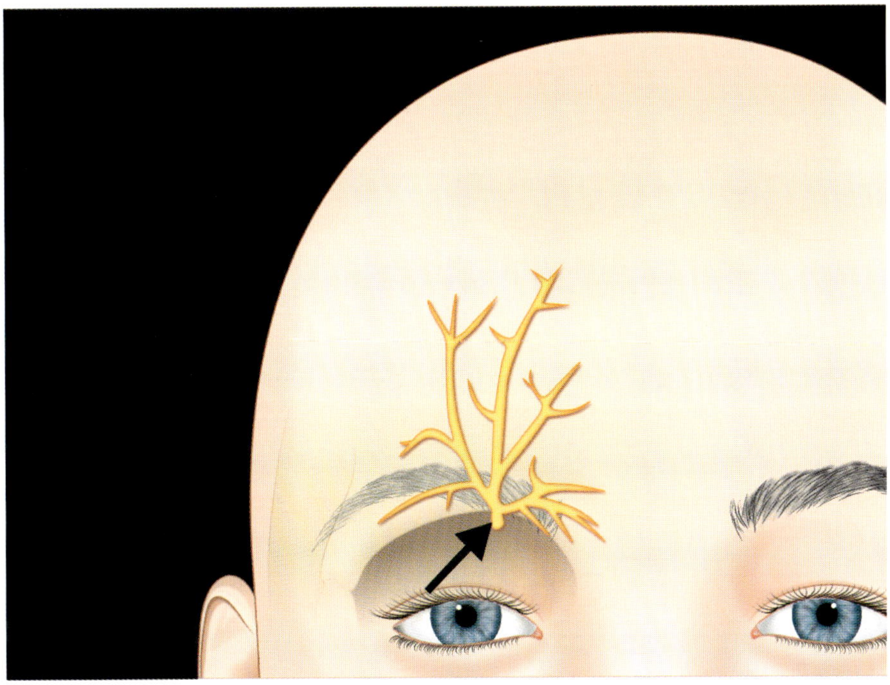

Figure 3.1

Supraorbital nerve at the mid-pupillary line present deep at the supraorbital notch. Infiltrating lidocaine around this nerve will anesthetize one-third to two-thirds of the anterior scalp.

property and hence used for either tumescent or local anesthesia. A ring block anesthesia is given over posterior aspect of scalp at the lower margins of the marked donor area (Fig. 3.1). Injections are given with an insulin syringe or 1 ml syringe with 30G needle via continuous wheal approach or multiple wheal approach. Approximately 0.05–0.1 ml is injected at each site to make a small elevation. The ring block is followed by infiltration of the scalp with tumescent solution in the same plane to achieve hemostasis and turgidity.

A small device known as vibrator can be used to alleviate the intensity of pain, along with ice pack compresses. The total dosage should always be monitored to prevent toxicity.

We list the practical issues in anesthetizing the patient, which one often faces while conducting hair transplant.[2]

The ideal layer for injection of vasoconstrictors is just below the dermis and above the galea. Injecting below the subgaleal layer (needle tip will be felt scrapping the bone) which is relatively avascular, increases the risk of periorbital edema due to the fluid tracking inferiorly in the subgaleal plane.

- The arterial supply to the recipient scalp courses up from below like spokes from rim of a wheel. The nerve supply differs; the supraorbital nerves supply most of the anterior one-third to two-thirds of the recipient area. These structures exit the skull deep to the eyebrow and run superiorly. Once these nerves are blocked, bulk of the frontal recipient site is blocked.
- *Epinephrine (tumescence in the scalp)*: The medication must be placed along the path of blood vessels (subcutaneous plane) and in a large enough concentration to produce vasoconstriction.
- Tumescence also helps in separating the galea from the subcutaneous layer and thus provides extra protection to deeper vessels and galea during surgery.
- In the donor area, the neurovascular supply runs from inferior to superior, and ring blocks need to be done only below the inferior aspect of planned harvest zones, at the level of occipital protuberance.
- *Staging of injections*: It is important to not inject anesthesia, epinephrine and tumescence in an area which is not to be operated in the next 2 hours of surgery to avoid wearing off of the effects before the slits are made. This applies to both donor area and recipient sites. Recipient sites need not be infiltrated earlier than 10–15 minutes prior to incision creation.
- Intradermal injections produce wheals and are often painful, thus should be ideally injected in numb scalp or through the painless anesthetized zone.
- The dilution minimizes the risk of side effects if tumescence is accidentally injected into the vessels.

- New recipient site bleeding and pain is often a clue that anesthesia may soon begin to fade and needs top up.
- If patients complain of frontal headache, the culprit may be excessive pressure on the scalp from elastic gauze bandage placed around the scalp to absorb fluids or incomplete hairline anesthesia. Loosening of bandage, repeating ring block and supraorbital block is recommended.
- Incomplete late donor anesthesia can be addressed by reinjecting the anesthesia 2–3 cm inferior to the area of pain.
- Use of vibrator and contact cooling along with injections for local anesthesia decreases the pain significantly. This occurs because vibration closes the gates of pain pathway to the brain through presynaptic inhibition.
- Use of bupivacaine is limited due to its potential cardiac toxicity. The maximum dosage of bupivacaine in adults in 175 mg. Ropivacaine produces less reduction of left ventricular pressure than bupivacaine. Ropivacaine is one of the safest long-acting local anesthetics in peripheral nerve blockade and carries the potential to replace bupivacaine in future.
- Doctor should be capable of tackling all emergencies in hair transplantation like vasovagal syncope, hypoglycemia, seizures, an attack of myocardial infarction, cardiac arrhythmias, hypertension and hypotension, allergic reaction and anaphylactoid reaction. Surgeon should have an emergency tray ready all the time along with 100% oxygen available in the clinic. A basic training in basic life support and use of automated external defibrillator should be given to all doctors and medical staff of the clinic.

PAIN MANAGEMENT

Hair transplant is a painful procedure, if one does not take adequate measures to alleviate the pain. The following concepts and techniques should be kept in mind before giving local anesthesia:

- Use as small needle as possible. We use 32G insulin syringe.
- Remember the principle of pricking the skin: slow and releasing it very slowly. Rapid injection of anesthesia in subcutaneous tissue causes pain.
- There are two main techniques of giving ring blocks. One is multiple wheal technique (Fig. 3.2) and another is continuous wheal technique (Fig. 3.3). In multiple wheal technique a 30G to 32G needle is used to form a subcutaneous wheal at every 5 odd cm along the ring. After waiting for onset of anesthesia, the needle is inserted intradermally medially and laterally through each wheal. Surgeons should have the habit of withdrawing plunger of the syringe after every prick.

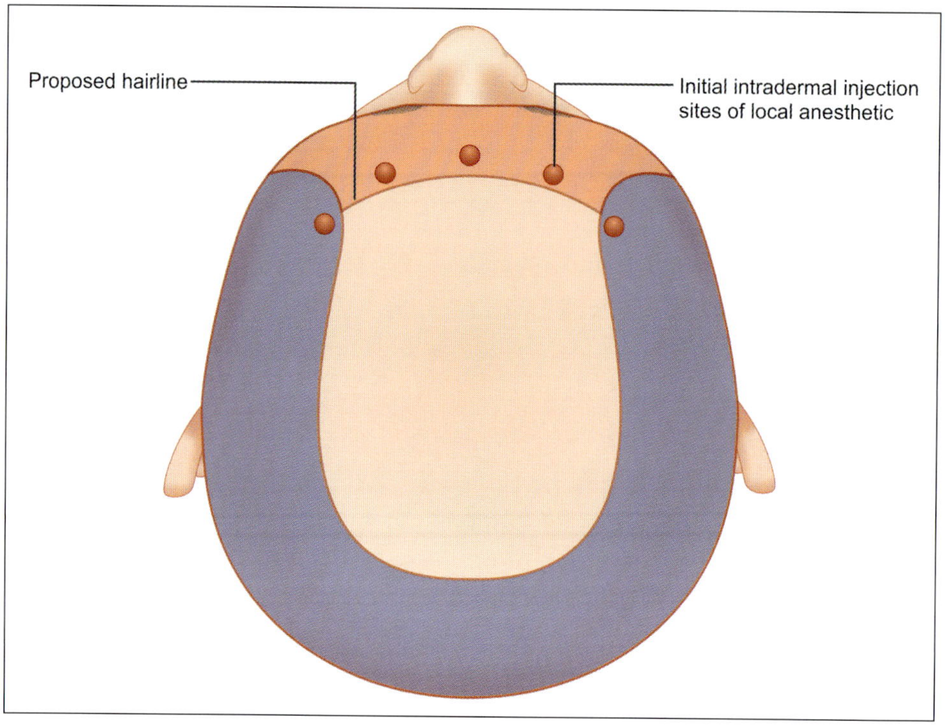

Figure 3.2

Multiple wheal technique.

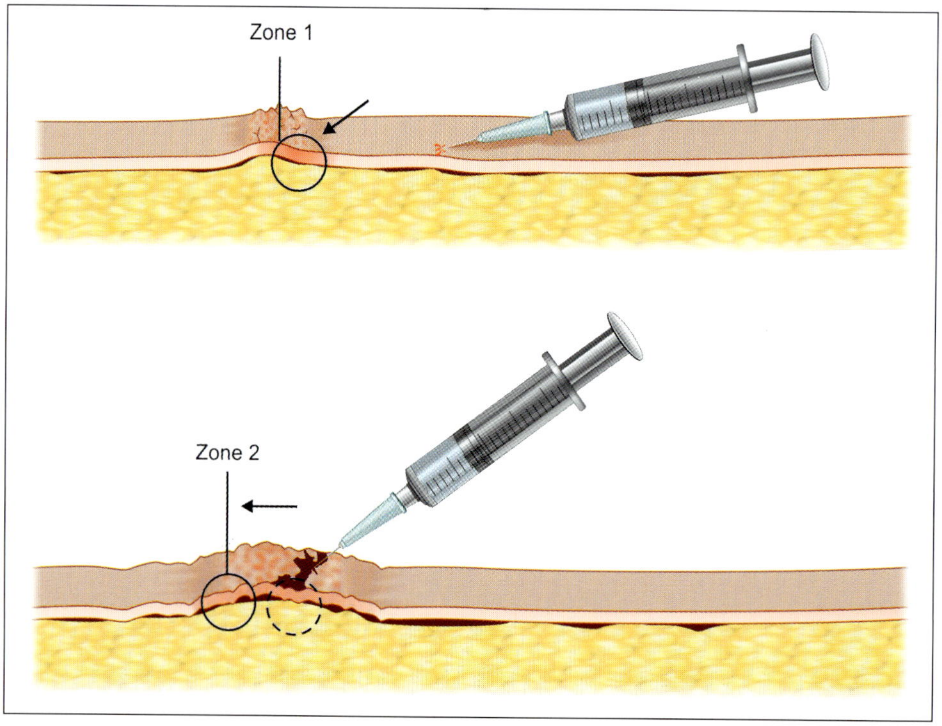

Figure 3.3

Continuous wheal technique.

In continuous wheal technique, 1 ml of anesthetic solution is injected in the dermis till blanched wheal forms. The next prick is given through the wheal, along the ring, by advancing the needle by 2–3 mm. Thus a raised boundary wall of ring block is created. If given ideally only the first prick is felt.

Another technique of giving a block is by 18G spinal needle which is inserted fully at the midpoint of donor or recipient area. The anesthetic solution is slowly advanced through the length as the needle is gradually withdrawn.

- During the course of extending the local anesthesia in the donor region for ring block, the first needle prick should be in the slit from where graft has been extracted, subsequent needle pricks should be inserted from the anesthetized site to the nonanesthetized site.
- Intradermal injections are painful and should be given only when the region is completely anesthetized.
- Using vibration and ice packs further reduces the pain and we use it extensively for injecting local anesthesia.
- Using longer syringes helps as well, since it can reduce the number of pricks.
- Buffering of solution by adding 8.4% sodium bicarbonate neutralizes local anesthetic (which are weak bases as hydrochloride salts in acidic forms). The anesthetics, lignocaine and bupivacaine are buffered in ratio of 9:1 and 50:1 respectively thus reducing the burning pain due to charged anesthetic molecules. However buffering of solution is associated with high incidence of postoperative edema.
- Warming the anesthetic solution using dry heat or warm water bath at 37°C reduces the pain.

Comments by Dr Robert Haber

There are two basic goals for local anesthesia for hair restoration. First, we want it to be effective so our patient does not feel the pain associated with cutting. This requires an understanding of anesthetic types, their rapidity of onset, duration of action, as well as sensory nerve distribution. Second, we want the anesthesia administration itself to be as painless as possible, as that is what the patient will remember most. Mastering the art of painless anesthesia is crucial for all hair surgeons, and this chapter reviews important elements. Oral or intravenous sedation is not always necessary but certainly helpful, while using buffered solutions, small needles, slow injection speed, vibratory pain blockade and properly selected anesthetic agents all play important roles toward the goal of painless anesthesia.

SUMMARY

Importance of pain minimization guarantees that the patient will return for a second sitting, if required.

- Use of midazolam for its sedative, anxiolytic and amnesic actions.
- Tumescent solution containing another type of anesthetic is injected to prolong the duration of anesthesia and to provide tumescence without crossing the safe therapeutic value of each drug.
- Bupivacaine or lignocaine can be used as the primary local anesthesia.
- Methods to minimize pain of local anesthesia administration includes: using the smallest gauze needle possible, use of buffer, use of vibrator and ice packs while pricking.

REFERENCES

1. Bradley W. Anesthesia. In: Unger W, Shapiro R, Unger R, Unger M (Eds). Hair Transplantation, 5th edn. New York: Informa Healthcare Publishing; 2011. 232-9.
2. Elliott V. Scalp anesthesia and hemostasis for FUE. In: Lam SM, Jr Williams KL (Eds). Hair Transplant 360, 1st edn. New Delhi: Jaypee Brothers Medical Publishers (P) Ltd. 2016;4: 84-97.

CHAPTER 4

Designing the Anterior Hairline

Pradeep Sethi, Arika Bansal, Abhinav Kumar, Sarita Sanke

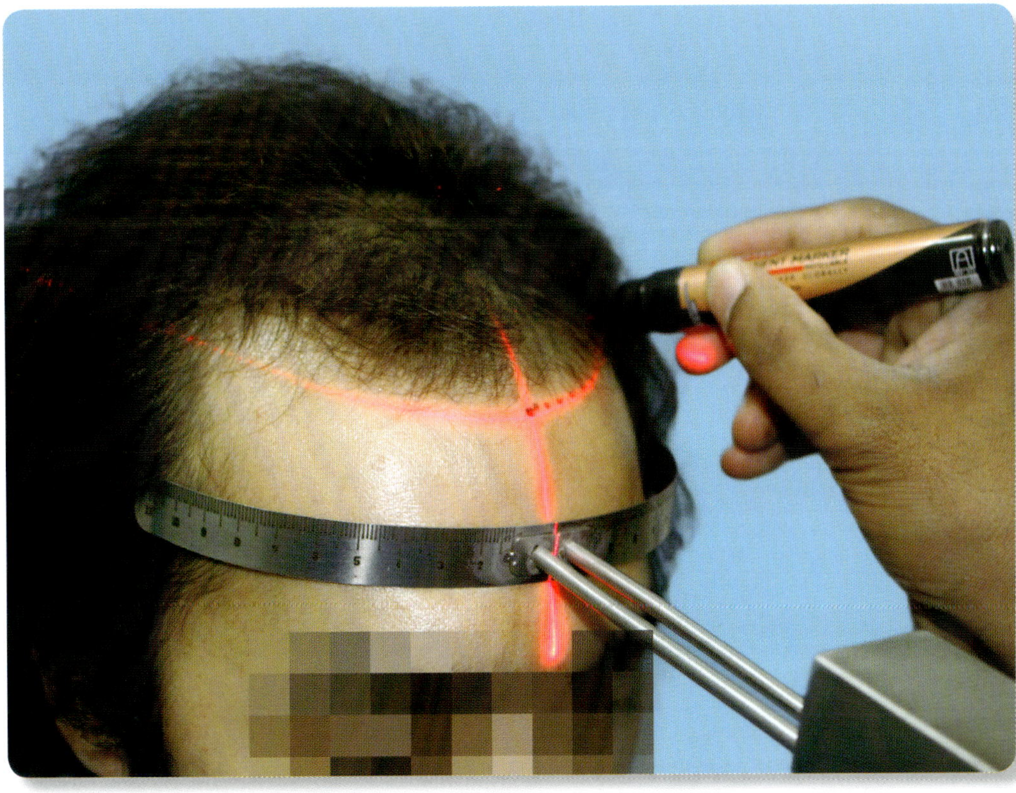

No two faces on earth are similar!

Every face contains two eyes, one nose, two ears, one forehead, two cheek bones, chin, two eyebrows, one mouth and one hairline! Every face is a permutation and combination of each of these components. It is customized to one individual. The anterior hairline is the gateway into the face. It is the most important aspect of the aesthetic part of the hair restoration surgery. It needs to be done aiming to reproduce a near natural hairline.

INTRODUCTION

Frontal hairline is one of the most important aesthetic feature of scalp hair and plays an important role in assessing the age of the patient. Recession of anterior hairline is almost always a part of androgenetic alopecia, and sometimes in cicatricial alopecia like frontal fibrosing alopecia, traction alopecia (especially in females these two can also be one of the causes).

Restoring the anterior hairline in a patient is challenging for any hair transplant surgeon. The three major goals of a surgeon would be to give a natural appearance to the hairline, maintain the symmetry grossly and thirdly the aesthetic appearance should be such that, it should make the patient look younger (Figs. 4.1A to E).

Five types of anterior hairline shapes have been mentioned by Sirinturk et al.[1] These include the round, M type, rectangular, bell-shaped and triangular (Figs. 4.2 to 4.6). Males usually have M type hairline, while females have round or rectangular hairline.

A. *Round:* This hairline is suited for a wider head with mature stable temporal hair. It shows convexity throughout the design.
B. *M type:* Severe frontotemporal recession is present.
C. *Rectangular:* Horizontal frontal line with minimal frontotemporal recess. This hairline design will consume more grafts but it is a more natural form of hairline and helps in restoring the original youthful look of the early twenties.
D. *Bell-shaped:* Large frontal height than normal. It is meant for a narrow head and it conserves grafts and has temporal recession.
E. *Triangular:* Hairline moves down from frontal to temporal area nearly straight.

ANATOMICAL LANDMARKS OF ANTERIOR HAIRLINE

Hairline designing is not pure mathematics where you just know the various anatomical points on the face and scalp and draw a line joining them to create a hairline. The unique selling point of a beautiful hairline is the inability of the

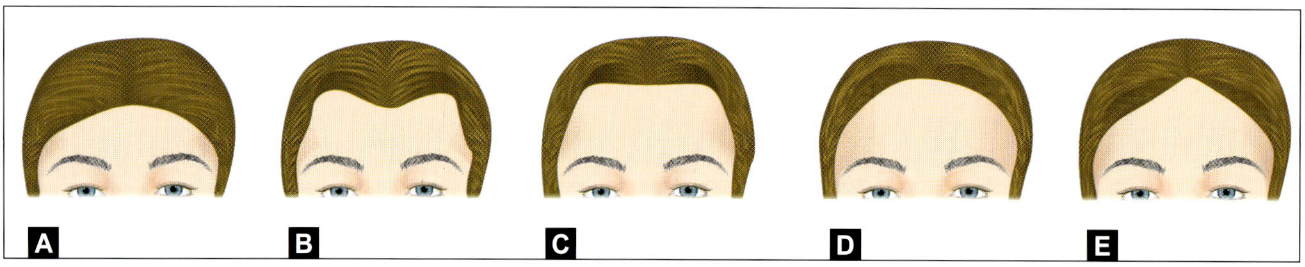

Figures 4.1A to E

Different designs of the anterior hairline.

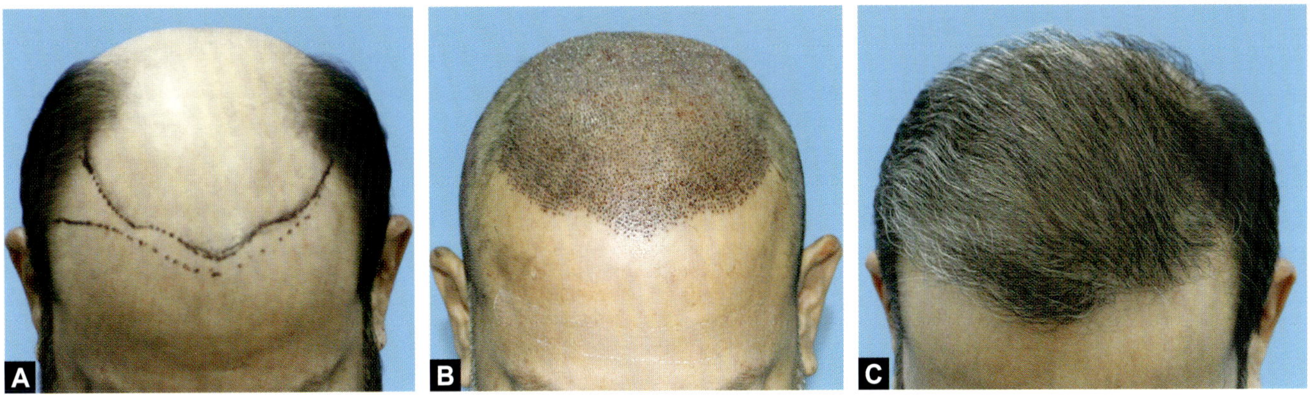

Figures 4.2A to C

Pictures depict a round hairline for a person with wider head.

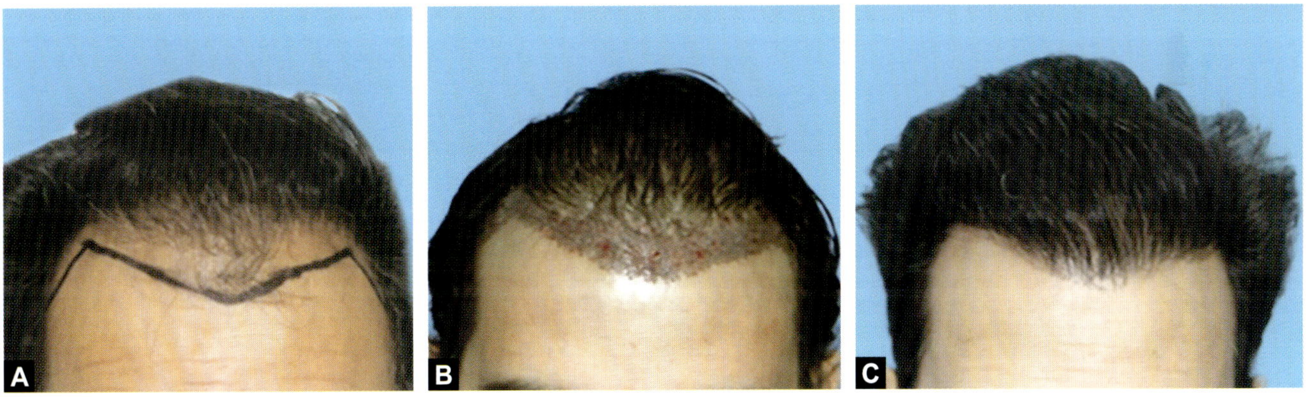

Figures 4.3A to C

Triangular hairline.

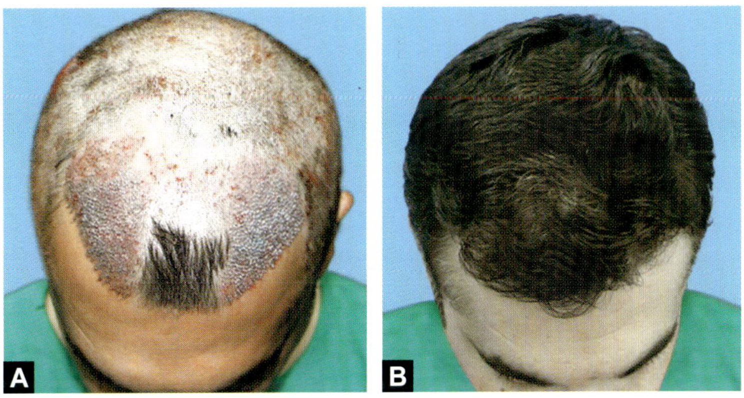

Figures 4.4A and B

A rectangular hairline—we make this hairline in people where we see a rectangular face with flat forehead.

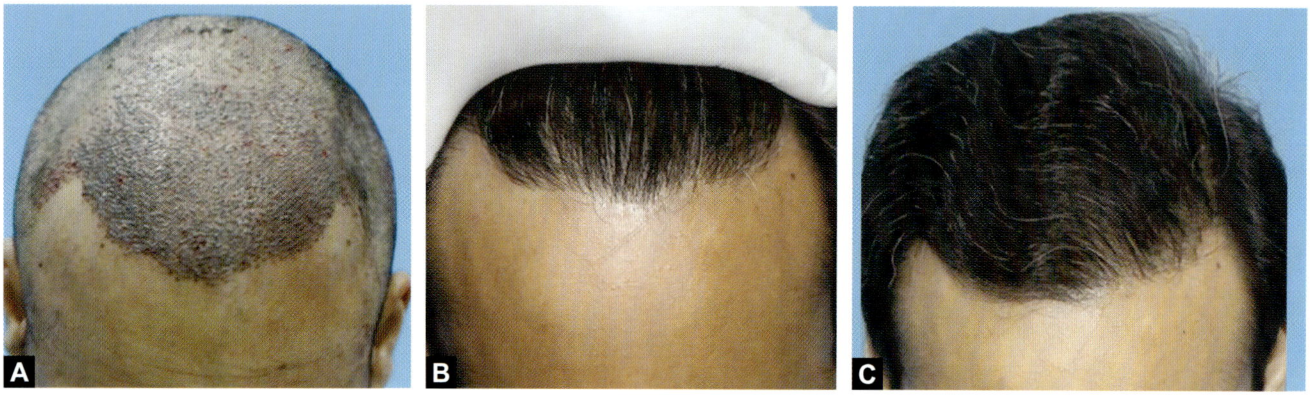

Figures 4.5A to C

Another variant of rectangular hairline with three small peaks.

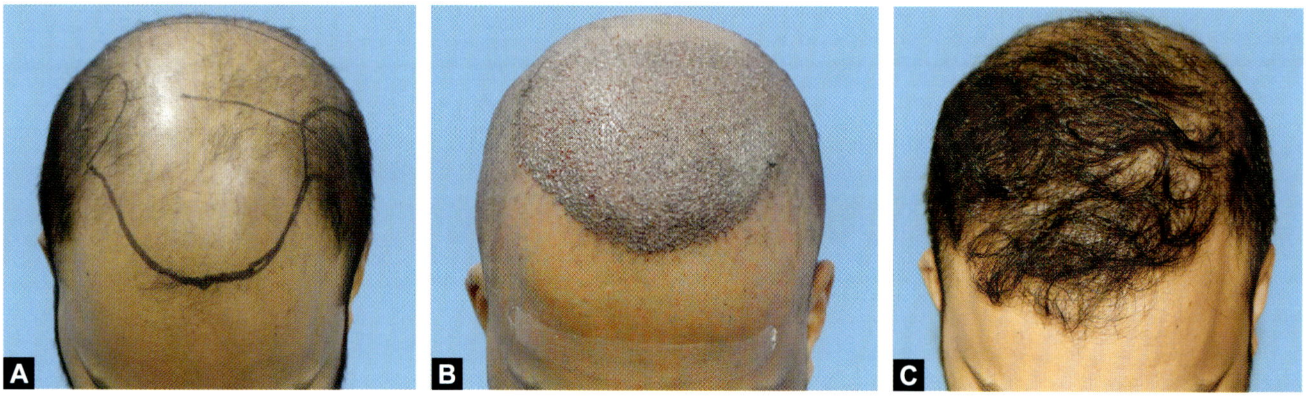

Figures 4.6A to C

A bell-shaped hairline in a male with its post-transplant results after 5 months.

onlooker to detect that you have got a transplant! It is only possible when the hairline does not hit the person's eyes as something unnatural or weird. A young hair transplant surgeon should use all his observation of natural hairlines to give the best possible hairline to his patient.

However, a basic understanding of landmarks is important (Figs. 4.7 and 4.8).[2]

Mid-frontal point (MFP): It should be marked on the vertical line from glabella to trichion. The forehead height (from trichion to glabella) is usually 6-6.5 cm. But for surgical lowering of hairline, the MFP should be marked usually at a height of 7–10 cm. However, this varies from person to person with different types of face contour.

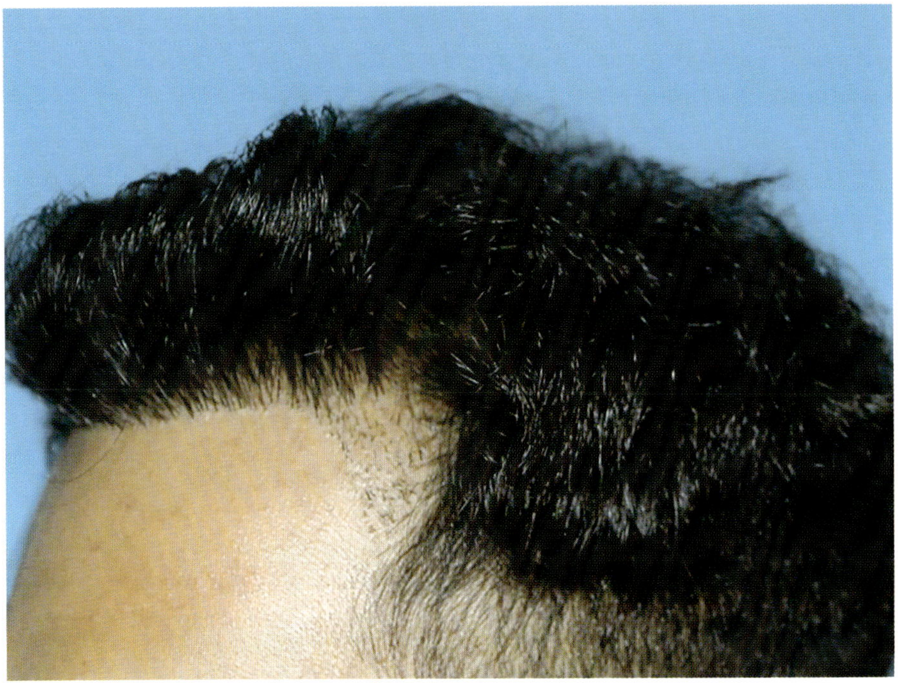

Figure 4.7

Image depicts a hairline which arches down from the MFP (mid frontal point) to MTP (mid temporal point) instead of arching upward. Always cross check the side views of the hairline to avoid such mistakes.

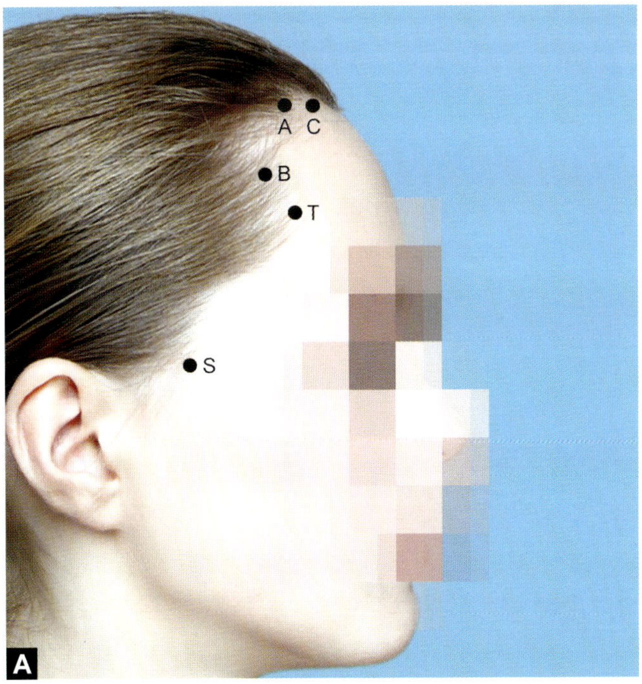

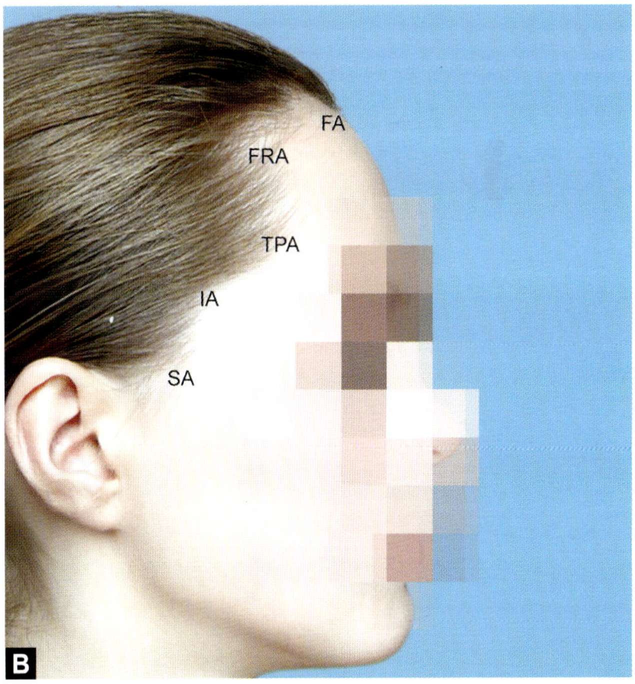

Figures 4.8A and B

Anatomical landmarks of the anterior hairline. A, C, B, T, S are the exact point where FA, FRA, TPA, IA and SA are located (Point A to C: FA; Point B: FRA; Point T: TPA; and Point S: SA).
(FA: frontal area; FRA: frontotemporal recess area; TPA: temporal peak area; IA: infratemple area; SA: sideburn area)

Frontotemporal angle (FTA): It is always located on a line drawn vertically from the lateral epicanthal folds. A line drawn from the MFP to the FTA should always slope slightly upward when viewed from the side. If the line arches down, it will look like an artificial hairline from side view. If patient wants the hairline to be more aggressive, the line from MFP to FTA can go flat but it can never arch down.

Frontal area (FA): Also known as widow's peak or central peak. It is an inverted triangular area, with its peak at the center pointing downward. This peak also known as mid-frontal point (MFP) forms reference point for determining the symmetry of the hairline, and the height of the hairline.

Frontotemporal recess area (FTR): The two other points of the triangle above form the FTR area. It lies on a line drawn vertically from the lateral epicanthal fold (Fig. 4.9).

Temporal peak area (TPA): It is the temporal area hairline pointing anteriorly toward the angle of eye.

Infratemple area (ITA): The area just below the TPA is the infratemple area and is concave in shape.

Mid-pupillary point is the point where the hairline starts to recede back, just behind the MFP (Fig. 4.10).

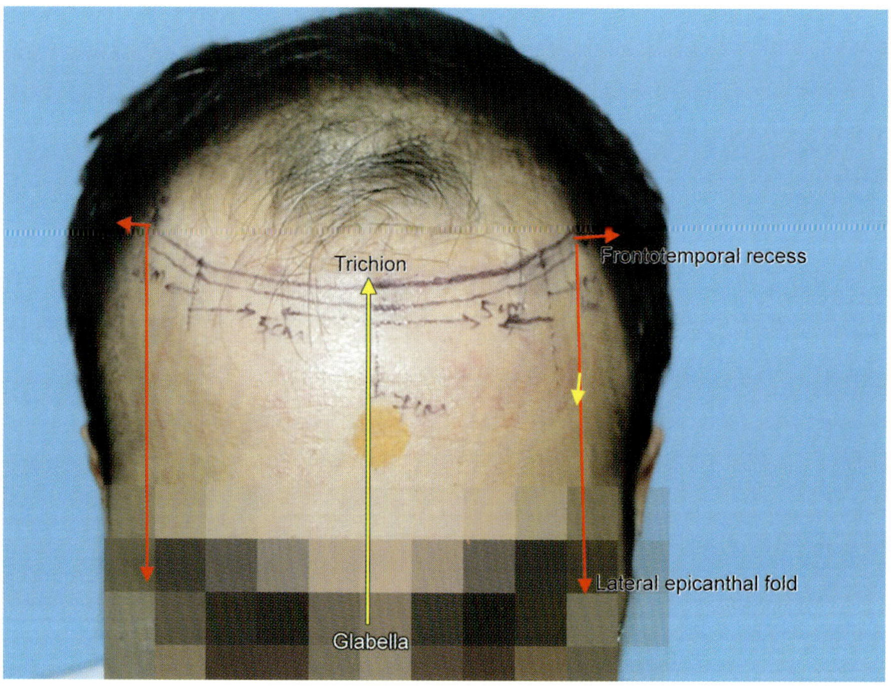

Figure 4.9

The yellow line depicts the forehead height from trichion at top to glabella at root of nose. The frontotemporal recess always lies on the red line extending vertically upward from lateral epicanthal folds.

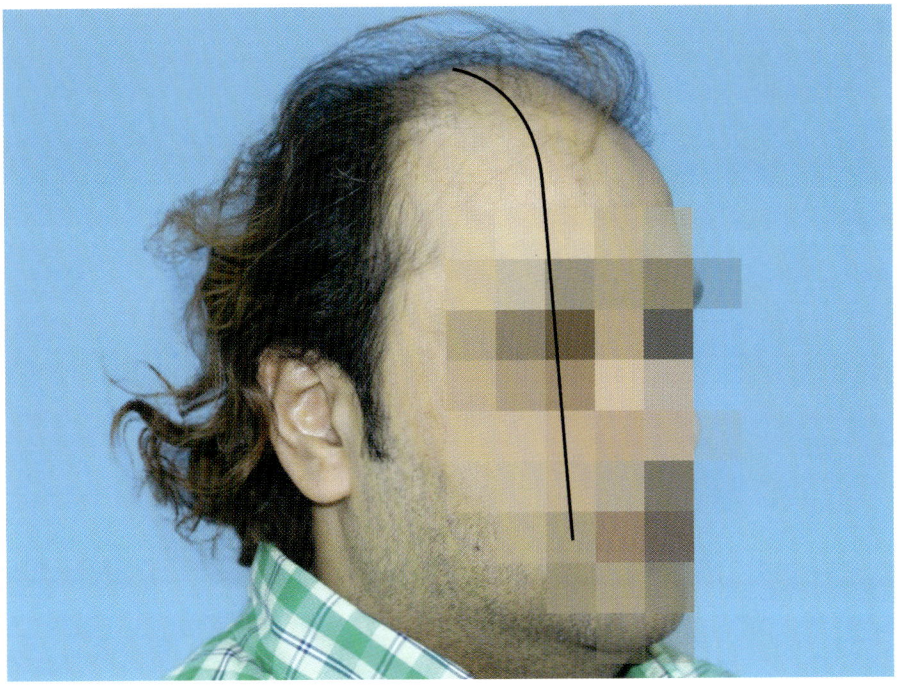

Figure 4.10
Mid-pupillary point.

Drawing the Hairline

After knowing the anatomical points, the hairline design starts with marking the mid-frontal point. Mid-frontal point can be kept anywhere between 7 cm and 10 cm from the glabella.[3] Doctors often fall into the trap of patients who are young and wish to keep the hairline very low at 7 cm or even at 6.5 cm, in spite of having a bigger head and family history of Norwood grade 7 baldness. Keeping a low hairline will make the patient repent in later years of his life when there is progressive loss of the hair behind and lateral to the reconstructed hairline, making the anterior transplanted hairline look unnatural. However, keeping the hairline too high will also not give satisfaction to the patient, so it is important to find the right distance of mid-frontal point from the glabella, which will ensure a consistent look of the patient throughout his rest of life. One way of deciding the mid-frontal point is the intersection between horizontal and vertical planes (Fig. 4.11).[3] Another way of deciding this point is to use a flexible scale and measure the distance from glabella and then mark the MFP followed by using a laser-assist hairline design device to mark the hairline (Fig. 4.12).[4]

After determining the mid-frontal point, the location of frontotemporal angle needs to be determined. It can be determined by drawing a line from lateral epicanthus of the eye back toward the point where it meets the temporal hair.[3]

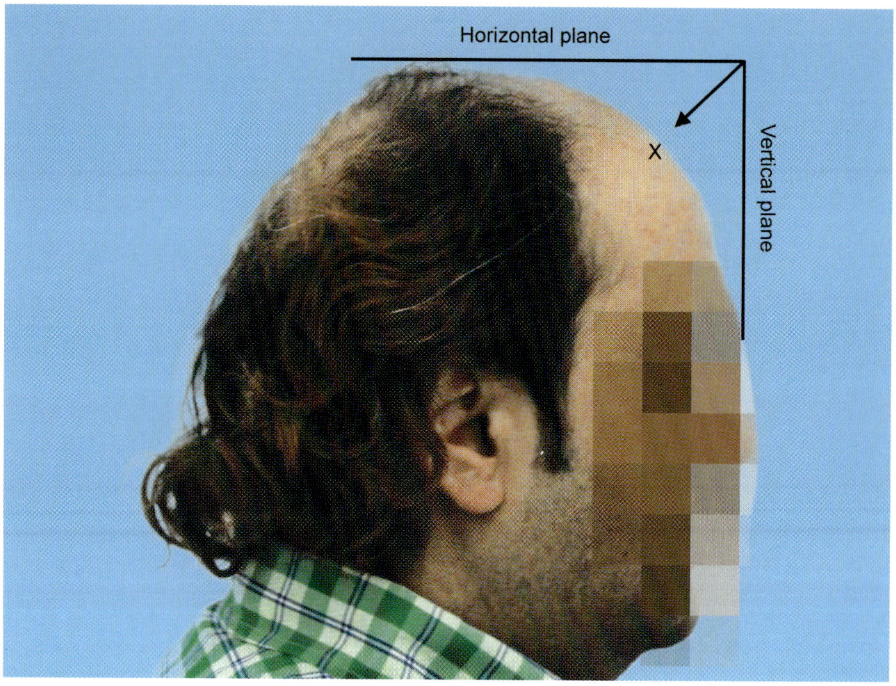

Figure 4.11

The point where the horizontal and vertical planes intersect is marked as mid-frontal point (MFP).

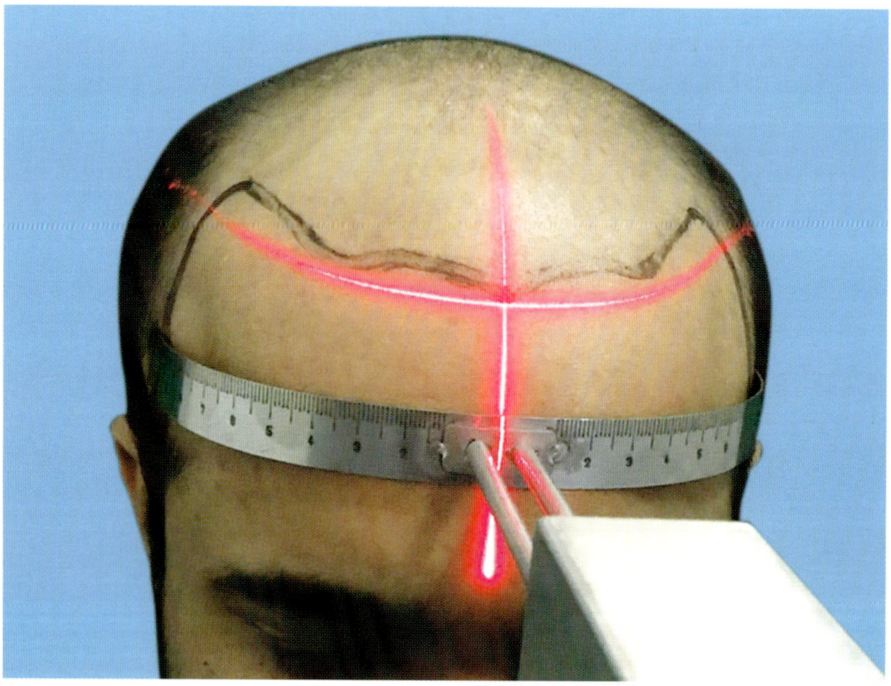

Figure 4.12

Laser-assist hairline design device which is being used to make a hairline, to ensure the symmetry of the hairline. Tracing your hairline along the laser beam is not necessary for a good hairline!

In case of severe degree of baldness where there is no temporal hair, visualizing lateral or parietal hump is important.[3] The lateral hump is a semicircular area of hair which bridges the lateral fringe and the mid-scalp region. It is present in Norwood Grade 6 baldness and is absent in Norwood grade 7 baldness. Visualizing this hump in Norwood grade 7 gives the lateral epicanthal line a target to intersect.[3] They usually meet near the top of the hump and lateral hump usually becomes the inferior border of frontotemporal angle (Fig. 4.13).[3]

Another visualization technique is drawing a line parallel to the side burn, and the point where it meets the lateral epicanthal line, is the location of frontotemporal angle (Fig. 4.14).[3]

After drawing the hairline, the patient should be shown the mirror in which he can visualise his to be the reconstructed hairline. One should remember that the image, which a patient sees in the mirror, is 2D image of the hairline and may ask for some corrections which do not fit into surgeons' imaginations.[5] Disconnect between the surgeons' imagination and patient's imagination has to be explained to the patient. The surgeon should also look at the hairline from a distance and from the back by making the patient look upward. One should remember that recession of the left and right temple is never identical, so slight asymmetry in hairline drawing is acceptable and provides naturalness in the look.

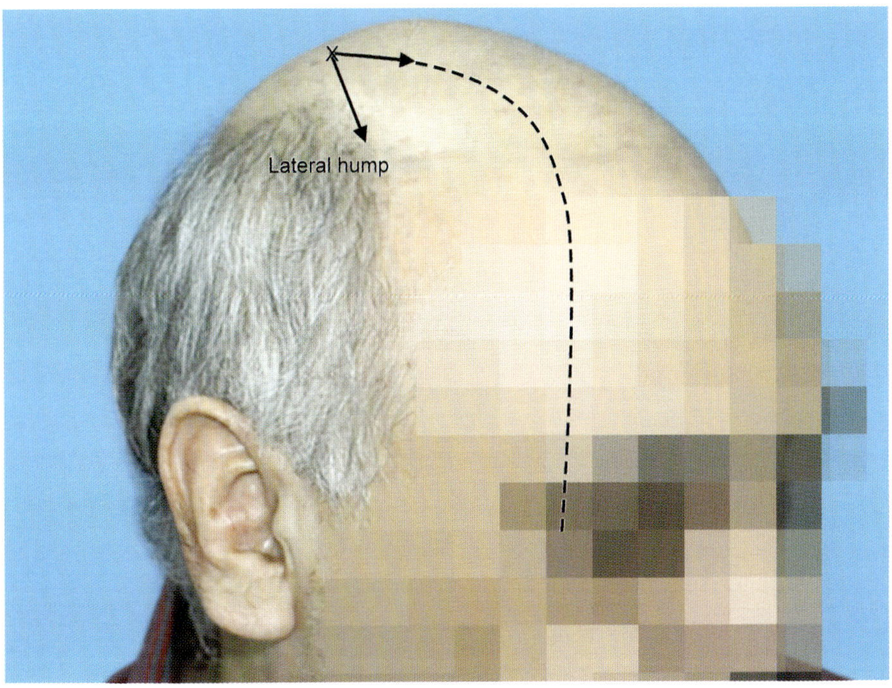

Figure 4.13

Intersection of the lateral epicanthal line with the upper border of the "lateral hump" gives the frontotemporal angle.

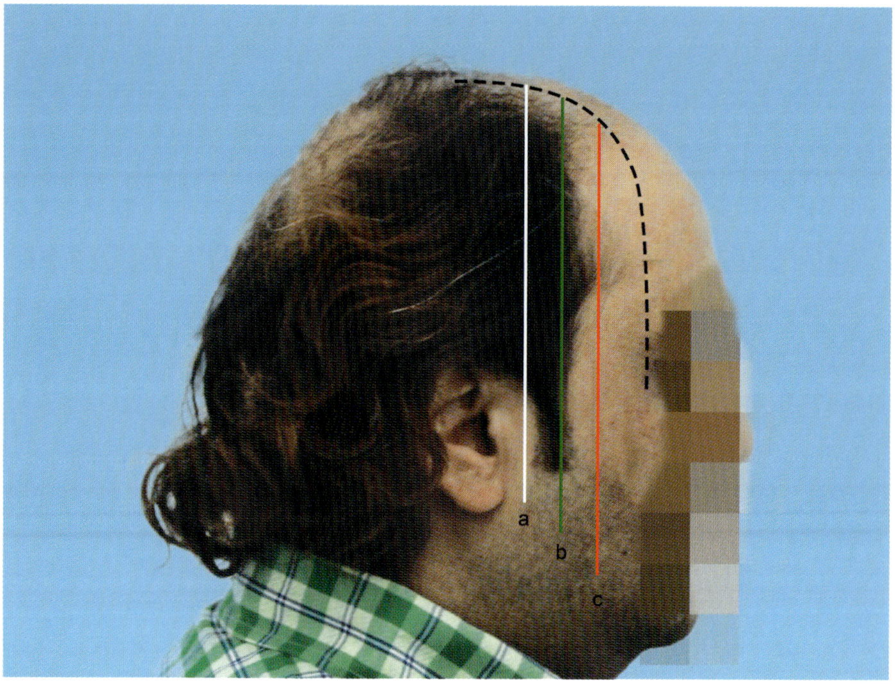

Figure 4.14

A line is drawn parallel to the side burn, and the point where it meets the lateral epicanthal line, is the location of frontotemporal angle.

HAIRLINE DESIGNING

After drawing the hairline, which is acceptable to both the surgeon and the patient, one can proceed with the surgery. The surgeon must evaluate and re-evaluate the symmetry, shape and position of hairline from all possible angles, i.e. from the front, with the head bent downward and from behind.[5] However, few patients may not agree to surgeon's designed hairline and will insist for a lower hairline, it can be done by creating a widow's peak which creates an illusion of a lower hairline.[3] A widow's peak is recommended in a conservative bell-shaped hairline. Some patients ask to fill the frontotemporal angle. Instead of filling the angle, the whole frontotemporal angle can be brought forward.[3] A hairline which looks symmetrical to the surgeon may look asymmetrical to the patient in the mirror because he is seeing himself in the mirror which distorts the 3D image of the surgeon to 2D image of the mirror due to asymmetry of the skull.[5] The surgeon should try to reach a middle path regarding the hairline design, before going ahead with the procedure.

Anterior hairline should always be constructed keeping in mind two zones: (1) transition zone (TZ) and (2) the defined zone (DZ) (Figs. 4.15 and 4.16).

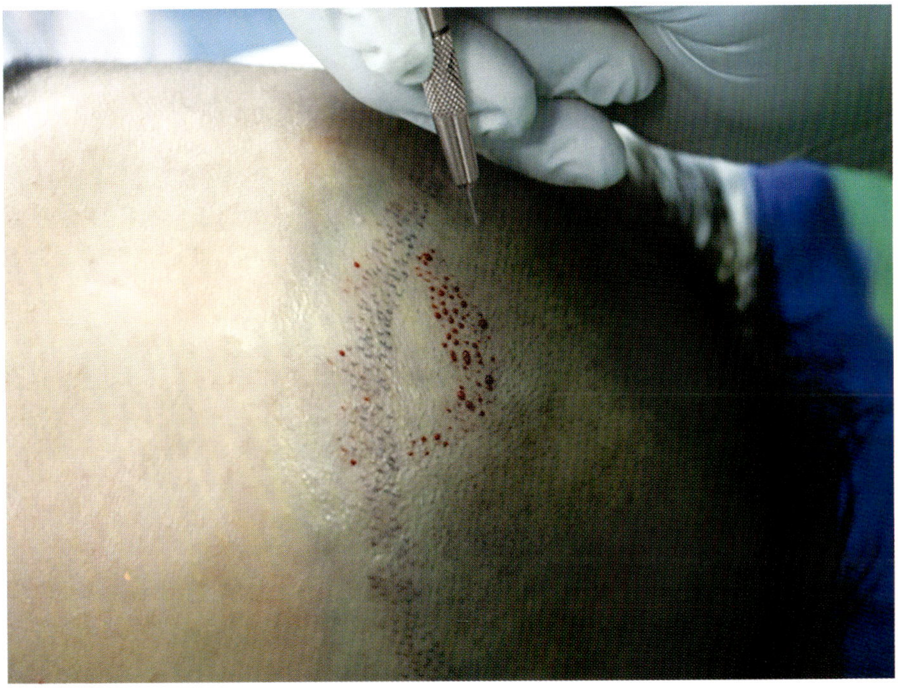

Figure 4.15

The image depicts the angle of the needle while slit making.

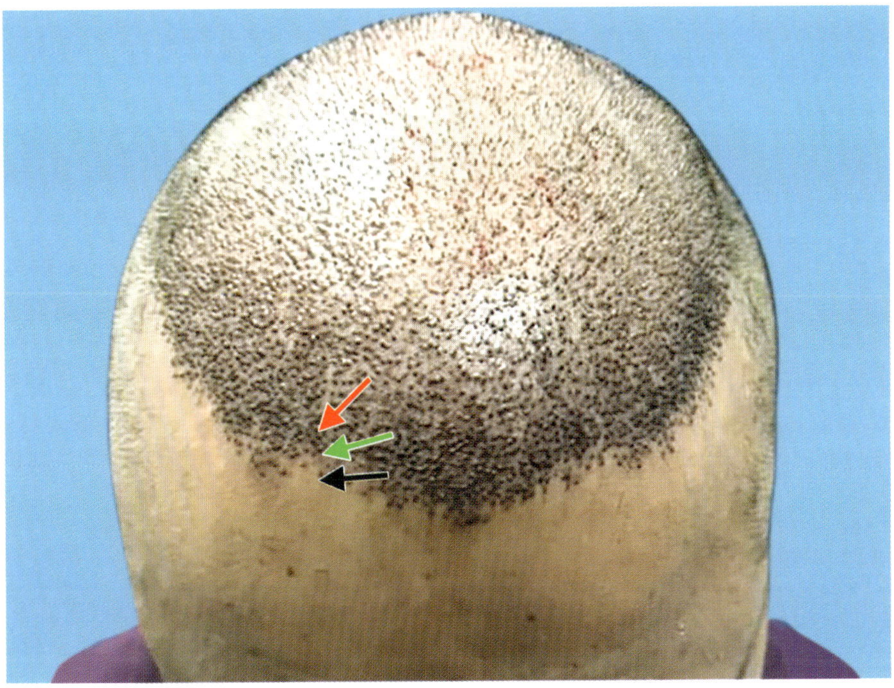

Figure 4.16

Red arrow: Defined zone area with more densely packed grafts. *Green arrow:* Transition zone area with 1–2 hair follicle grafts. *Black arrow:* Irregular anterior border showing microirregularities.

Transition zone (TZ): Most anterior area of frontal line (anterior 0.5–1 cm area of the scalp), where density of hair is less and consist of irregularities. Density of hair should be sparse here. It should be initially irregular and ill-defined and then become more defined as it progresses to the defined zone (DZ). Single follicle hair graft should be planted in the initial 0.5 cm, to give the hairline a softer look. This should be followed by 2 follicles hair graft posteriorly. These hair should be placed in a zigzag pattern, to give it a natural look and not in a straight line.

Microirregularities: Tiny irregularities are usually made in the transition zone comprising of small triangular clusters of single graft hair follicles. These irregularities are known as microirregularities and can be made out only on close observation.

Macroirregularities: The anterior hairline is not a straight line but a curvaceous one. These curves can be made out from a distance and are known as macro-irregularities.

Defined zone (DZ): Defined zone area just behind the TZ, where density of hair increases. The hair in this area should look more dense, fuller and defined. Two-follicle and 3-follicle hair grafts should be planted in this area. The angle of the hair should be 30–40° to the scalp. The direction of frontal hair should usually point forward. As you move posteriorly, the angle should be increased to 40–50°.

Frontotemporal hairline: A mild recession in the FTA should be maintained in males to give a natural look. However, females are an exception where the recession should not be present. The hair are grafted similarly as in TZ and DZ. The angle should be 10–20°, and the direction of hair should be pointing inferiorly towards ear.

RECIPIENT SITE CREATION IN HAIRLINE

Creating hairline zone is an art, which should be mastered if one wants to be a successful hair transplant surgeon. The doctor should improve his hairline design after seeing every result of his previous transplants. He has to compete with himself to find flaws in his previous hairline to keep improving in giving excellent results. The art and science of slit creation after drawing the hairline has equally important role in giving fabulous hairlines in patients. There are some basic guidelines, which should be followed.

- All recipient sites should be aimed forward in a parallel or slightly converging pattern.[5]

- Vellus hair and miniaturized hair provide the hint about the angles and directions during slit making and plantation of grafts.
- The density along the hairline and central forelock should be higher than the rest of the areas. It should be dense but not overdense as forelock is a site for recipient site necrosis. Few surgeons extend the forelock posteriorly making it an oval region instead of a circular zone, so that the onlooker cannot see through the vertex from the front and in oblique view.[5]
- The presence of macroirregularities and microirregularities along the hairline. Macro-irregularities are equally important, they provide waviness to the hairline.[5] They may or may not be present in a good hairline. Hairline should never be sharp and straight.
- Microirregularities further amplify the unevenness. The peaks of micro-irregularities should be nonsharp, nonuniform, with uneven density present at unequal interval.
- The first two to three rows of slits should be soft, behind this, slits should be constructed in dense manner in an *interlocking* pattern (Figs. 4.17A and B).[5]
- Addition of free floating sentinel hair away from zone of microirregularity further adds to the asymmetry.

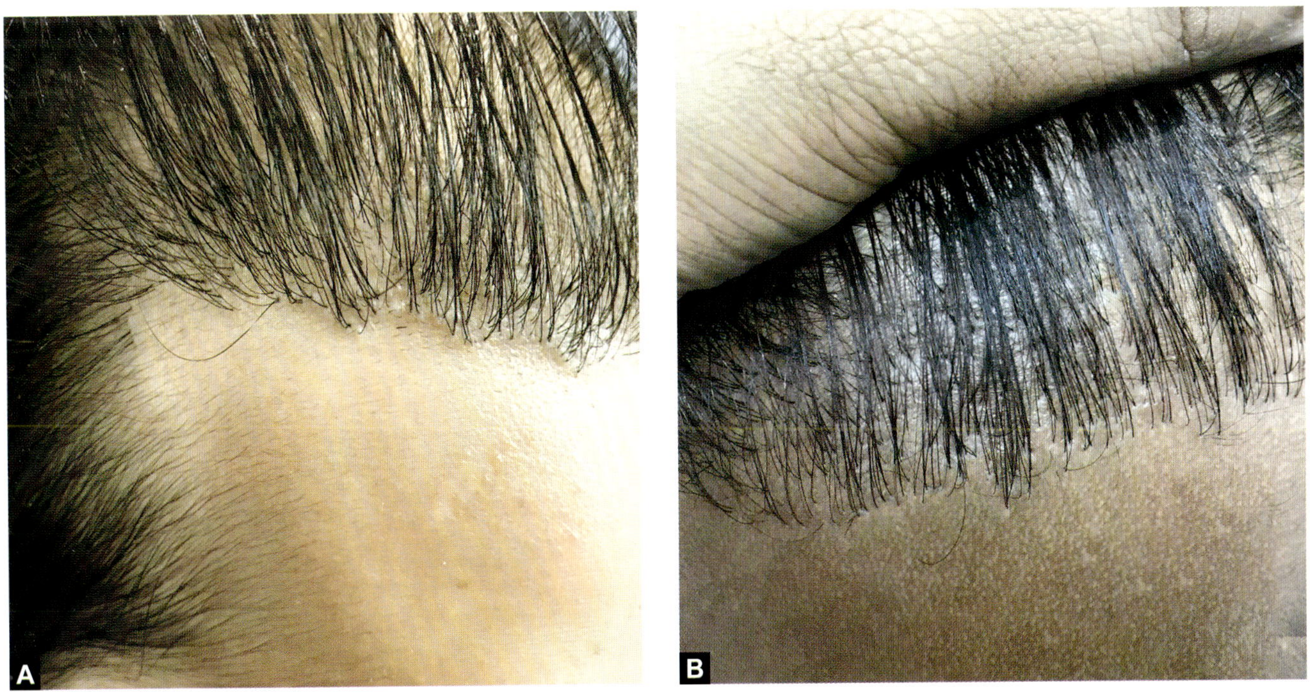

Figures 4.17A and B

A non-interlocked hairline with "see through effect" and parallel stalking (predictable linear arrangement).

- Single hair should be placed in the zone of microirregularities. Around 200–300 hair provide sufficient softness to the hairline (Fig. 4.18).
- There can be variation in the above approach depending on cases. Limited number of grafts is the biggest issue. Sometimes we do violate the scientific principles of hairline design like making FTA lateral to the lateral epicanthal line in case of Norwood grade 7 and in cases where the head size is big.
- In African origins, the hairline does not possess macro- and microirregularities and is extremely straight with little frontotemporal recession.
- The lateral end of the hairline can be drawn back as a continuing convex arc or can end with a slight flare. If the lateral aspect of hairline ends with a slight flare, it has to be supplemented with a more anterior temple reconstruction compared to the hairline which ends with the tail moving backward (Figs. 4.19A and B).

STEPWISE DEMONSTRATION OF SLIT MAKING WITH CREATING THE HAIRLINE

The stepwise demonstration of slit making with creating the hairline is shown in Figures 4.20 to 4.24.

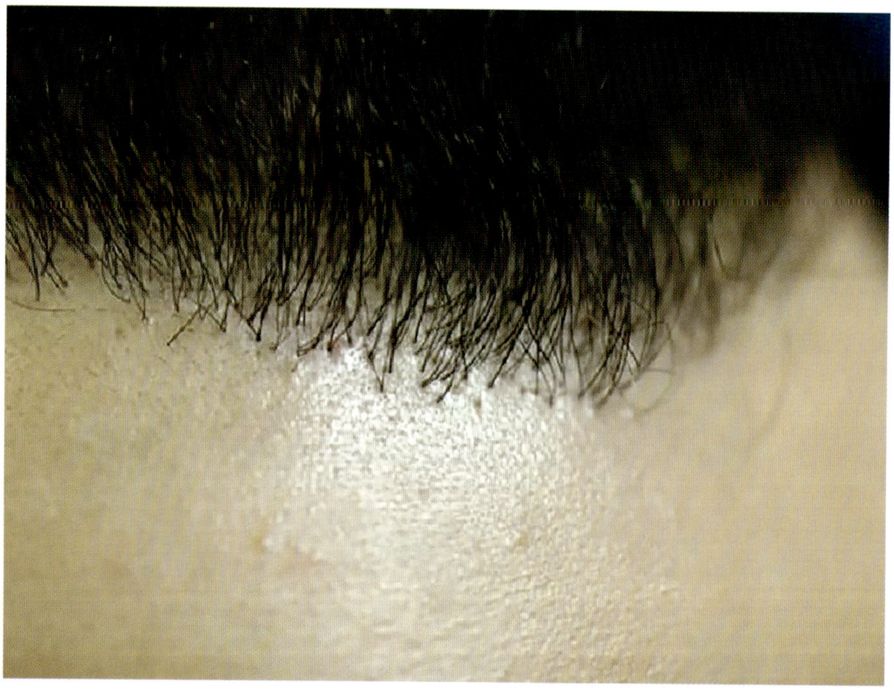

Figure 4.18

Presence of double hair follicles in the anterior border of hairline and in the transition zone. Careful scrutiny of the follicles for the hidden telogen hair in the graft by the doctor or the senior most assistant should be done.

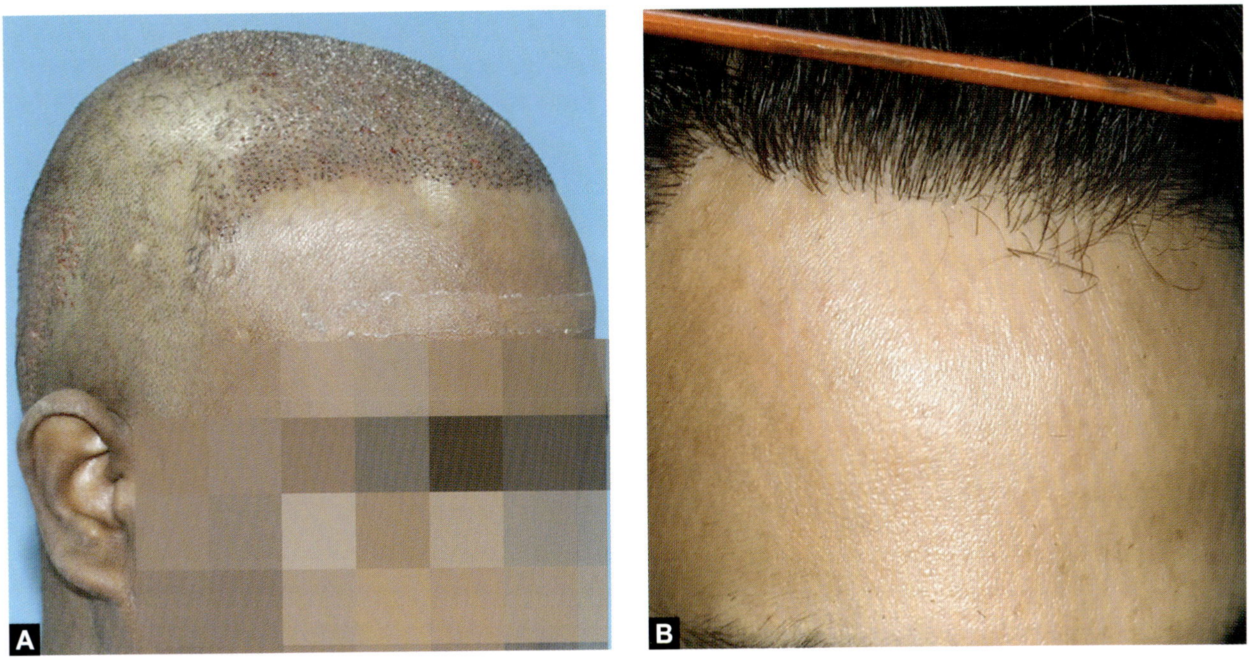

Figures 4.19A and B

(A) Hairline ending with lateral flare; (B) Note the lateral flare of the hairline.

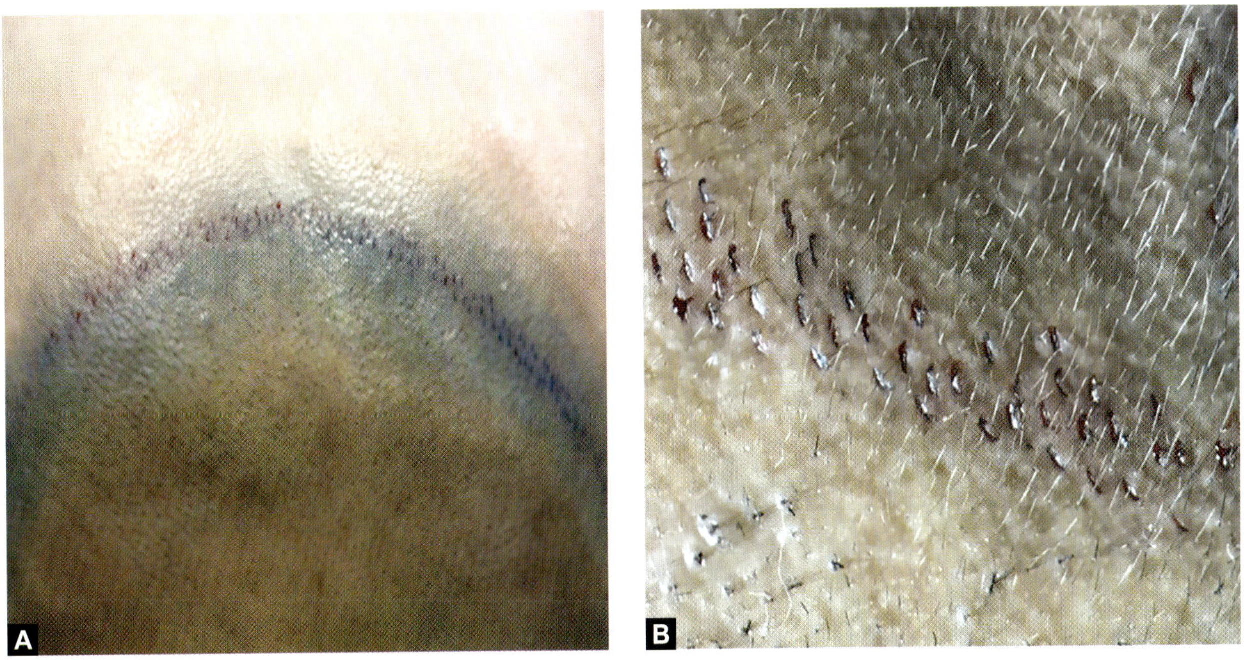

Figures 4.20A and B

(A) Step 1A—it involves creation of 1 hair site (three rows), which are made on the hairline drawn with marker. Slits which are made here are sagittal and follows a nonlinear pattern for interlocking effect. They are made with 20G needle; (B) Step 1B—the horizontal distance between two one-hair site should not be same and height of peaks of microirregularity should be different.

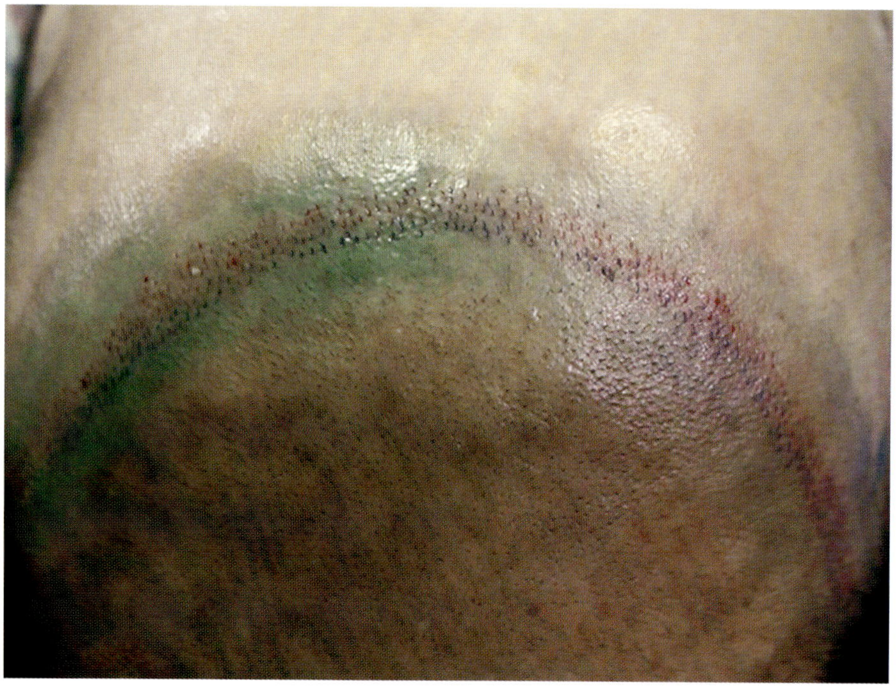

Figure 4.21

Step 2—it involves further strengthening of hairline by creating a fourth row behind the first two lines along with creation of microirregularity with blunt and small irregularly-shaped peaks.

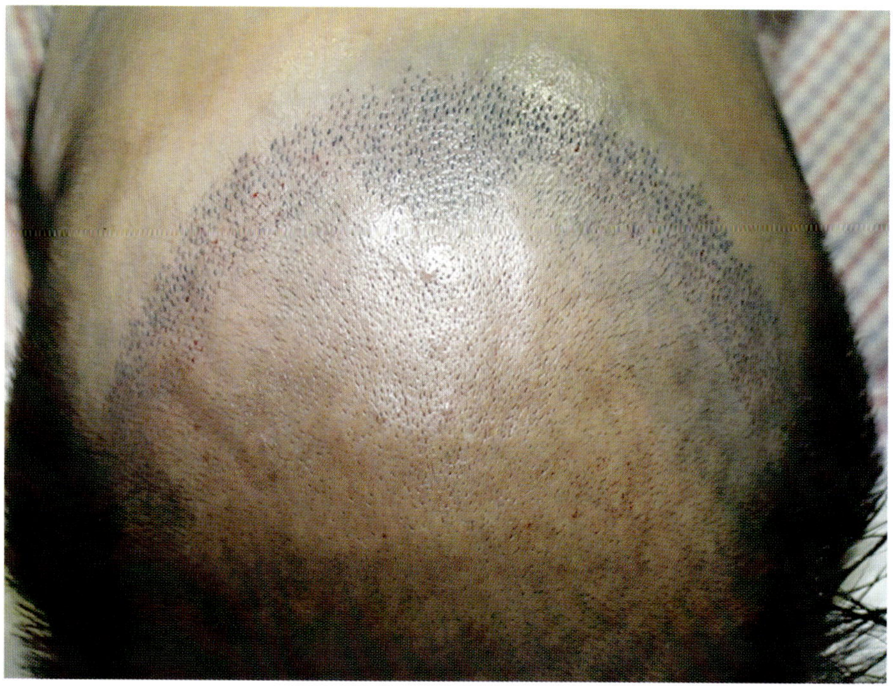

Figure 4.22

Step 3—creation of additional 4–5 rows of sagittally-oriented slits behind the first four rows along with creation of 2 hair sites in central forelock.

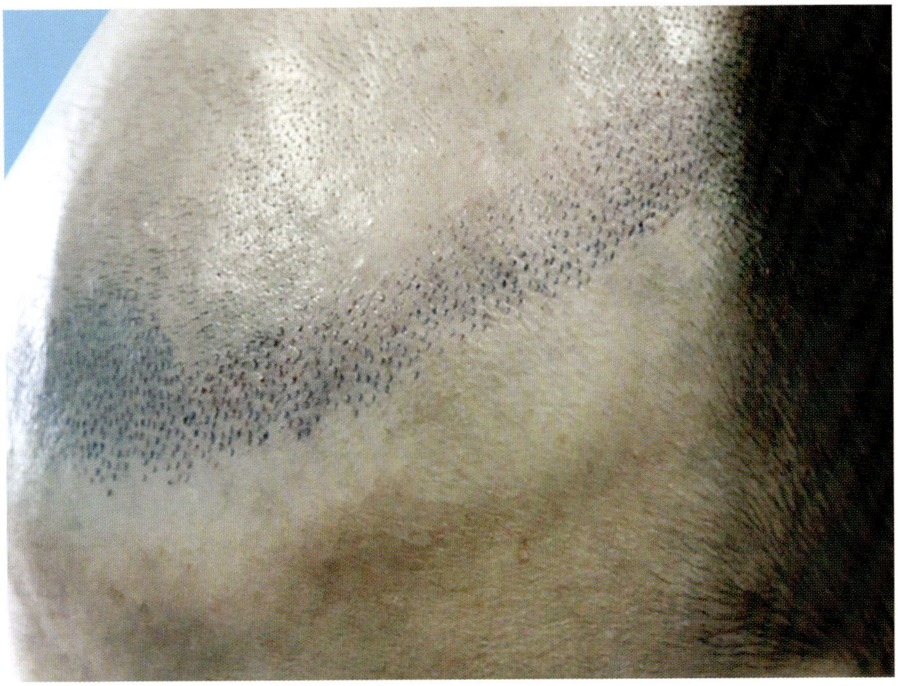

Figure 4.23

Step 4—creation of microirregularity with blunt peaks of different heights with their location being just above the prominence of the frontal bone on the forehead.

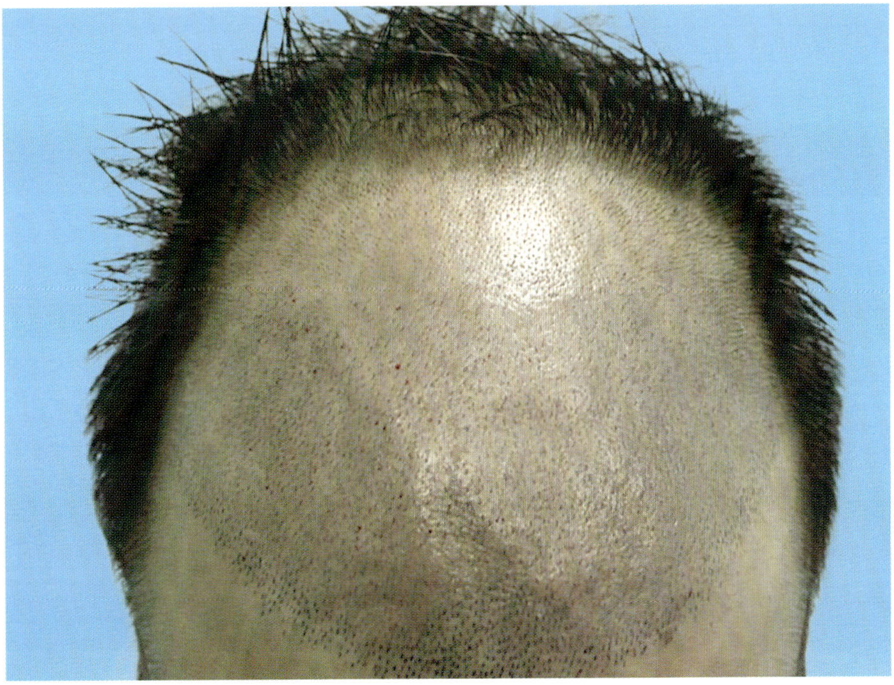

Figure 4.24

Step 5—after creation of first 6–7 rows of hairline along with creation of microirregularities, slits with correct angles and direction should be made behind the hairline zone.

ARTISTRY IN HAIRLINE CREATION

Recreating a Cowlick or Preserving the Pre-existing Cowlick

Cowlick is a radiating spiral of hair, which is usually present in female hairlines but is also sometimes found in male hairlines.[5] Preserving the cowlick or creating a cowlick is an art worth mastering as it imparts fabulous naturalness to the hairline. It is usually present in the midline of the hairline. Many parts of cowlick grow even in backward direction (Figs. 4.25A to D).

Bringing Artistry into Hairline Creation

Hairline creation needs much more than just knowing the distance from glabella and making a good symmetrical line with right frontotemporal angles.

For example, here shows what passion in hair transplant is all about (Figs. 4.26A to F). Our surgeons created an amazing result in the first transplant they did with the following patient as shown in the pre-existing reconstructed hairline. With greed for more, both patient and surgeon mutually agreed to further improve the hairline and to make that hairline from good to amazing.

Hairline designing is a job of the surgeon who is also an artist. He has to use his imagination and foresee the result as each and every slit he creates will determine the look of the patient. At the same time he has to keep in mind the limitation of number of grafts. The following hair transplant result of a single patient demonstrates the importance of creating an amazing hairline and why one should imagine and reimagine the hairline for a patient before going ahead with the procedure. He should spend maximum possible time in slit creation (Figs. 4.27A to D).

SLIT CREATION[6]

Slit creation is a blind procedure. One should be aware about the blood supply and vascular supply of the scalp before proceeding to slit creation. It can be created in two ways: coronal slits and sagittal slits, or a mix of two types at various sites. Slit creation is an art of digging the soil to create space for implanting trees while moving through a jungle.

1. Right depth of slit is essentially the first thing to be kept in mind, since any incision that penetrates too deeply may damage the blood supply to the scalp that may cause decrease perfusion to scalp distal to injury and may result in necrosis and there may be no growth of hair. Use of tumescence, which is a mixture of lidocaine, epinephrine and normal saline causes puffing up of scalp along with vasoconstriction, thus minimizes the risk of necrosis by decreasing the chance of vessel injury.
2. *Needle versus blade:* We have used both needle and blade in our hair transplantation method during slit making. Slit making through needle is

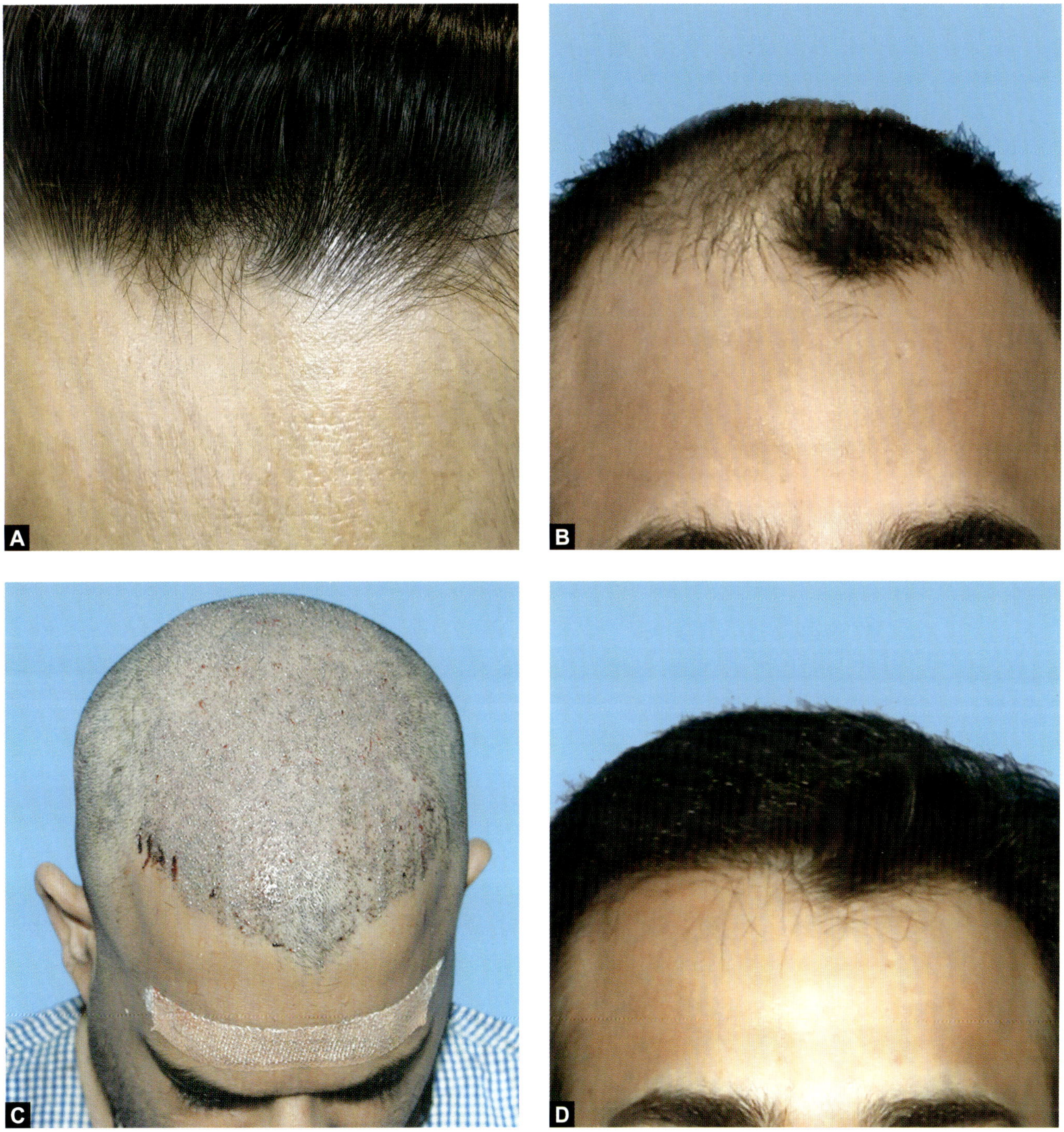

Figures 4.25A to D

(A) A classical cowlick; (B to D) Note the beautiful cowlick which has been preserved while restoring the patient's hairline. It is a bunch of hair which grows in different direction from the rest of the hairline. Preserving the cowlick even further enhances the naturalness of the hairline. It also creates an illusion of lower hairline.

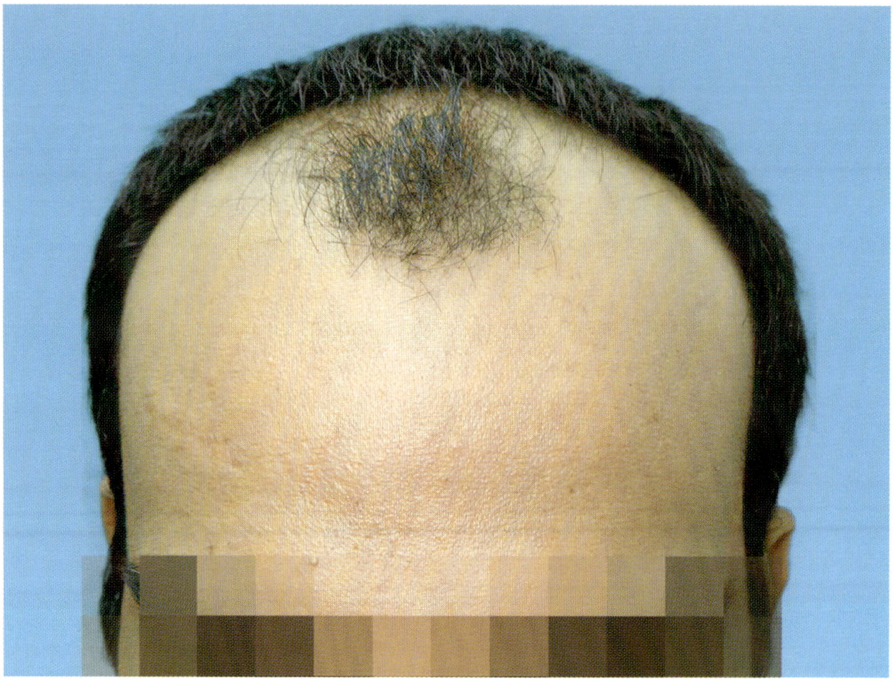

Figure 4.26A

The appearance of patient before hair transplant.

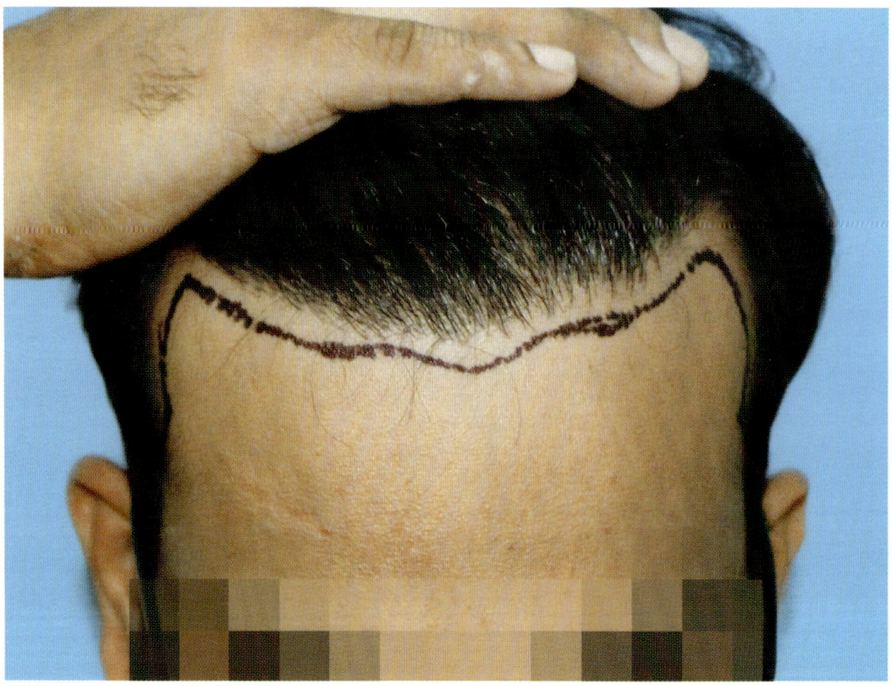

Figure 4.26B

After first transplant which we did in the year 2014, both patient and surgeon decided to lower the hairline in year 2017. The new hairline was drawn as shown in the figure.

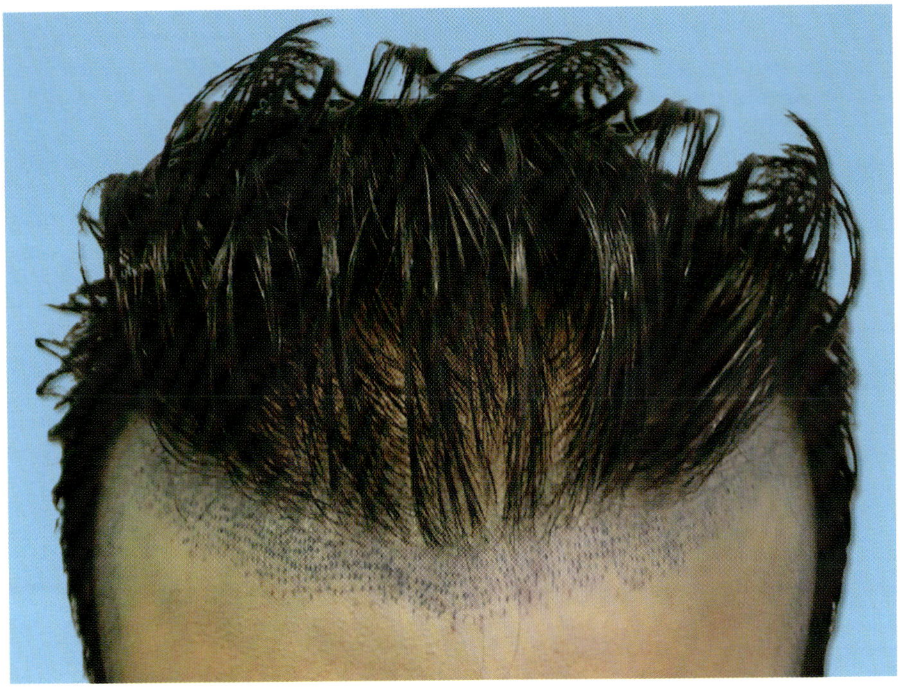

Figure 4.26C

Slits were created for hairline lowering.

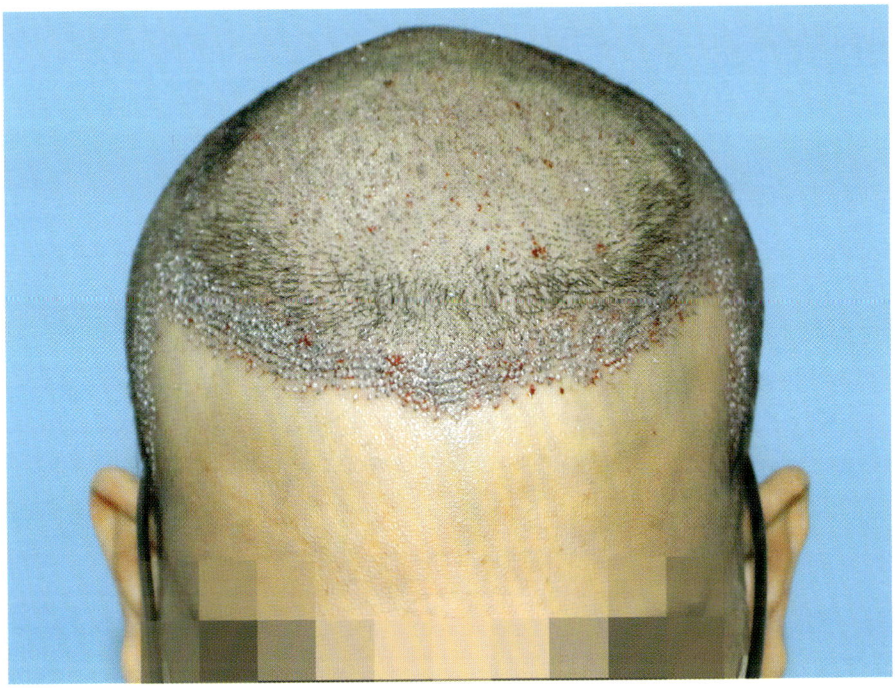

Figure 4.26D

Postoperative image with graft placed in the these slits.

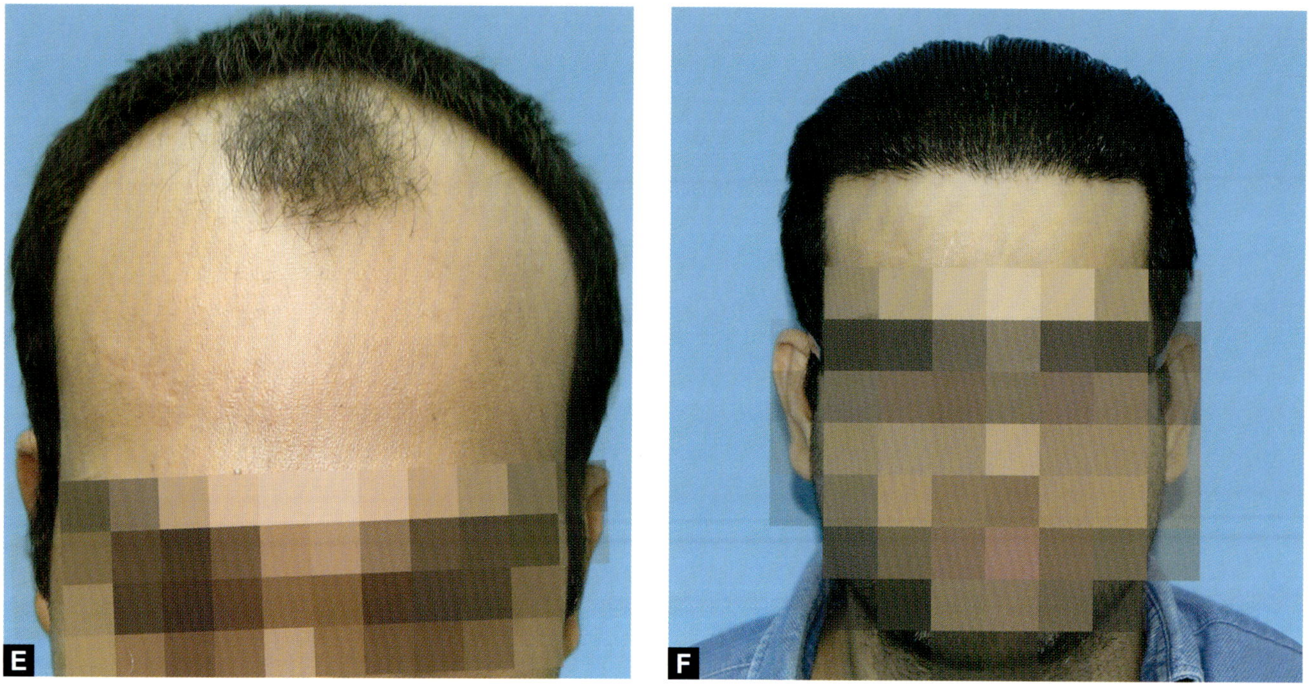

Figures 4.26E and F

Final, before and after photograph of the patient.

effective, cheaper but more tiring method since needle needs to be changed after every 100–150 slits. Another point, needle being tapering at the tip needs to be penetrated a little deeper than blade to provide adequate space for the follicles. Using 20G needle in hairline, but 1.0 mm punch instead of 0.95 mm or 0.9 mm punch for punching of graft may stifle the graft in the slits, so it is essential to match the slit size with punch size for smooth implantation of the grafts. Slit making behind the hairline can be made with a 19G or 20G needle depending on the type of punch used. The *CTS (cut to size)* blade being of uniform width, more sharp, having better ergonomics is more convenient for slit making, however being more sharp, the visibility of slits during implantation is lesser than the slits by needles (Fig. 4.28).

3. Using good lighting and magnification and proper shaving is extremely crucial since wrongly angled needles or blade during slit making will damage pre-existing hair. This may lead to massive effluvium or shock loss. The sagittal angled slits being parallel to the grafts have lesser risk of damaging hair follicles.
4. *Coronal slits versus sagittal slits (Fig. 4.29)*: First of all as authors of this book, we want to clarify that we are seeing brilliant results from both sagittal slits and coronal slits which we are creating during hair restoration.

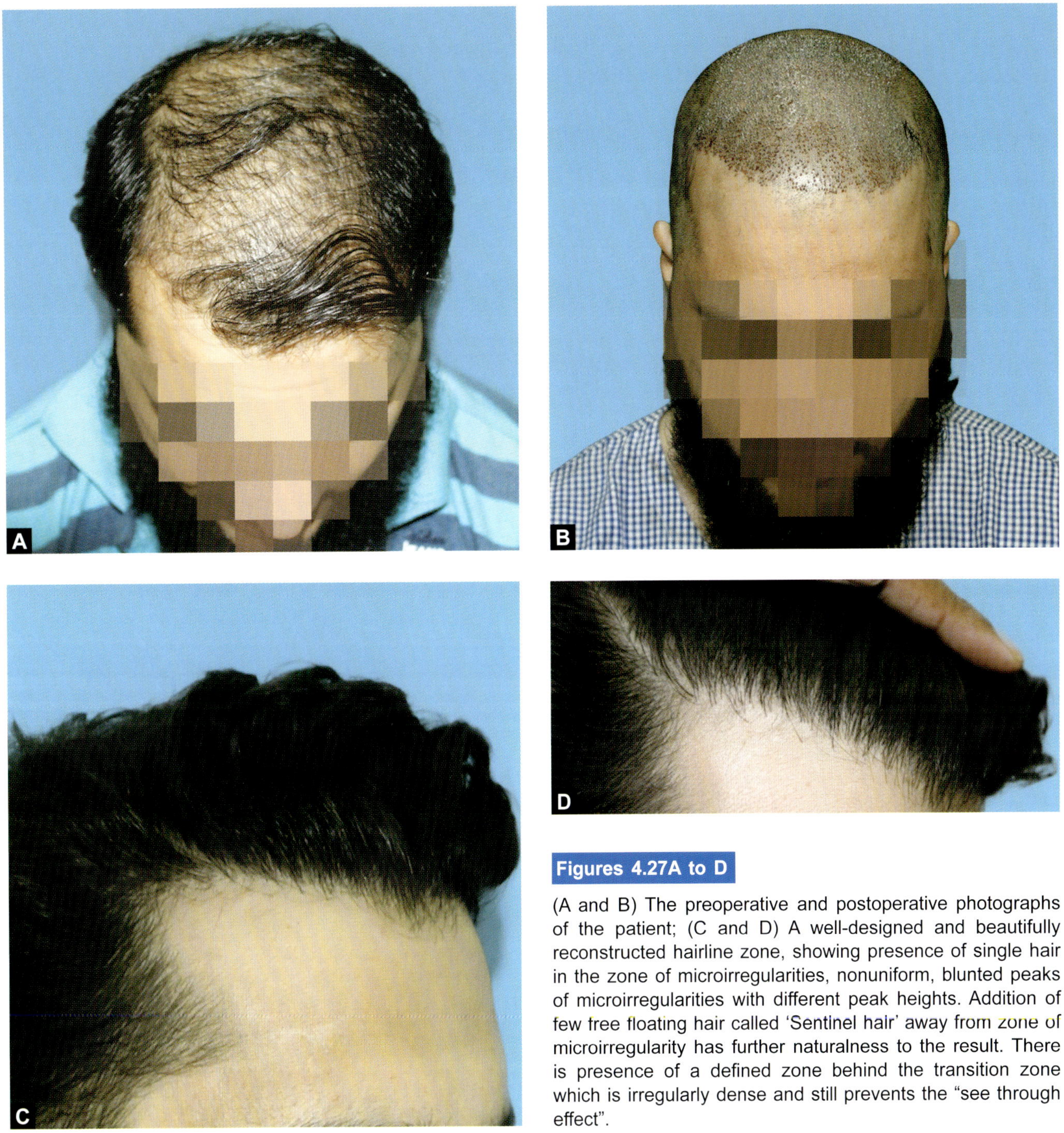

Figures 4.27A to D

(A and B) The preoperative and postoperative photographs of the patient; (C and D) A well-designed and beautifully reconstructed hairline zone, showing presence of single hair in the zone of microirregularities, nonuniform, blunted peaks of microirregularities with different peak heights. Addition of few free floating hair called 'Sentinel hair' away from zone of microirregularity has further naturalness to the result. There is presence of a defined zone behind the transition zone which is irregularly dense and still prevents the "see through effect".

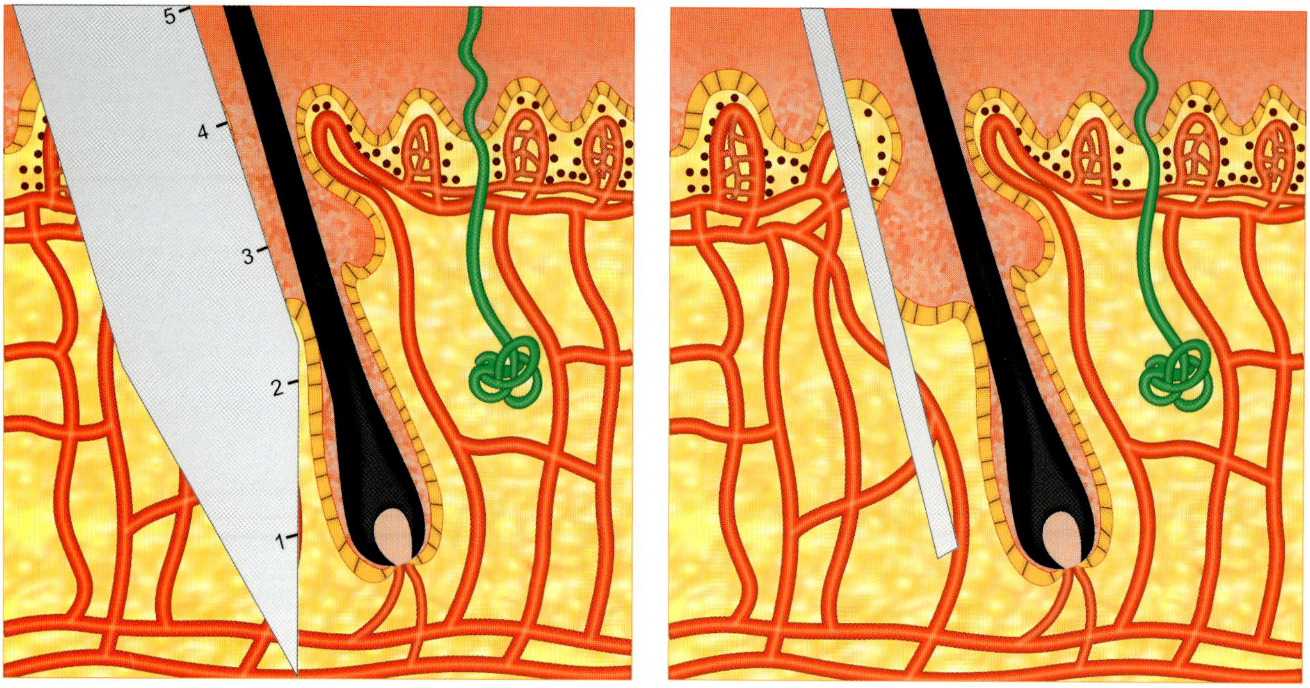

Figure 4.28

Needle has to pierce far deeper to create adequate space for the implanted roots, thus may cause more vascular damage than the CTS blade which has to reach just at the level of neighboring hair root.

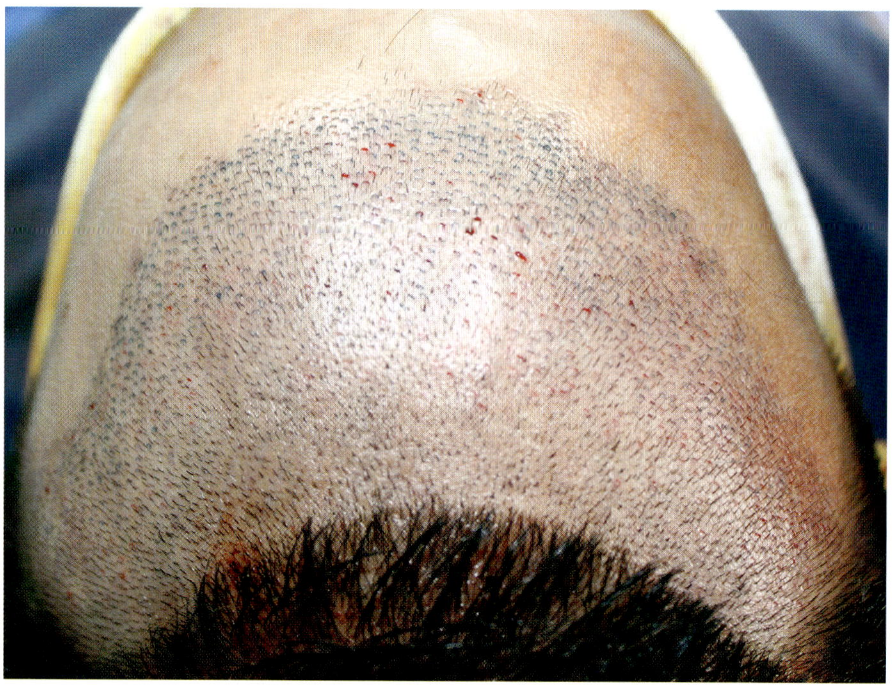

Figure 4.29

Coronal angled slits.

One surgeon prefers sagittal slits and the other surgeon prefers coronal slits. We wish to enumerate various pros and cons of both types of slit making, but there is no such study to confirm the superiority of one over the other.

- Sagittal slits are made parallel to the direction of hair growth while coronal slits are made at right angle to the direction of hair growth.
- Theoretically, coronal slits are better since the hair exit the scalp beside each other compared to sagittal slits where hair exit the scalp behind each other leading to linear appearance of grafts. However, such observation holds true when one views the hair head on, sagittal oriented hair may give an illusion of higher density when viewed from side of scalp. Coronal slits are also angle resistant as the hair does not slide in the slits and change its angle after implantation of grafts.
- Needle having a far less sharper surface compared to blade will produce vascular damage at only at its lower point, thus nullifying the hypothesis of more vascular damage with needle. Practically the authors have found no difference in the results with both the types of slit making and have achieved fabulous results with both.[7]

The process for making slits at frontotemporal angle is shown in Figures 4.30 to 4.32.

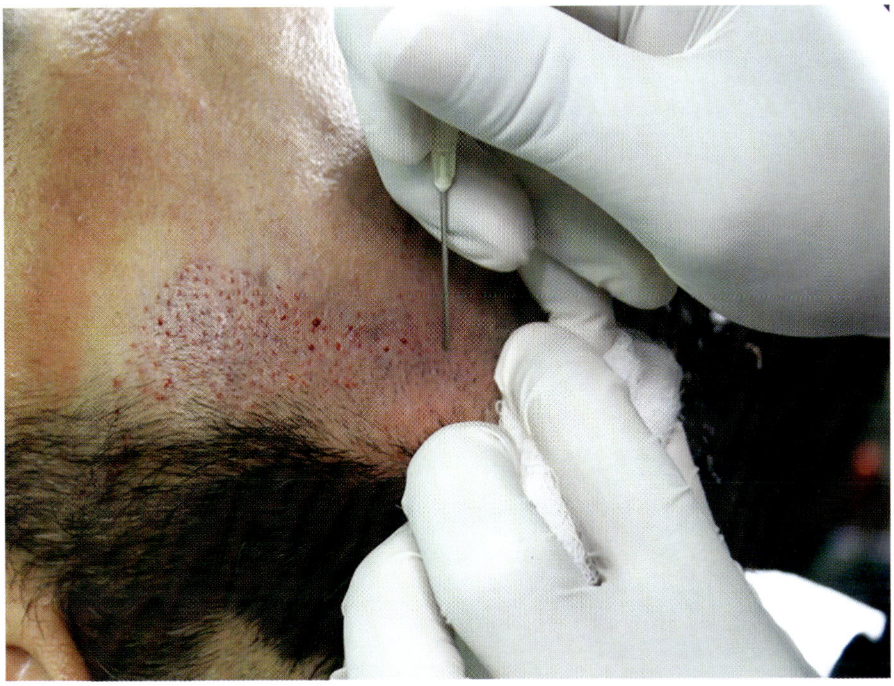

Figure 4.30

There is subtle change in direction of hair at frontotemporal angle. The slits which are medial to frontotemporal angle should be preferably directed slightly medially.

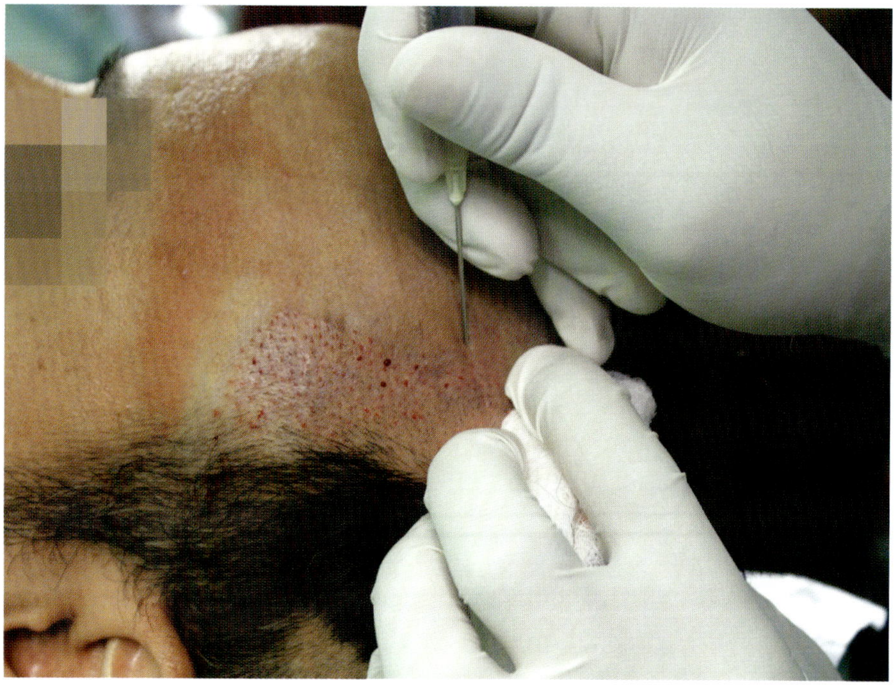

Figure 4.31

The hair which needs to be implanted exactly at frontotemporal angle needs to be directed in the direction of frontotemporal angle so slits are made exactly in the direction of frontotemporal angle.

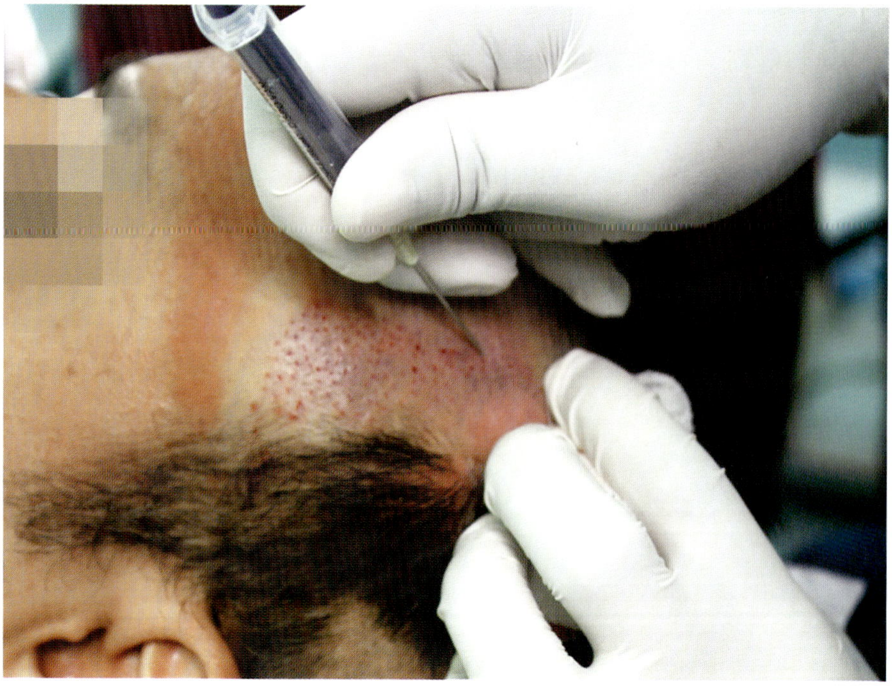

Figure 4.32

If we are constructing the temple then the slits immediately lateral to the frontotemporal point needs to be directed laterally and inferiorly.

A WRONG ONE!

Case 1

Making a wrong hairline is relatively easier than making a correct one. We present an example of patient who got hair transplant done at one center. A lot of blunders were committed in his case (Figs. 4.33 to 4.37).

Case 2

We present another case of wrongly done hair transplant where surgery was done without taking into consideration, the landmarks on the face (Figs. 4.38A to C).

IMPLANTATION OF GRAFTS AT THE HAIRLINE

Care should be taken to implant single grafts in the zone of microirregularity and in the first few rows. The grafts should be checked before implanting to avoid the mistake of *implanting double grafts with one telogen hair*, which can be missed occasionally. Implantation of grafts in proper direction and angulations is as important as making the slits correctly. The technician doing the implantation of the grafts should be aware of the angle and angulations of slit making; else implantation should be done by the surgeon himself. The implanters should be pushed into the slits at correct angles and should reach adequate depth.

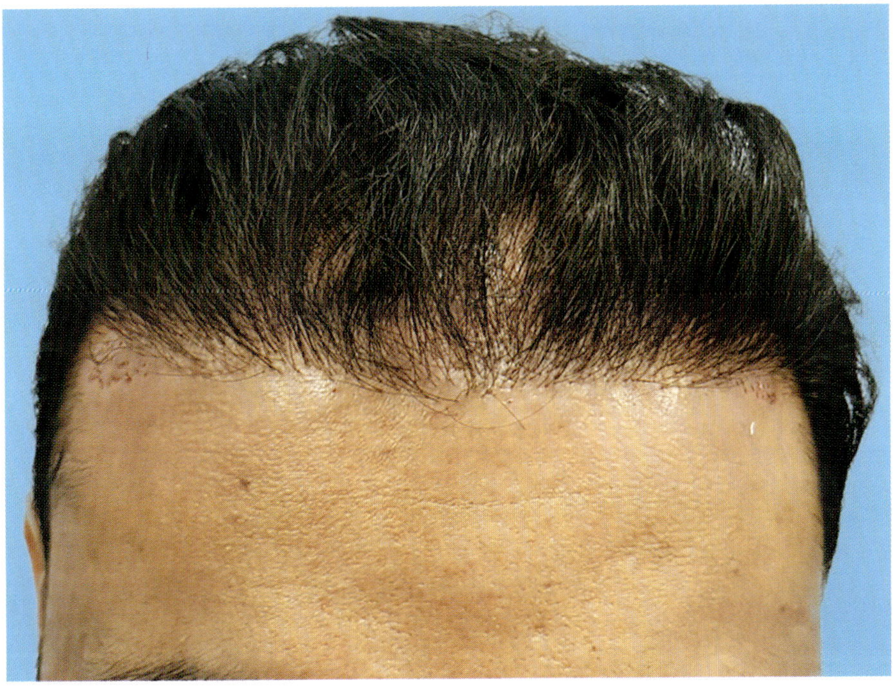

Figure 4.33

Image depicts a hairline of a patient which has been wrongly made. (Let us find out what is wrong with it!)

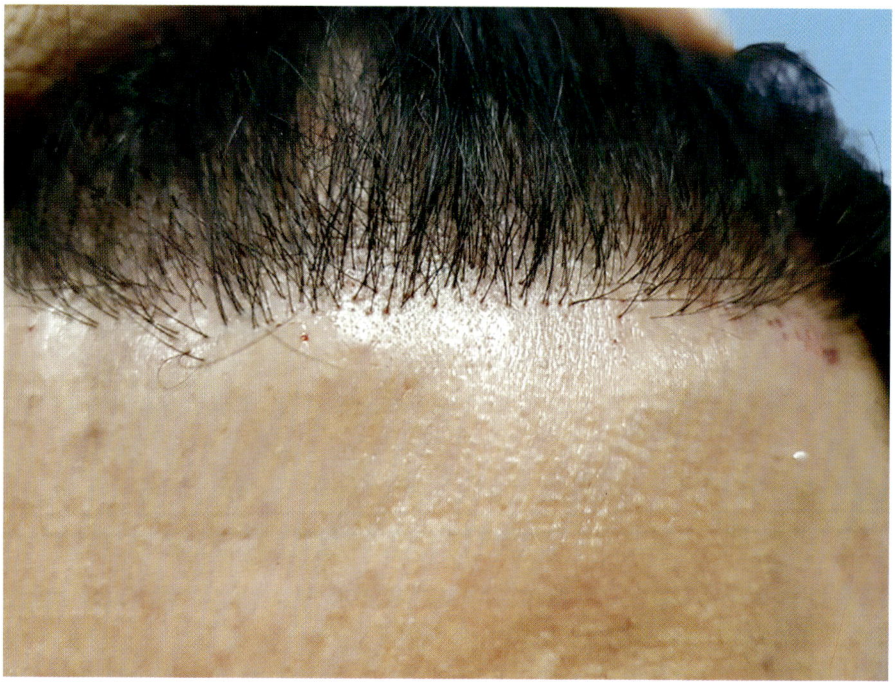

Figure 4.34

Grafts with multiple follicles are placed at the hairline. The element of micro-irregularity is missing. The sentinel hair are present.

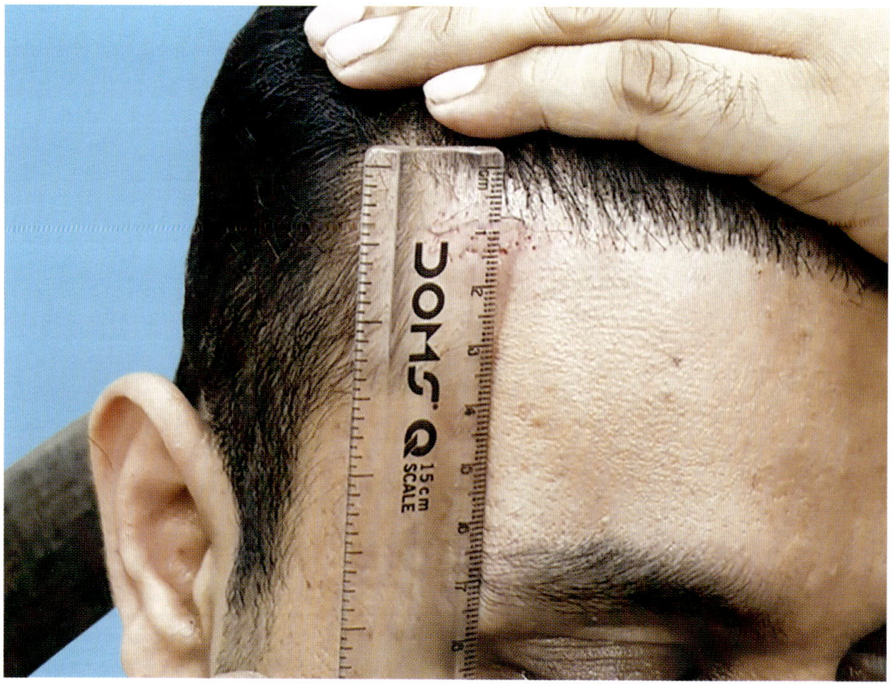

Figure 4.35

The frontotemporal angle is lateral to the lateral canthus of the right eye. In this case the hairline has been kept very low and frontotemporal angle is at wrong place.

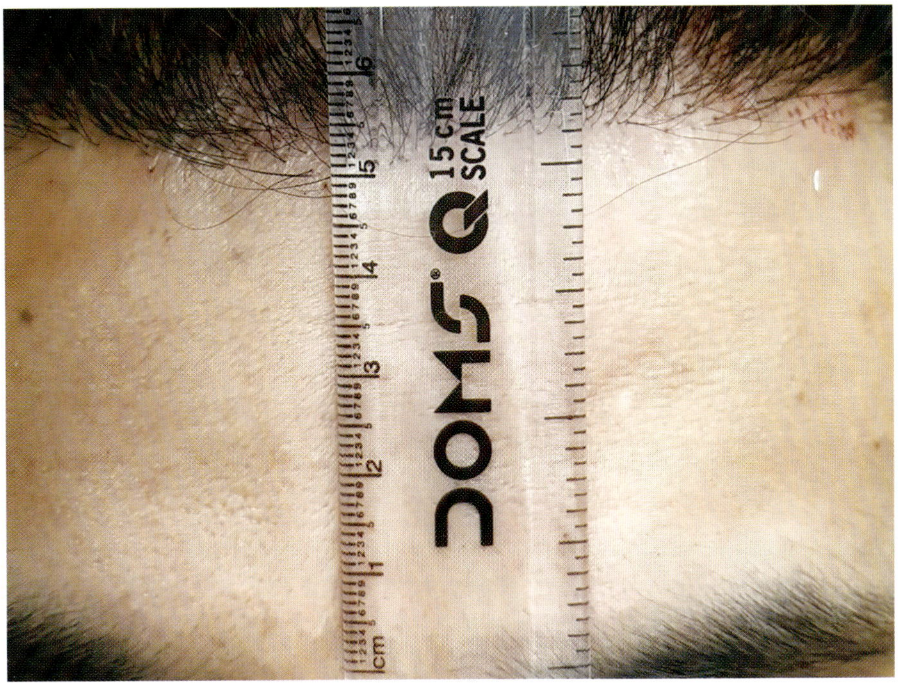

Figure 4.36

They made the mid-frontal point at 5 cm from the glabella which is a blunder. The hairline looks straight with filled and laterally placed fronto-temporal angles which makes the forehead look small like a female.

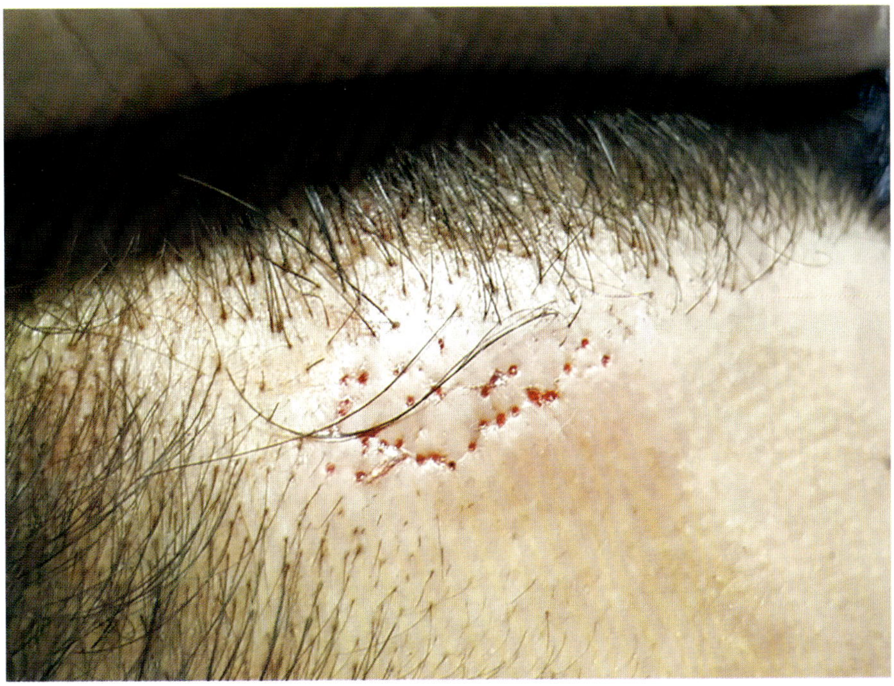

Figure 4.37

In fact they filled the frontotemporal angle and we had to extract those grafts twice by the sharp serrated punch.

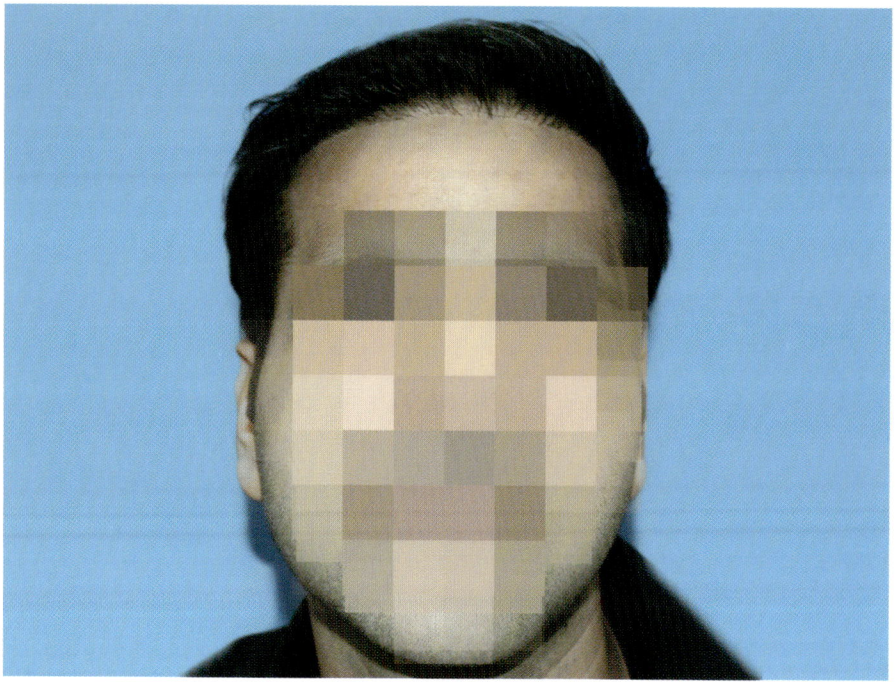

Figure 4.38A

This patient came to us for corrective hair transplant. He was 21-years-old, who had Norwood grade II baldness. He went for hair restoration as advised by his doctor at 21 years of age. The hairline in his case was made at 6.5 cm from the glabella. The shape of the hairline was round which does not suit his face and forehead. The reconstructed hairline is sparse and extremely sharp due to absence of micro- and macroirregularity.

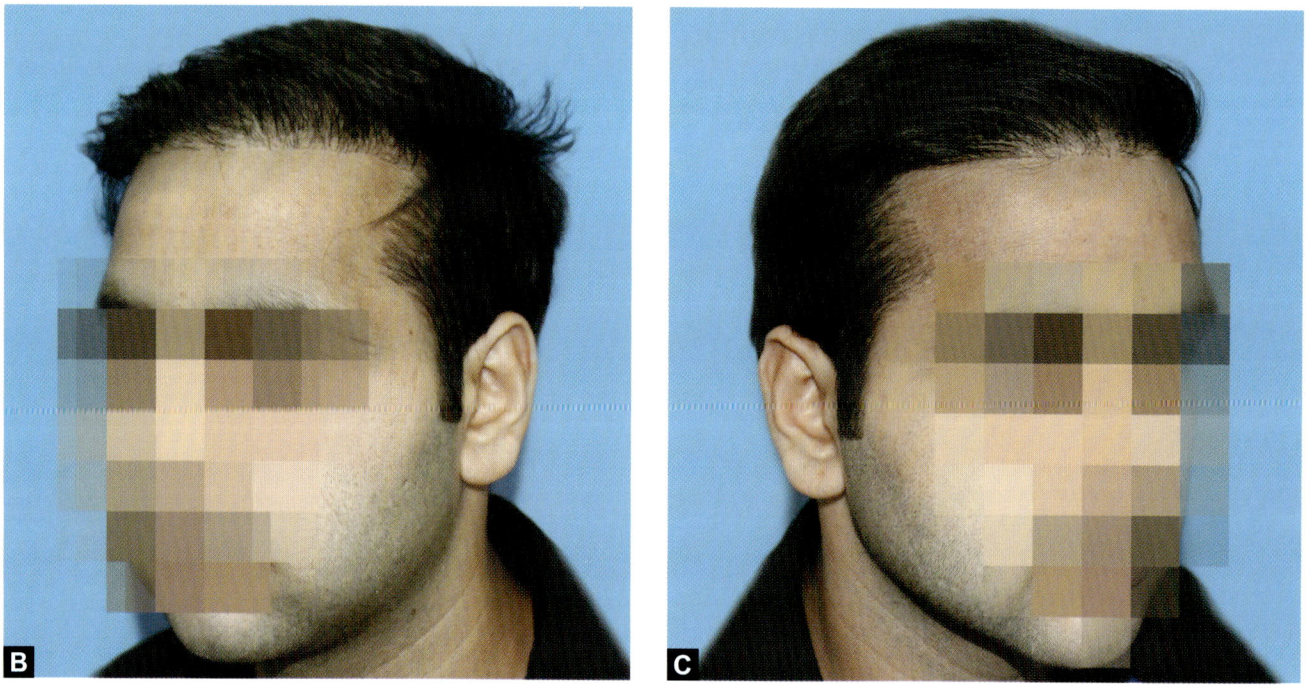

Figures 4.38B and C

The hairline curves downward at the frontotemporal angle instead of going up or staying at the same plane as mid-frontal point. The frontotemporal angles are lateral to the scientifically accepted landmark, making it look unaesthetic. Temple reconstruction should not be done in a case of 21-year-old person due to unpredictable nature of baldness. The temple hair needed more acute placement.

The orientation of implanters should match the type of slits, which are made, i.e. coronal or sagittal. The grafts should be pushed from the epidermal end during unloading of the grafts. There should not be excessive manipulation of grafts during unloading. Touching the roots should be avoided at all cost.

CONCLUDING THOUGHTS

Designing the hairline in a balding patient requires a lot of expertise. The doctor has to foresee the result in the patient. A higher hairline can be made low but not vice versa. This principle should always be kept in mind by young surgeons. The surgeon should keep in mind that a very well designed dense but low hairline may need temple reconstruction as well. Learning the art of hairline designing is complete only when doctor develops the knack of understanding the facial features and tries to fit the hairline according to his face.

We thank Dr Robert True for putting considerable effort in a very short duration of time for correcting some glaring mistakes.

Comments by Dr Anil Kumar Garg

The anterior hairline (AHL) is a most important aspect of hair restoration. The reconstructed hairline should look natural. It requires fusion of art and science. Sometimes it is difficult for a novice surgeon to reconstruct hairline as it needs visual perception and imagination.

Few factors of hairline are location, shape, size and internal distribution. The location means a distance of AHL from the glabella. There are few criteria as described in this chapter but we shall also consider the age of the patient, his present grade of baldness, family history of baldness and various donor area availability.

Very common demand by the patient is low hairline or a hairline where it was when he was 18 years of his age. A common rule is—*higher hairline is better than lower hairline, the reason being you can always lower it but not vice versa.* Hair loss is a progressive phenomenon with limited donor hair follicles supply. The shape of hairline depends on size and shape of head and this depends on ethnicity. Details have been described in this chapter.

There is a need to explain patient is that anterior hairline is basically where hair falls after styling but not from where hair is ejecting and this is usually 1–2 cm below from where hair is ejecting. This explanation can certainly convince the patient who asks to lower hairline. Another graft economical methods of lowering hairline are mentioned in the chapter.

There are landmarks for designing of hairline. They are—the mid-frontal point (distance from glabella to trichion), frontotemporal point, temporal peak point. The criteria for these points have been nicely explained in the chapter and they are yet gold standard to locate them. Joining of all these points makes a hairline skeleton. There is a relation between temporal peak point and mid-frontal point. As the mid-frontal point recedes so as temporal peak point recedes. If a vertical line is drawn from the mid-frontal point and temporal peak point on a side profile picture of face the distance between both lines should be less than 3 cm. Similarly, the hairline recedes parallel to a horizontal plane of the forehead. The internal distribution of anterior hairline zone like transition zone and the definite zone has been described in this chapter. So far as on date, the criteria of hairline design have been same.

My opinion about hairline design is that aesthetics of the face is a definite proportion of one structure to another, and somewhere the mathematics lies behind the aesthetic.

Evidence suggests our perception of physical beauty is based on how closely the features of one's face reflect *phi* (the golden ratio) in their proportions. Meaning, all faces perceived to be beautiful, each different from the other and are united in their adherence to the golden ratio. By that extension, it must certainly be possible to use a mathematical parameter to design anterior hairline on all faces. We all know Leonardo da Vinci concept of facial dimensions that is the *rule of 1/3*.

All matured male hairlines show a mid-frontal mound with either side frontotemporal deepened bald area called frontotemporal angle (FTA) and two temporal peaks (TP) in the temple area. In an attempt to decode this pattern, a face with an aesthetic hairline was chosen and its anterior hairline was marked. Then using animation software, the 3D image was converted to a flat 2D image (without changing distances and maintaining facial proportion). It was observed that the angulated male hairline pattern was translated into a rectangle (Figs. 4.39A and B).

A face having a broader forehead has a shallow frontotemporal angle and a curved forehead has a deeper frontotemporal angle. Hence, it can be said that the curvature of one's face/forehead is reflected in one's hairline.

Considering these two observations, the author came up with a method to design an anterior hairline in patients of male pattern baldness. The method is flexible and takes into consideration the grade of baldness, head shape and size, ethnic variations and patient's personal requirements. The surgeon's artistic mind can also be incorporated in this method. The result is an aesthetic anterior hairline, which looks natural and appeals to the patient's satisfaction.

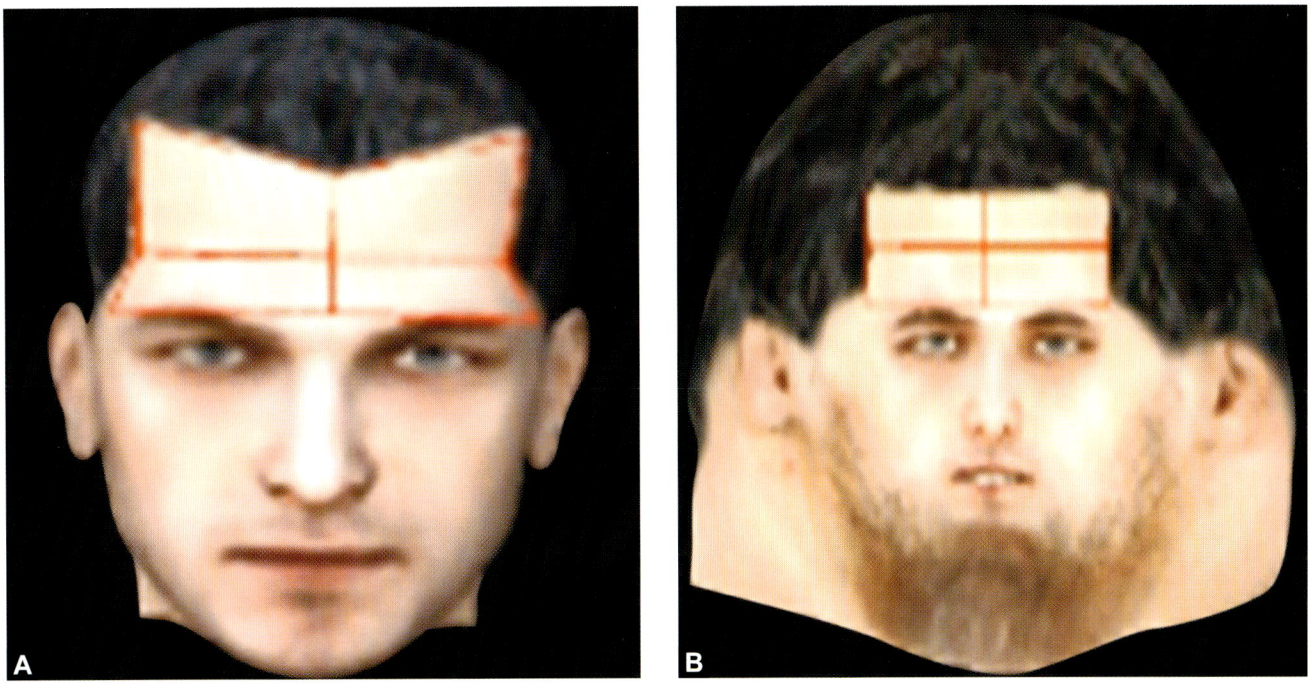

Figures 4.39A and B

(A) Three-dimensional image of anterior hairline on face; (B) Two-dimensional image of face.

Methods

Instruments needed are a flexible measuring tape and a skin marker.

1. Reference point A at glabella is taken in between eyebrows.
2. Mark points E and E′ on either side near lateral canthus 8 cm from point A in the horizontal plane.
3. Mid-frontal point B is marked 8 cm (or ±1 cm depending upon the grade of baldness) from glabella (point A) in the mid-vertical plane.
4. The frontotemporal points (points C and C′) are marked on the frontotemporal area at a distance of 8 cm in a horizontal plane from point B and at a distance of 8 cm in a vertical plane from lateral canthus points E and E' (depending on the grade of baldness and patient's choice, there can be variation of 1 cm). So, the frontotemporal point is the point of intersection of two lines taken 8 cm in from the mid-frontal point B and 8 cm from the lateral canthus point E.
5. The temporal peak points (D and D′) are marked in temporal area on a line joining the frontotemporal peak points (C and C′) to the lateral canthus points (E and E′). This line makes an anterior border of the temporal triangle. The temporal peak points D and D′ are taken slightly more than halfway toward the lateral canthus usually 5 cm from frontotemporal points C and C.′

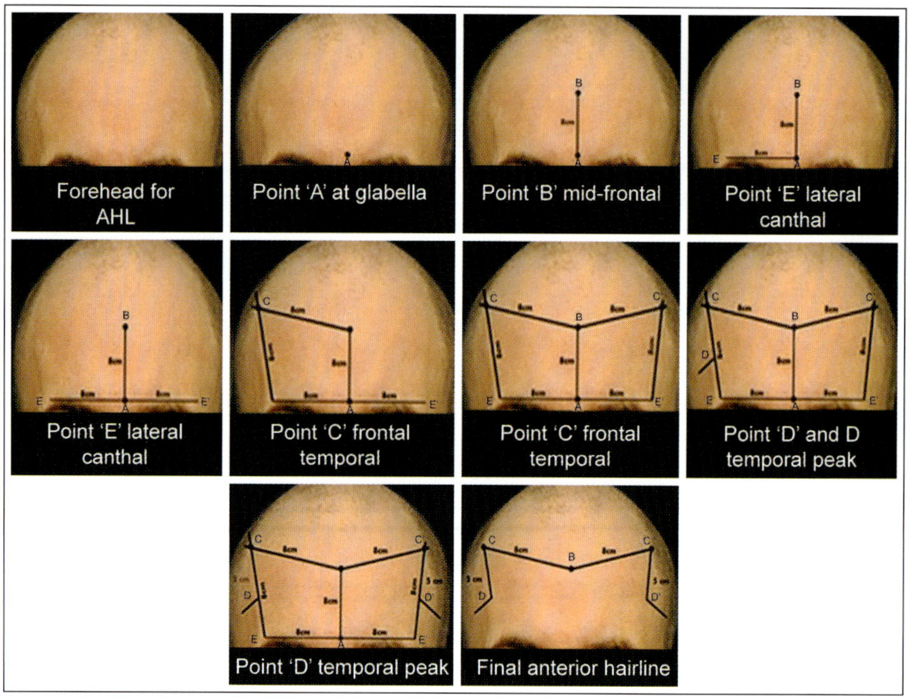

Figure 4.40

Steps to design anterior hairline in cases of male pattern baldness.

If existing temporal peak points and/or the temporal fringe are touching the line joining the frontotemporal peak to the lateral canthus points, then reconstruction of the temporal peak point is not required.

All above points are joined as follows:

1. *Reconstruction of the anterior hairline:* Points B to C on one side and B to C′ on the other side. So, the line joining C to B to C′ is the anterior hairline.
2. *Reconstruction of the temporal triangle:* Join point C to point D. These are the anterior temporal lines. Repeat on the other side.

Now draw a line from point D downward posteriorly to join the remaining temporal hair of the sideburn. This completes the temporal triangle. For clarification see Figure 4.40. All distances are on the surface of the forehead, taken by a flexible measuring tape. The distances are as follows: AB—8 cm, AE—8 cm, BC—8 cm, CE—8 cm, CD—5 cm.

Commentator's View on Hairline Designing

In male pattern alopecia, there is deepening of the frontotemporal area followed by the recession of the mid-frontal point. There can also be thinning of the temporal fringe and then receding of the temporal peak point. In further stages of baldness, there can be lowering of the parietal hump. These events take place in proportion to one another so we need to reconstruct them, maintaining the same proportion in which they have receded so a natural characteristic is maintained. Anterior hairline receding is parallel to the transverse plane of the forehead, the FTP recedes in a vertical canthal line and the MFP and TP also recede in proportion. The frontotemporal angle recedes more than the mid-frontal point.

There are a few established criteria for placement of the mid-frontal point. One is a range of 7–11 cm from the glabella. Another is the junction of the horizontal surface of the scalp and the vertical plane of the forehead. The third is 1/3 face height as the face is divided into three equal parts. The 7–11 cm distance decision depends on the grade of baldness and availability of donor area and patients preference. In a patient of grade VII baldness maximum distance, 11 cm was not accepted by any of our patients. While in the author's method the range is 8 cm ± 1 cm. This is a relatively much narrower range to decide. The Norwood grade of baldness distance is less than 8 cm while in higher grades the distance is 8 cm or more. In very rare cases, the distance is more than 9 cm. Now we can harvest nonscalp donor hair and the technique is also improved so the availability of donor hair is increased. This makes it possible to lower the hairline up to 9 cm even in grade VII patients. In our series of grade VII patients, the maximum distance of MFP to glabella (AB) is 9 cm, which was well accepted. The option of more than 9 cm was not accepted by anyone.

An aesthetic hairline looks parallel or slopes upward when viewed from the side. The apex of the frontotemporal angle lies on the vertical canthal line. The created frontotemporal point should not be lower than the mid-frontal point, and should not be placed posterior to a line drawn vertically from tragus. The FTP should be located anterior to the pretragus line. The existing method of locating the FTA is a line drawn from the lateral epicanthus superiorly and then posteriorly to meet the existing temporal hair. In mild-to-moderate degrees of hair loss, it works well, but in more severe degrees of hair loss, where the temporal hair has receded and the lateral fringe has dropped, finding this point will be very difficult because there is no temporal hair with which the lateral epicanthal line can intersect. Visualizing and recreating the “lateral hump” can help in this situation. So, in the existing method designing of the FTA and anterior hairline needs a lot of criteria and measurements.

As per the author’s approach, a single measurement of 8 cm ± 1 cm from two references point is sufficient to locate all important landmarks needed to design the anterior hairline. To place the FTA, two measurements are needed. One is 8 cm in a horizontal plane from the MFP and the other is 8 cm from a point E near the lateral canthus in the vertical plane. The intersection of these two measurements is the FTA. This frontotemporal angle is in the vertical canthal line, above the mid-frontal point, anterior to the pretragus line and the angle was acute. After the growth of transplanted hair, it was a natural-looking angle. This also facilitates automatically how much the parietal hump has to be lifted. All the existing criteria have already been incorporated and taken well into account, there is no need to remember this separately. This we have done in more than 431 patients and realized it is a much simpler method to follow.

The placement of the temporal peak point is a point where two imaginary lines intersect. One line from the base of the nose to the mid-pupil and the other line from the mid-frontal point to the ear lobeline. Practically it is not easy to draw such lines. It requires imaginary visual perception and experience. In the author's approach, it is very convenient to locate the temporal peak point. The temporal peak point lies over the line joining the frontotemporal point and the lateral canthus point, usually 5 cm below the FTP. It is noteworthy that number 8 and 5 are numbers of the Fibonacci sequence and the ratio between 5 and 8 is the golden ratio *phi* (1.618) and both are Fibonacci numbers. These numbers and this ratio are found everywhere in nature. This was also seen when we converted 3D image of a face to a 2D face image.

Marking hairline zones is the same as described by Shapiro. The author's method makes a skeletal frame of the complete anterior border of the hair-bearing scalp separating the face. There is always flexibility for the surgeon's artistic view as well as for patient's preference. As for racial/ethnic and shape and size of the head, these are concerns all taken into account by this method. A flat forehead will have a flat anterior hairline while a more curved forehead will have an oval or round anterior hairline.

Comparison of the design of the anterior hairline and the placement of the temporal peak point by the author's method was done by the existing method. The placement of the mid-frontal points and the frontotemporal points by both the methods were located at a nearly same location, the difference was in the anterior location of the temporal peak point. When Mayer's method was followed, the temporal peak point was more anteriorly placed on the forehead while in the author's method, the point was average 0.6 cm posterior to the Mayer temporal point. The Mayer's temporal point looks better on a young face with a lower anterior hairline. Also, it requires more grafts to be used for temporal reconstruction. The difference is Mayer's method considers only the size of the face but not the curvature of the forehead and face.

The follow-up results of patients are shown in Figure 4.41.

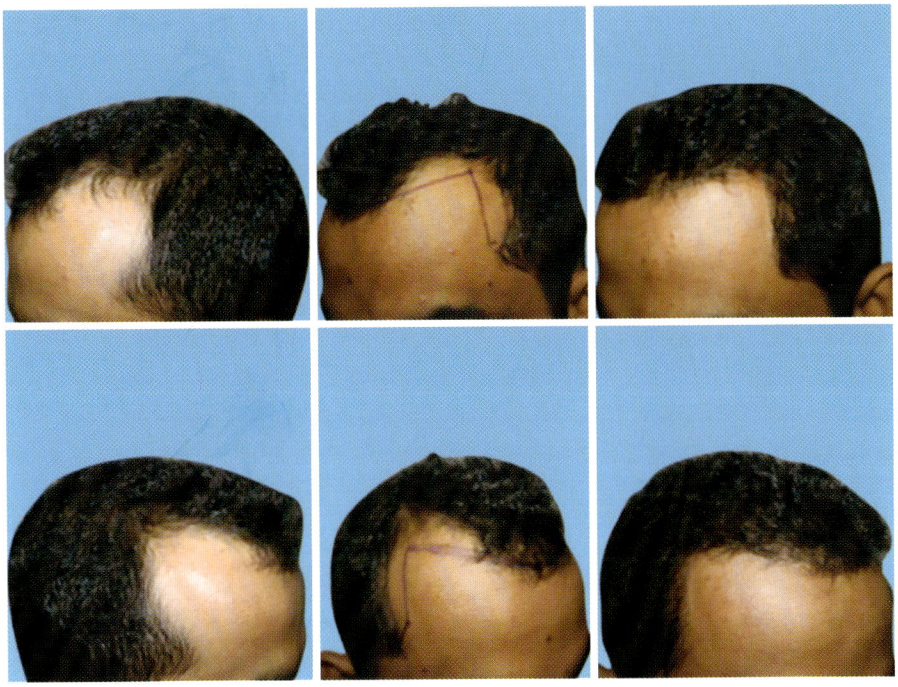

Figure 4.41

Follow-up results of patients.

SUMMARY

- Different hairline shapes are suited for different faces.
- The donor availability is a major criteria in deciding the hairline.
- Hairline symmetry should be checked with laser-assist hairline device, with naked eye (from front and back) and via photograph.
- There will always be some discrepancy in what patient sees in the mirror (2D image) and what you see in naked eyes (3D image).
- Minute asymmetry with gross symmetry in hairline is to be sought to provide naturalness.
- As known already, hairline is not a line rather a zone in itself, hence inclusion of macro- and microirregularities is important to bring artistry in the hairline.
- Implantation of only single hair follicles for the first 0.5 cm is done to give the hairline a softer look.

REFERENCES

1. Sirinturk S, Bagheri H, Govsa F, et al. Study of frontal hairline patterns for natural design and restoration. Surg Radiol Anat. 2017;39(6):679-84.

2. Park JH. Novel principles and techniques to create a natural design in female hairline correction surgery. Plast Reconstr Surg Glob Open. 2016;3(12):e589.
3. Shapiro R. Principles of creating a natural hairline. In: Shapiro R, Unger W, Unger R, Unger M (Eds). Hair Transplantation, 5th edn. New York: Informa Healthcare Publishing; 2011. 374-82.
4. Eliyahu R. Path D laser-assist hairline design device—a new product [Internet] United States. Cole Instruments. 2013 July 18 [2017 February 27]. Available from: https://www.coleinstruments.com/path-d-laser-assist-hairline-design-new-product
5. Lam M. Hair transplant operative 360. In: Lam M (Ed). Hair Transplant 360 for Physicians, 2nd edn. New Delhi: Jaypee Brothers Medical Publishers (P) Ltd.; 2016. 67-180.
6. Martinick J. The Recipient Site. In: Shapiro R, Unger W, Unger R, Unger M (Eds). Hair Transplantation, 5th edn. New York: Informa Healthcare Publishing; 2011. 351-6.
7. Garg AK, Garg S. Decoding facial esthetics to recreate an esthetic hairline: a method which includes forehead curvature. J Cutan Aesthet Surg. 2017;10:195-9.

CHAPTER 5

Temple, Hump and Mid-scalp Reconstruction

Pradeep Sethi, Arika Bansal, Abhinav Kumar

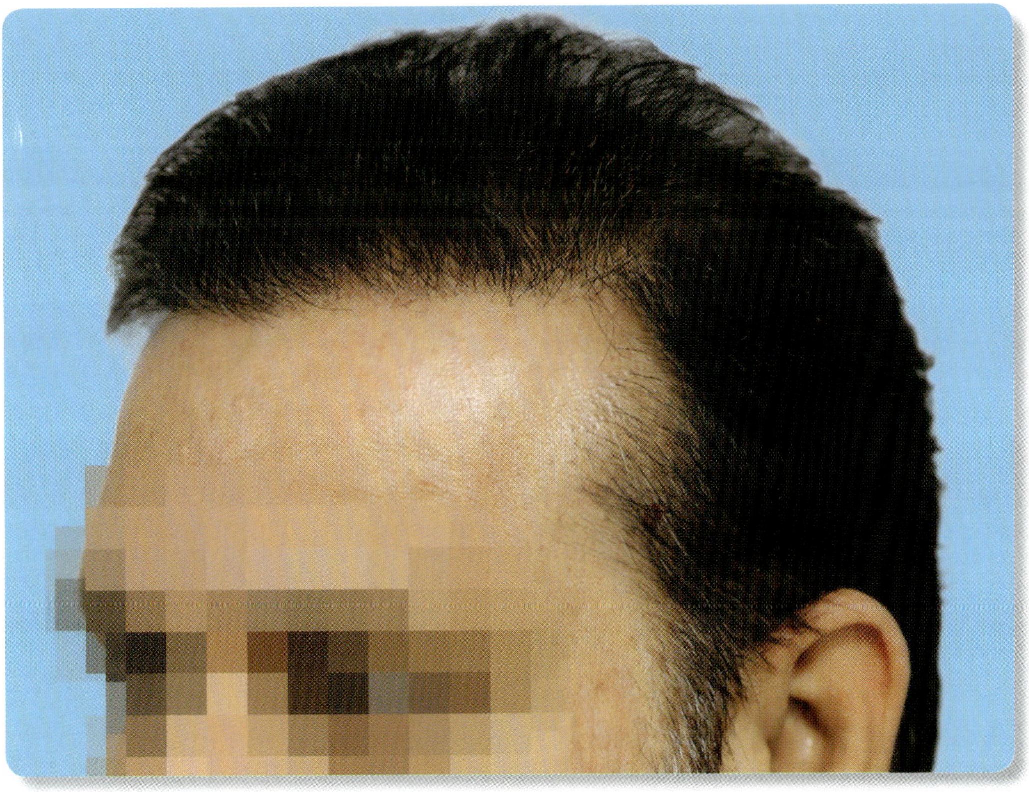

A washed out temple point makes a forehead bigger and hence the bald look. With proper planning a small number of appropriate grafts can give a very great look with reduced hairless area of the forehead. If not done well it can be catastrophic!

INTRODUCTION

Temple construction is an art worth mastering. For an aesthetically designed hairline, a good temple reconstruction is the key. If one is full-fledged into hair transplant and is doing hair restoration passionately, he will never be satisfied without creating great temples. Temple reconstruction is an advanced surgical technique. One should not be doing temple reconstruction in early years of practice. Temple creation gives a balanced look. If you restore hairline without restoring the temples and they recede with age, the hairline may look odd later.

On the other side, like the crown, temple reconstruction is an extremely difficult thing to master. One should do it only after doing hundreds of surgeries independently and seeing their complete results. The angles in the temples need to be extremely acute.[1] Sometimes one makes a very aggressive hairline and temples may consume a lot of grafts which may leave vacant areas on the mid-scalp or insufficient donor for future correction. One has to develop critical thinking for creating those beautiful temple points. It can be learnt by observing hairline and temples of every person who is coming to you for consult.

THUMB RULE

The degree of recession of the temporal hairline should match with recession of anterior hairline. Temple–hairline balance is the key to great artistic results (Figs. 5.1A to C).[2]

HOW TO DESIGN A TEMPLE?

There are three aspects of temple reconstruction: (1) upper temple, (2) temple and (3) temporal point (Figs. 5.2 to 5.4).[2]

The hairline at the temple should complement the anterior hairline. For beginners, they should try to keep the hairline high as they are not proficient in temple reconstruction and so that it eliminates the need for hair transplant at temple. The patient may insist on a low and youthful hairline but the young surgeon should know his limitations and should refuse patients with such demands or take assistance from senior surgeons. A high hairline can always be lowered but not vice versa.

CREATION OF RECIPIENT SITES OF THE TEMPLE

Temporal region has major vasculature so it is important to give sufficient tumescence to minimize damage to underlying blood vessels.[1] The anesthesia process may be very painful at temporal region so use of vibrator and slow

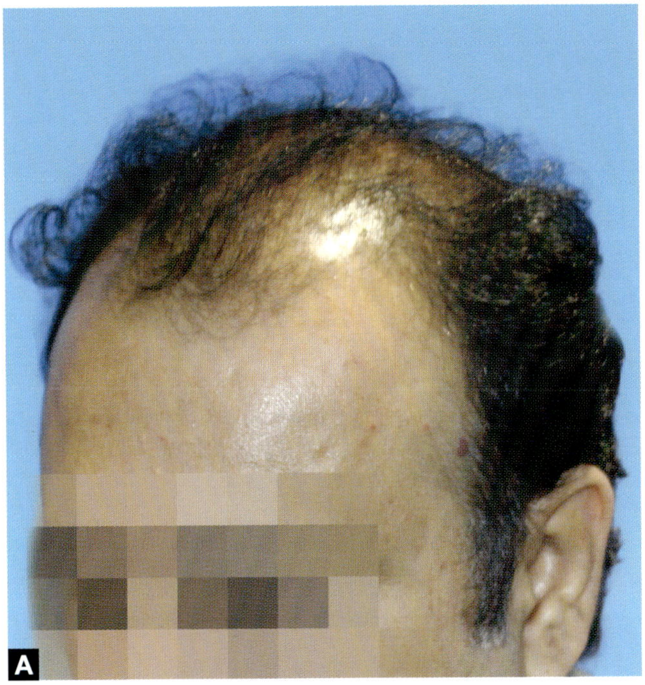

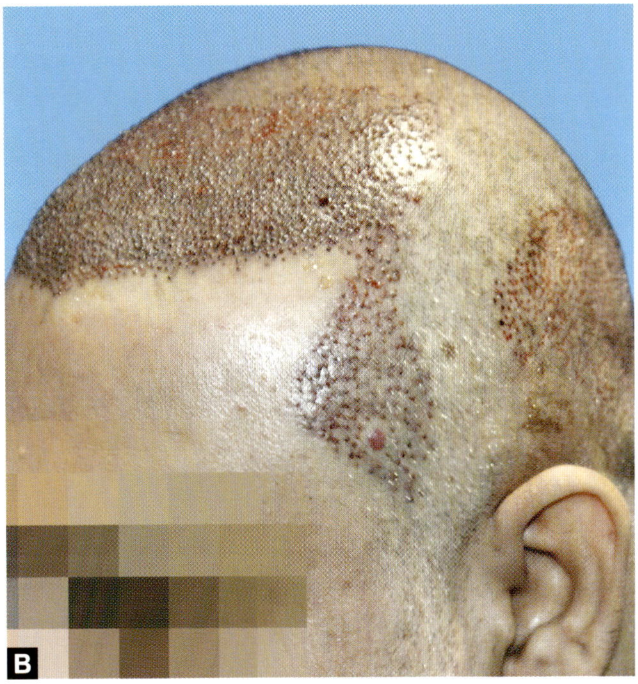

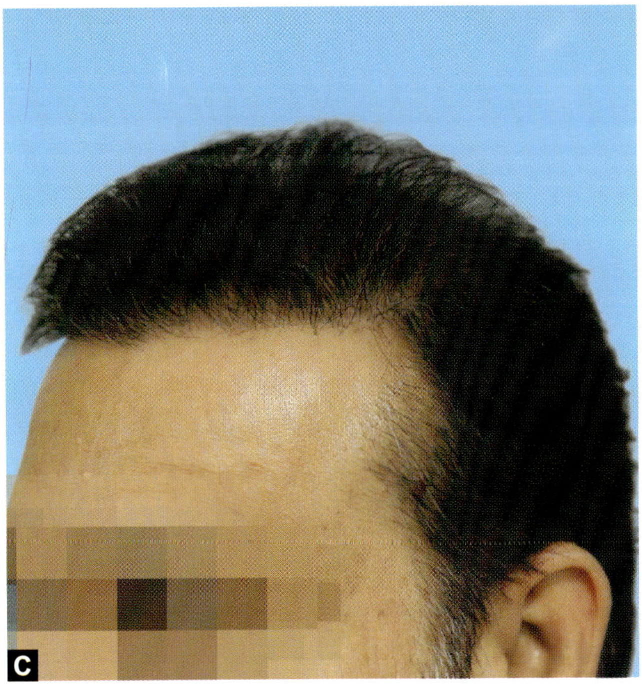

Figures 5.1A to C

Stresses upon the importance of temple reconstruction, a beautifully created temple adds to the youthfulness if done correctly and complements the hairline. *Note the direction of hair in the temple and the temporal point.*

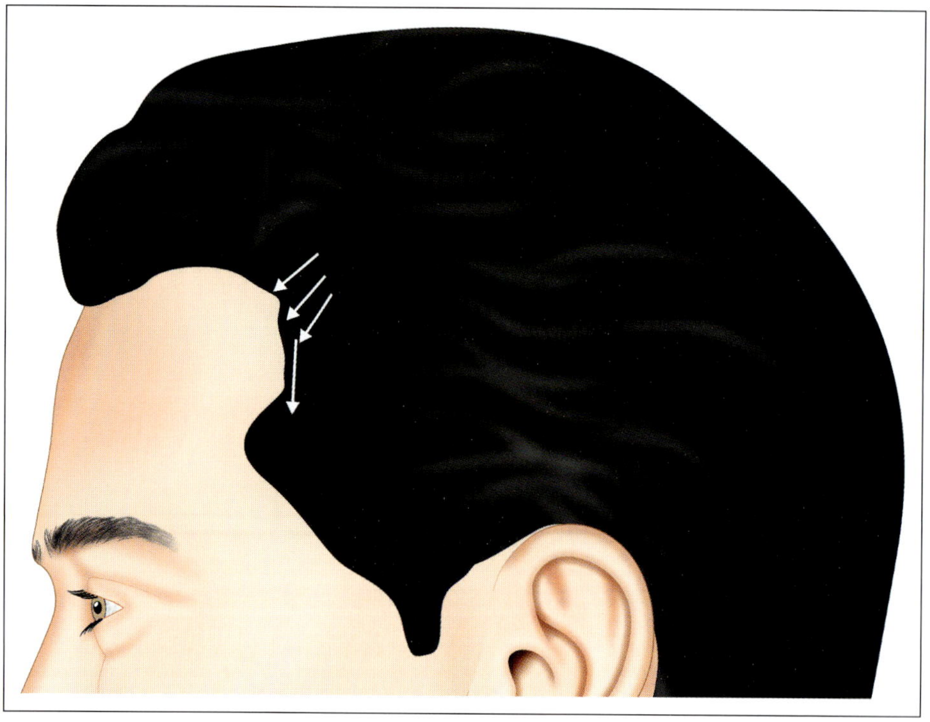

Figure 5.2

Upper temple. The lateral most portion of hairline ends at the upper temple. The natural upper temple hair curves slightly anteroinferiorly. Unlike the hairline, the angles in the temple region need to be very acute (<10°).

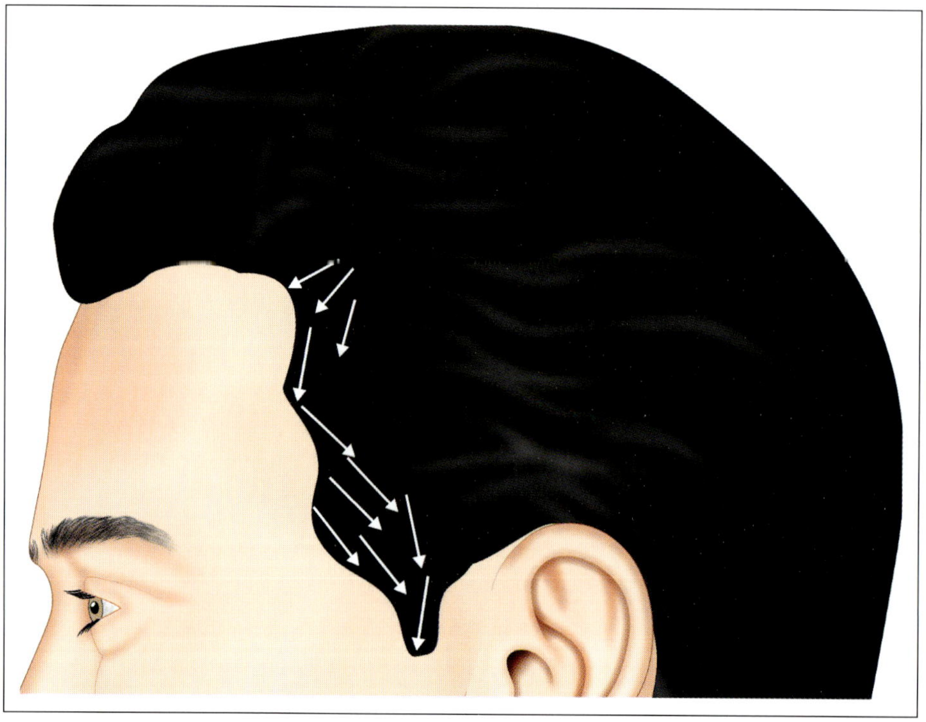

Figure 5.3

Temple. An ideal temple is an area in which hair sweeps anteroinferiorly, then changes direction to posteroinferiorly and then goes inferiorly again at the lowest point. A nonbalding person may not be having an ideal temple and may not fit into the diagram shown above, but it is important to observe hundreds of nonbalding persons to understand what a beautiful temple is all about.[3]

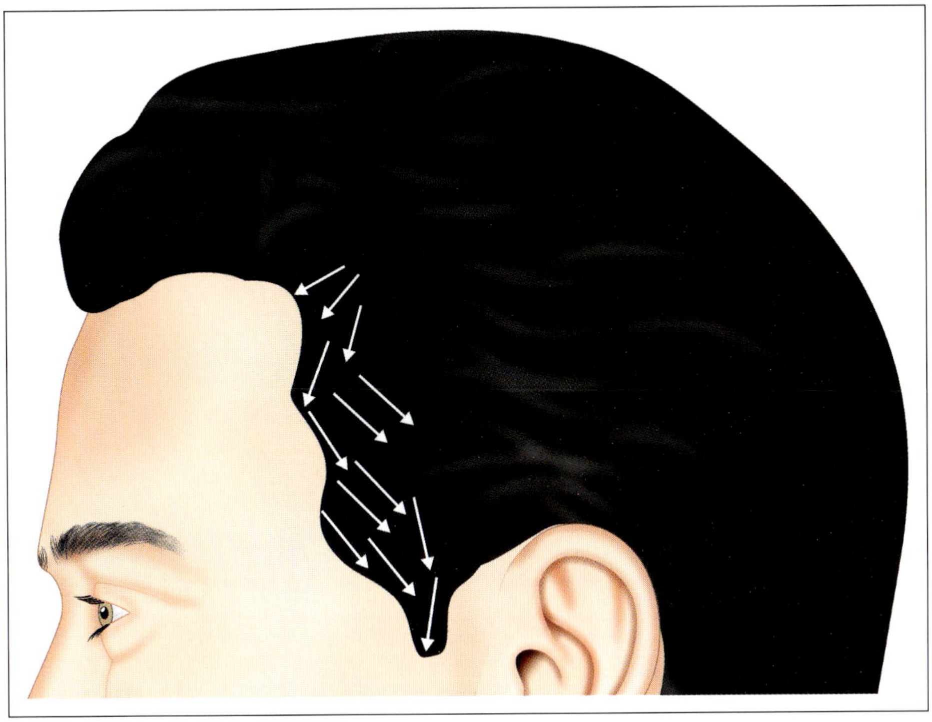

Figure 5.4

Temporal point. It can be theoretically determined by one line drawn from the tip of the nose through mid-pupil and the second line drawn from the earlobe to the trichion. It is the point where the temple hair's direction changes from anteroinferiorly to almost completely posteriorly and then going inferoposteriorly. Usually a temple can be constructed with or without temporal point. For a small extension of frontotemporal recession, 80–100 grafts are needed on each side while full-fledged temple reconstruction with temporal points needs 150–250 grafts.[1]

injection technique is must. Secondly, the skin at the temple is lax as compared to the rest of the scalp, so sufficient countertraction is needed while slit creation.[1] The depth should be adequate as lax skin may result in creation of slits of inadequate depth, in which the graft may not survive.[1] Thirdly, needle of right sizes should be used; either 20G or 21G needle should be used to place single or double grafts. Slits made with 19G or 18G needle may result in sliding out of the grafts. *The grafts needed for temple hair reconstruction should ideally be single and less pigmented.* The patient should wear and remove the surgical cap very carefully and should not sleep on the sides after the surgery.

IMPLANTATION

We use SAVA™ implanters in our direct hair transplantation technique. Hair at the nape of the neck or above the ears are an ideal choice as they are single and less pigmented. One should always note the presence of reverse thinning (at the nape of the neck) while selecting hair from these areas, as such hair should not be chosen. *The curly hair should be avoided as they will not curl upon the skin.* Beard hair should never be implanted on the temple. Chest hair, if straight and thin can be taken for temple reconstruction. They have to be placed at an extremely acute angle of 5–10° by an expert surgeon assisted by expert technicians (Figs. 5.5 to 5.8).

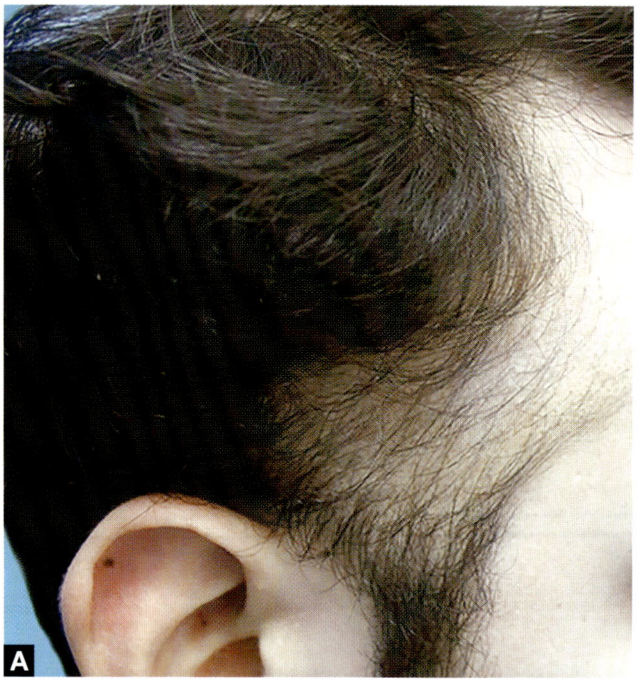

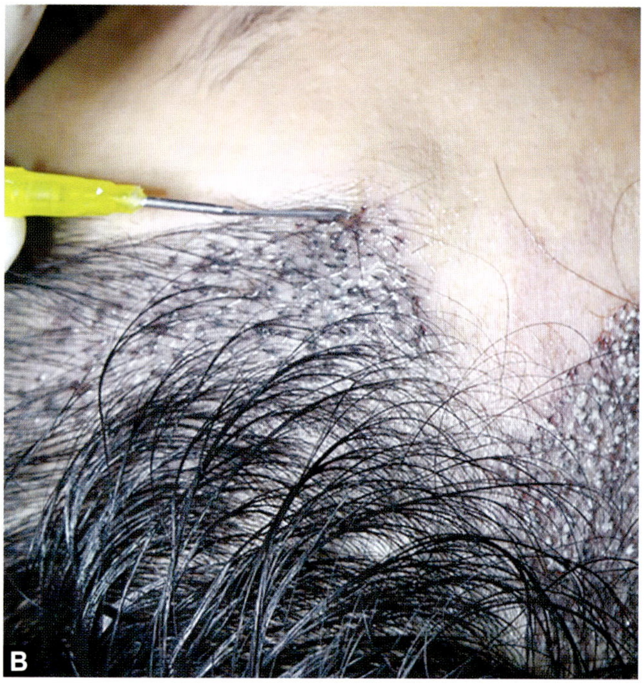

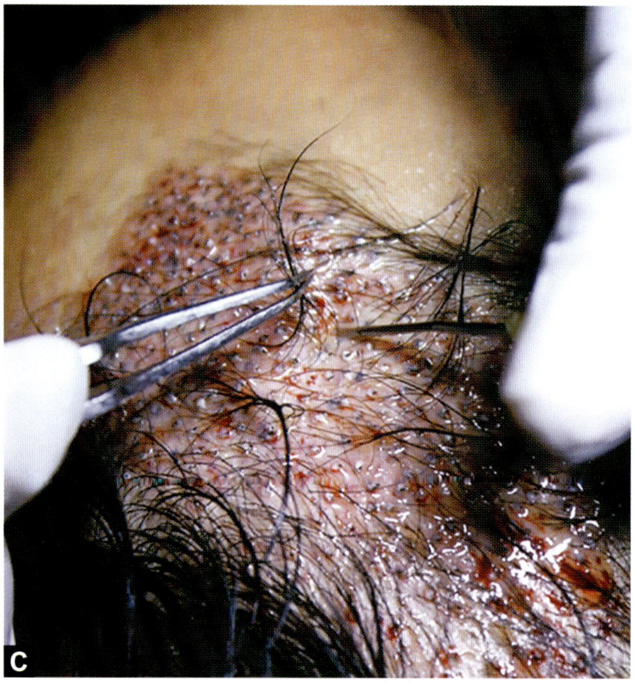

Figures 5.5A to C

(A) Presence of traction alopecia at the temple. Such type of alopecia is seen in people who wear turban. The traction alopecia in temple has reached the superior part of the ear. Due to some amount of scarring of scalp in traction alopecia, the depth of the slits should be adequate to ensure graft acceptability. This can be achieved by giving sufficient countertraction while making the extremely acute slits at the temple; (B) The angle of the implanters while implanting the grafts at the temple point in the same patient of traction alopecia. The neighboring hair provide guidance regarding the direction and angulations of the grafts. The frontotemporal angle and hairline is present in the right side of the photograph. The grafts are directed posteroinferiorly, thus the implanters need to be directed anterosuperiorly; (C) Direction and angle of implanters at various sites of temple during implantation in patient of traction alopecia. The grafts are directed posteroinferiorly.

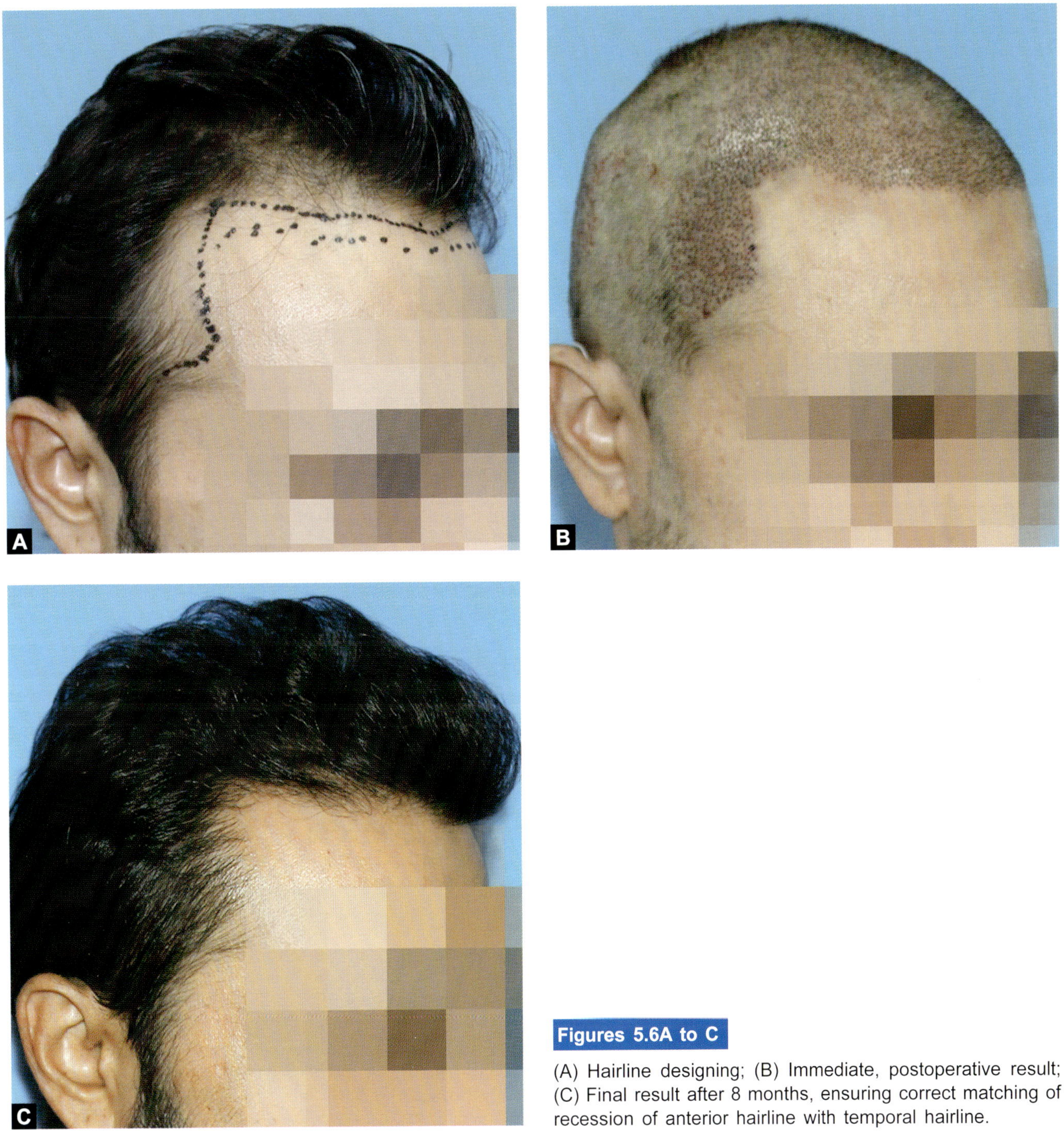

Figures 5.6A to C

(A) Hairline designing; (B) Immediate, postoperative result; (C) Final result after 8 months, ensuring correct matching of recession of anterior hairline with temporal hairline.

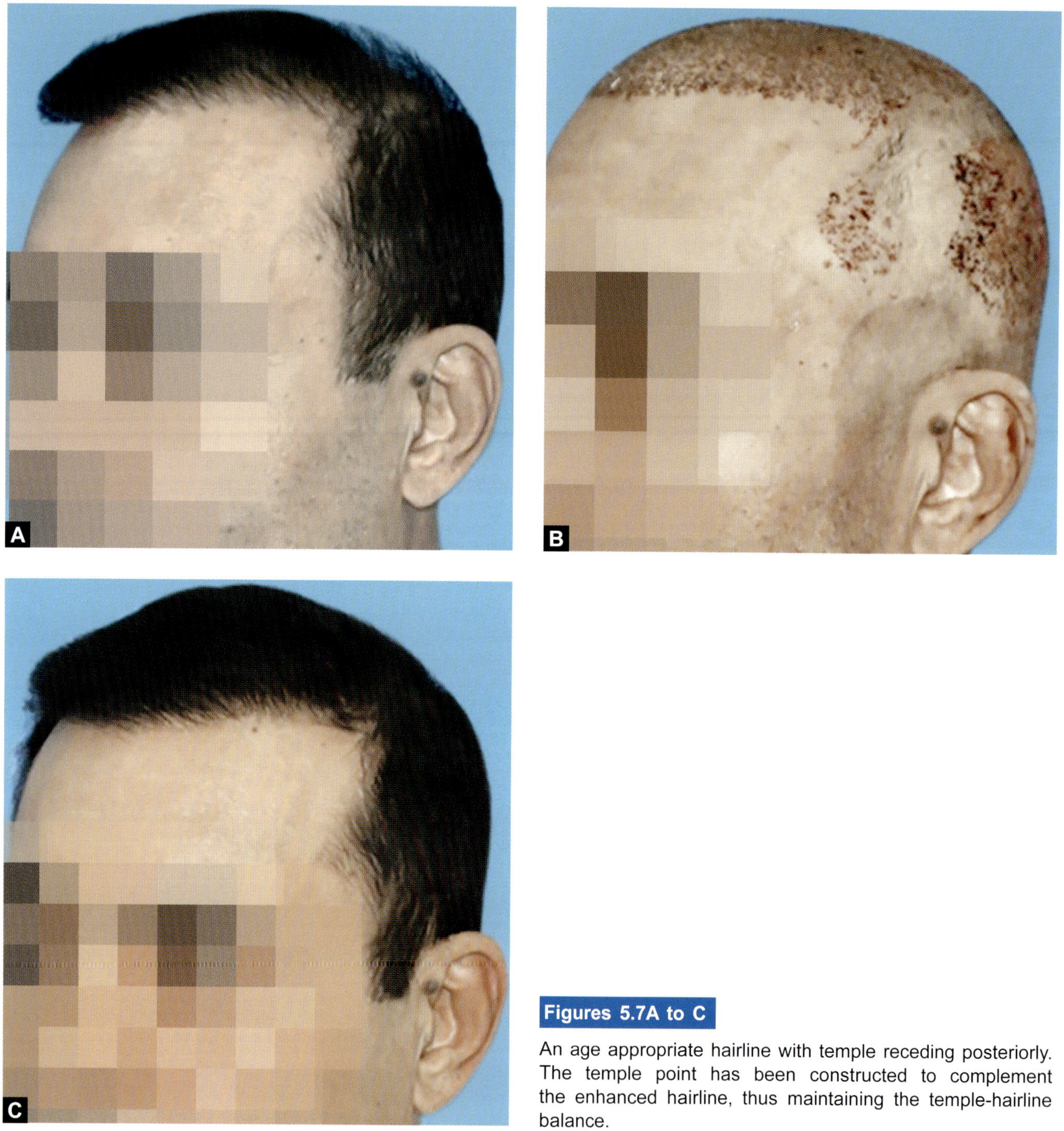

Figures 5.7A to C

An age appropriate hairline with temple receding posteriorly. The temple point has been constructed to complement the enhanced hairline, thus maintaining the temple-hairline balance.

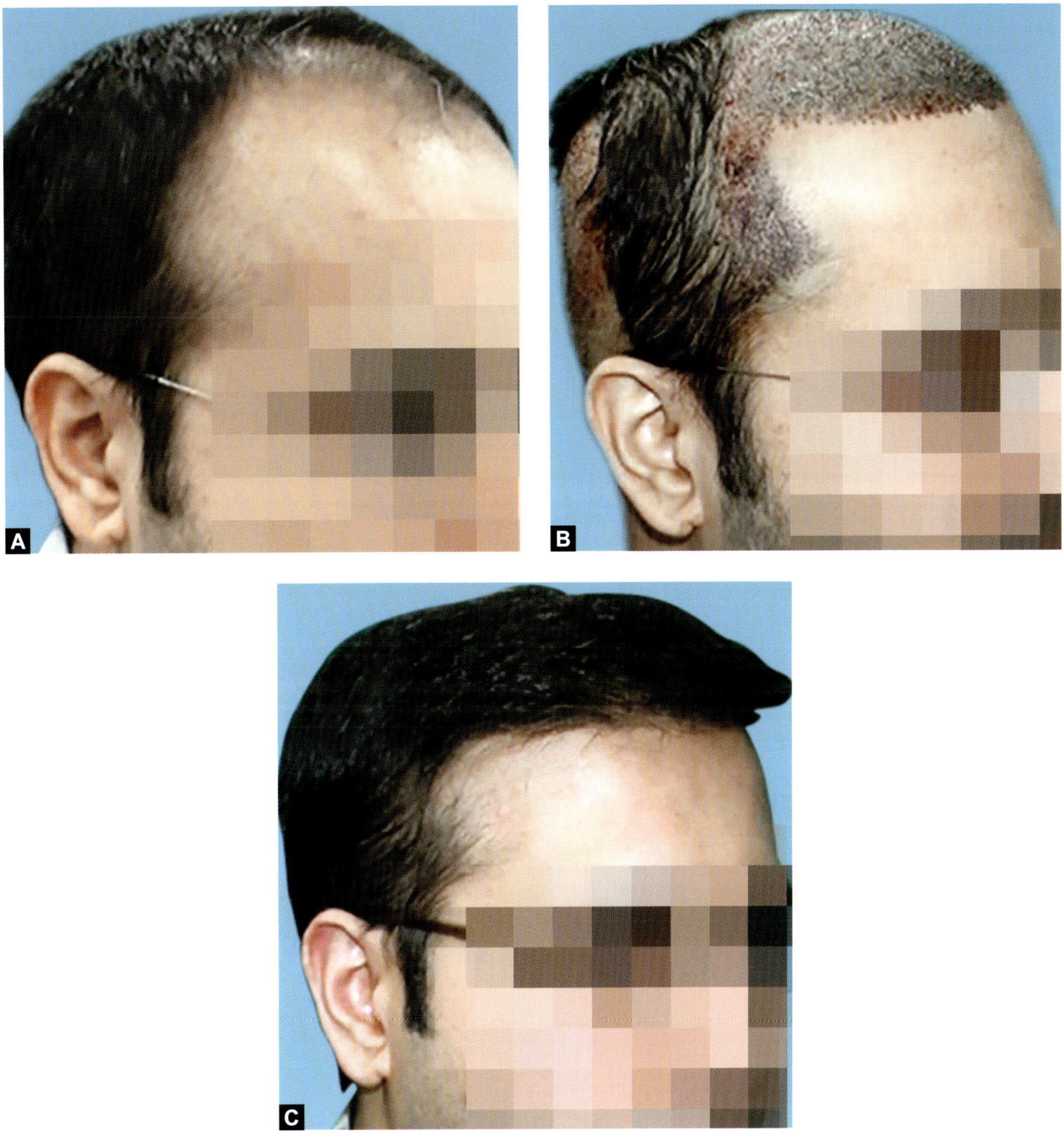

Figures 5.8A to C

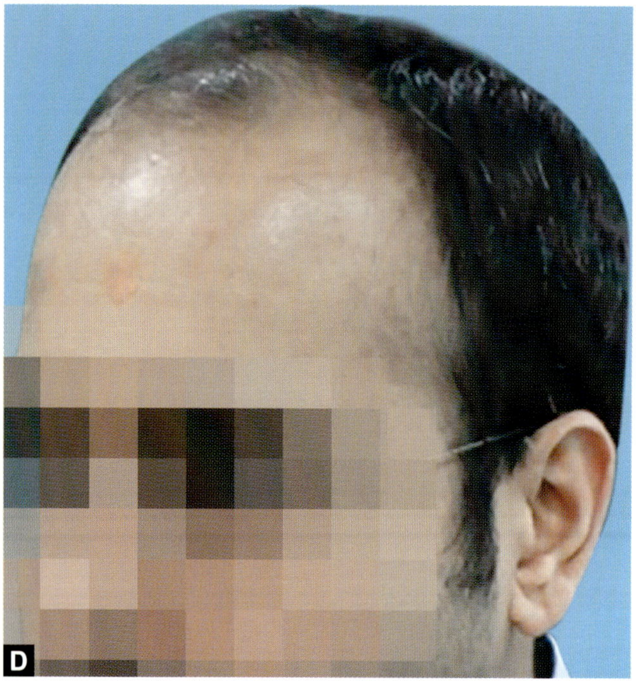

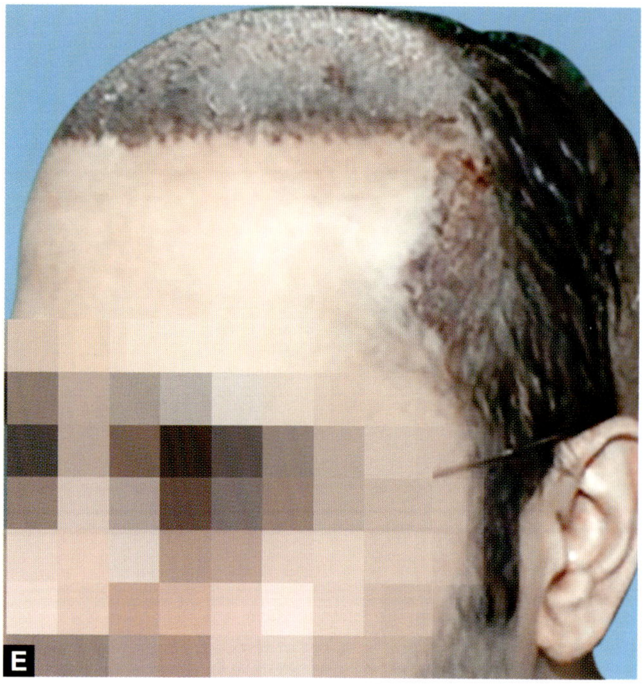

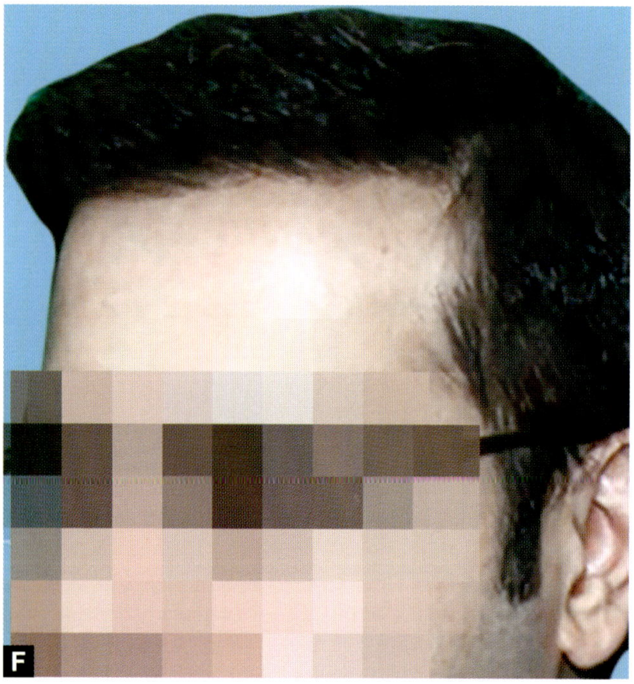

Figures 5.8D to F

Figures 5.8A to F

This series of photographs has been added to emphasize the fact that hairline creation and temple creation should always look natural and should take into consideration: the age of the patient, the degree of baldness, and the degree of baldness on his paternal sides and maternal sides. An aggressive temple was constructed for this patient as he was young. If only hairline reconstruction would have been done in this patient without temple reconstruction, then the hairline would have looked like a "toupee". The hairline tends to ascend from mid-frontal point to frontotemporal point and then merges smoothly with the reconstructed upper temple. The upper temple where the hair are directed anteroinferiorly merges with the temporal point, where the hair direction changes to posteroinferiorly. Both right and left temporal point should be absolutely symmetrical and possess same magnitude of recession and hair density. Here we implanted 250 grafts per side. A promise regarding application of minoxidil and intake of finasteride is must in such patients to ensure limited progression of baldness.

A WRONGLY CONSTRUCTED TEMPLE (FIG. 5.9)

The temple had been reconstructed in this patient to complement the enhanced hairline. The surgeon was able to successfully create a beautiful hairline. However, during construction of temple, he committed few mistakes. He failed to create the

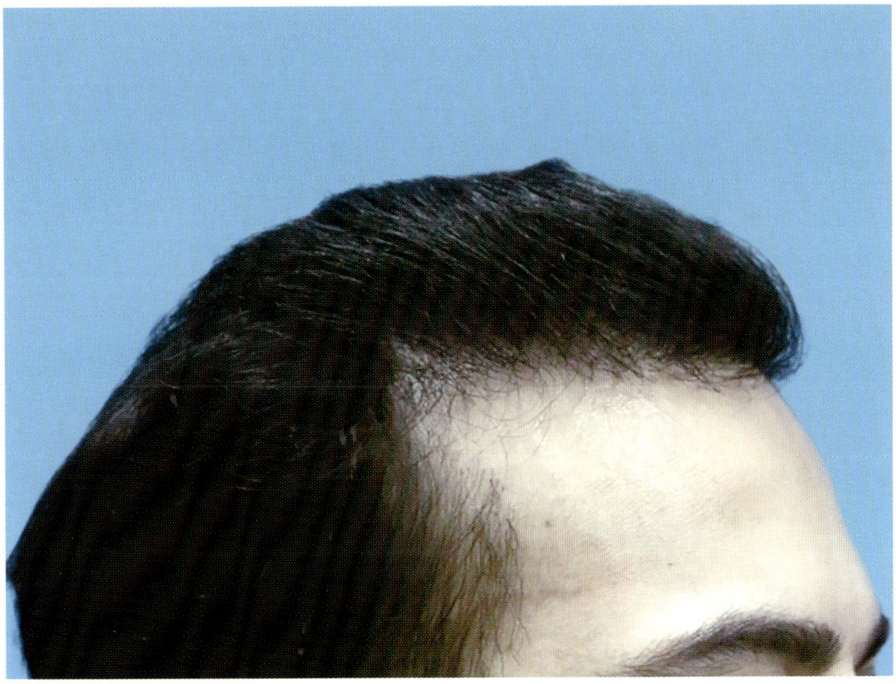

Figure 5.9
A wrongly constructed temple.

upper temple which is more important than the lower temple or his grafts at the upper temple did not grow. The direction of temple hair at temporal point and lower temple is inferior instead of posteroinferiorly. The density of temple region is relatively lesser compared to natural temple. This means that a lot of temple hair planted did not grow due to extremely superficial slits. There is absence of any temporal point. However, surgeon was knowledgeable enough to choose lightly pigmented hair and implanted them at super flat angles.

HUMP RECONSTRUCTION

Hump is defined as the semicircular region of scalp where the lateral border of mid-scalp meets the temporal region.[2] The hump is identified by a vertical imaginary line drawn through the lateral canthus of the eye.[1] The hair on the hump may go during the progression of baldness. Patient coming for transplant in Norwood grade V and Norwood grade VI has a hump and hump is the last part of temporal hair to recede.[2]

Patients with intact hump, who underwent transplant more than 4,000 grafts should continue with oral intake of finasteride and topical application of minoxidil to retain their hump. Such patients are at risk of progression of baldness which may lead to development of rim of baldness around the transplanted zone after loss of hair in the hump.

Hump location also helps in deciding the frontotemporal angle. Visualizing the hump creates a target for the lateral epicanthal line to intersect.[2] A vertical line drawn parallel to external auditory meatus intersects the lateral epicanthal line, this is usually the site of frontotemporal angle.[2] The lateral hump usually becomes the inferior border of frontotemporal angle.[2] However, we violate this principle in certain cases where our frontotemporal angle may pass through the middle of the hump. Only scalp grafts need to be implanted in the hump, as they need to merge with the temporal hair and the hump is the region of parting of scalp in many patients. They are usually implanted densely with scalp grafts. The recipient sites during the hump recreation are angled forward in order to merge with mid forward directed mid-scalp recipient sites but these recipient sites gradually change their direction to downward as these recipient sites merge with the hair in the temporal region.[1]

MID-SCALP RECONSTRUCTION

Mid-scalp is defined as a region located posterior to the hairline, anterior to the crown and medial to the two laterally located humps.[1] Mid-scalp is a relatively large region of scalp which needs a lot of grafts depending on the head size.

The density in the mid-scalp can be graded with maximum possible density at the hairline zone and immediately behind the hairline (Figs. 5.10A and B). The density decreases gradually as one approaches the mid-scalp. Scalp to hair contrast is one thing to be kept in mind in such people.

Patient with dark skin and/or with dark hair may need lower density of grafts for adequate coverage compared to patient with fair skin with dark hair. Patients with curly hair may be satisfied with less density compared to those with straight hair.

There can be differential implantation on mid-scalp with more density on the side of parting compared to density on the other side which will be hidden with long hair from the other side. This approach is used when we have limited number of grafts to play with.

We often mix beard grafts with scalp grafts in mid-scalp. One thing which needs to be kept in mind is the principle of donor dominance where character of hair at the transplanted zone resembles that of the donor zone (Fig. 5.11).

TEMPLE RECONSTRUCTION IN TRACTION ALOPECIA

Due to prolonged use of turbans since childhood some people develop a unique pattern of hair loss. In this pattern, there is symmetrical regression of hairline, regression of temple and side locks of scalp. Slowly and steadily there is washout of complete hairline including the fronto-temporal angles, the temple and the

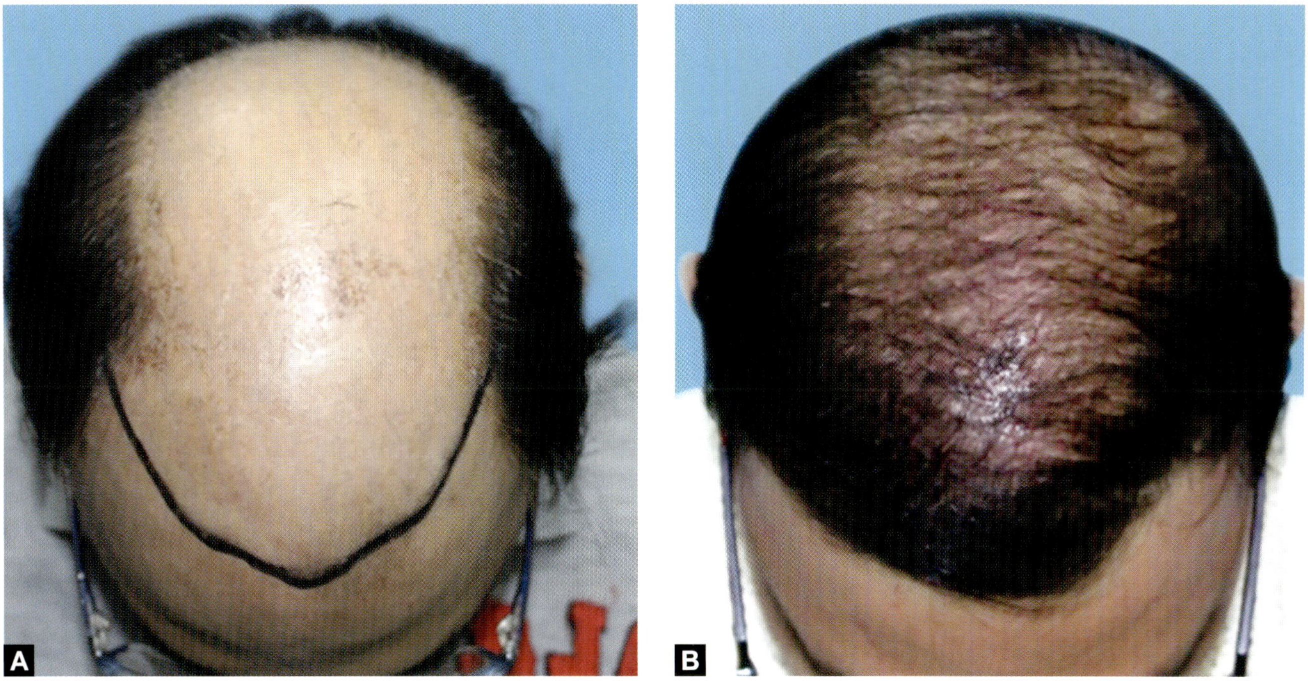

Figures 5.10A and B

The above set of photographs shows presence of graded decrease in density as one approaches the crown from the hairline. We had implanted mostly beard hair in the mid-scalp while hairline and crown were implanted with scalp grafts in single surgical visit in this patient. This is the reason for less than optimum density in the mid-scalp since beard grafts are mostly single haired grafts. Figure 10B is of a patient 5 months after transplant. The beard grafts sometimes grow late so there is still scope of improvement.

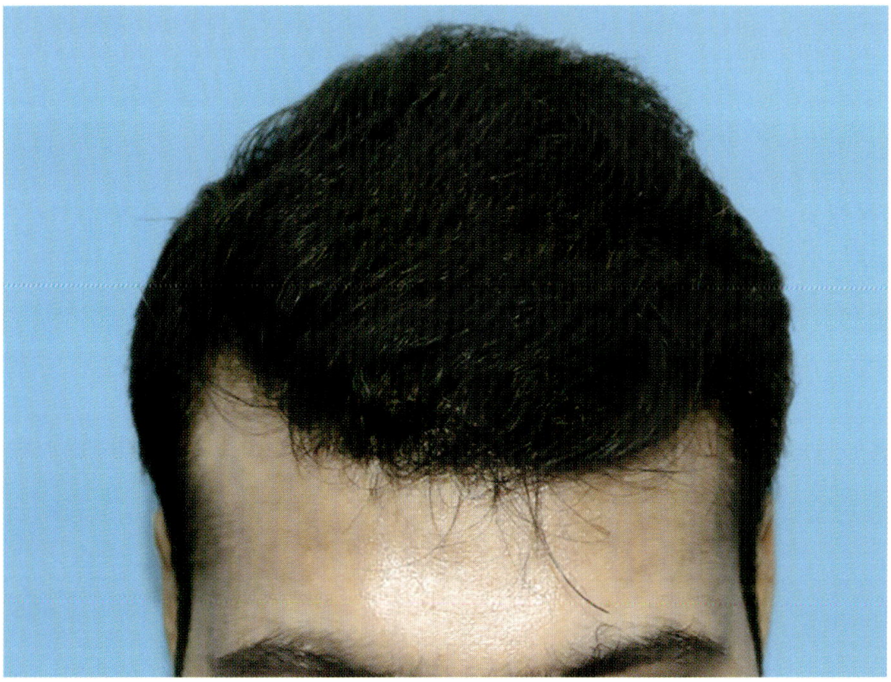

Figure 5.11

The mid-scalp grafts are made of mostly beard grafts which can be identified by their curl and waviness.

sidelocks. The regression of temple may reach up to the superior aspect of ears (Figs. 5.12A and B).

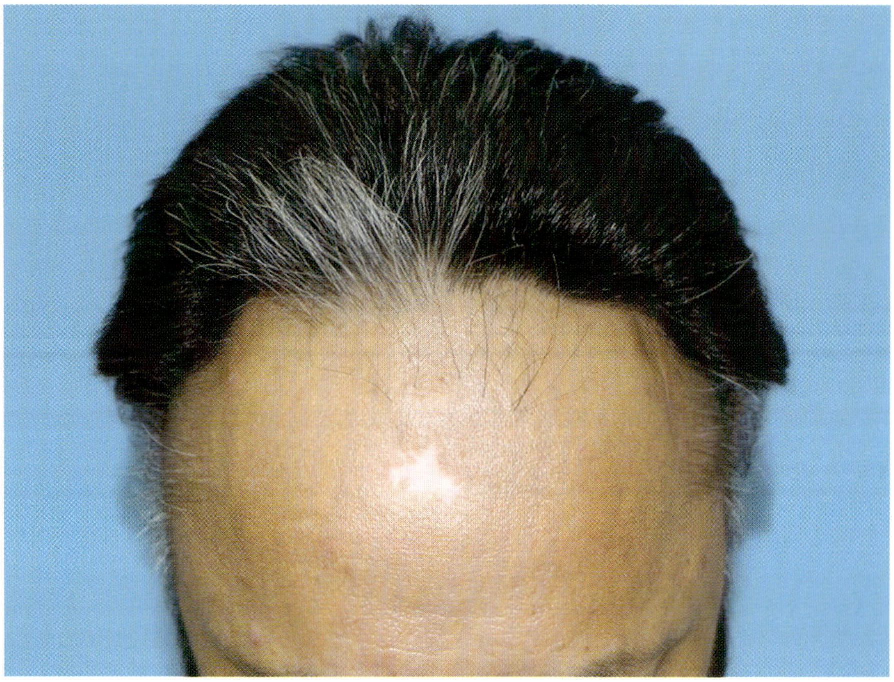

Figure 5.12A

Regression of hairline and washout of frontotemporal area including the frontotemporal angles.

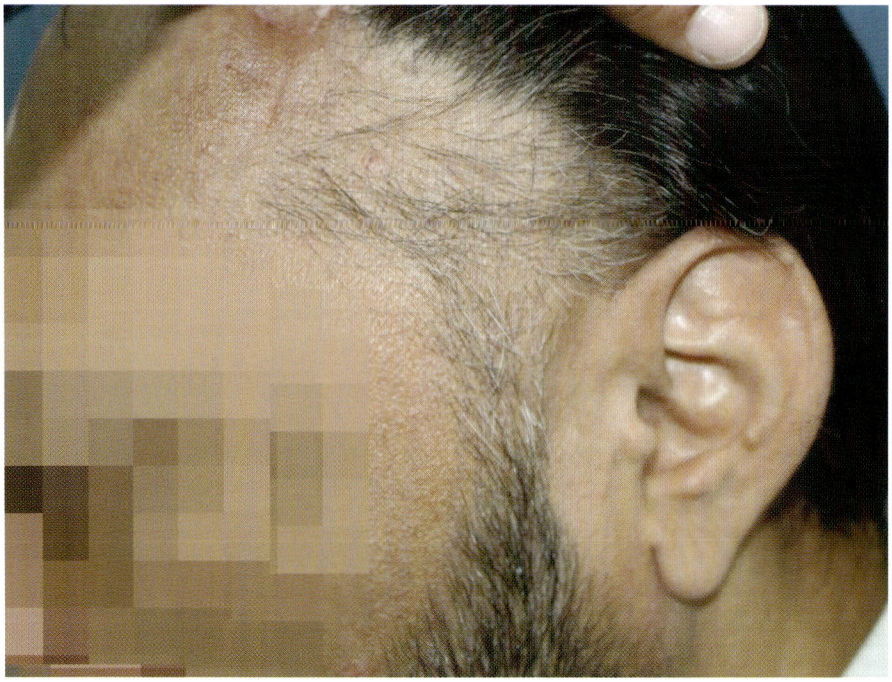

Figure 5.12B

There is complete washout of temple and upper 1/3rd of side locks. The effect of traction is seen up to the superior aspect of ear.

Reconstructing the hairline and the temple requires full understanding of "direction" and "angles" of the hairline, upper temple, temporal points, the lower temple, and the side locks (Figs. 5.13A to I).

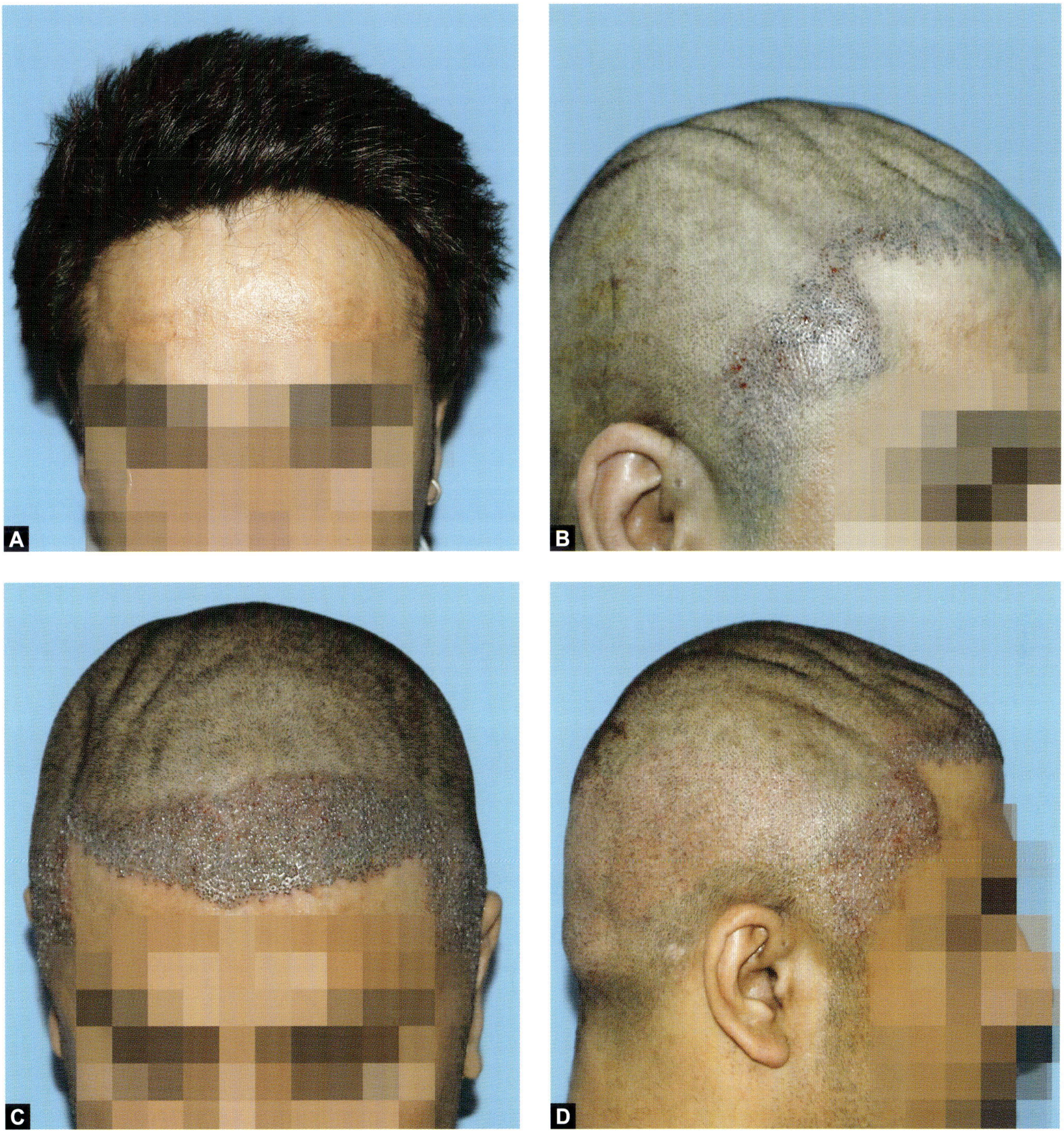

Figures 5.13A to D

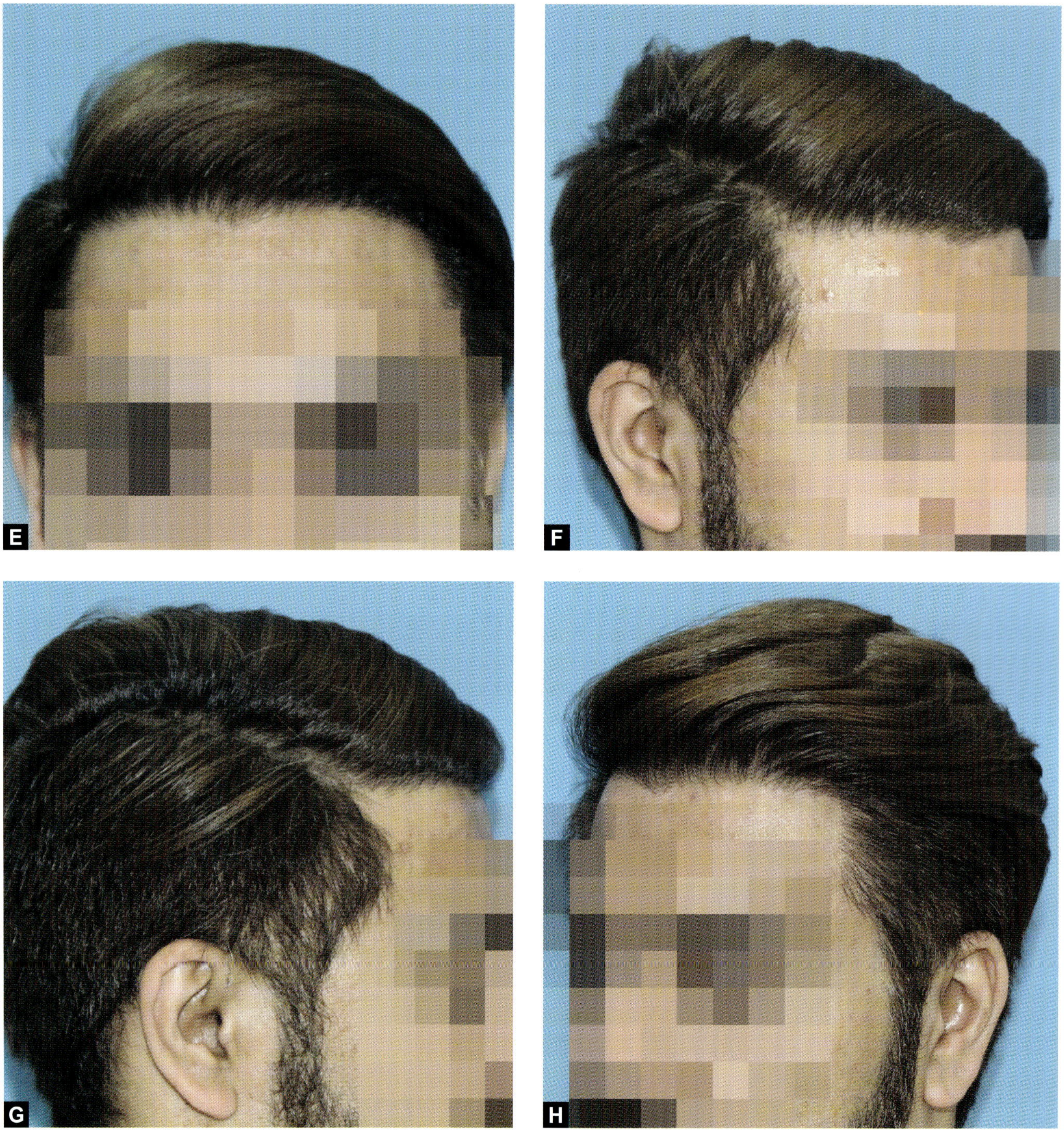

Figures 5.13E to H

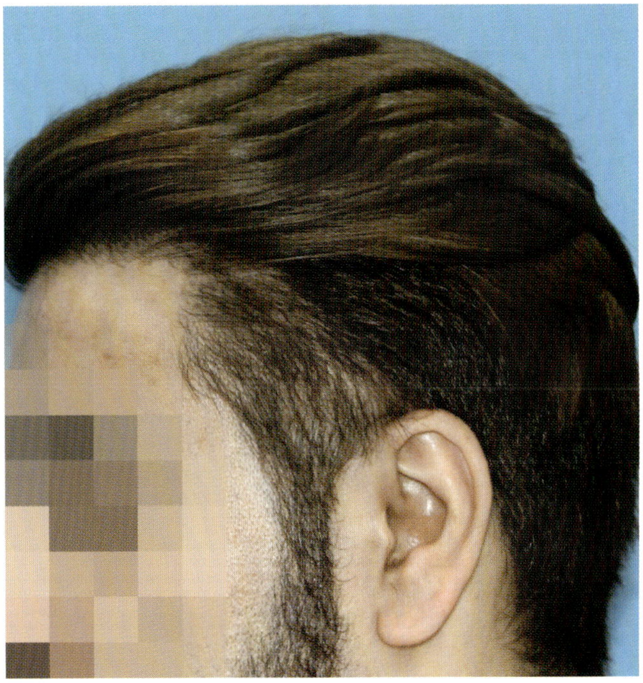

Figure 5.13I

Figures 5.13A to I

The series of photographs shows the case of hairline and temple reconstruction and its result after 1 year of surgery. A finer look at the changing direction of temple hair will help a surgeon in constructing a beautiful temple. The hairline and temple have been aggressive in this case with hairline balancing the temple. Effort should be made to fully correct the temple (instead of under correction) as the risk of androgenetic alopecia is extremely low.

CONCLUDING THOUGHTS

Temple reconstruction is an art worth mastering as it greatly improves the look of the patient. However, the new surgeon should master the hairline reconstruction first and always listen to his inner conscience while deciding the hairline as much lower anterior hairline may fetch him more money but reduces the chance of correcting his mistakes. A wrongly constructed temple may spoil all the goodwill he has generated by creating a great hairline and will also waste significant number of grafts which could have been used somewhere else. Correcting such temple will need extraction of wrongly implanted hair and reimplantation of hair with correct angles. Hump reconstruction is equally important, the surgeon should spare some scalp grafts for hump reconstruction. The graft should be placed in relatively less dense manner in mid-scalp compared to the hairline and the crown.

SUMMARY

- Temple is a part of anterior hairline and rules of microirregularity applies to temple as well.
- Temple reconstruction should be done only when it is absolutely necessary as maintaining the temple-hairline balance is essential.
- Temple reconstruction should not be done below 25 years of age due to the risk of progression of baldness.
- Temple area has hair pointing in different directions and following the same is important.
- Slits and implantation of grafts in temple are done at 5 to 10° to the skin surface.
- Anterior two lines of temple also requires implanting of single follicle grafts.
- The grafts from the nape of the neck or above the ears are preferred as they are often single and less pigmented.
- It is necessary to observe and assist in many temple reconstruction cases to learn the art.

REFERENCES

1. Lam SM. Hair Transplant Operative 360, 2nd edn. New Delhi: Jaypee Brothers Medical Publishers (P) Ltd.; 2016. 146-54.
2. Shapiro R. Principles of creating a natural hairline. In: Unger W, Shapiro R, Unger R, Unger M (Eds). Hair Transplantation, 5th edn. Philadelphia: Informa Healthcare; 2011. 375-6.
3. Lam SM. "http://www.youtube.com/watch?v=6FnIHZnv71k" www.youtube.com/watch?v=6FnIHZnv71k

CHAPTER 6

Designing the Crown

Arika Bansal, Pradeep Sethi, Abhinav Kumar

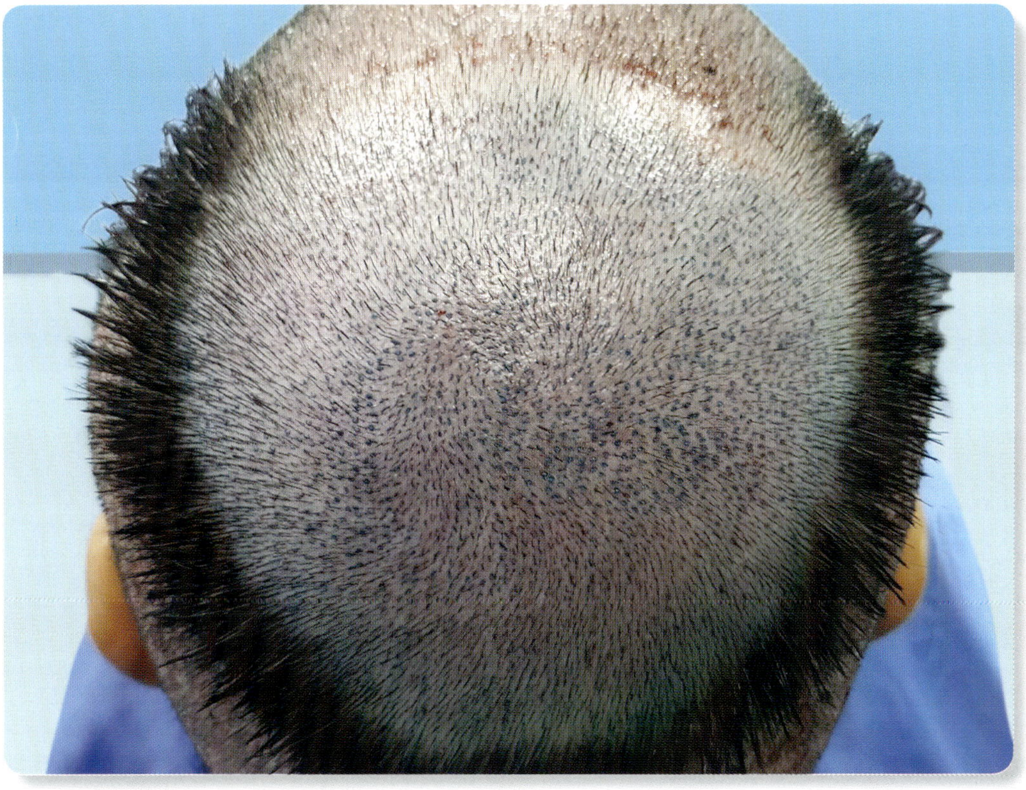

The next important area in aesthetics of hair restoration after anterior hairline is crown. Crown is a Black hole, where a lot of grafts can sink before giving an acceptable density to be appreciated by the patient and the physician!

INTRODUCTION

Crown hair transplant is a challenging art to master. The anterior part of the crown is called vertex and is the highest point of cranial vault. Choosing a right patient for crown reconstruction is very important. Thinning in the crown becomes visible with even 10–20% loss of hair density. A young patient who is having a progressive baldness and undergoes restoration of crown should be counseled about the increase of baldness in the crown if he does not continue with finasteride and minoxidil. It may then appear like a rim or halo of baldness around an island of hair (Fig. 6.1).

Crown is an area which is not given importance by surgeons or even the patients if they need hairline restoration. Generally maximum number of grafts are planned for the hairline, frontal and mid scalp and only 1,000–3,500 grafts are left for the crown. For treating a fully bald crown in a grade VI bald patient, 4,000–6,000 grafts would be needed for full coverage. Ideally a crown needs a higher number of grafts than what is actually implanted. People with higher grade of baldness (Norwood grade VI and grade VII) at an early age, who desire complete coverage in a single visit, but have limited number of grafts should opt for a higher hairline to allow for crown coverage and also ensuring sufficient scalp reserve to treat the inevitable progression of baldness.

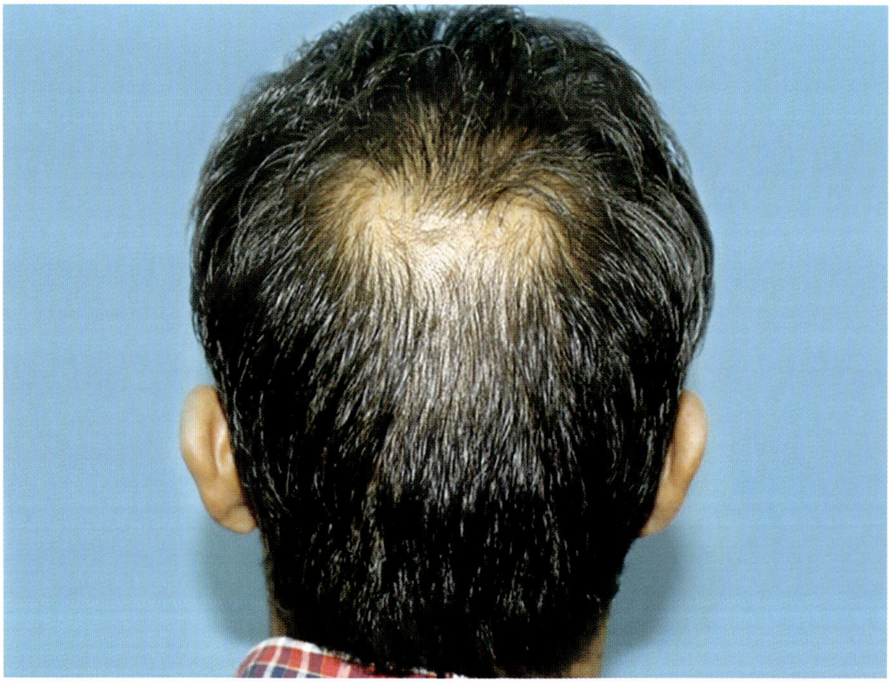

Figure 6.1

A half-moon shaped *halo* around the transplanted hair due to progression of baldness. The patient was irregular with daily intake of oral finasteride and did not apply minoxidil.

EVALUATION OF CROWN[1]

The surgeon has to understand the pattern of natural growth of existing hair, the angle of their growth, number of whorls, the presence or absence of coronet and direction of whorl/s. He may have to create a completely new whorl on the bald scalp.

- The first thing to know are the patterns of natural hair growth in the crown. Ziering and Krenitsky[2] found five distinct patterns in a study of 534 patients (Fig. 6.2). A clockwise whorl ("S" pattern), an anticlockwise whorl ("Z" pattern), a combination of two clockwise whorl ("DSS" pattern) and a combination of a clockwise and an anticlockwise whorl ("DSZ" pattern), and finally a diffuse pattern. He did not find double anticlockwise pattern. Evaluation of vellus hair in a balding patient may guide in finding the center of the whorl in a patient. In the absence of any remnant of a native whorl, it is better to create single whorl off-center and it should match the direction of parting of hair.
- The second thing to notice is the pattern of vertex hair loss. It can be a round or oval pattern, or kidney-shaped pattern or coronet pattern which is a smaller circle or semicircle below the oval pattern (Fig. 6.3). Surgeons should not miss this coronet during crown reconstruction as it may appear like a balding halo below the actual crown few years down the line after crown reconstruction (Fig. 6.4).
- The third thing to understand is the different angulations of hair to be transplanted in the crown. Crown is conceptually divided into four parts: (1) center of crown, (2) vertex transition point, (3) upper arc, and (4) the lower arc (Fig. 6.5). The center of the whorl needs higher number of grafts for giving a natural appearance as fanning of grafts from the center will always give less

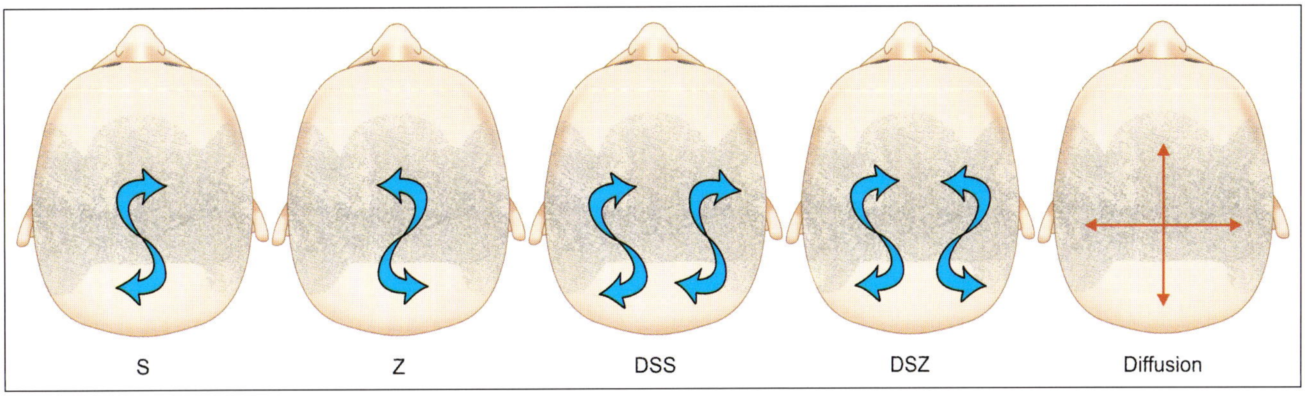

Figure 6.2

Different patterns of natural hair growth in the crown.

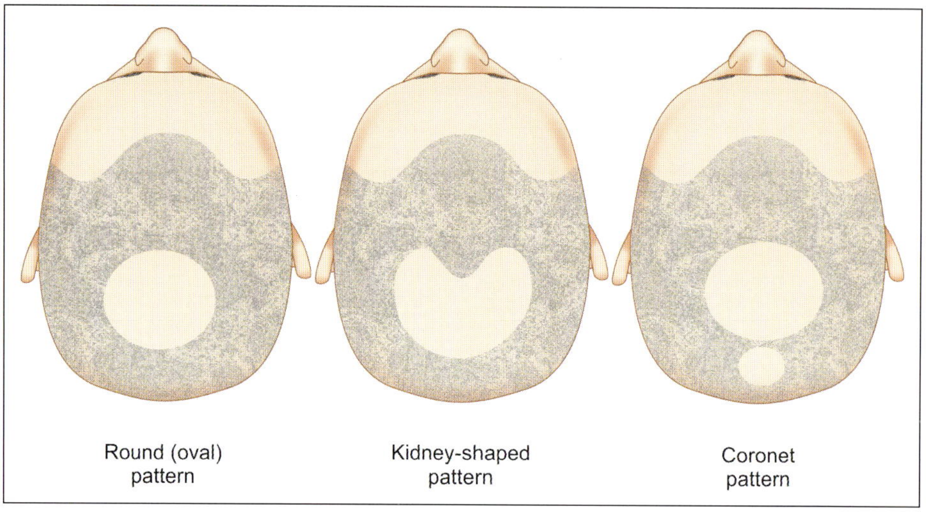

Figure 6.3

Patterns of hair loss in crown.

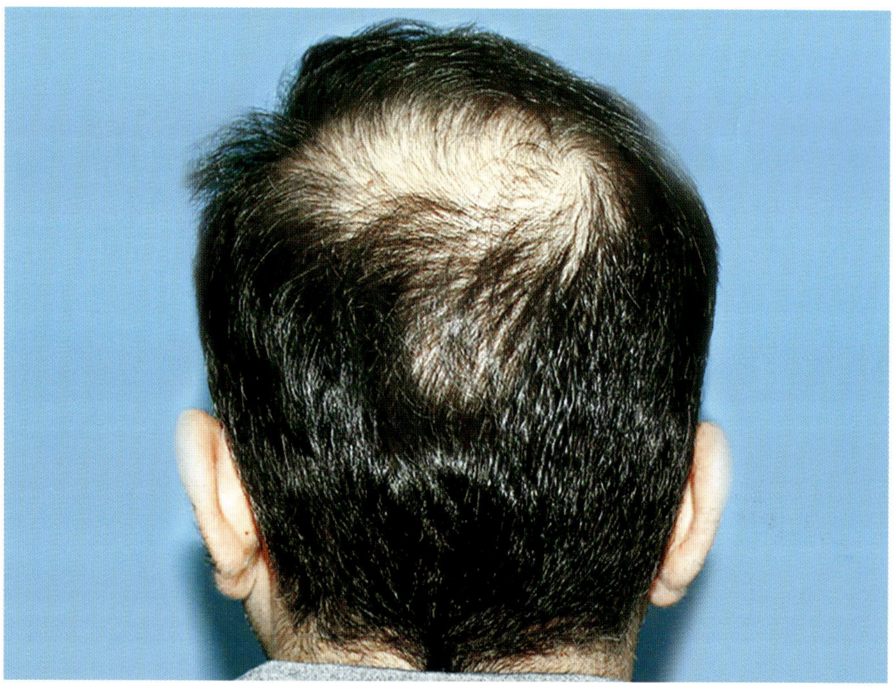

Figure 6.4

The coronet should not be missed. No extraction of donor hair should be done from the coronet as it lies in the temporary zone.

than satisfactory density. Some authors recommend a lower density at the center of the whorl. The upper arc should have the maximum density with double and triple grafts since it also covers the lower portion of crown. The high density of the upper arc covers the lower arc and significantly decreases

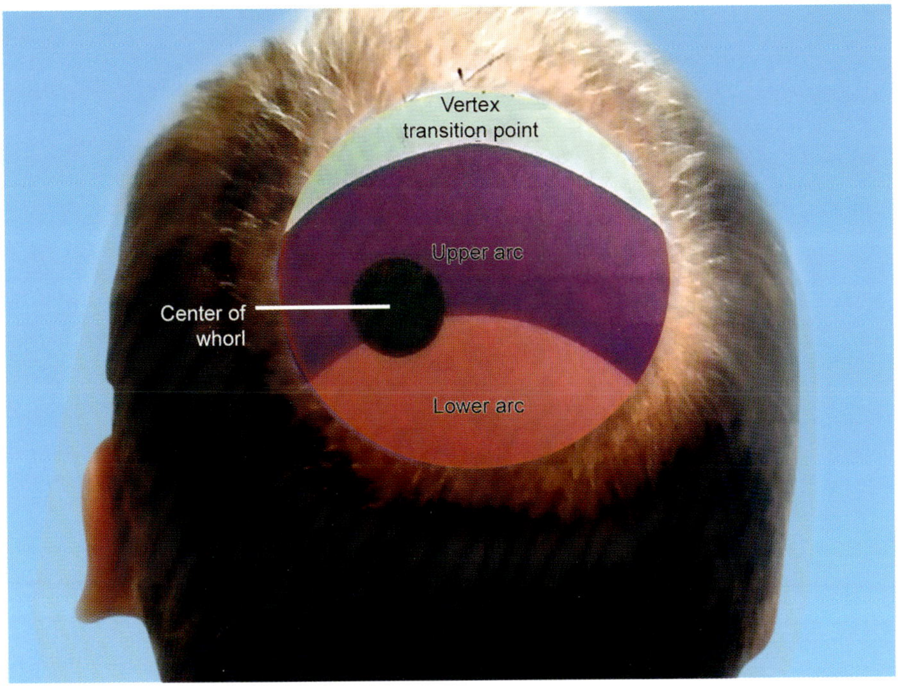

Figure 6.5

Division of the crown into four parts: (1) center of whorl, (2) vertex transition point, (3) upper arc, and (4) the lower arc.

the see-through effect of the lower part of the crown and gives an illusion of high density in the lower arc. The upper arc extends upward, so it also improves the visual density of posterior part of mid-scalp.

Slit Making in the Crown[1]

The surgeon must be aware of the "angle" and "direction". The angle of a recipient site refers to the anterior-posterior tilt of the site relative to the scalp. The direction refers to the left-to-right rotation of the recipient site. The angles of slits should be around 30° in the vertex transition point, 45° in the upper arc, 70–90° in the center of the whorl and 30° in the lower arc (Fig. 6.6). The angle becomes higher but remains acute as we approach the center of the whorl thus giving the lifting effect of the transplanted hair creating a more rounded scalp from lateral view and also allows bouncing of the hair on crown (Figs. 6.7 and 6.8). Similarly the angle starts decreasing as we move toward the periphery of the lower arc to as low as 20°. Close examination of direction and angles of preexisting miniaturized hair while slit making by using loupes with 5X magnification helps us in creating slits with correct angles and directions.

The Figures 6.9A to H depict various angles of slit creation on the crown and pictorially elaborates the art of slit making.

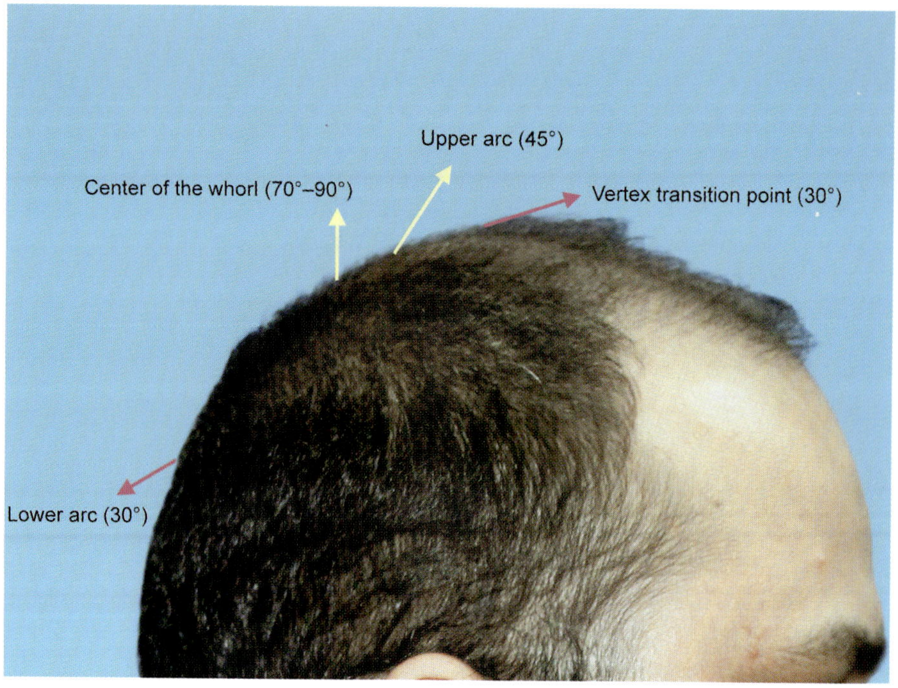

Figure 6.6

Angles that should be maintained while making the slits at various sites of the crown.

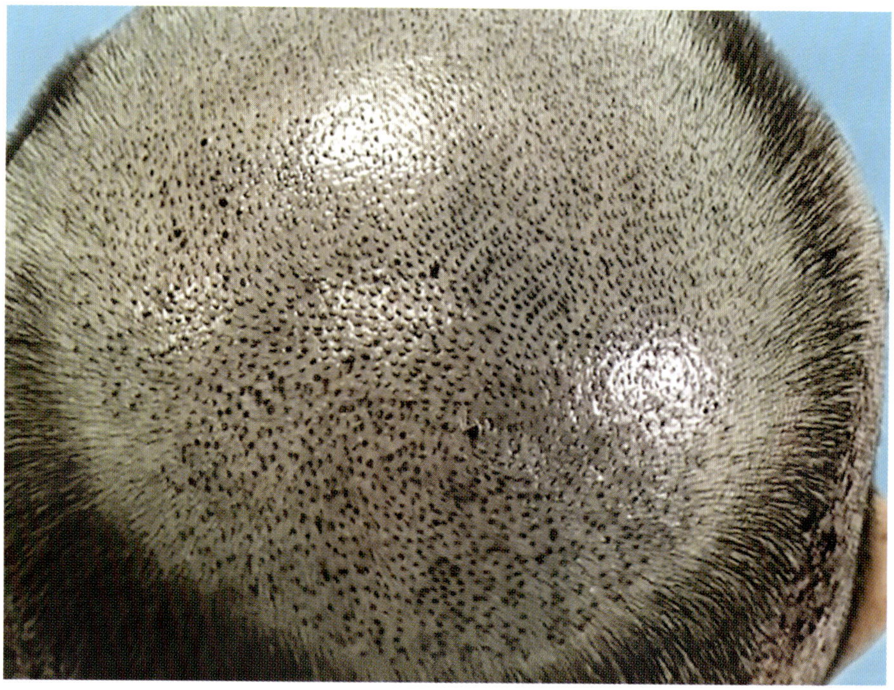

Figure 6.7

Slit creation in crown in a patient with Norwood grade VII baldness with counter-clockwise whorl in the center with radial fanning. The number of slits created in the upper arc is much higher than the lower arc. The radial fanning was done for smooth merging with the grafts of the mid scalp and lateral part of the scalp.

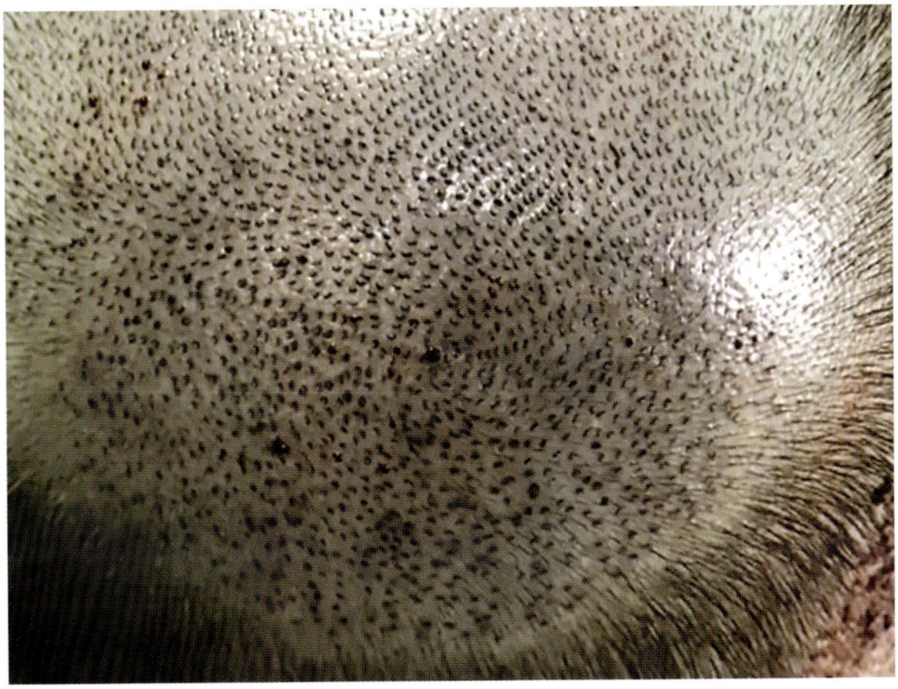

Figure 6.8

Figure shows closer view of the center of the whorl with every slit in a slightly different direction. The slits have been created using 20G needle. The angles of slit in the center of whorl were kept at 70–80°. The angles became more acute, nearing 45° along the radials of the whorl. The angle of slit creation further decreased to 20–30° as we approached the periphery of the whorl. Implantation has been done with the use of dull needle implanters of different sizes to accommodate single or multiple grafts. The graft excision was done with 0.9–0.95 mm sharp serrounded punches.

Correct directions and angles of slits helps us in creating a natural crown, which is rounded in profile view and shows the whorl in right direction. The preexisting hair in the crown are also not neutralized by a different direction of the transplanted hair (Figs. 6.10 to 6.16).

CASE STUDY 1

A 27-year-old male presented to us for hair transplant in the crown. Initially we insisted on medical management considering his age and progressing diameter of his bald patch of the crown. But on repeated insistence we had to take up his case for transplantation as he had to be in public glare all the time. Consent was taken mentioning about the remote possibility of shortage of scalp grafts for hairline and mid scalp in case he experiences higher grade of baldness in future. As shown in Figures 6.17A to D, he has a right-sided clockwise whorl, his donor was good in density, and his scalp had good elasticity.

Attention was paid to avoid any damage to any preexisting hair even if they were on the verge of becoming vellus hair.

Comments by Dr Robert True on this Case

I am sorry it sounds as though you let your clinical judgment be dictated by a desire to please the patient, even though he does not know better. Never a good decision.

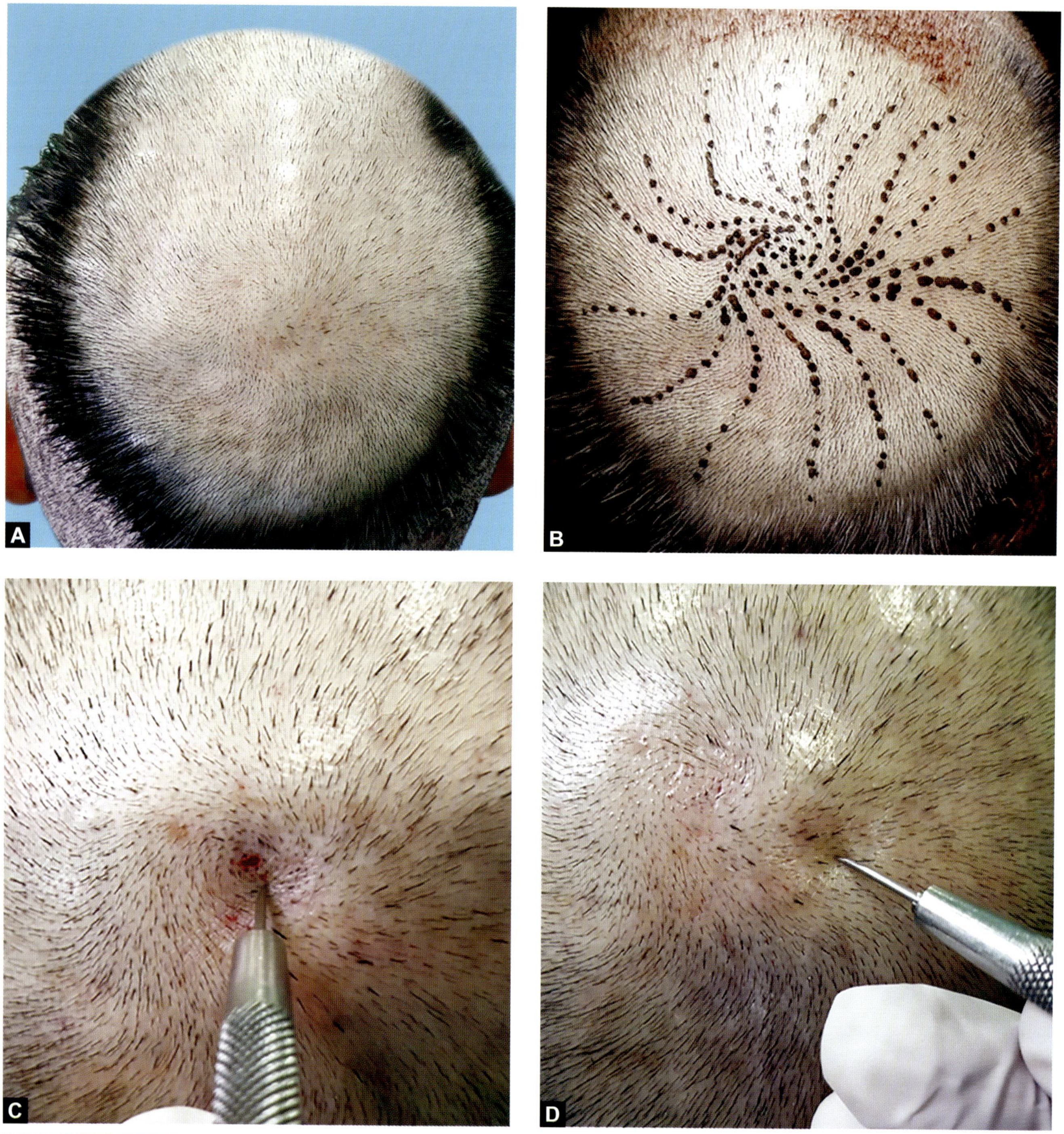

Figures 6.9A to D

(A) A balding crown, where we implanted few hundred grafts few years ago. The baldness progressed over time and the client came for hair restoration on the crown; (B) We designed counter-clockwise whorl in the center with radial fanning. We planned to reconstruct his original crown; (C) The next few pictures will depict the angles at which we had made the slits in the crown in these patients. The angles at the center of the crown were at 80–90°; (D) As one move from center of the whorl to the periphery, the angles of the slits starts become more acute. At this point we have made the slits at 45°. Also note the direction of the needle which matches with the direction of the miniaturized hair.

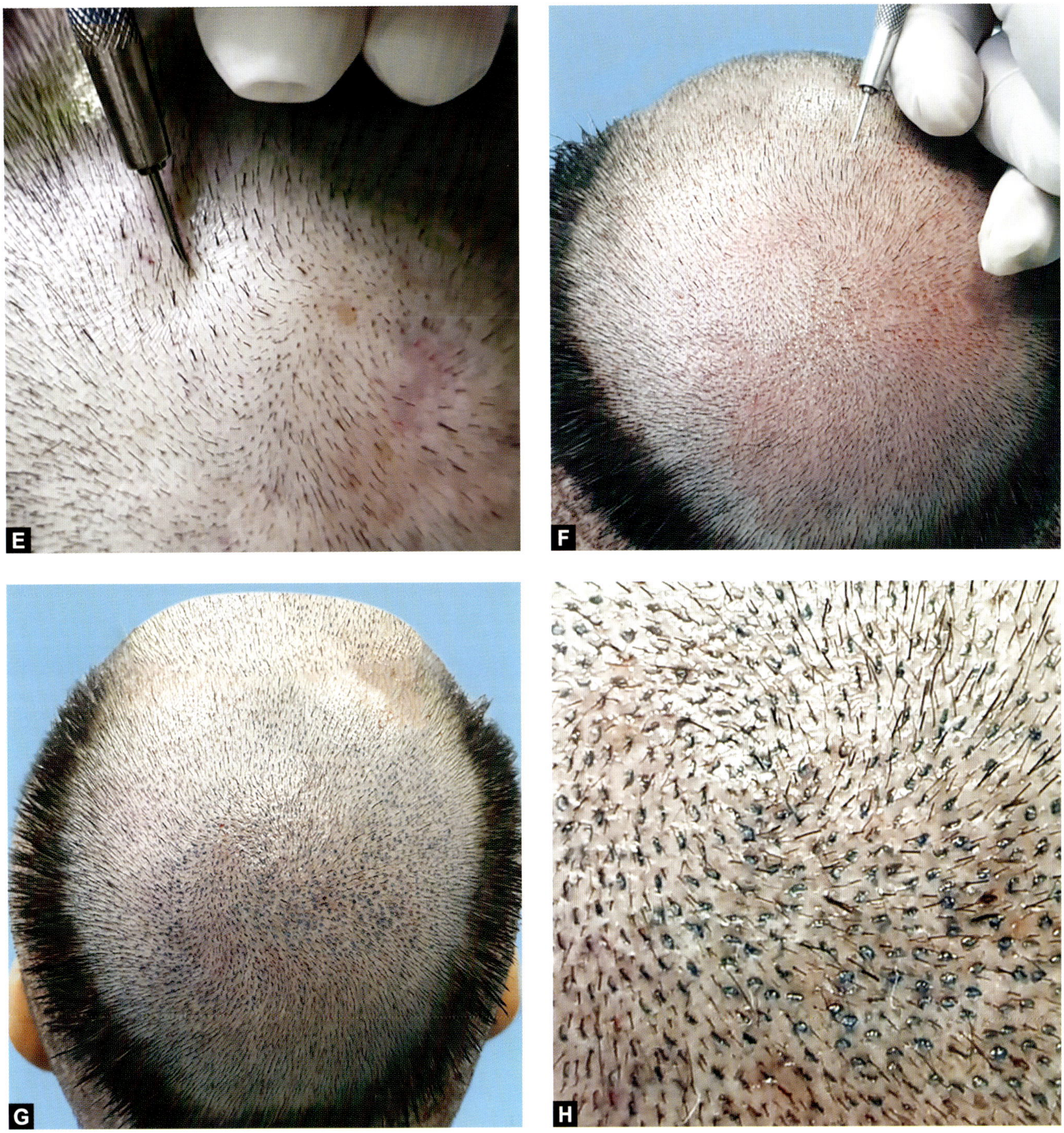

Figures 6.9E to H

(E) Note the direction and angle of slits at the superolateral aspect of the crown; (F) At the vertex transition point, the angle and direction of slits become acute and forward to ensure smooth merging with the preexisting hair; (G) The appearance of crown after slit making; and (H) The magnified view of center of the anticlockwise whorl. The technician implanting the grafts should be aware of the direction and angles of slits in direct hair transplantation. It is advised to do the implantation under 5X magnification. The direction and angles of implanters will match with the angles and directions of slits.

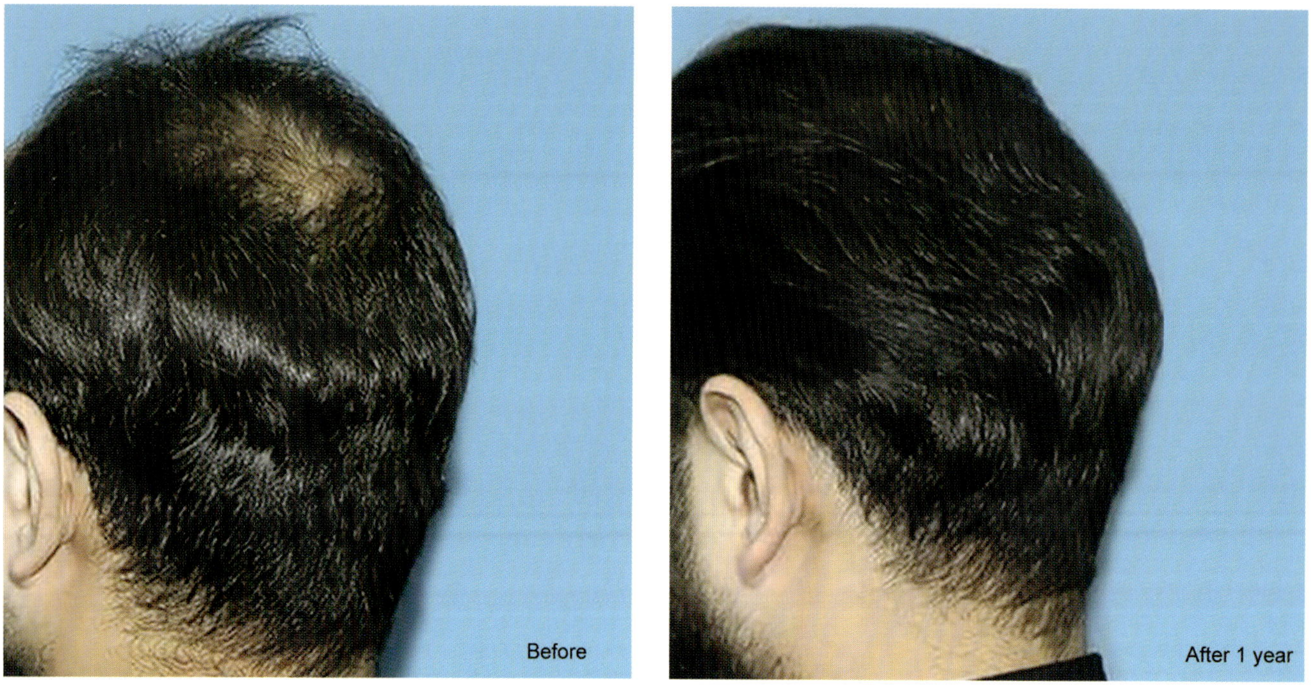

Figure 6.10

This picture illustrates the rounding effect of crown from a profile view due to implantation of grafts at less acute angles in the whorl (around 45–80°) during crown hair transplant which gives a lifting effect to the nearby hair thus maintaining the contour of the crown.

I think this is hardly a remote possibility; rather, it is a highly likely probability. I do not approve of transplanting the crown before the front and mid scalp has been transplanted in patients under 35 years of age. Over the coming years of your practice you will see why?

CASE STUDY 2

Fanning Technique

A 40-year-old man with limited number of grafts due to failed previous hair restoration surgery wished for low hairline and crown coverage to make him look young in spite of having a big head size and a very large crown. This problem forced us to adopt unconventional approach for crown restoration. The client had a crown of very large diameter requiring a minimum of 3,000 grafts for successful restoration (Figs. 6.18A to C). However, we gave an illusion of successful coverage with 1,200 grafts without conventional approach (as the donor area was compromised by previous surgery punch scars which limited extraction of grafts for the crown). The grafts were fanned out in a whorl like fashion to diminish the visibility of scalp.

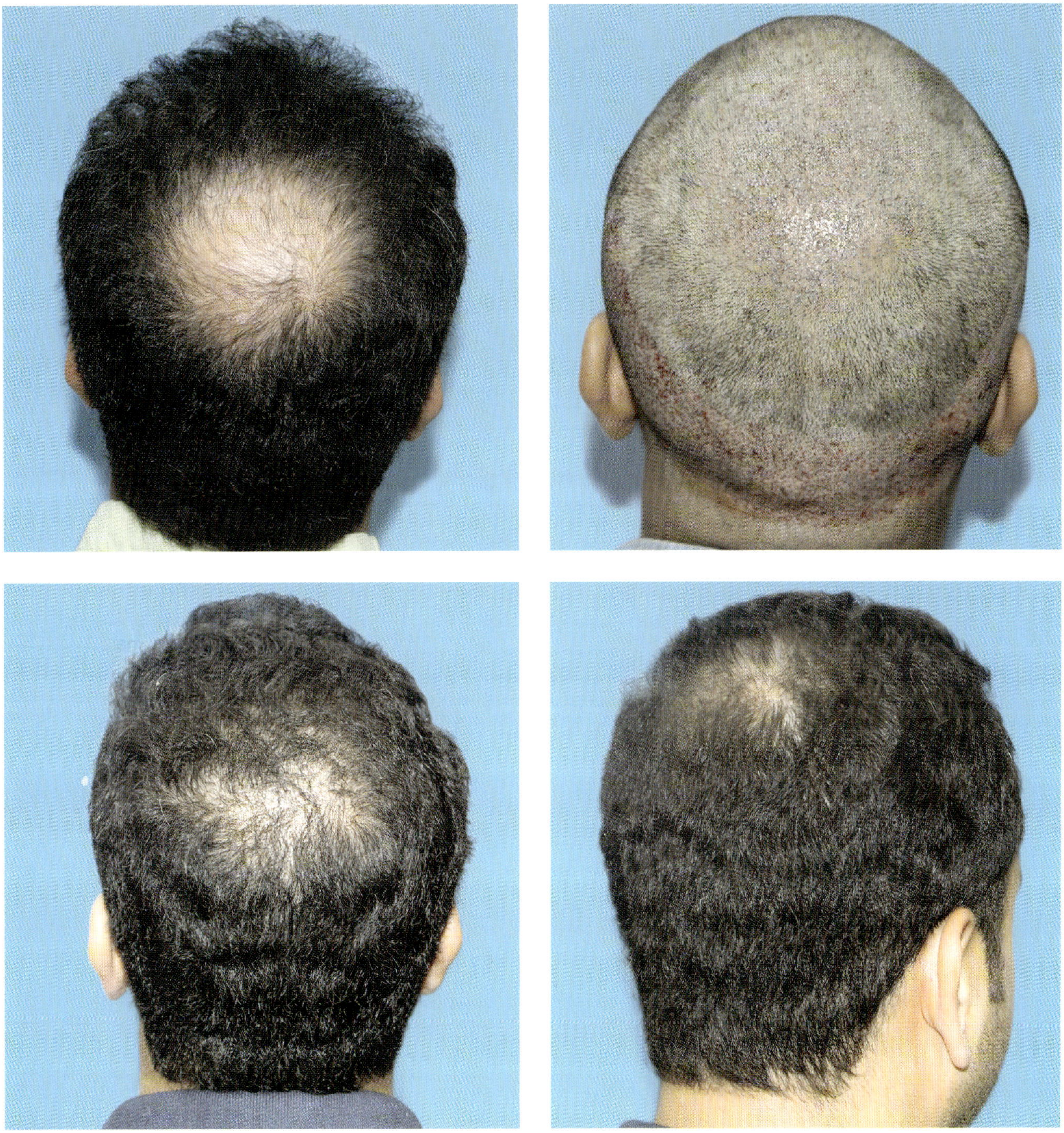

Figure 6.11

Figure shows crown restoration using direct hair transplantation method—the crown has retained its clockwise whorl pattern and it has completely merged with the posterior part of mid-scalp. The center of the whorl is less dense as compared to the periphery. The pattern of preexisting whorl is retained.

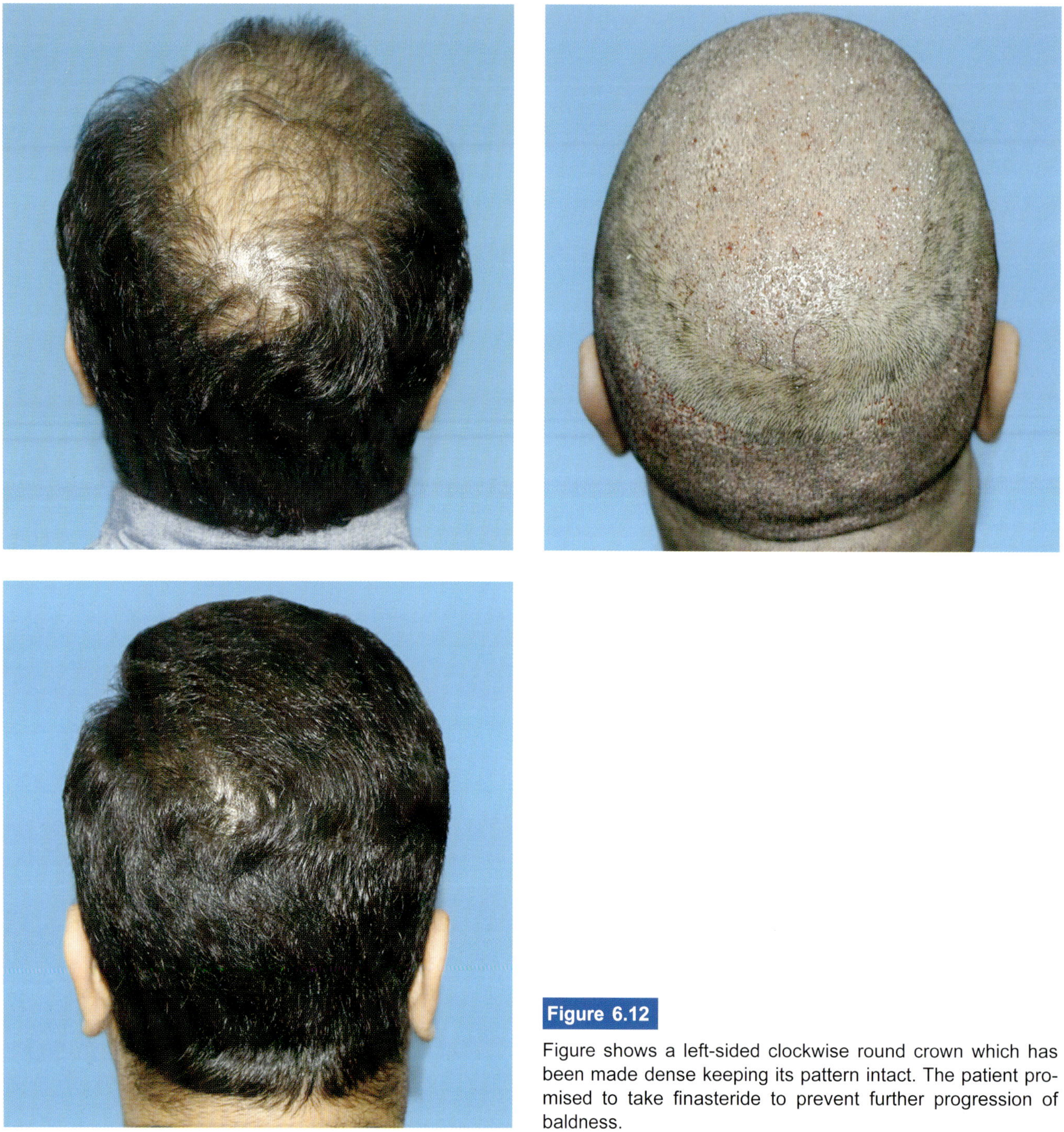

Figure 6.12

Figure shows a left-sided clockwise round crown which has been made dense keeping its pattern intact. The patient promised to take finasteride to prevent further progression of baldness.

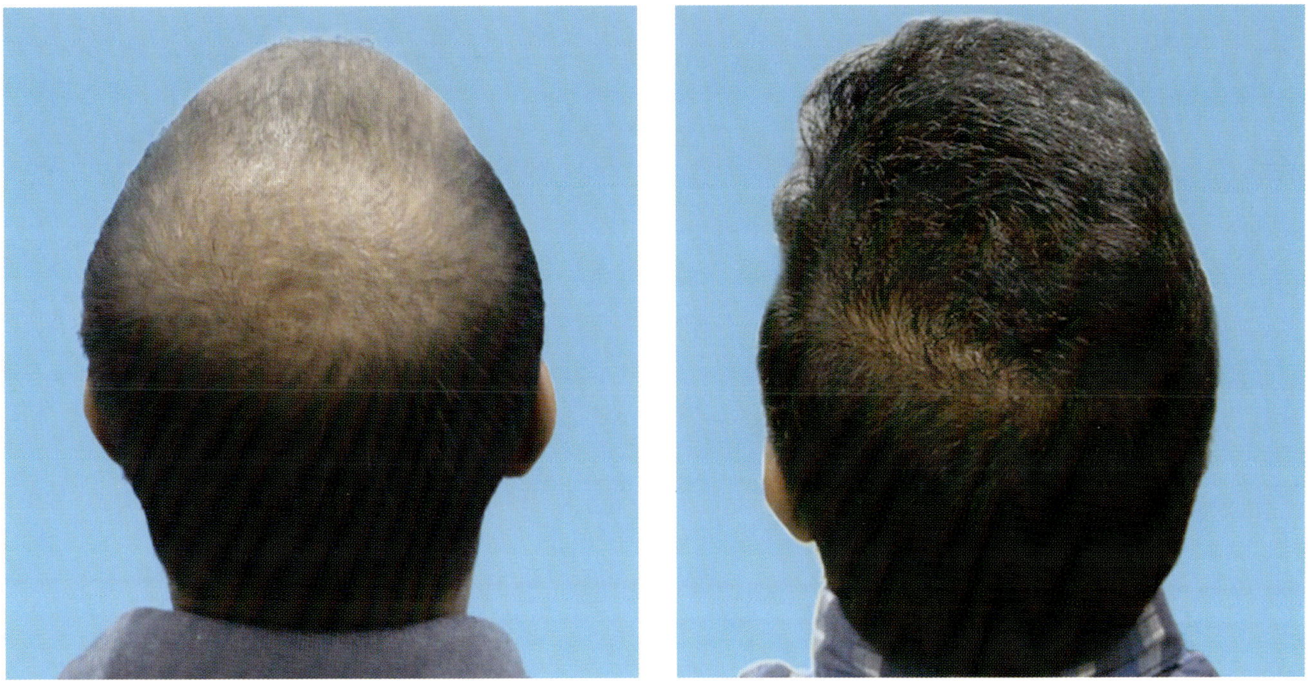

Figure 6.13

Figure shows reconstruction of an oval-shaped crown. The patient was of Norwood grade 6.

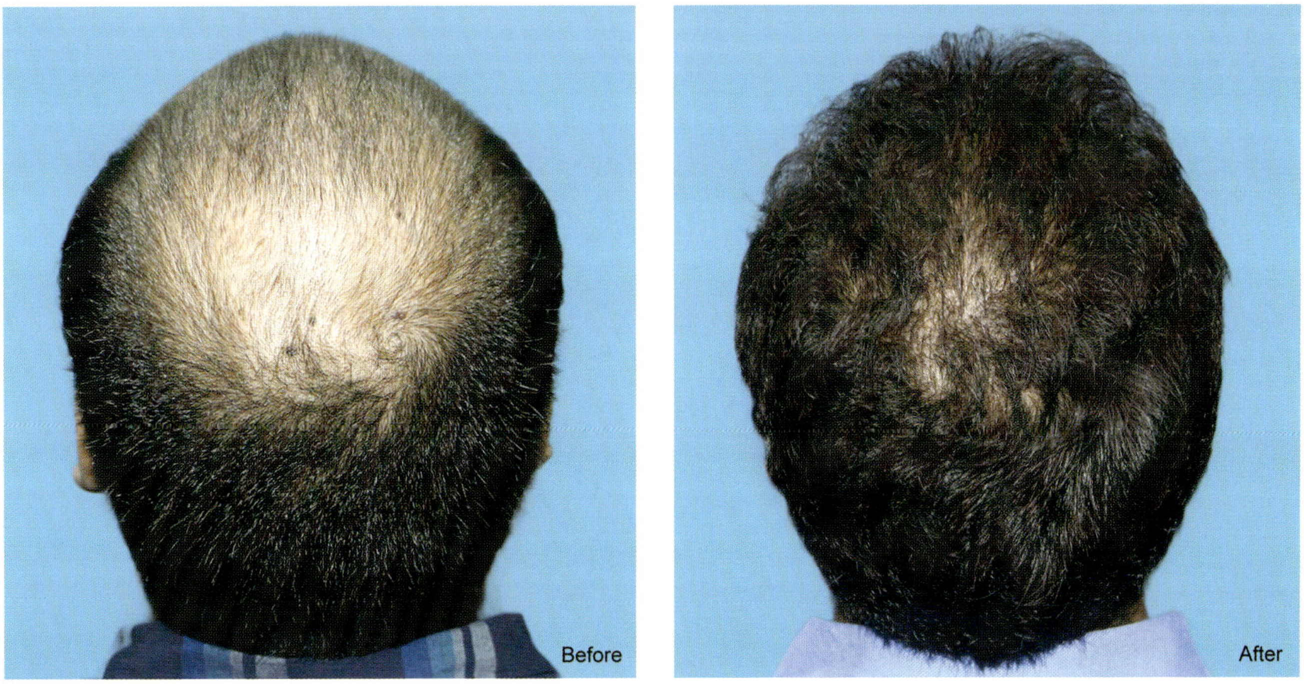

Figure 6.14

Figure shows creation of central whorl with the use of 2,000 grafts in a young patient. The crown merged nicely with the vertex and the occipital part of the scalp. This patient is advised to apply minoxidil and take oral finasteride to slow down further progression of baldness.

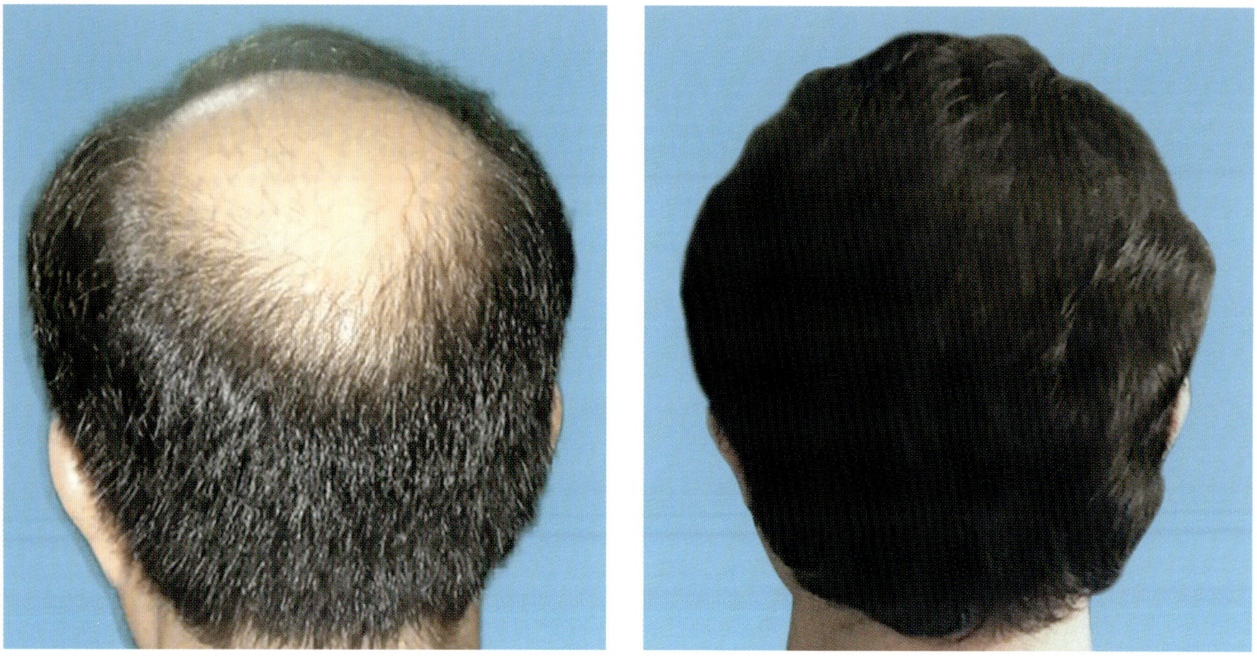

Figure 6.15

Crown reconstruction in a patient where instead of whorl creation in the lower arc, a fall has been created in the lower arc which grows downward to merge with existing hair in the occipital part of the scalp.

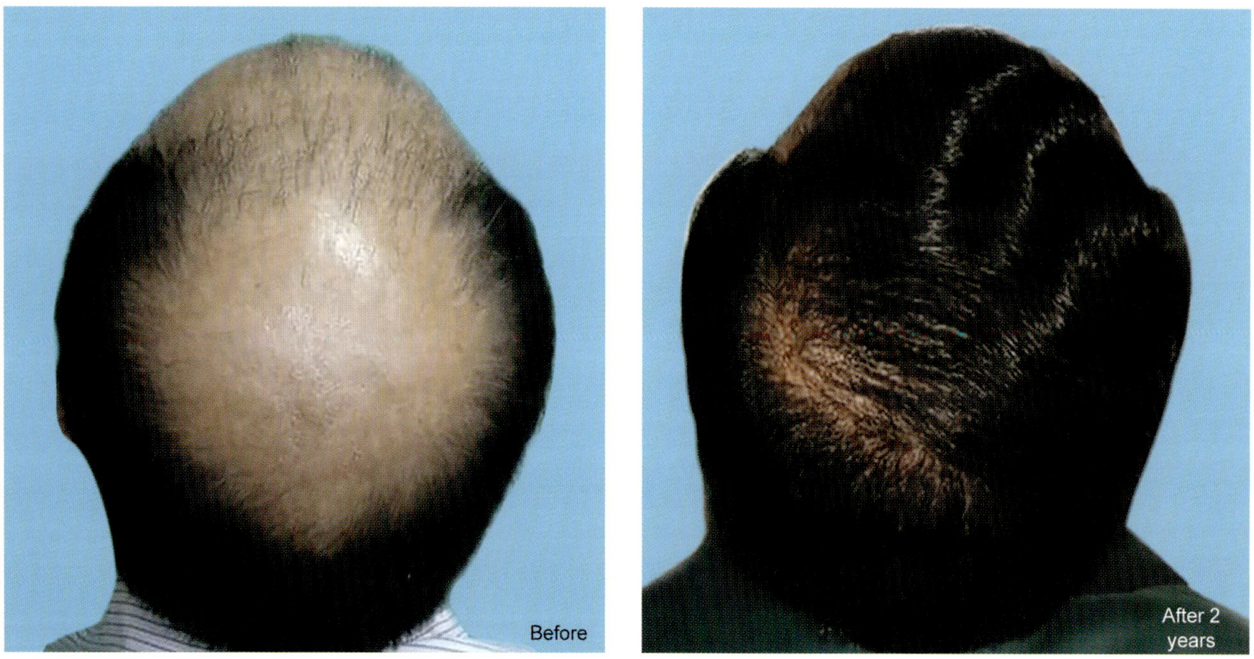

Figure 6.16

Roof view of a patient with complete crown reconstruction with around 5,000 grafts in a 55-year-old patient. The left-sided crown which has been created matches the parting side of the patient with center of the whorl less dense and higher density on the upper arc. The lower arc merged of with the occipital scalp hair. The knowledge and imagination of the surgeon along with preexisting vellus hair helped us in creating this whorl.

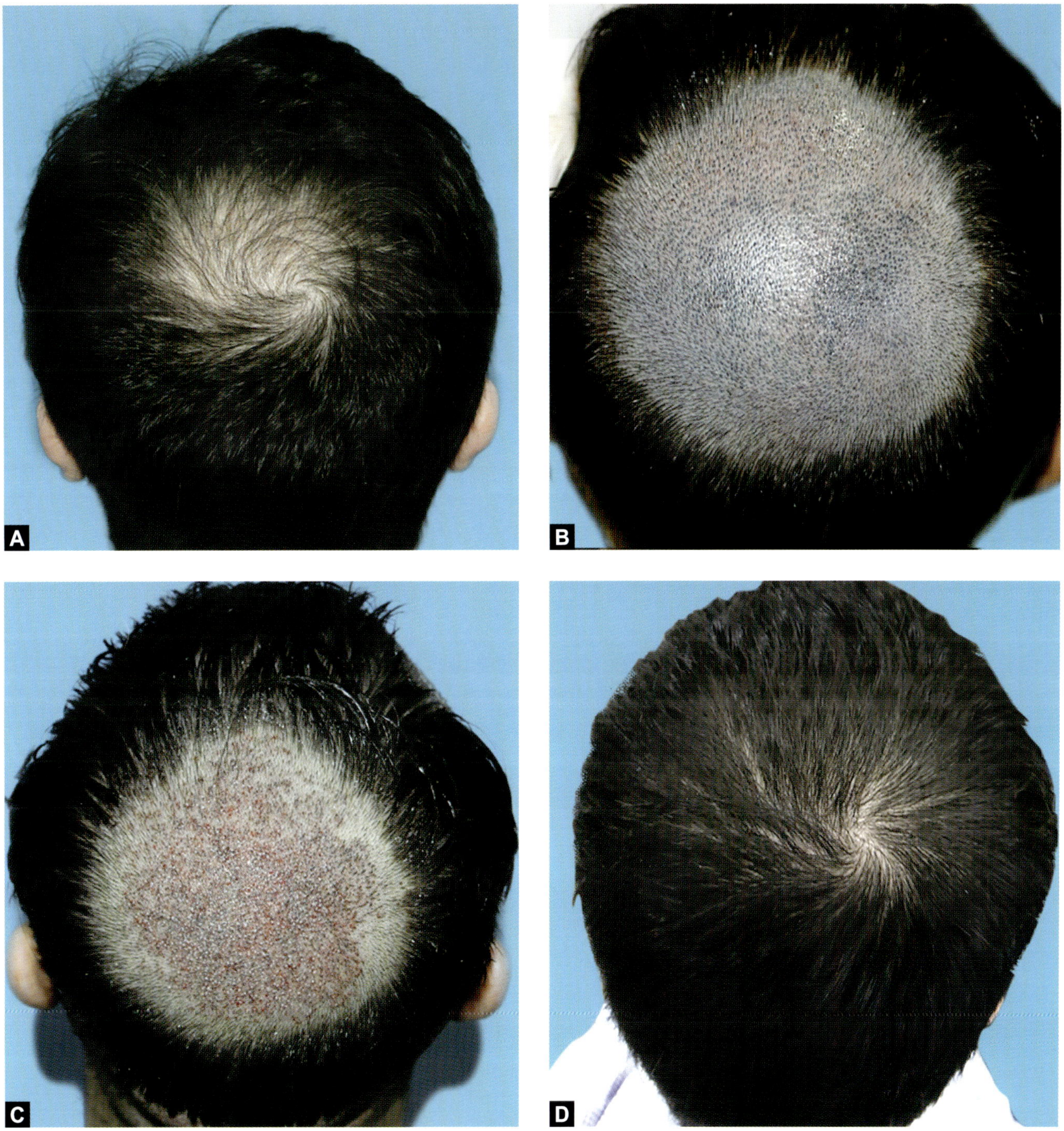

Figures 6.17A to D

(A) Right-sided clockwise whorl. His donor area is good with thick caliber hair; (B) First we trimmed much larger areas of the scalp considering his progressive baldness and presence of hair which were in the process of miniaturization in the periphery of the crown. This was done to create enough slits in the periphery to reduce the risk of development of rim of baldness within few years of transplant in case patient becomes non-compliant with the medication. Slits were created under 5X magnification keeping in mind the preexisting whorl. Attention was paid to avoid any damage to any preexisting hair even if they were on the verge of becoming vellus hair; (C) A total of 2,000 grafts were placed in the pre-made slits. Postoperative instructions were followed properly by the patient; and (D) This is the result after 5 months. Further improvement in density is expected since complete result comes in 8 months to 1 year.

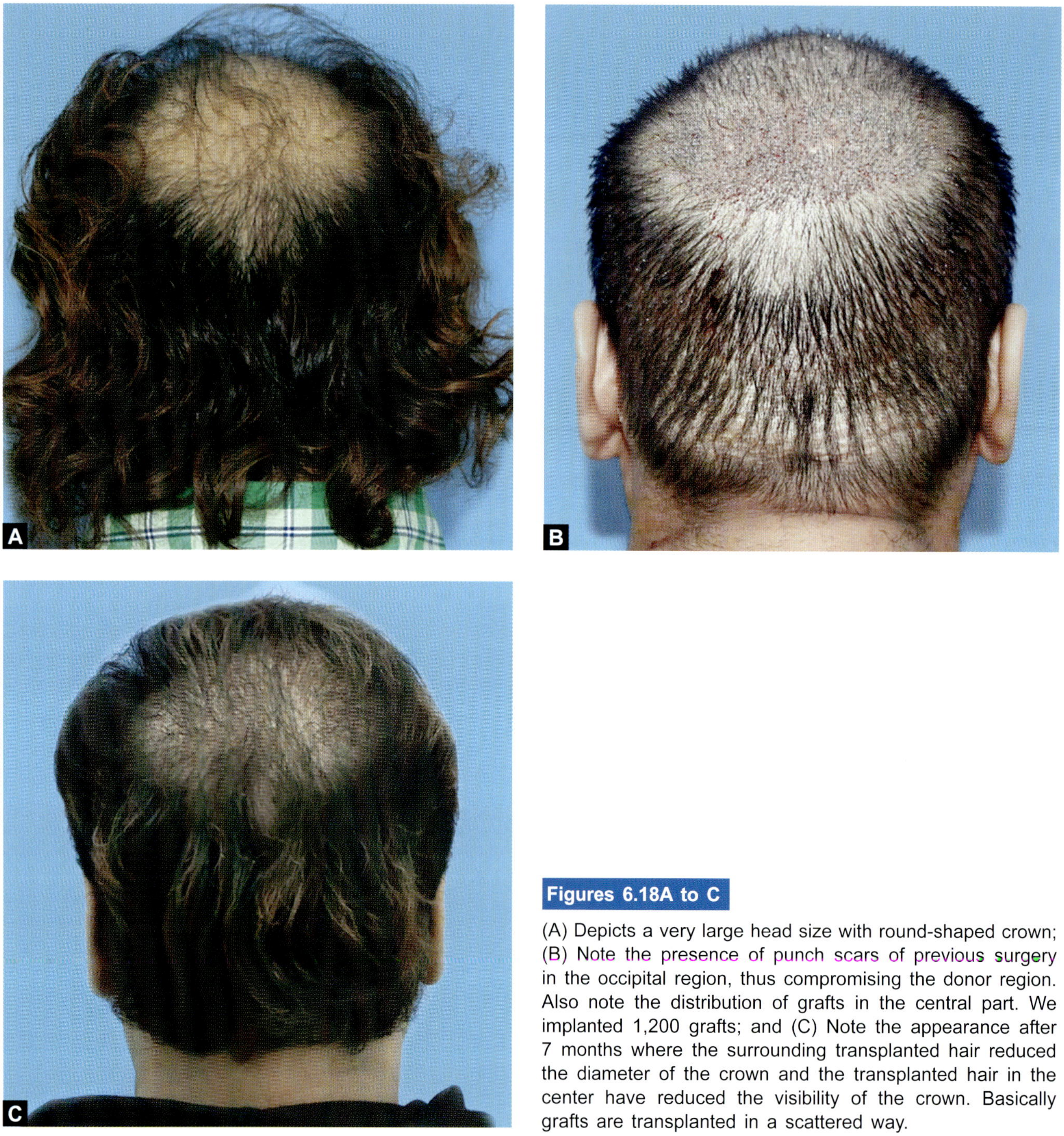

Figures 6.18A to C

(A) Depicts a very large head size with round-shaped crown; (B) Note the presence of punch scars of previous surgery in the occipital region, thus compromising the donor region. Also note the distribution of grafts in the central part. We implanted 1,200 grafts; and (C) Note the appearance after 7 months where the surrounding transplanted hair reduced the diameter of the crown and the transplanted hair in the center have reduced the visibility of the crown. Basically grafts are transplanted in a scattered way.

CONCLUDING THOUGHTS

We sincerely hope that hair transplant surgeons will get an idea about the finer aspects of crown reconstruction. The crown is equally important part of patients' overall appearance and effort should be made to restore the hairline as well as the crown with the use of scalp and beard grafts.

Comments by Dr Bessam Farjo

The crown is a dilemma in terms of when and how to treat. Crown hair loss progression around a transplanted area will potentially result in a pattern that does not occur in nature with an island of hair surrounded by ring of baldness. Early life attempts at transplanting the crown when it is less stable, carries higher risk of this unnatural pattern.

Beginner surgeons are less equipped to make this judgment. Early treatment with nonsurgical options such as medications, lasers or PRP, and stabilizing the crown should buy the surgeon time and avoid having to make a decision about transplanting the crown in the first place.

SUMMARY

- Crown thinning becomes apparent with just the loss of 10–20% hair.
- Presence of vellus hair guides the surgeon in recreating the pre-existing whorl. If that is not the case, a whorl should be created off center matching the direction of parting of hair.
- The concept of dividing the crown into four parts; the center, vertex transition point, upper arc, and lower arc is done and each segment is implanted with proper planning.
- Slit making in crown should be done under highest magnification for positioning the hair at correct angle.
- Surgical assistants who do implantation of grafts in crown should be aware of the implantation angles.

REFERENCES

1. Lam SM. Hair Transplant Operative 360, 2nd edn. New Delhi: Jaypee Brothers Medical Publishers (P) Ltd.; 2016.156-63.
2. Ziering C, Krenitsky G. The Ziering whorl classification of scalp hair. Dermatol Surg. 2003;29(8):817-21.

CHAPTER 7

Body Hair Transplant

Arika Bansal, Abhinav Kumar, Pradeep Sethi

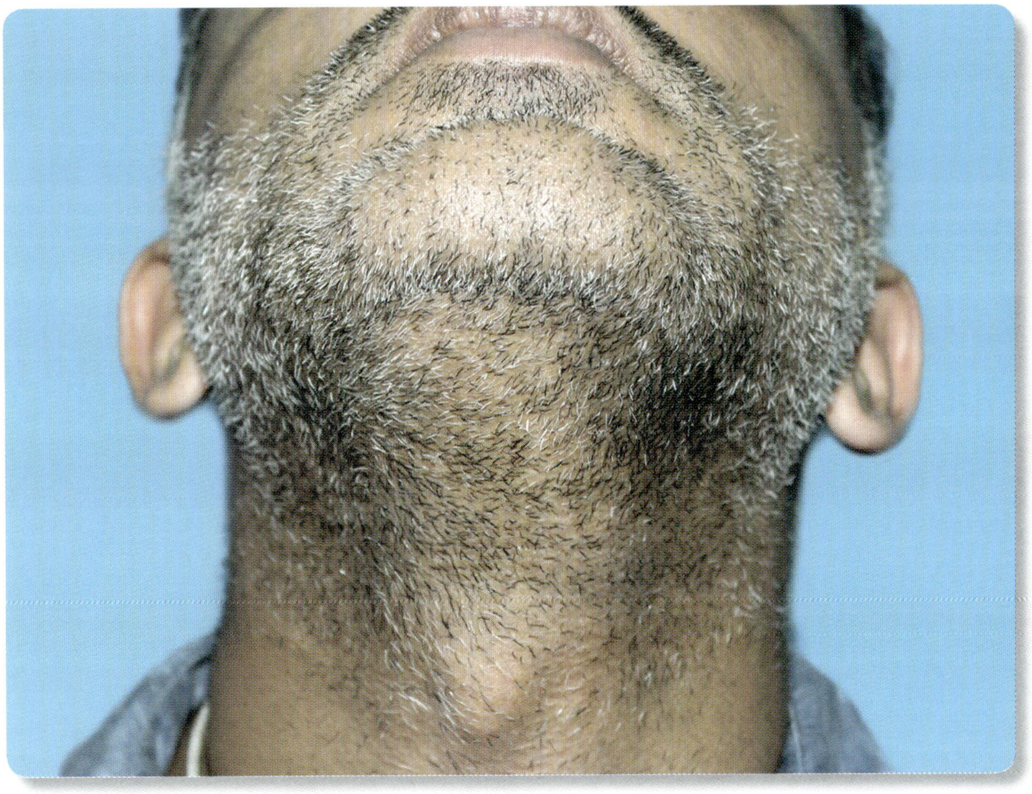

Where ever there is a will, there is a way! With increasing demands to cover the advanced grades of the baldness, body hair are the next resources to tap for. But the behaviour and hair cycle of hair of different areas are different. With a complete knowledge and experience of different body hair, physicians should try body hair whenever there is a need. A smart way of mixing the beard hair, which are mostly wiry, single, with long anagen phase with the scalp hair can give coverage of larger areas.

INTRODUCTION

Beard is a source of over 3,000–5,000 extractable grafts in a good donor thus should be considered the second best resource after scalp grafts for hair transplantation. Our chapter will deal with mainly beard hair as one rarely needs to go beyond beard hair (like chest and leg hair) as a donor for hair transplantation.

Features of Beard Hair

Beard hair are easy to extract. They are resistant to the effect of male hormone. Beard can be straight or wiry. A wiry beard can look out of place in the scalp, so should be mixed intelligently with scalp hair.

Beard can be safely implanted 2 cm behind the hairline. It can be mixed with scalp hair to increase density. In case of limited number of scalp grafts, it can be mixed with scalp grafts to make the crown denser. Beard hair usually do not follow the curl inside the skin, so the external curl should be ignored while directing the punch.

Beard grafts should not be implanted in the hairline, in the hump and in the temple as their texture and caliber is different from scalp grafts. It should never be implanted in the crown in isolation.

INDICATIONS FOR BEARD HAIR TRANSPLANT

Beard grafts can be used in advanced grades of baldness which may require beard for complete coverage in single sitting. Beard can be used as a donor in case of failed follicular unit transplant (FUT) or follicular unit excision (FUE) surgeries where the donor grafts have been exhausted. Beard can be used in case of cicatricial alopecia where scalp donor is inadequate.

SCALP GRAFTS VERSUS BEARD GRAFTS

Anagen phase of beard hair is much shorter than scalp hair. The anagen phase of beard hair is 1 year compared to 2–6 years of scalp hair. About 30% of beard hair are in telogen phase at one point of time compared to just 15% scalp hair.[1] Beard grafts have a root of bigger diameter compared to scalp grafts and they lie more superficially in the epidermis. The length of the beard hair varies from area to area. The length of moustache hair is shorter, while the length of neck beard hair is longer (Fig. 7.1A).

Beard Hair Extraction

Part Preparation

- Beard should be shaved 3–4 days before harvesting to select only the anagen hair.

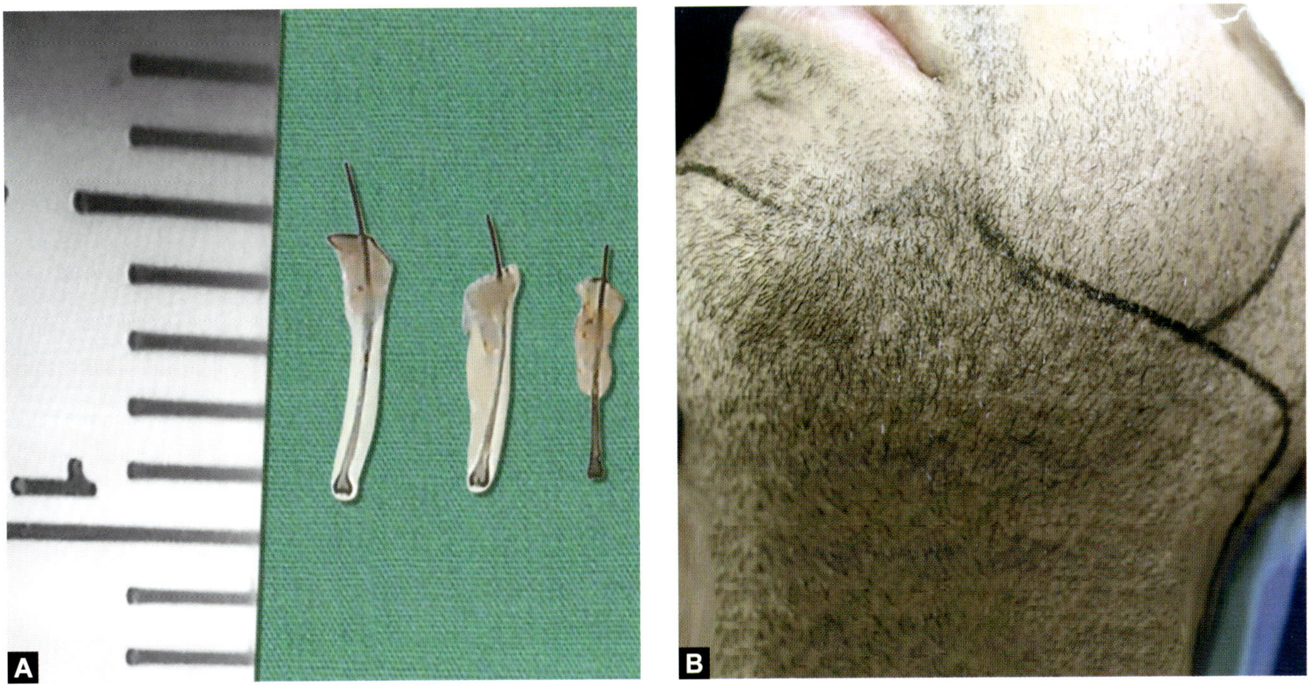

Figures 7.1A and B

(A) Varied length of beard hair in different areas of the beard; and (B) Demarcation of beard. Please note that we have gone above the jawline in this patient and have even included the side locks for extraction of grafts. Normally the extraction is done below the jawline in the shadow region of the face.
Courtesy: Dr Chiara Insalaco (Fig. 1A).

- Dyeing of the beard should be done if they are gray to ensure correct loading into the implanter and to avoid implanting the grafts upside down.
- Proper demarcation of beard should be done to separate "to be scored" dense region and sparse region. It is also done to avoid going beyond the planned areas of extraction which often happens due to the limited visual field of the loupe (Fig. 7.1B).
- Cleaning with antiseptic.

Anesthesia[2-4]

Ring block is given during anesthesia (Fig. 7.2). Giving anesthesia in beard is a relatively more painful process. Using vibrator to suppress the pain, giving alprazolam preoperatively or applying topical anesthetic (eutectic mixture of lidocaine and prilocaine) at least forty minutes before starting the extraction process can decrease the memory of painful beard extraction significantly. The vessels in the neck should be kept in mind while injecting local anesthesia; one should inject slowly to minimize the pain.

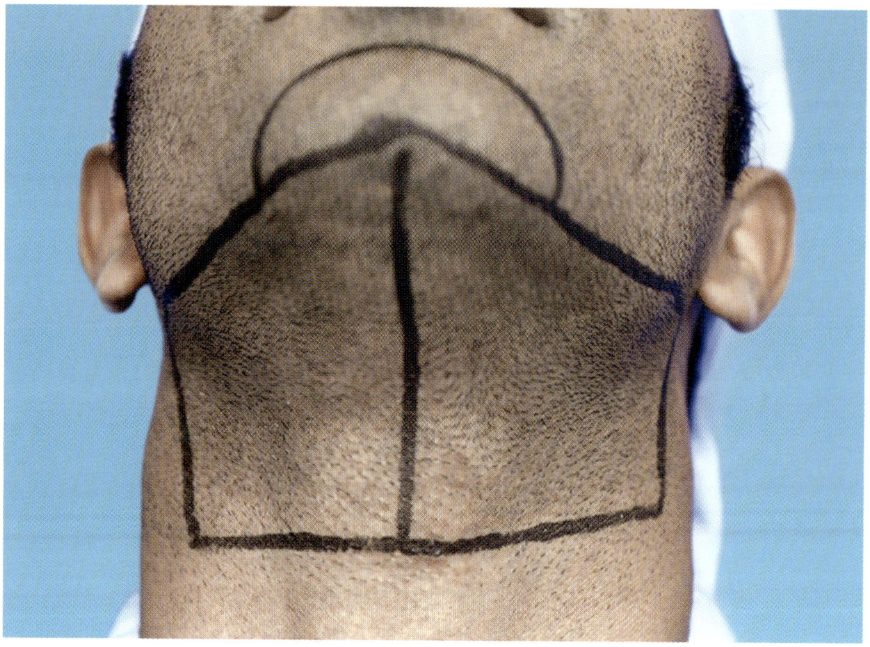

Figure 7.2

Design of ring block for beard anesthesia and demarcation of the "to be harvested zone". This patient's beard was harvested in the past as well.

Infiltration anesthesia with anesthetic mixture of 1% lidocaine with adrenaline (1:100,000) can be used, after defining the donor area in the body. Tumescence mixture used is with 30 ml normal saline with 0.25 ml adrenaline (1:2,000,000) to achieve the necessary tissue turgor. Beard hair grows over thicker soft tissue with no bony prominences underneath as compared to scalp hair; hence more tumescence may be required to produce adequate tissue turgor. The tumescence disperses very rapidly in the soft tissue. It is more important for the assistant to stretch the skin of the neck and face in the opposite direction for proper scoring of grafts. Use of tumescent anesthesia helps in harvesting from a larger body area without exceeding the permissible limit. Some surgeons also use bupivacaine due to its longer duration of action. While adverse reactions with bupivacaine are rare, at higher dosages or if accidentally injected in blood vessels it has the potential to cause ventricular tachycardia or fibrillation, which may be refractory to treatment.

Scoring of Grafts

A proper stretching of skin by the assistant or the surgeon is needed for accurate scoring of grafts. Position of patient in beard extraction is left lateral decubitus, right lateral decubitus, and supine with neck hyperextended (Fig. 7.3A).

I have felt that scoring of beard grafts is easier than scalp grafts with sharp serrated punches especially in chin region. The grafts in the chin region are aligned at obtuse angles and easily extractable. It is important to score only the anagen hair which can be identified by the epidermal blush when viewed under 4X to 5X magnification. The punch should be centered on this epidermal blush and not the hair. The curl of the hair should be ignored in beard grafts.

Efforts should be made to score as deep as possible when the grafts are longer as beard grafts are comparatively more fragile compared to scalp grafts. Scoring angles are extremely acute and there is variation in direction of beard in lower part of neck from one region to other. There may be presence of whorls in beard. Capability of surgeon to extract such grafts is an important factor. A gentle jerk with forester is all that is needed for extraction in the chin and jawline, but more force is required in other areas of the neck, hence thin beard grafts should be scored deep to minimize the extraction force. Rarely there are multiple hair in beard grafts which if handled carefully will grow.

Selecting the right punch size and ensuring the sharpness of punch for beard extraction is critical. The beard grafts are more prone to desiccation and ischemia. A blunt punch will cause abrasion of the skin surface and graft burial due to continuously changing direction of beard hair. The blunt punch will abrade the skin before hitting the surface with full force. One should be cautious while extracting from a beard whorl where direction of each beard keeps changing. Secondly the beard contains much lesser fat compared to scalp graft thus they are prone to damage by heat and poor graft handling. Selecting a slightly bigger punch is beneficial. We have observed that punches ranging from size 0.75 mm to 0.9 mm leave almost invisible scars. We prefer to use a slightly larger punch size of 0.8 mm to ensure good graft survival on scalp. A special caution is needed in dark skinned patients who are planned for beard extraction.

Retaining the Beard Aesthetics

Maintaining beard aesthetics is another challenge as patients want to give beard for hair transplant, but still want to retain at least 50% of the beard without any significant scar in the beard region or patchy hair loss.

One should always demarcate the extraction zone from the nonextraction zone. The extraction at the jawline should be nonlinear, alternate in a zig-zag or undulating pattern to prevent the emergence of demarcation line (Fig. 7.3B).

Maximum extraction can be done from the chin region below the lower lip, it contains the highest density of beard with grafts of maximum caliber, thus having the highest chance of survival. Almost 100% of the beard can be extracted in the lower part of the neck but one should assess its quality before going ahead with the extraction process as they are thinner and fragile compared to other grafts.

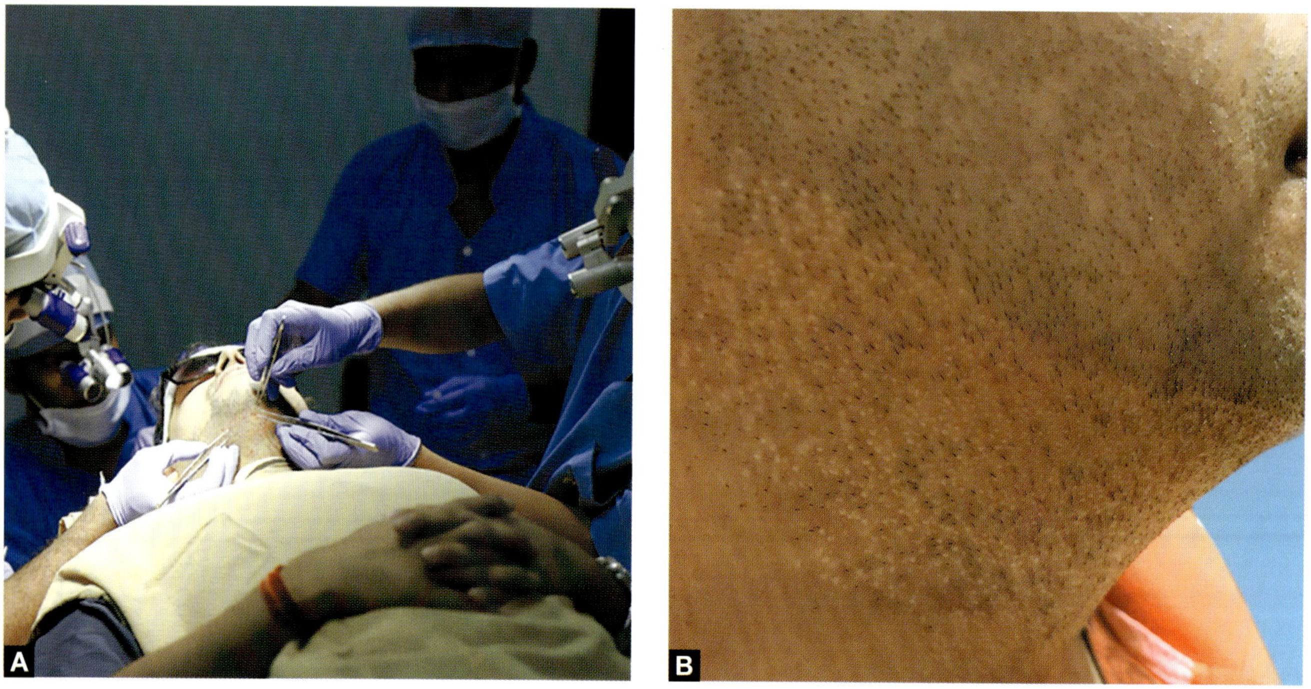

Figures 7.3A and B

(A) Position of patient during scoring of grafts and the extraction process. Most of the grafts at the jawline and chin can be extracted with single forcep if scoring of grafts is proper; and (B) The straight line which demarcates the extracted zone from the non-extracted zone is well evident. One should be careful while extracting above the jawline as it is the visible part of face. The area below the jawline comes in the shadow area. Note the development of linear hypopigmented scars which has developed due to continuous extraction in the beard by sharp serrated follicular unit excision (FUE) punch. One cannot predict the development of hypopigmented scars in the beard. The extraction should be noncontinuous in a zig-zag or slightly undulating pattern above the jawline.

Noncontinuous extraction should be done below the jawline keeping in mind the aesthetics of beard region (Figs. 7.4 to 7.6). Extraction from posterior part of the side-burns can be done. *Side-burns, being a transition zone from scalp to beard have characteristics of both scalp and beard* (Figs. 7.7A to C). Grafts on side-burns on clinical examination look like beard grafts but when they grow they look similar to the scalp hair.

Punch size and sharpness of punch is critical in beard as they contain little fat. A blunt punch may generate too much heat resulting in damage of the graft. Effort should be made to extract beard which are in anagen phase. They are darker in color and are thicker compared to their telogen counterpart.

A beard can be curly, wavy or straight. A curly beard needs a slightly larger punch size of 0.8–0.9 mm to avoid follicular transections. A straight or wavy beard can be managed with 0.75–0.8 mm punch; however adequate fat should surround the beard to ensure regrowth at the recipient site.

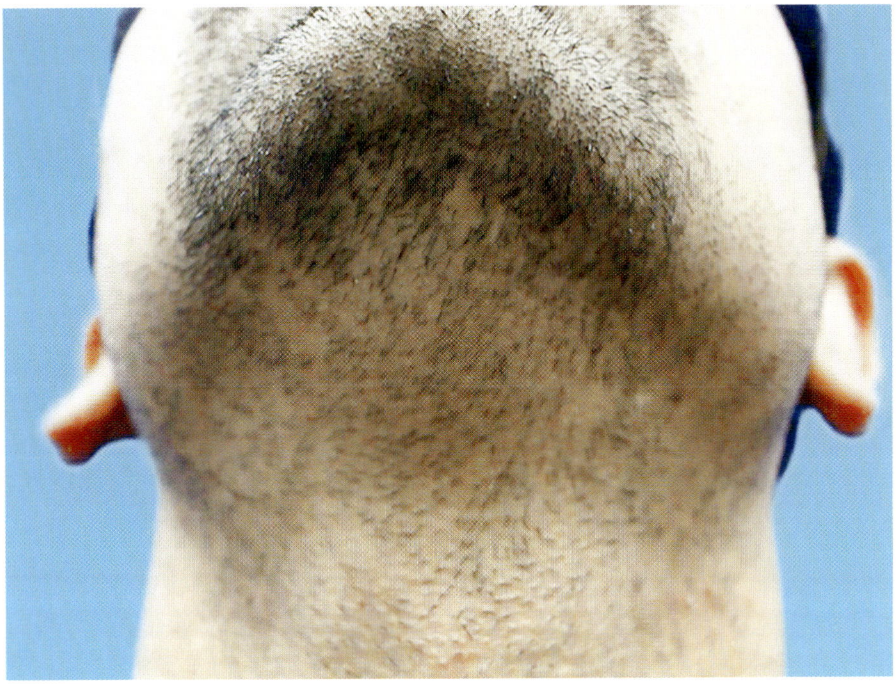

Figure 7.4

Sparse beard with good density in the chin region. We had already extracted 1,000 grafts from the beard in the previous surgery. Complete and continuous extraction can be done in the lower part of the neck. Area below the chin region was already sparse and patient was ready to sacrifice the full beard in the shadow region of the neck, so complete extraction was done below the jawline with a 0.8 mm sharp and serrated punch. In the previous surgery the extraction was made with a 0.9 mm blunt punch.

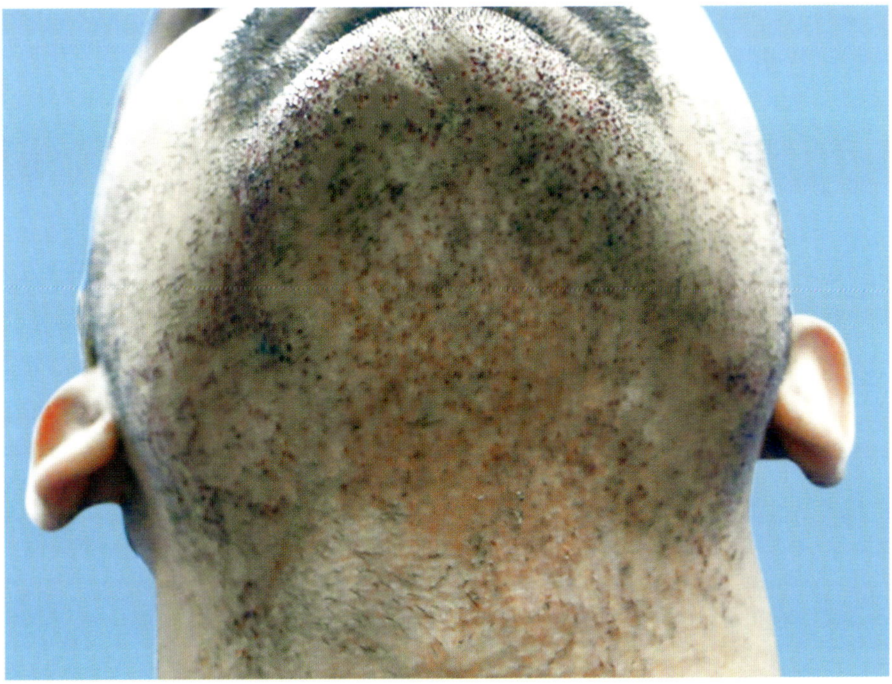

Figure 7.5

The immediate postoperative picture. The red dots show the site where extraction has been carried out. We extracted extensively keeping in mind the symmetry and the variable density of beard at various sites.

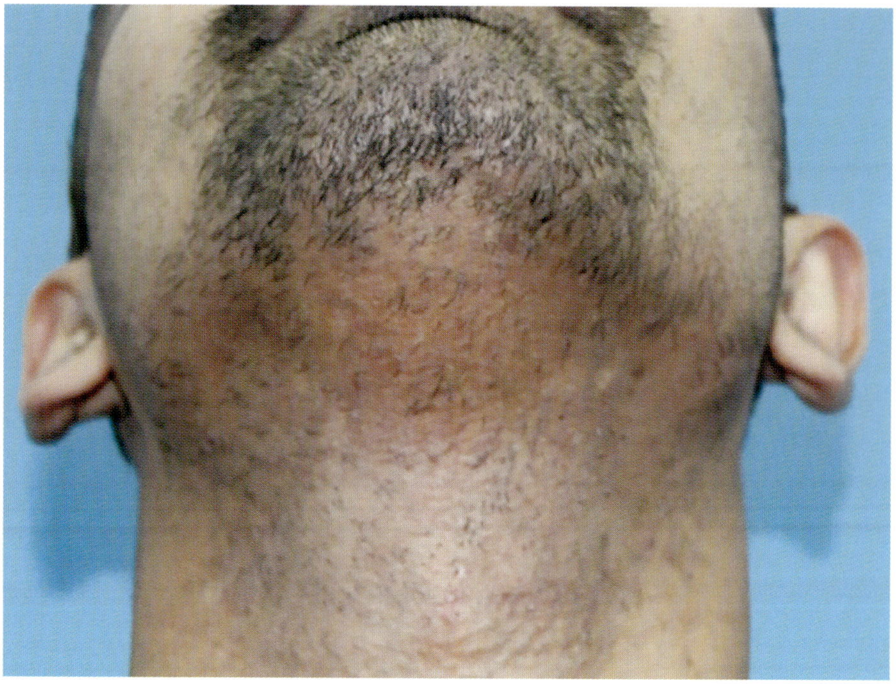

Figure 7.6

Depiction of the same regions 7 days after extraction. Note the absence of any significant scar, uniform spread of the sparse beard after the extraction and absence of demarcation line. A total of 2,000 grafts have been extracted from this beard in two sessions. Thus, this case is a case of over-extraction from beard. The patient does not wish to keep any beard in future.

Complications of Taking Beard as a Donor

The most common complication is postinflammatory hyper- or hypopigmentation. Which can be minimized by using the sharpest and smallest possible punch. Hypopigmentation cannot be predicted even after using the best suited punch. We have seen that hyperpigmentation fades over time with use of topical depigmenting creams and sunscreen.

Another complication is development of linear scars due to continuous punching (Fig. 7.2). Another common complication is due to over extraction from one site leading to development of alopecia areata like patches.

Due to excessive injection of tumescence and local anesthesia, there is temporary paresis of facial muscles. It happens because the motor marginal mandibular nerve passes along the jawline and is compressed due to excessive fluid injected in that region (Fig. 7.8).

We have observed that in certain cases that, scalp hair grow while beard hair fails to grow leading to poor density in the recipient sites.

CASE STUDY 1

We conducted a mega session of extraction of 7,000 grafts over 2 days. We had to extract around 3,000 grafts from the beard. We present this case to demonstrate how beard aesthetic is retained even after extracting 3,000 grafts (Figs. 7.9A to F).

The results after 7 days.

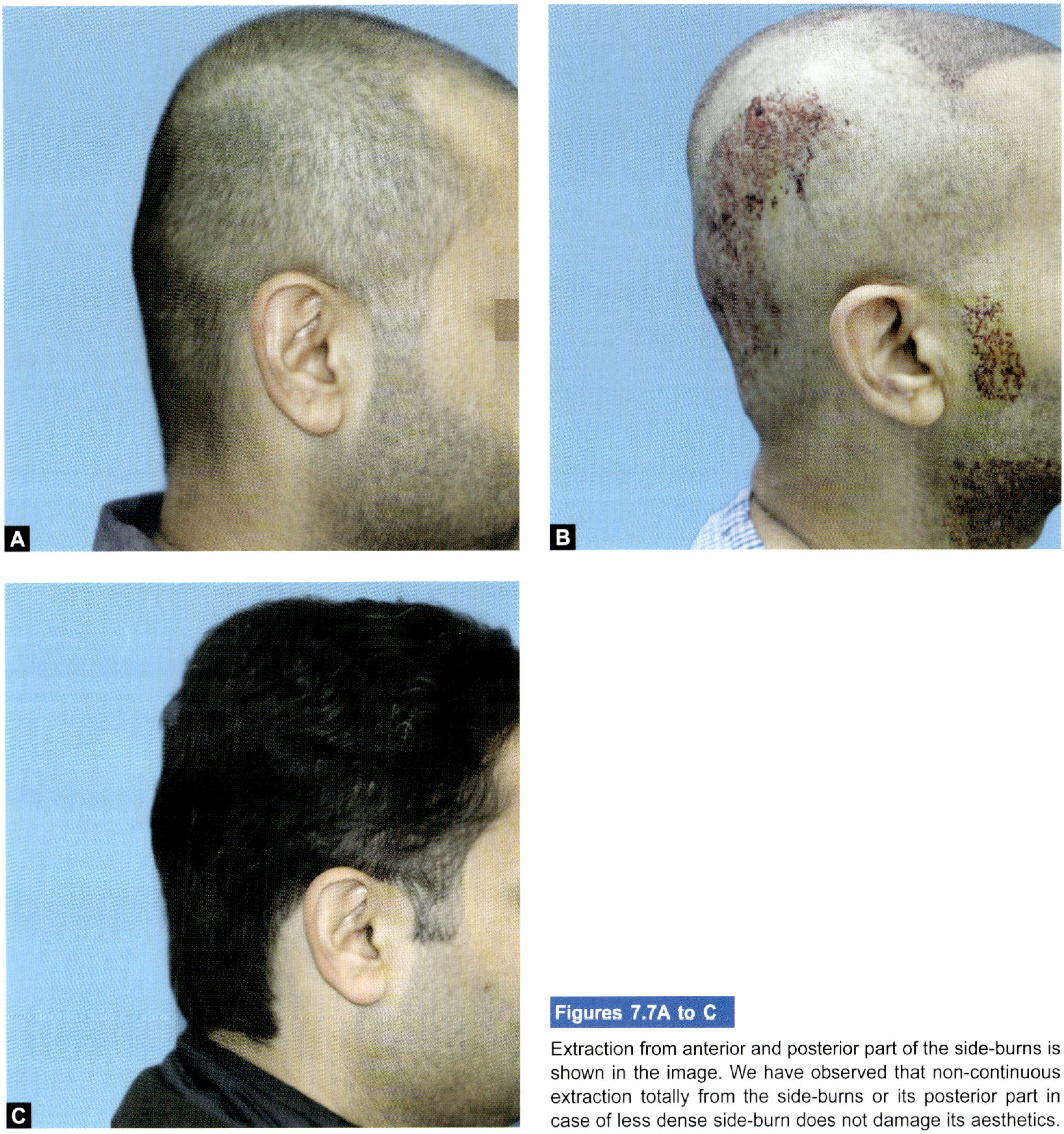

Figures 7.7A to C

Extraction from anterior and posterior part of the side-burns is shown in the image. We have observed that non-continuous extraction totally from the side-burns or its posterior part in case of less dense side-burn does not damage its aesthetics.

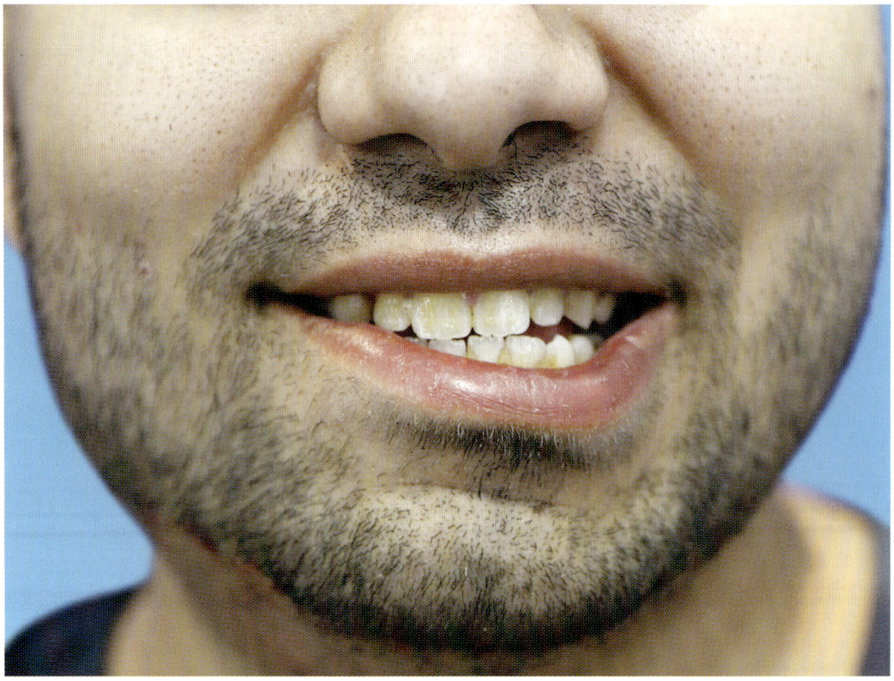

Figure 7.8

Facial paresis due to injection of anesthesia and tumescence.

CASE STUDY 2 (FIGS. 7.10A AND B) AND CASE STUDY 3 (FIGS. 7.10C AND D)

Chest Hair Extraction

Extracting chest hair is tough. They have high transection rates as grafts are at extremely acute angles. The extraction should be periareolar. The middle one-third of the chest should not be punched as there is tendency to form hypertrophic scars. Chest with dense hair growth and people who shave their chest regularly are preferred for chest hair extraction. Chest should be shaved 7–10 days before surgery to select only anagen hair (Figs. 7.11A to D).

Comments by Dr Chiara Insalaca

Beard is an important resource of hair. There are particular cases where we need the help of body hair to perform our hair restoration. The main reasons are the following: poor donor area; run out donor area due to previous hair restorations; we can use beard hair to treat and cover strip scars; and when the recipient area exceeds the donor area. The advantages of beard hair are that they are thicker and wavier than scalp hair, so they can give more coverage to the bald area. At the same time, because of their different nature it is better to use them from the mid-scalp up to the crown. A hairline could look fake and unnatural, so it is always better to use scalp hair for it. Recently, I studied the beard characteristics of some patients.

My study shows:

- Average number of hair per graft (calculated density) = 1
- Average follicular unit density (number of follicles per cm^2) = 65
    - Average hair density (number of hair per cm^2) = 70
- In conclusion the beard is the best body hair source to use in those cases where the body hair is not enough.

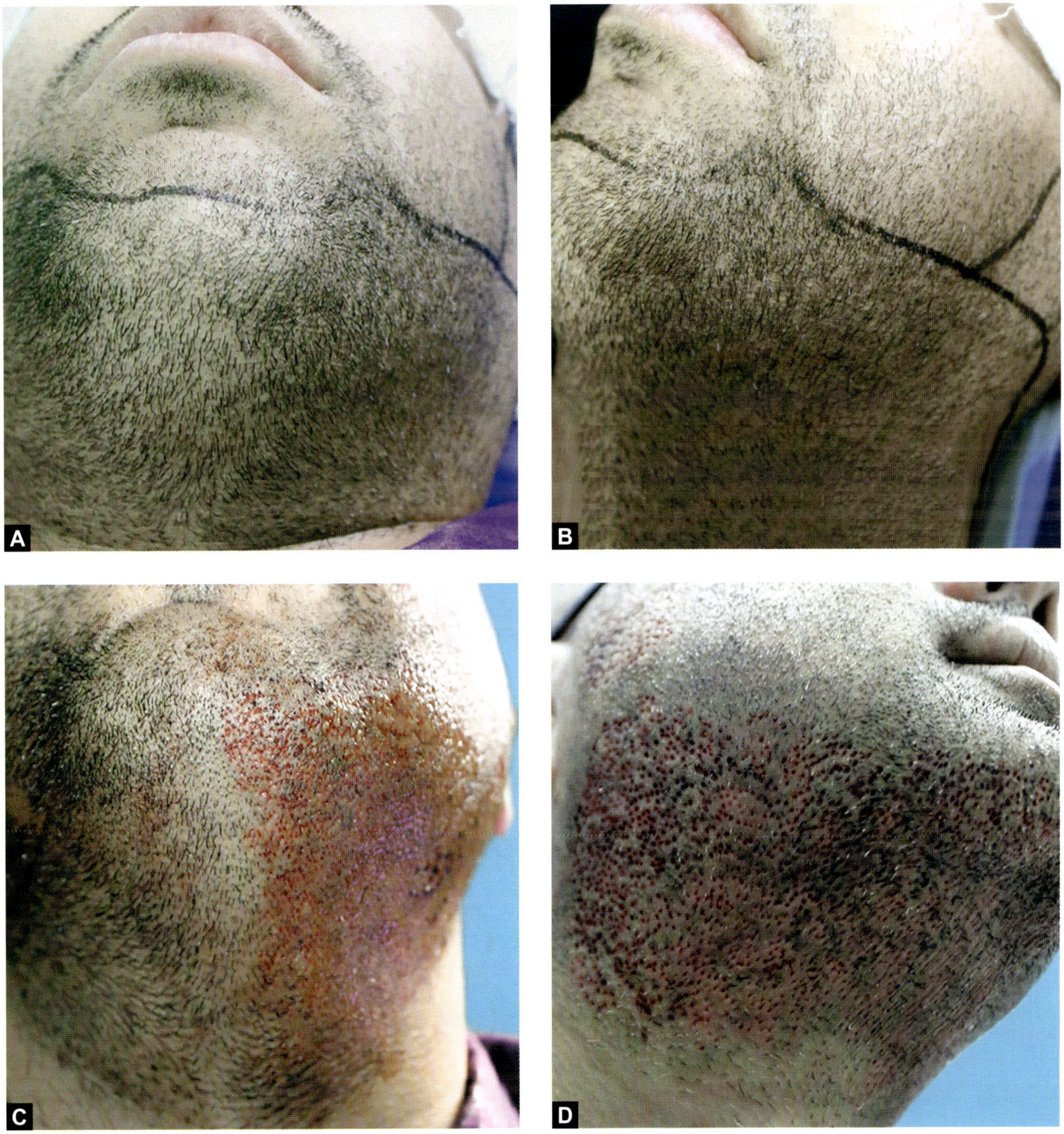

Figures 7.9A to D

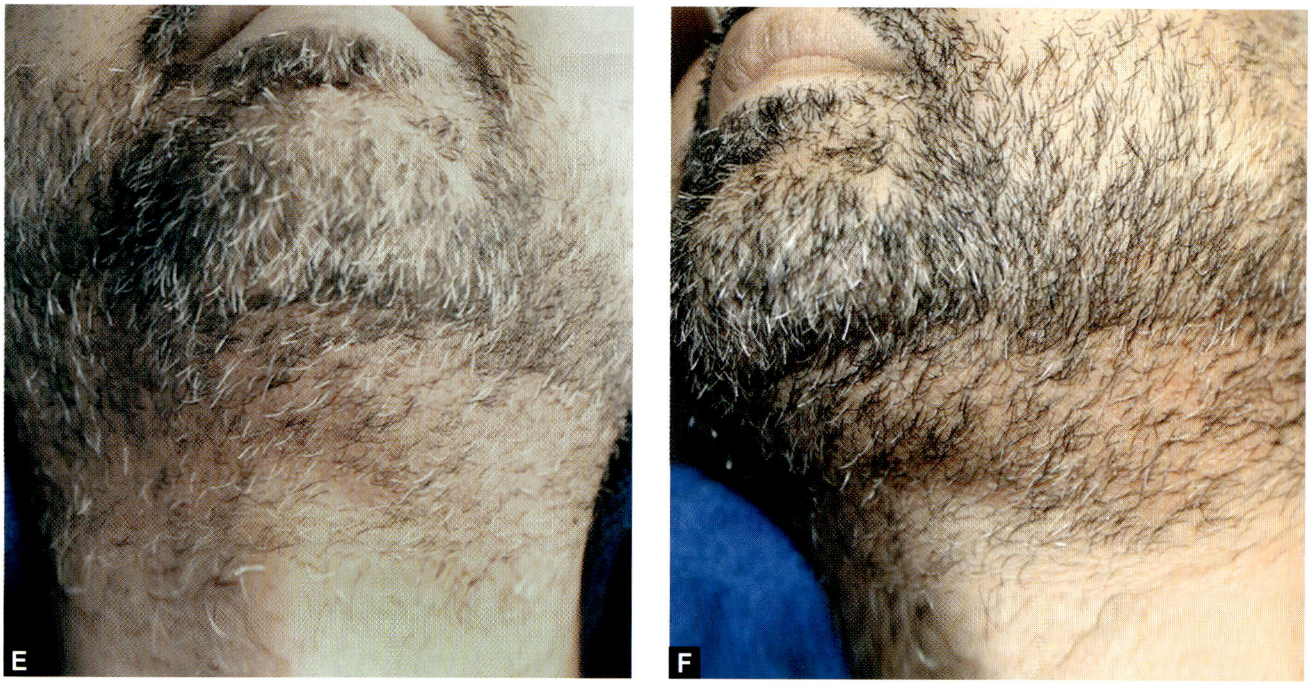

Figures 7.9E and F

Figures 7.9A to F

(A) Demonstration of a very dense beard where extraction of more than 3,000–4,000 grafts is possible. We planned to extract 3,000 grafts over a period of 2 days; (B) We even planned to extract 200 grafts from each of the side locks. We went above the jawline for beard extraction in this patient. We clearly demarcated dense beard zones from the non-dense beard zones; (C) On day 1: we extracted from the left half of the beard using a 0.8 mm serrated sharp punch. We went above the jawline only in areas where density was high to maintain the symmetry in beard density; (D) Note the close noncontinuous extraction which we did in this patient. It may look scary at present, but we took sufficient caution. Our punching density was high in areas with higher beard density and low in areas of low density; (E) Postoperative picture of the same beard on day 7. Things to note in this picture are the absence of patchy hair loss, uniform beard density below the jawline and absence of any visible beard scar following punching; and (F) Demonstration of the jawline where density of beard has uniformly reduced. There is no demarcation line separating the dense extracted zone from the nonextracted zone. There is absence of any redness. Even after extracting closely, there is absence of any patchy loss of hair.

Comments by Dr Arvind Poswal

Being the inventor of beard hair to scalp hair transplant, there is no standard number of extracting grafts. We had patients from Orientals, from Koreans who hardly have 100-200 hair in total.

On the other hand, we have used about 6,873 FU beard hair grafts from a patient of German descend—patient nicknamed Argentine underwent 11,460 FUSE grafts procedure in year 2008 (using 2,000 scalp, 6,873 beard including 207 moustache grafts, 2,285 truncal and 302 armpit donor grafts) (Figs. 7.12A and B).[5]

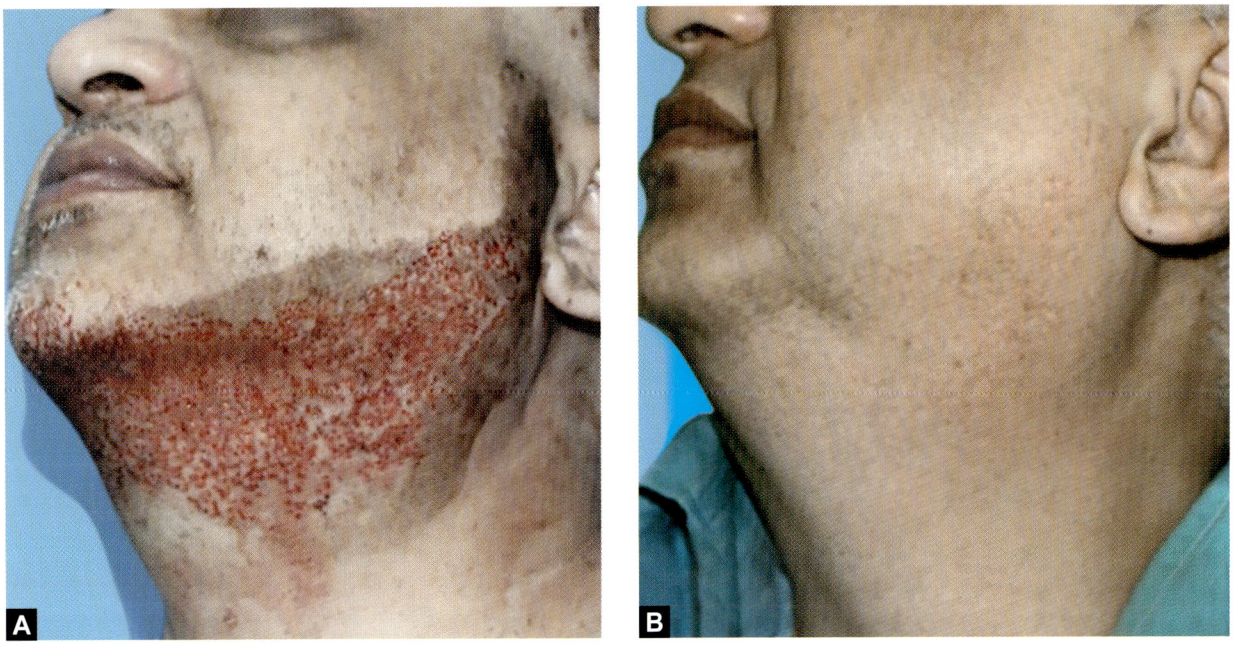

Figures 7.10A and B

The dreadful postoperative photograph of a patient of Norwood grade 7 patient where we extracted 3,210 beard grafts with 0.8 mm sharp serrated punch. The photographs below it are after 6 months of hair transplant. It may seem a case of over extraction to lot of surgeons but patient did not wished to keep beard in future and it was impossible to give full coverage in this Norwood grade 7 patient in single sitting.

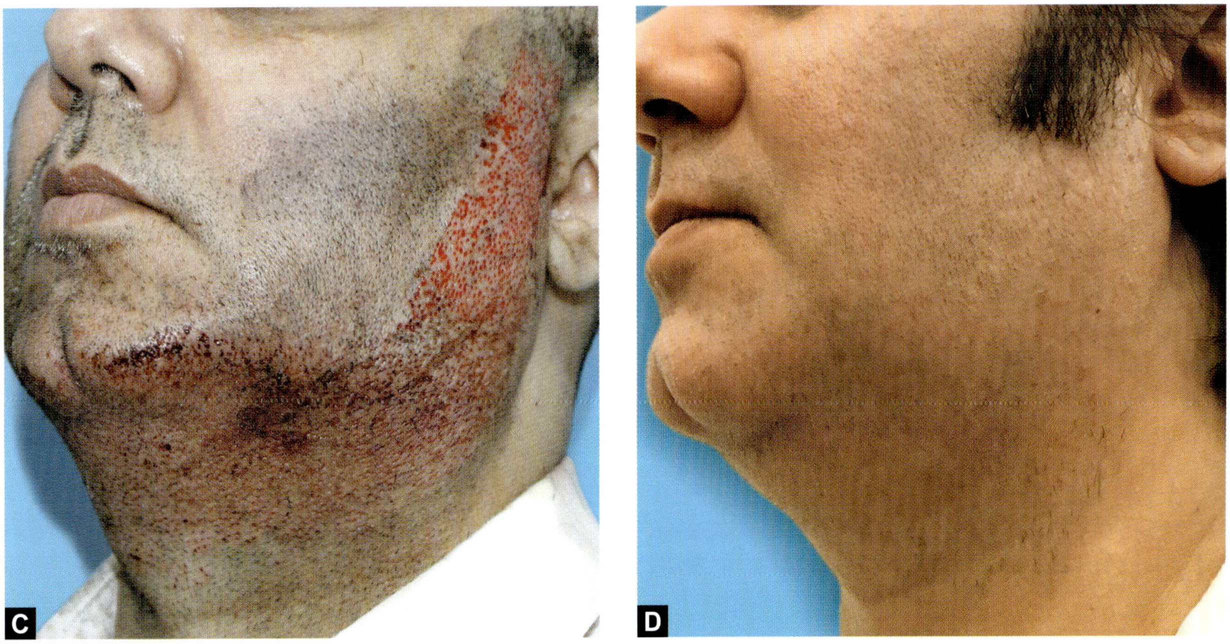

Figures 7.10C and D

Immediate postoperative and 6-months postoperative photograph of a beard region of a patient with compromised scalp donor due to previous failed hair transplant. A total of 3300 grafts from beard and side-burns were extracted. The postoperative photograph after 9-month shows visibly no scar even after attempting 100% beard extraction.

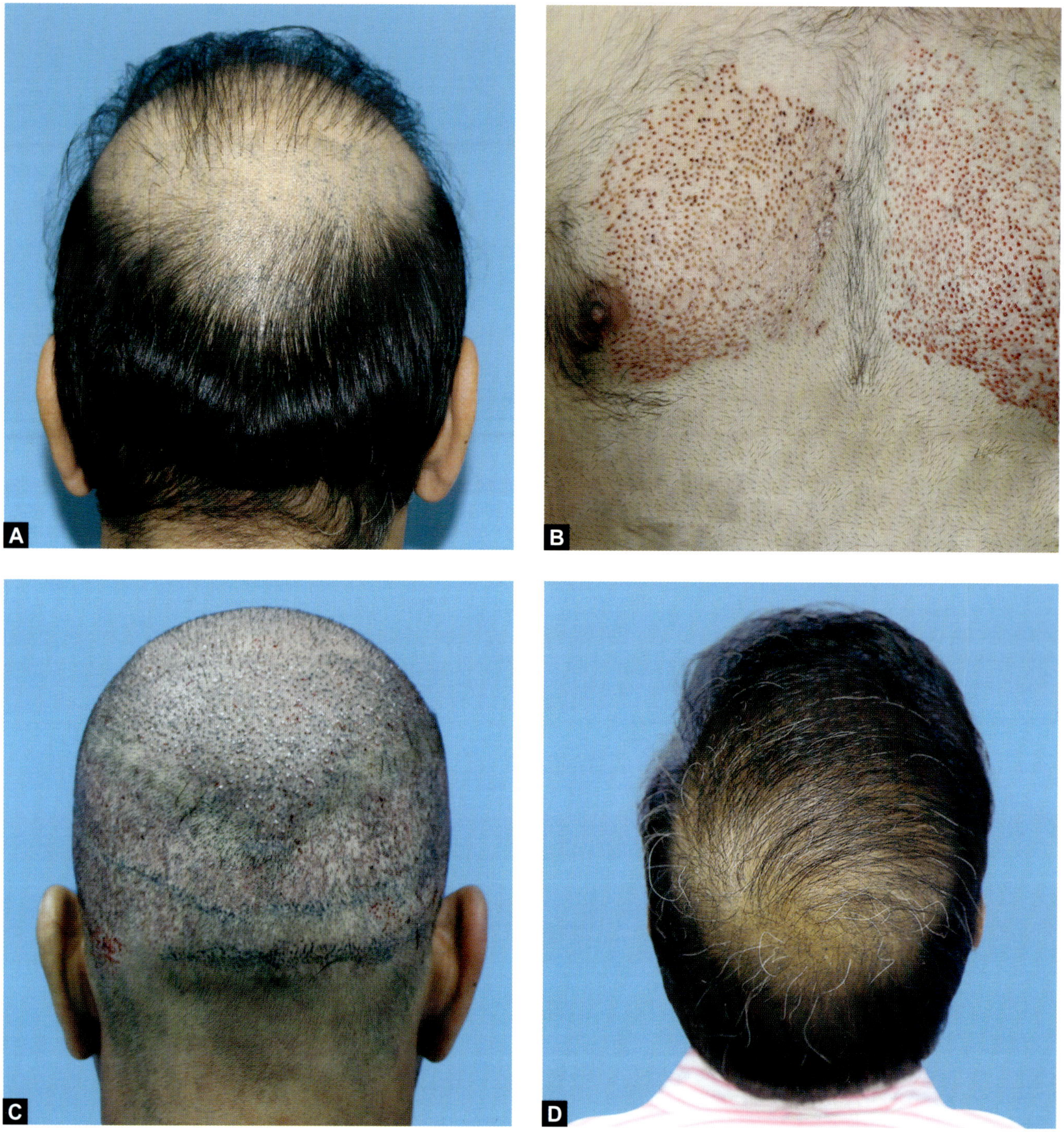

Figures 7.11A to D

Series of images to show a case where we took extensively from chest (2000 grafts) due to depleted scalp donor (two FUT and one FUE). We implanted chest grafts in the crown and the hump. The remaining part of the scalp was implanted with predominantly beard graft (3500 beard grafts) and only 800 scalp grafts. Only 50–60% of the chest grafts have grown as shown in the image with good growth in rest of the scalp.

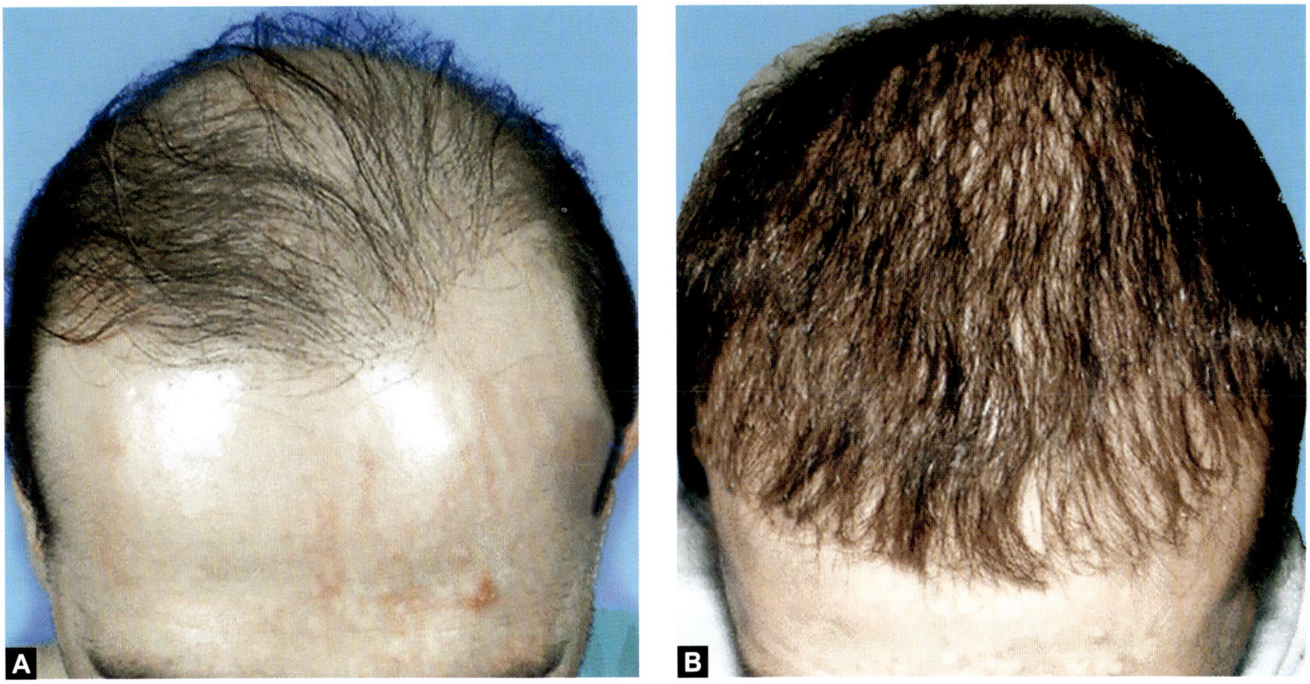

Figures 7.12A and B

The patient underwent 11,460 FUSE grafts procedure in year 2008 (using 2,000 scalp, 6,873 beard including 207 moustache grafts, 2,285 truncal and 302 armpit donor grafts).

View worldwide discussion on online consumer forum: http://www.hairsite.com/hair-loss/board_entry-id-53760-page-45-category-2-order-last_answer-descasc-DESC.html

I agree with the author, that the beard grafts being thicker in diameter should not be used in the front few rows of hairline. But we have also come across patients whose beard hair is almost similar to scalp and after transplant it has given them a thicker, fuller look. So, it is necessary to evaluate.

Being the inventor of body hair to scalp transplant Dr Arvind Poswal has formulated the guidelines of BHHT (body hair to head transplant).

These guidelines are based on our follow-up observations in patients:[6]

- Preshave the body donor areas 3–5 days before the extraction. It is a simple step and very helpful to pinpoint the actively growing hair that need to be used.
- Use only the body donor hair in active growing phase for purpose of transplant. Do not use telogen hair.

- Assume the transplanted body hair will retain their original characteristics (length, caliber, color, predisposition to graying, curl, anagen/telogen percentages, and hair growth cycles).
- Factor in the impact of growth cycles and characteristics of the body donor hair proposed to be transplanted.
- Mix the various body as well as scalp donor hair in any particular area of scalp.

Comments by Dr Anil Garg

Beard is a good source of donor hair follicles if they are present and patients give consent for it. The density of beard hair varies from person to person. The growth of beard hair is dependent on androgen which is an advantage in androgenetic alopecia. It is not necessary that every individual we can harvest 5,000 hair follicles. In the present era of the body, image youngster likes to have a beard and many of them come for reconstruction of beard.

Advantages are they are thicker in caliber as compare to the scalp and often curly. This characteristic of beard hair gives more visual density when implanted.

We need to extract beard from the shadow area.

On the day of extraction, beard hair length shall be 2 mm and if white then dye them. Beard hair shall be shaved 3–4 days before the day of hair transplant for easy identification of anagen hair.

Tumescence anesthesia is preferred over regional and or ring block. It is advisable to use local prilocaine gel application before 1 hour and then tumescence anesthesia. Injection midazolam or oral sedation also help.

During extraction, select anagen hair, the epidermal blush is a diagnostic sign of anagen hair.

The depth of scoring is just 2–3 mm is enough as you score the beard grafts pops out easily. Extraction either by a single step or two step may be required if they are adherent. Forced extraction may lead to extraction of only hair shaft leaving behind rest of follicle which may give cyst or folliculitis.

Extraction rules are same as of scalp FUE. Every third or fourth hair follicles should be extracted. Overharvesting should be avoided (pictures shown here are of overharvesting which in any case should not be done).

The facial nerve, facial artery, and carotid artery should be kept in mind during extraction of beard.

Beard hair follicles are delicate and more sensitive to ischemia. It is preferable that graft out body time shall be minimal and no touch to root or use of implanters is preferred.

Hypopigmentation, folliculitis and cyst formation, facial paralysis may be as a complication of beard hair follicle harvesting. It is better we explain to the patient the above possible complications during surgery. All precaution should be taken to minimize or prevent side effect.

It is strongly advisable that in any area beard hair shall not be implanted alone. These hair follicles shall always be mixed with scalp hair follicles.

Chest hair follicles extraction is more demanding technically because their exit angle is acuter and lies in more fatty tissue. Only 20% chest hair are in anagen phase. To select anagen hair follicles for extraction advise shaving of chest 7–10 days prior to extraction.

Dr Robert True has given hair density index for selection of patients for chest hair follicles extraction.

Thickness, density and length are parameters to decide for suitability of chest hair follicles extraction.

Use of prilocaine gel and tumescence anesthesia with sedation, small bore needle, ice pack, and vibrator can effectively control the pain of infiltration of anesthetic agent.

Comments by Dr Hyun-Wook Baik

I experienced that beard is very good donor area with very few scar problems than every doctor is worrying. This is the best review about body hair transplant I have ever seen. I hope that lots of doctors stop under correcting recipient area by using body hair and give more happiness to patients by reading this review.

SUMMARY

- Beard is a good reserve of large number of grafts and considered the second best source after scalp grafts.
- It can be safely implanted 2 cm behind hairline with intelligent mixing thereafter is key.
- Special care is needs to be taken while administrating anesthesia due to presence of numerous vessels in neck.
- Pain during anesthesia is a major concern. Soft hands and skilful hands are of prime importance.
- Use of tumescent and more importantly stretching of skin by an assistant is required for efficient graft extraction.
- Use of sharp, serrounded punch of the right size is critical to score grafts. Blunt punch can give rise to ugly scar.
- The healing of beard is extremely fast after surgery.

REFERENCES

1. Saxena K, Savant SS. Body to scalp: evolving trends in body hair transplantation. Indian Dermatol Online J. 2017;8(3):167-75.
2. Nurein H, Mohanty S. Anesthesia in FUE. In: Saxena K, Saxena D (Eds). FUE Hair Restoration Major Procedures Minor Incisions. Mumbai, India: Cosmazone Pvt Ltd; 2012. 47-52.
3. Behroozan DS, Goldberg LH. Dermal tumescent local anesthesia in cutaneous surgery. J Am Acad Dermatol. 2005;53:828-30.
4. Mysore V. Body hair transplantation: case report of successful outcome. J Cutan Aesthet Surg. 2013;6:113-6.
5. Dr. A's. (2016). Sub Gallery Argentine. [online] Available from http://fusehair.com/portfolio-posts/sub-gallery-argentine/. [Accessed April, 2018].
6. Dr. A's. (2016). Body Hair Transplants (FUSE). [online] Available from http://fusehair.com/body-hair-transplants-fuse/. [Accessed April, 2018].

CHAPTER 8

Art and Science of Scoring of Grafts

Abhinav Kumar, Arika Bansal

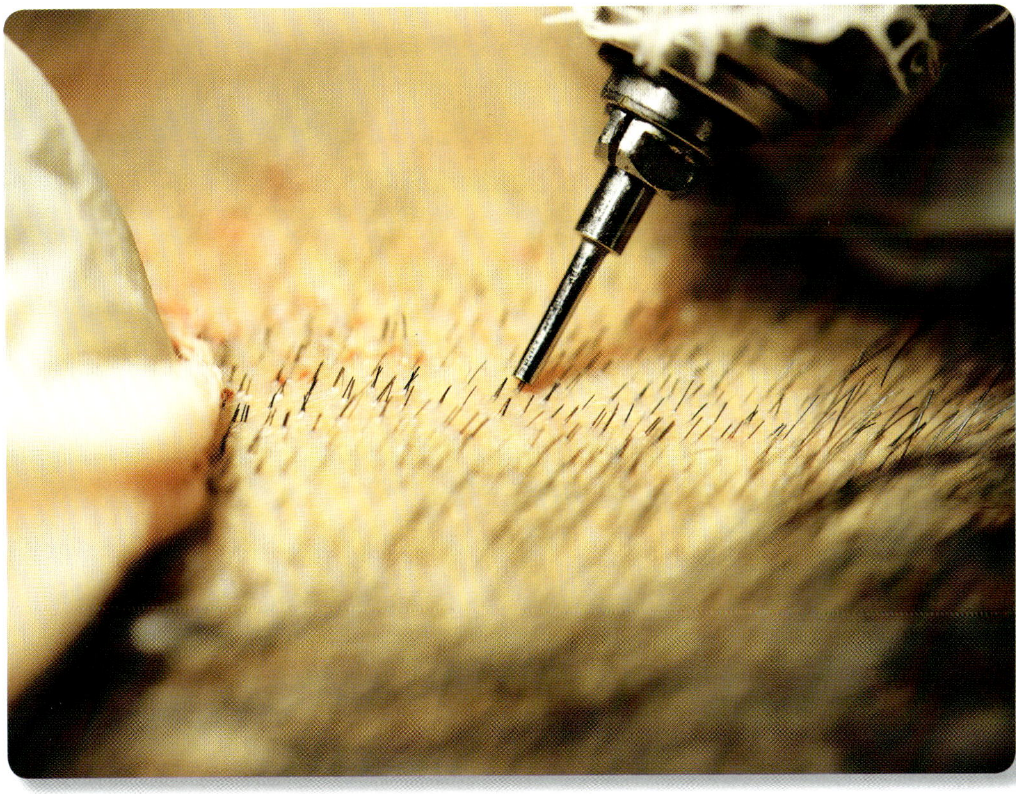

Mankind has evolved from Stone Age to 21st century with the help of instruments! The thinking and creative minds of physicians and scientists all across the world aim to maximize the procedure in terms of providing comprehensive results of aesthetically acceptable complete coverage of the bald area, adequate density and long lasting results and without damaging the donor cosmesis. This is only possible by choosing right kind of updated instruments.

INTRODUCTION

Scoring of grafts is the key to successful hair restoration surgery by follicular unit excision earlier called follicular unit extraction (FUE) or direct hair transplantation (DHT). We briefly outline the steps of successful and optimum extraction from scalp during FUE surgery.

DONOR EVALUATION

Donor area should be evaluated at the time of preoperative workup. The surgeon should estimate the number of grafts, that he will be able to extract from scalp and beard and decide his approach accordingly. The total number of grafts which can be extracted from scalp and beard should be estimated. Presence of previous follicular unit transplantation (FUT) scar, traumatic scars and FUE scars, presence of seborrhea and presence of retrograde thinning, along with variation of density in different parts of the scalp should be noted (Figs. 8.1 to 8.3).

Secondly, the surgeon should clearly demarcate the safe donor zone from nonsafe areas by examination of the extent of baldness of the patient and his family members. There may be areas of full density in the lower part of the crown which have not started thinning yet but may thin in future (Fig. 8.4). Areas where scarring is present should be demarcated and extraction should not be done around the scar.

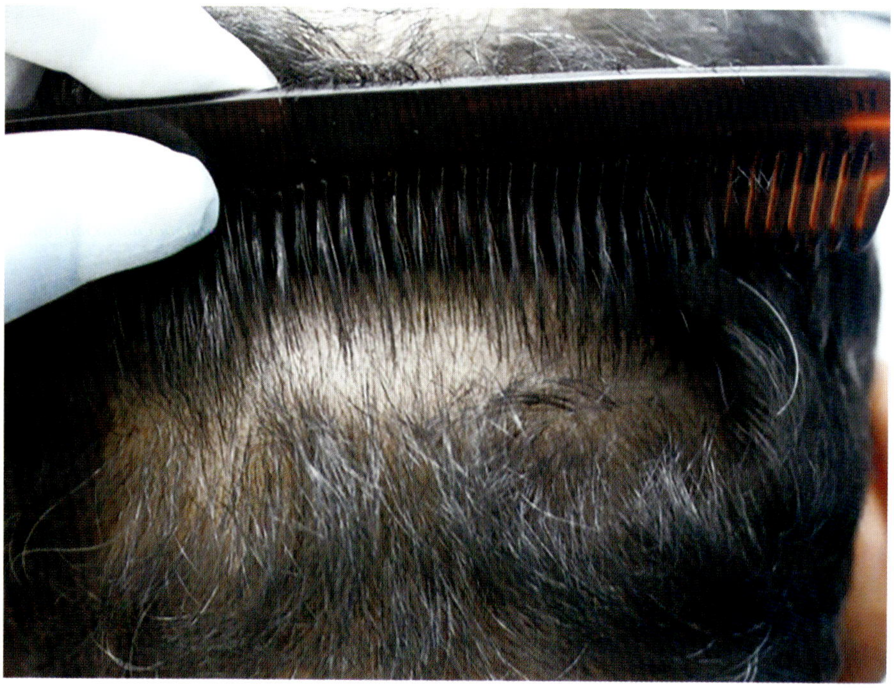

Figure 8.1

Donor assessment should be done to estimate the number of grafts which can be extracted from scalp and beard, which ultimately decides the position of hairline and density of slits to be made and area which can be covered on the scalp.

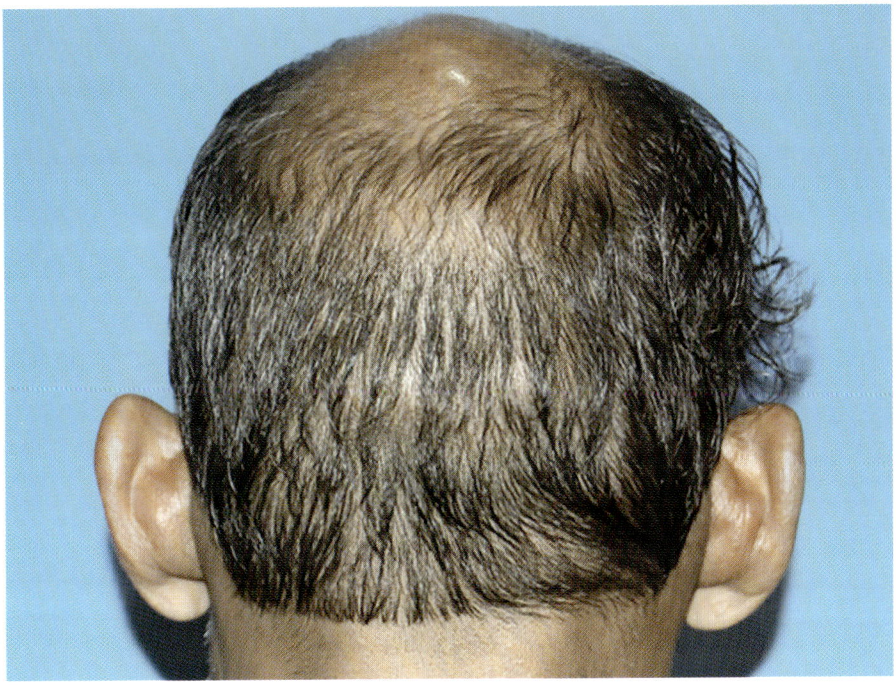

Figure 8.2

Depiction of a poor donor area. Note the "see through effect" in the center of occipital region over the occipital prominence compared to sides of the scalp. Such area should be clearly demarcated and extraction of around 1,500 grafts was possible maintaining the donor aesthetics in a single sitting in this patient.

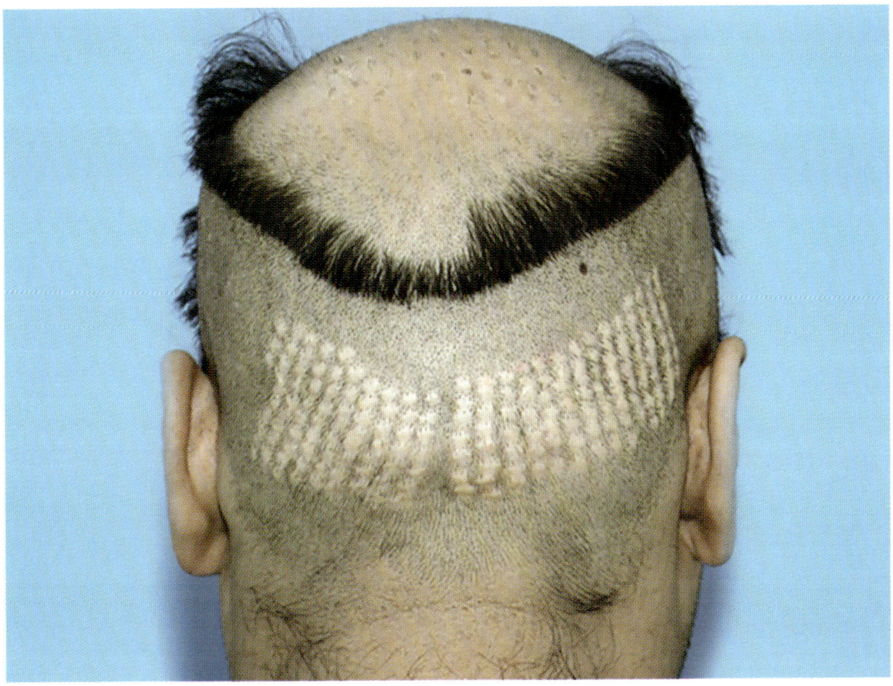

Figure 8.3

Presence of scars of punch grafting which was done long time back. Area between the punch scars should be spared for extraction of grafts to maintain donor aesthetics.

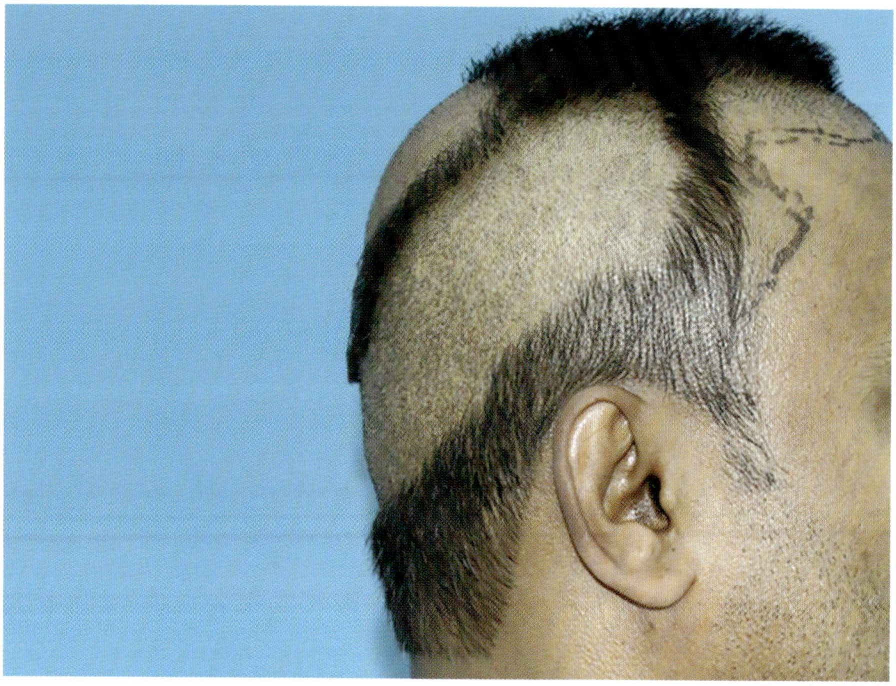

Figure 8.4

One should trim the patient in a scientific way before the surgery. This patient had come for second session of hair transplant on the crown, along with restoration of hairline. Note how the safe donor region is segregated from the unsafe zone by a rim of hair. Similarly the hair around the nape of the neck and just above the ear is spared as they were prone to retrograde thinning and had less density.

The areas where the surgeon notices retrograde thinning, i.e. thinning starting from the nape of the neck and progressing upward toward the vertex, should be avoided. The thinning is more prominent in the middle two-thirds of the posterior part of the scalp compared to lateral one-third (Figs. 8.5A to C).

After trimming of donor region, further evaluation should be done to assess the follicles under 4X to 5X magnification.

A donor scalp which may look voluminous without trimming may be having multiple follicle grafts present at distance or may be densely packed with closely grouped multiple follicle grafts. They may have only single or double follicle grafts with hair of higher caliber. There can be good density with hair of less caliber in donor scalp and poor density with hair of higher caliber.

TRIMMING

The length of hair should be 1.0–1.5 mm, just enough to notice the direction and angulations of hair under magnification after injection of tumescence.

Window trimming is usually done for those who opt for smaller surgery of up to 2,000 grafts or in females who usually need not more than 1,500 grafts for adequate

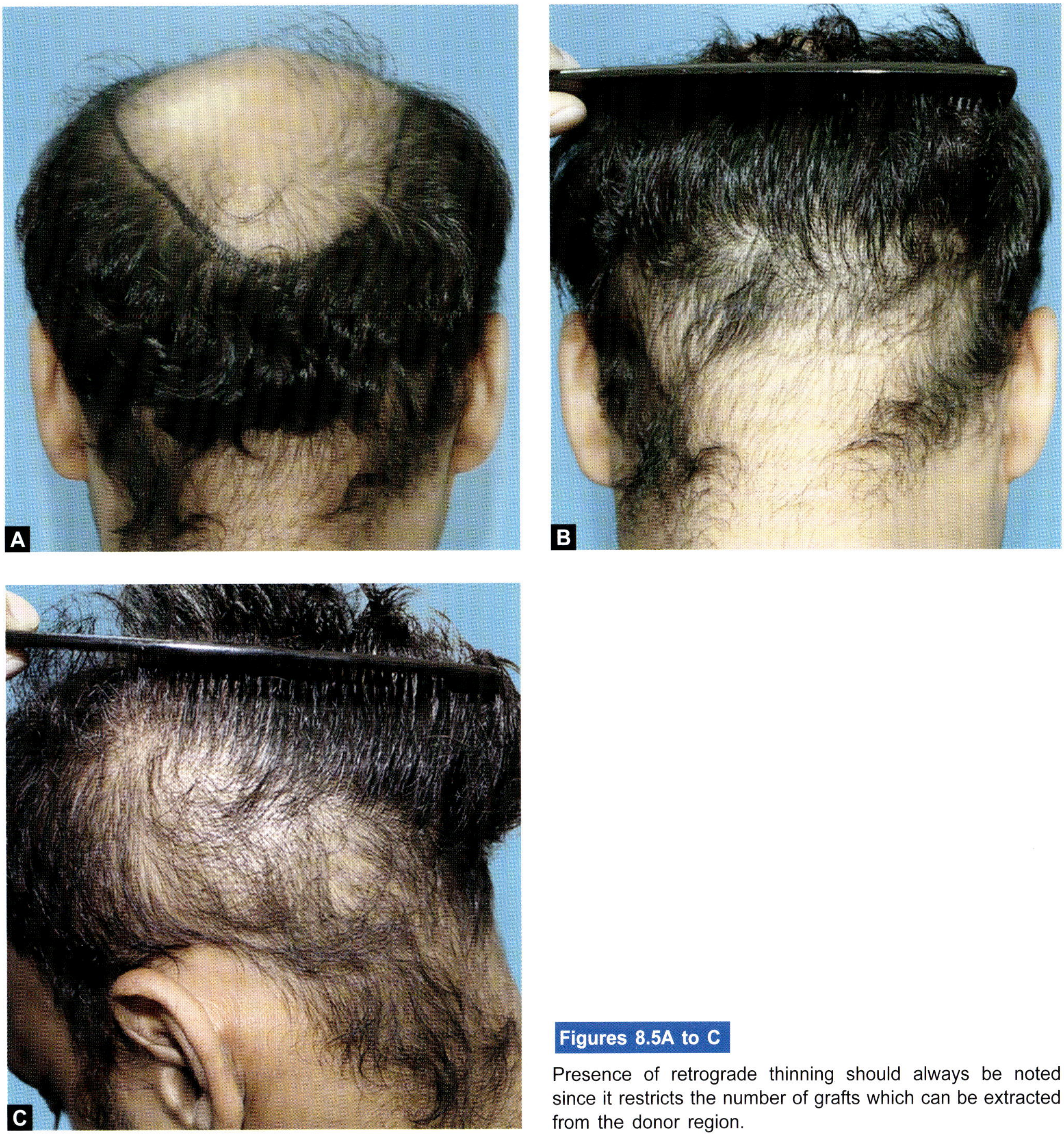

Figures 8.5A to C

Presence of retrograde thinning should always be noted since it restricts the number of grafts which can be extracted from the donor region.

camouflage of their female pattern hair loss. The males are advised to grow their hair long enough for avoiding appearance of bald patch from behind. The risk of over extraction with window trimming should always be kept in mind (Figs. 8.6 and 8.7).

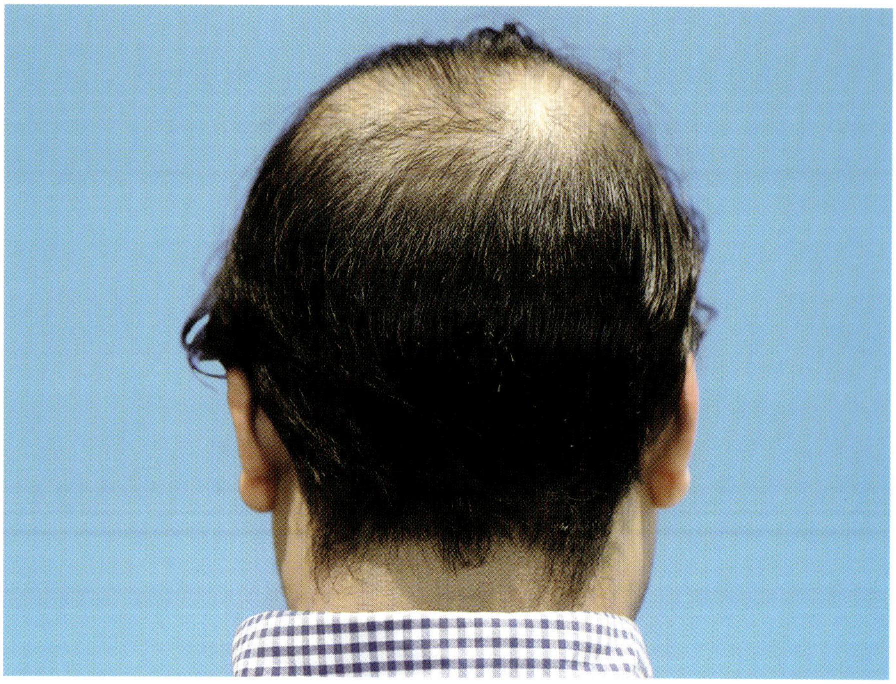

Figure 8.6

Demonstration of window trimmed patch which is covered by the long hair above it.

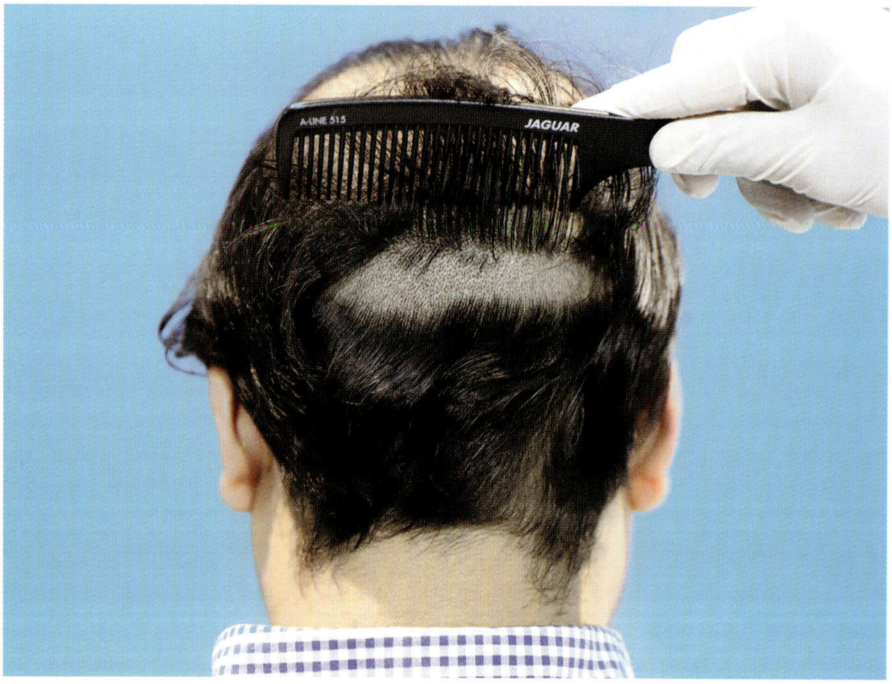

Figure 8.7

Window trimmed zone where direct hair transplantation has been done. Note there is always a risk of over extraction when such method is adopted. Care should be taken not to over extract from such area and extend or create another the window in case one falls short of grafts.

STERILIZATION AND ANESTHESIA

The scalp is cleaned with antiseptic scrub before the start of surgery. A repeat cleaning of the donor region with 7% povidone-iodine solution followed by its complete removal with normal saline is done. Anesthesia in the form of ring block is injected.

SCORING OF GRAFTS[1]

A smaller exit angle of the grafts potentially increases the trauma to the donor area because a punch directed at a steeper angle creates an elliptical wound that is significantly larger in area than a perpendicular punch is used for the same area.

As punch comes in contact with the skin and dissects through it and the dermis, the increased force of friction causes follicular displacement. This displacement of follicle increases the transection rates in hands of a new surgeon. This will increase the graft requirement by increasing the number of punch insertions needed to obtain target number of grafts thus hampering future FUE surgery (Fig. 8.8).

To increase the exit angle, 0.4 ml/cm^2 of normal saline needs to be injected to make the direction of hair follicle less acute to minimize transection rates. Even if we stretch the skin properly while scoring the grafts, there will be minimal skin deformation when the punch hits the skin resulting in nearly zero follicle movement.

In case of splayed follicles where the two follicles are not parallel to each other but diverge at lower one-third of the follicular unit, keeping the punch slightly off center toward the splayed graft, and limiting the depth of punching will help in getting intact follicles. If partial transaction still exists, one can increase the punch size to get intact grafts to 1.05 mm. A different approach is to change the punch type

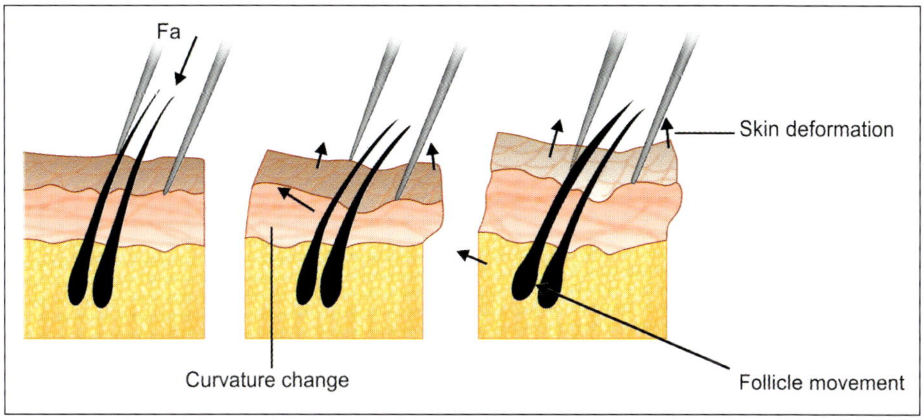

Figure 8.8

As punch hits the skin surface; it deforms the skin, which results in movement of follicle as shown in this Figure. This follicular movement can result in high partial follicular transaction in case of splayed follicles.

to Dr Jean Devroye's hybrid Trumpet punch. The flat punch has a sharp square-shaped external border, sharp enough to cut the scalp under pressure and low speed; however, the internal border cannot be sharp and has to be smooth in order to dissect the graft forward without cutting or transecting it (Figs. 8.9A and B).

Optimally one should use the smallest possible punch diameter that will encircle the intact follicle. FUE pioneers such as Dr Cole, Dr Robert, Dr Wolf, Dr Lorenzo and Dr Harris have developed a consensus that punch sizes between 0.8 mm and 1 mm leaves no noticeable difference in donor site appearance and excellent harvesting rates.[2] Harvesting devices include manual punches, mechanically-assisted devices, vacuum-assisted extraction devices and automated robotic-assisted devices.

The cutting edge of follicular extraction punches can be either sharp or blunt. The modern sharp punches advocate minimizing the thickness of these punches to reduce adjacent tissue damage. The sharp punch reduces mechanical force and torque that cause mechanical trauma to follicular structures and dermal tissue, thus reducing graft transection. Reduced mechanical force also reduces the risk of buried grafts.[2] The risk of burial of grafts are especially high in areas with high subcutaneous fat which are lower one-third of the safe donor region and the chest.

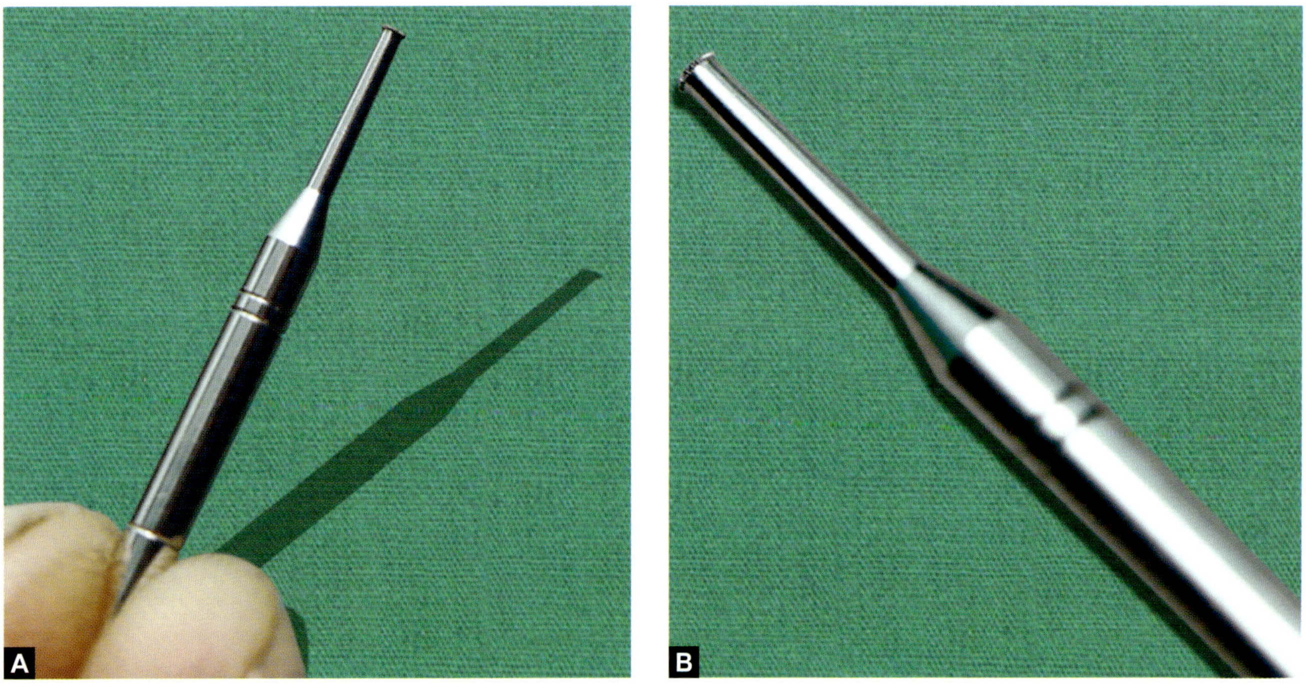

Figures 8.9A and B

The hybrid Trumpet punch designed by Dr Jean Devroye. It is a hybrid punch with a 90° outer edge and a smooth funnel-shaped inner edge. It offers the advantage of both sharp and blunt punch. It works like a dissection tool rather than a cutting tool.

An ideal sharp punch is a circular punch made of hardened stainless steel with sharp edge on outside and blunt inner surface to protect the follicle.

"Serrounded" punch developed by Dr Cole and "Triple wave" developed by Dr Rassman are serrated punches designed to reduce the cutting surface area thus reducing the friction and axial force required to penetrate the skin[3] (Fig. 8.10).

The depth of the incision should be limited to the minimum depth possible to obtain intact follicle without damaging the outer root sheath of hair. However, in case of beard extraction and cases where grafts are thin with minimal or poor quality fat, our personal experience is that one should score deeply to minimize the damage to the stem cells along the length of the grafts during extraction with forcep even at cost of slightly increased follicular transection. Disrupting the attachment of arrector pili muscle is generally required to make the extraction easy. Once muscular attachment is severed, the follicle can be removed in total. The punch penetration ranges from 2 mm to 3 mm. The physician must be aware of the changing harvesting parameters like hair directions, angle, depth of penetration and punch size as he moves from one donor area to other.[4]

Often, the narrowest portion of multi-hair follicle is at the surface and surface area of follicle may increase below the surface due to splaying. Limiting the depth of the punch will be useful. Using a larger punch or "Wind-O" punch by Dr John Cole may also be useful in preserving the multi-hair follicle. If a portion of dermal papilla is remained behind, there can be regrowth of the partial follicle.[3]

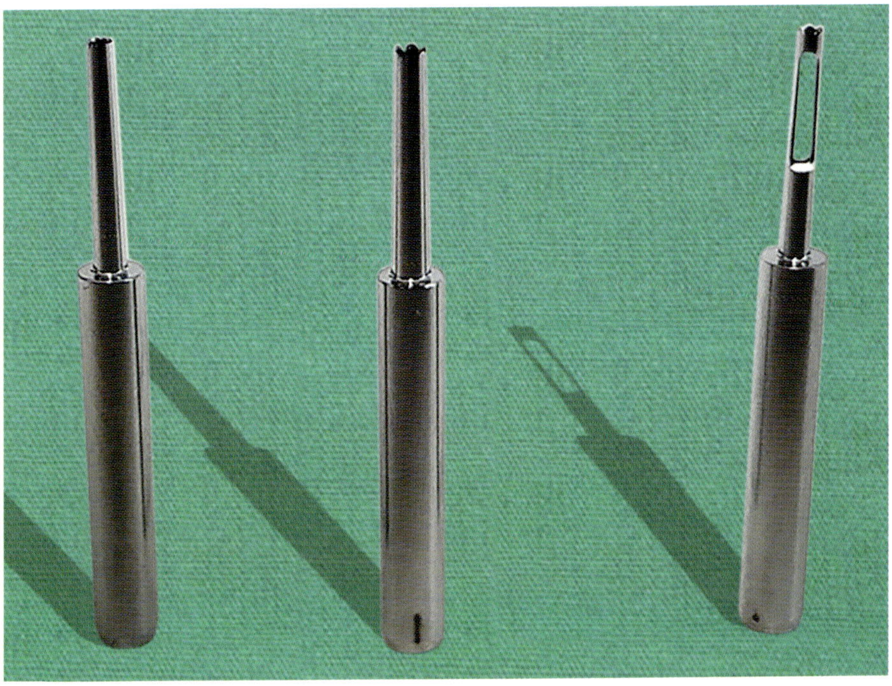

Figure 8.10

Three variants of sharp Serrounded® punches. The latest variant being the "wind-o" punch which minimizes the friction with the surrounding skin even further thus minimizing the heat generated.
Courtesy: www.coleinstruments.com.

Removal of the scored graft requires use of Jeweller's forcep. The physician should keep in mind that the bulge region of hair follicle can be compressed or traumatized while extraction. During extraction the graft should not be tightly held at the shaft.

Curly hair are prone to transections. Before committing for FUE surgery, a small trial of donor harvesting site is recommended. With very curly hair, it is recommended to use a larger punch (1–1.2 mm) to score the skin superficially. If the transection rates are high, it is helpful to use blunt punch. However, using sharp punch with minimal advancement (<2 mm) followed by extremely delicate two-hand removal technique will yield intact graft.[4] Use of hypodermic needle as describe by Dr Poswal for body hair extraction is useful in cutting the subdermal tissue and arrector pili muscles.[5]

Dr James Harris invented the blunt dissecting punch and methodology of tissue dissection is described as surgically advanced follicular extraction (SAFE)™ system (Fig. 8.11). Blunt punch requires greater physical force, that may damage the follicles and increases the risk of buried grafts but a sharp punch is usually unforgiving in hands of a new surgeon compared to a blunt punch and results in high transection rates. The theory behind this dissection method is the blunt punch follicular transection by acting as a wedge when dissecting the follicles from attached tissues. The punch and the dissecting technique direct the splayed follicles into the lumen of the punch thus reducing follicular transection.

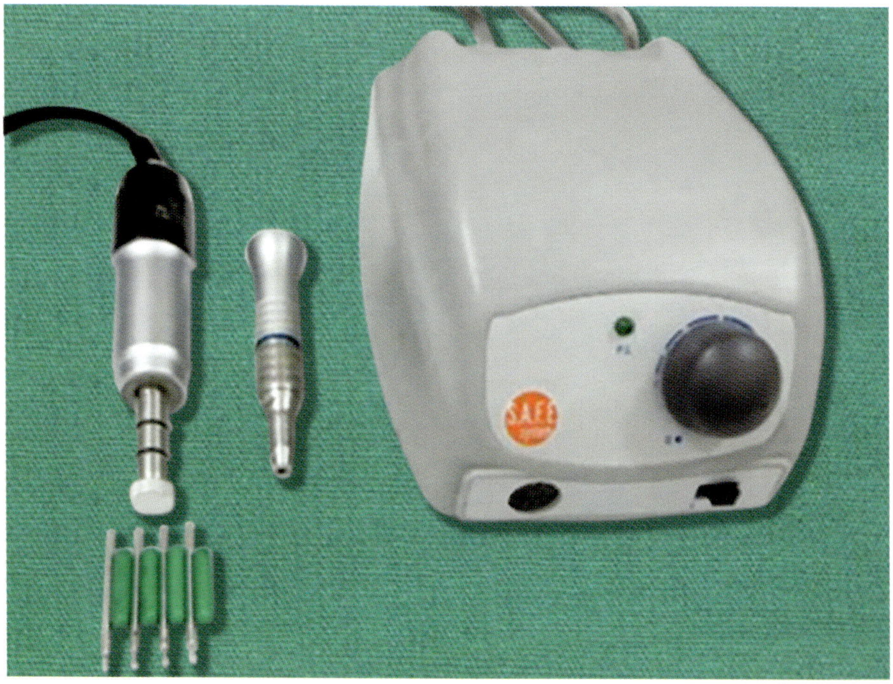

Figure 8.11

Surgically advanced follicular extraction (SAFE)™ system.

The first step requires a sharp punch to be centered over the exiting hair and skin is cut 0.3–0.5 mm depth. The second step involves inserting the blunt punch through the scored skin.[6]

An increase in punch diameter from 0.8 mm to 1 mm increases the surface area of scar by 58%, thus size of the punch should be carefully selected.[7] Using 1.0 mm punch may result in coalescing of holes, in case surgeon makes high density scoring to extract optimum number of grafts from scalp.

Beard and torso hair vary widely in angle and direction of hair emergence even in same patient. There may be whorls in beard and chest. Therefore, direction of punch must constantly be adjusted during extraction. The submental beard area and the torso subcutaneous tissue are generally soft and fatty, rather than fibrous, so there is little risk of popping and requires minimal jerk with Forester.

HOW WE DO IT?

We prefer motorized Programmable Power Cole Isolation Device (PCID)® (Fig. 8.12). The size of punch depends on few test grafts extracted.

- The minimum possible size of the punch which gives intact grafts should be selected. There should be sufficient fat around the grafts and minimum possible partial transaction.
- Requisite of a good extraction include:
  - Comfortable seating position
  - Right magnification of 4X to 5X and correct punch angles which is aligned with the graft orientation (Figs. 8.13A to D)
  - Sufficient but not excessive tumescence to decrease the angulations of graft and to minimize the bleeding
  - Proper stretching of skin when punch hits the skin surface to avoid burial of graft.
- The scoring should be as less deep as possible. Scoring it deep increases the risk of partial transaction, but in case of long grafts one may need to score deeper to cut the arrector pili muscles. The situation may become tricky when there are long and splayed grafts which decapitate with less deep punching and do not come out.
- It should be kept in mind that the graft angles and depth, along with orientation of graft changes as one moves from one donor region to another, so a depth which is adequate at one site of the scalp may not be adequate at another site. The depth of scoring needed to extract the grafts is higher at superior margin of safe donor area due to strong adherence of grafts just inferior to crown. Test grafts from new site should be taken out before going ahead with full-fledged punching.

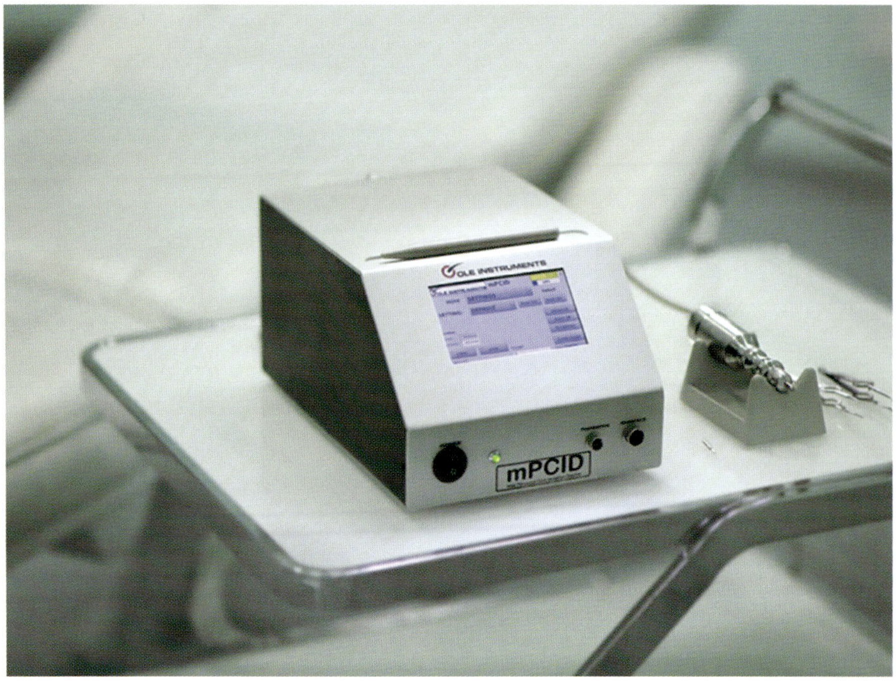

Figure 8.12

Programmable Power Cole Isolation Device (PCID)®. This device is used to extract grafts by fitting sharp Serrounded® punch.

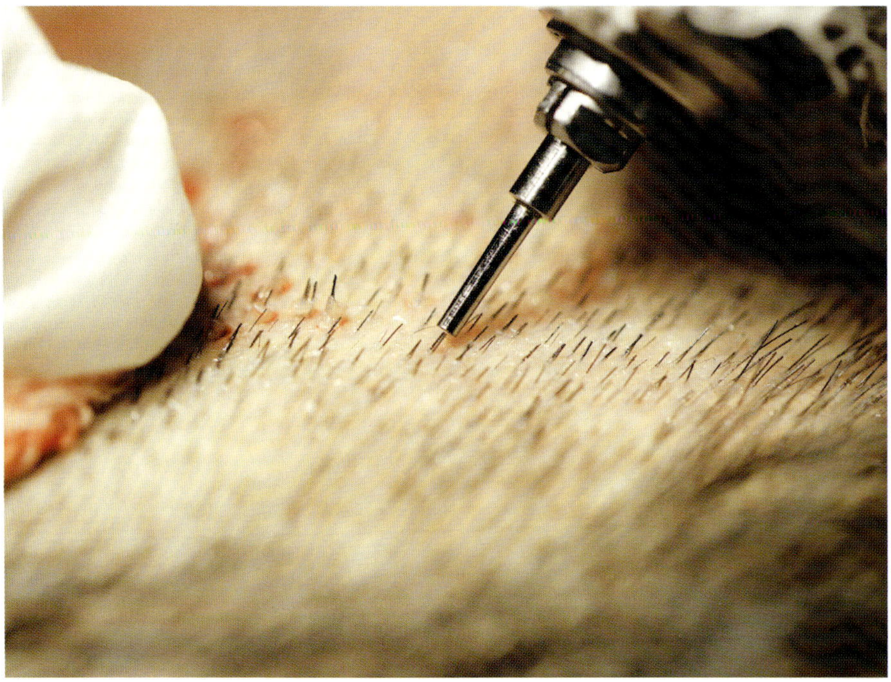

Figure 8.13A

Alignment—it means to place the shaft of the punch parallel to the target hair.

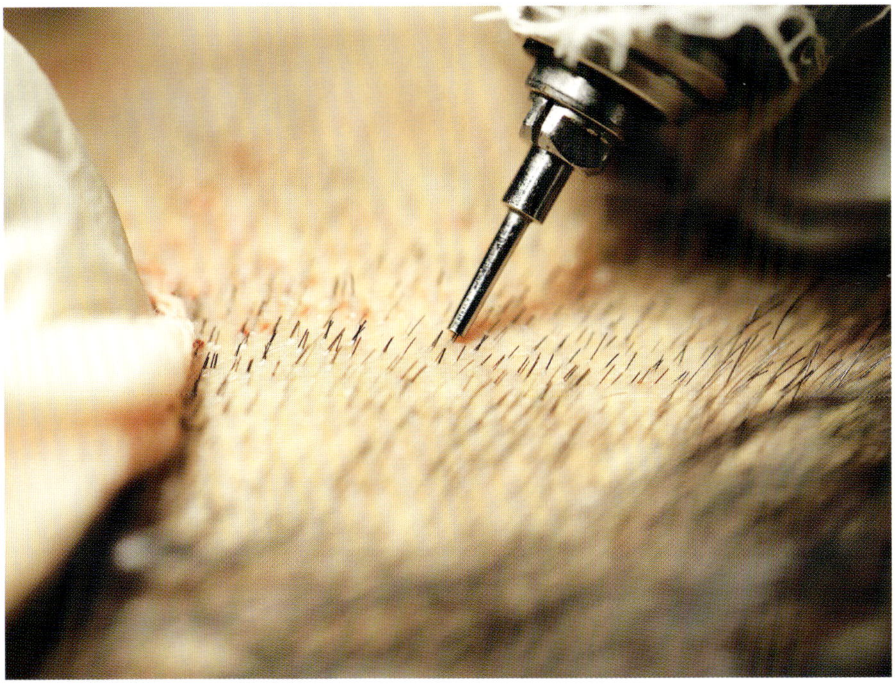

Figure 8.13B

Engagement—it refers to the point when the tip of the punch touch the skin surface.

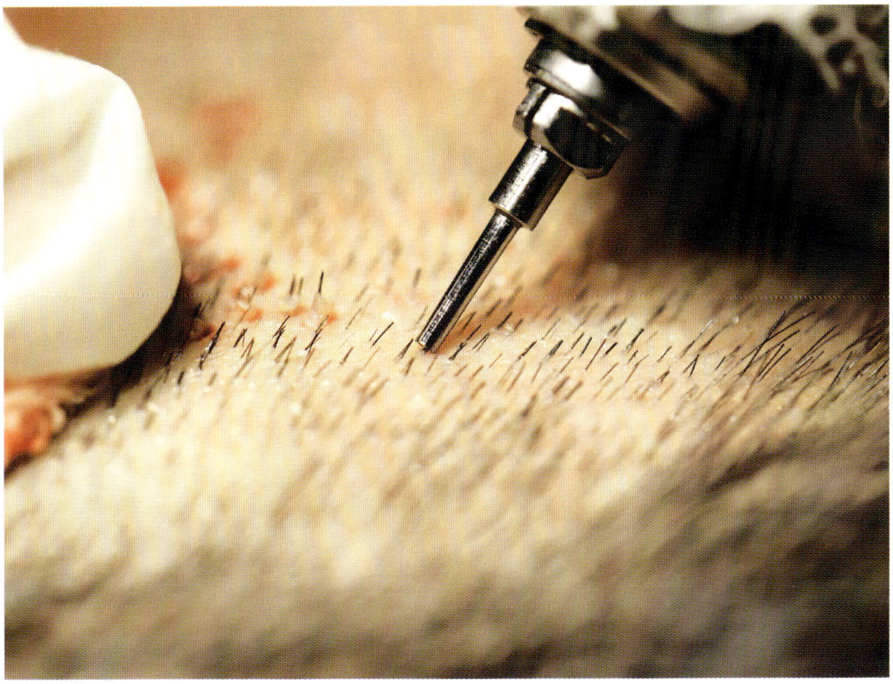

Figure 8.13C

Advancement—when punch is advanced into the skin to dissect the tissue around the grafts, it is called advancement.

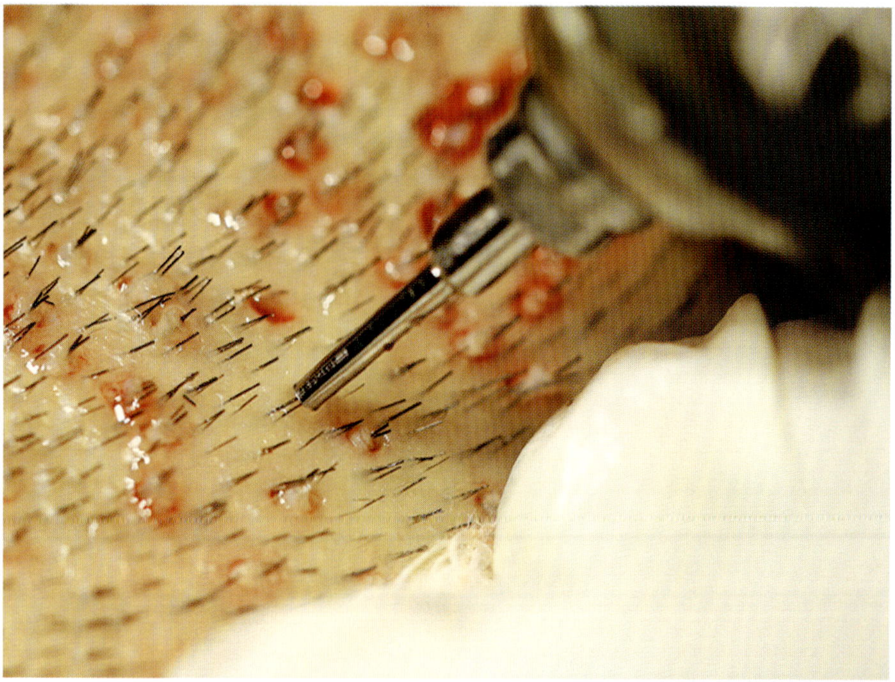

Figure 8.13D

Nonaligned punch—the shaft of the punch is not parallel to the direction of hair thus, leading to partial or complete transection.

- The depth of the graft changes when patient who has got previously conducted FUE session go for another session as fibrosis of FUE scar creates variable depth at various sites, leading to a highly difficult extraction process. Pre-existing FUT scar should be kept in mind while doing extraction. Scoring of grafts should be avoided as the direction of the hair just above and below the FUT scar may not be directed inferiorly due to the fibrotic process in the scar (Figs. 8.14 and 8.15).
- There can be splayed grafts, along with nonsplayed grafts, so selecting right punch size is important as choosing less than adequate diameter will lead to partial transaction of splayed grafts. It is equally important to inject saline intradermally to make the graft less acute angled.
- Always remember to note the heat generated while scoring of the graft, it can be assessed by touching the punch and heat of the motorized FUE device. A heated device may damage the graft permanently by damaging the stem cells in the bulge region even within grafts with sufficient fat and no follicular transaction.
- Naked grafts without inadequate fat around them may or may not grow.
- Focus on accurate and scoring at right depth consistently over higher speed of extraction.
- Keeping the grafts hydrated and free from blood is equally important by spraying chilled normal saline before the assistant transfers it into storage solution.

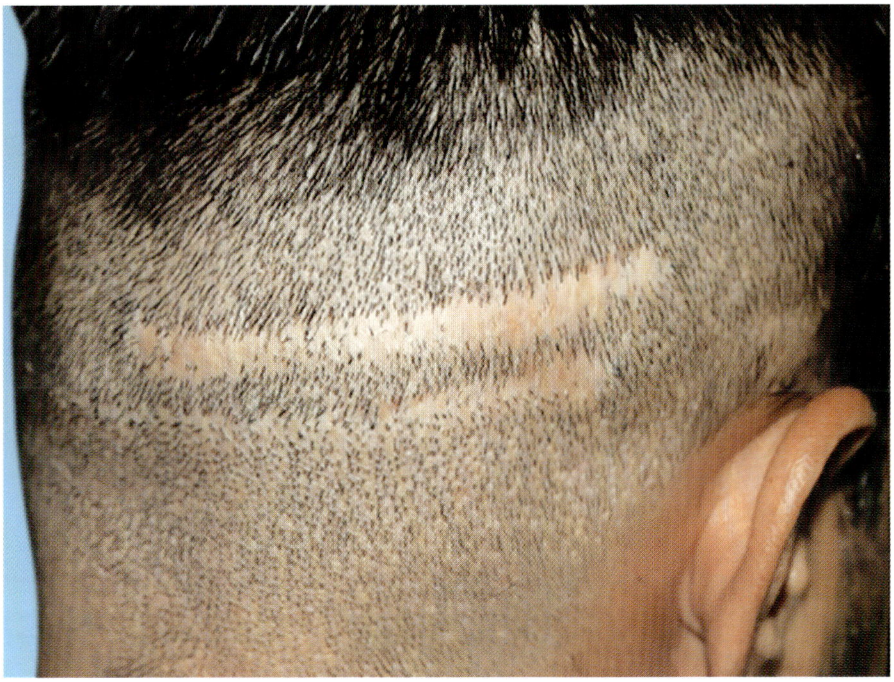

Figure 8.14

Demonstrates a wide follicular unit transplantation (FUT) scar. No extraction (follicular unit extraction scar marks are absent above FUT scar) was done just above the FUT scar as it makes the scar visible.

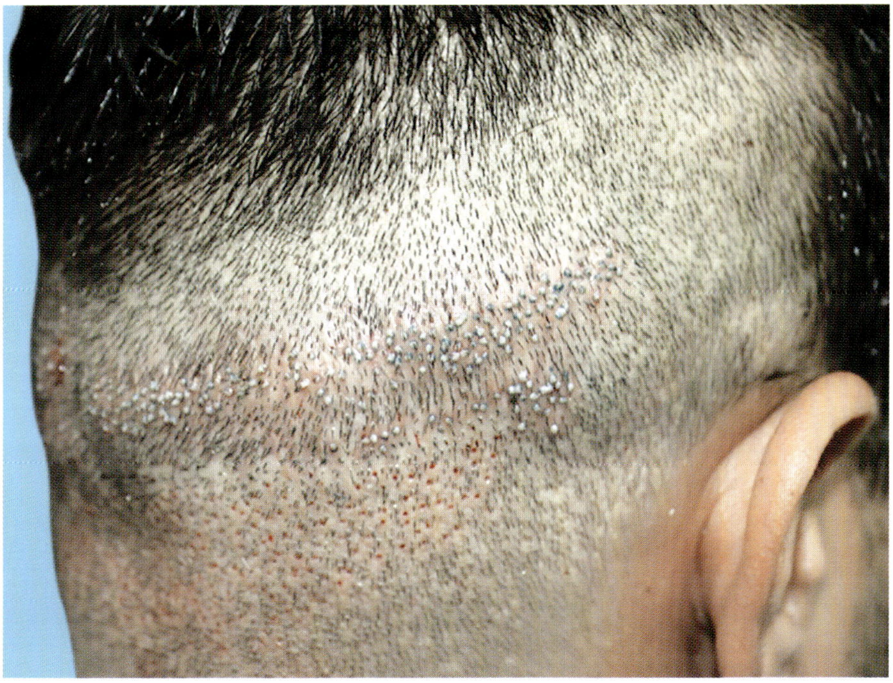

Figure 8.15

The FUT scar was repaired by implanting 500 grafts in those scars 3 months after doing hair transplantation. Repair of the FUT scar by implantation of 500 beard grafts.

- Accurate and uniform extraction from all donor sites on the scalp should be done; there is a greater risk of moth-eaten appearance if one makes non-uniform extraction.
- One should note that the follicular density and hair caliber in temporal region can be lesser than in the occipital region, so scoring density will be usually lower in temporal region.
- Use hair of nape of neck for temple reconstruction or eyebrow reconstruction.
- The sites where punching has been done in a previous FUE surgery, should not be punched as aggressively as compared to nonpunched areas to maintain uniform donor aesthetics.

SUMMARY

- Donor evaluation—To estimate number of grafts that can be harvested, the extent of baldness, previous FUT scar, traumatic scars, previous FUE scars and retrograde thinning of hair.
- Choosing the right punch in favor of getting intact grafts with enough surrounding tissue is important to ensure graft survival.
- Disruption of attachment of arrector pili muscle is required for easy extraction.
- Comfortable seating position, 4x to 5x magnification, correct punching angles, tumescence and proper stretching of skin are helpful for easy scoring of grafts.
- In case of previous FUT scar, scoring should not be done too close to the scar.
- Accurate and intelligent scoring from the safe donor area is to be done else there is a risk of moth eaten appearance due to over extraction.

REFERENCES

1. Zontos G, Rose PT, Nikiforidis G. A mathematical proof of how the outgrowth angle of hair follicles influences the injury to the donor area in FUE harvesting. Dermatol Surg. 2014;40(10):1147-50.
2. Cole JP. An analysis of follicular punches, mechanics, and dynamics in follicular unit extraction. Facial Plast Surg Clin North Am. 2013;21:437-47.
3. Rassman WR, Bernstein RM. Follicular unit extraction: minimally invasive surgery for hair transplantation. Dermatol Surg. 2002;28:720-8.
4. Boden SA, Jr Williams KL. Motorized FUE with sharp punch. In: Lam SM, Jr Williams KL (Eds). Hair Transplant 360, 1st edn. New Delhi, India: Jaypee Brothers Medical Publishers (P) Ltd.; 2016. 241-307.
5. Poswal A. Expanding needle concept for better extraction of body hair grafts. Indian J Dermatol. 2013;58(3):240.
6. Harris JA. New methodology and instrumentation for follicular unit extraction: lower follicle transection rates and expanded patient candidacy. Dermatol Surg. 2006;32(1): 56-61.
7. Zontos G. The physics of follicular unit extraction. In: Lam SM, Jr Williams KL (Eds). Hair Transplant 360, 2nd edn. New Delhi: Jaypee Brothers Medical Publishers (P) Ltd.; 2016. 47.

CHAPTER 9

Graft Handling

Abhinav Kumar, Pradeep Sethi, Sarita Sanke

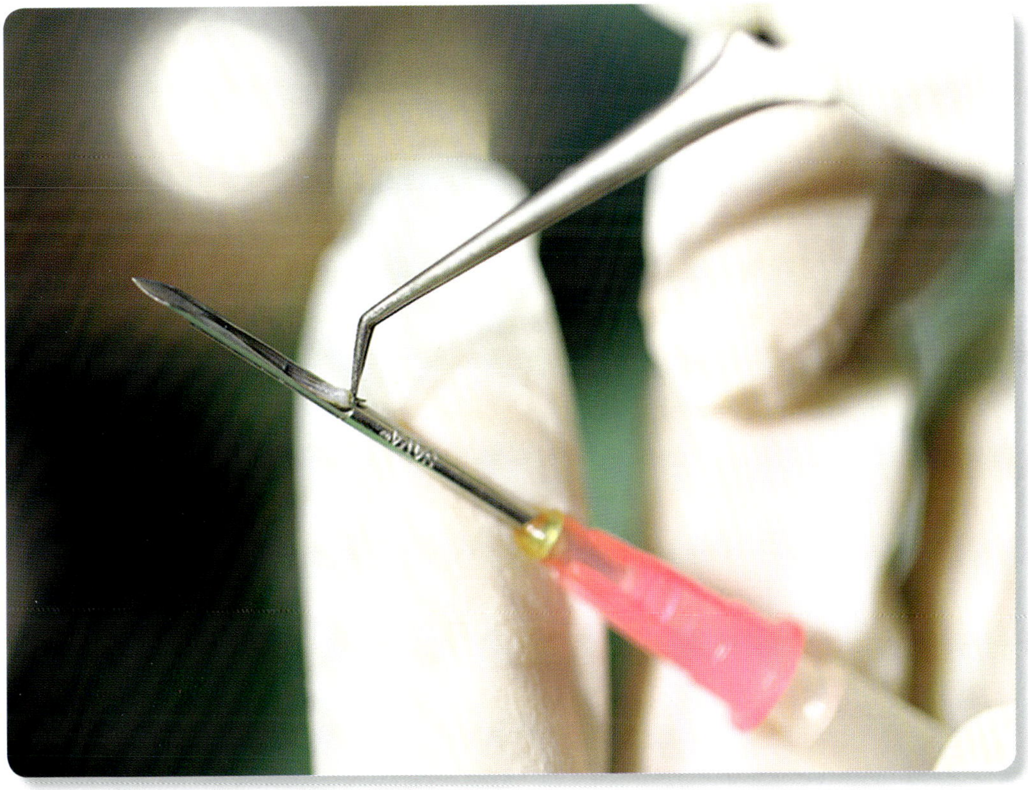

The results of the procedure ultimately depends upon the tenderness with which the grafts are handled. Each graft is a living being! The authors personally consider each graft as one human baby and not able to grow one graft means murdering one! When such diligence flows from the top of the crew, the rest of the support staff also get aligned to this thought process and ultimately the graft survival rate shoots up, which we all need badly, both patients and the surgeons.

INTRODUCTION

Graft handling is key to hair growth after scoring has been done by motorized punch or manual punch or after strip surgery. We believe that experienced assistants should be extracting the graft under high magnification of 4X to 5X.

Graft handling involves:

- Extraction of grafts
- Graft storage
- Loading of grafts
- Implantation of grafts.

EXTRACTION OF GRAFTS

There are many ways to harvest follicular unit excision (FUE) grafts from donor area. It depends on how surgeon performs hair restoration, in laying position or sit down position. In the first case, a straight or curved forcep is used to push the surrounding skin downward in order to expose the grafts. In the meantime the graft is held and extracted very gently.

In the sit down position technique the extraction is performed using specific forceps, such as Castroviejo and ATOE™ (Aide to extraction). The Castroviejo forcep grabs the graft directly inside the scored site, and the ATOE™ holds the top of the graft, this method facilitates extraction of grafts. This method facilitates easy graft removal with minimum depth extraction. The use of ATOE™ facilitates minimizing follicular injury. Up to 25 grafts can be extracted at one time with ATOE.

The steps of extraction of grafts by forceps are illustrated below:

- The grafts are held firmly from the tip with a straight forester (Fig. 9.1).
- The straight or a curved forester with a grip is used to push the surrounding skin around the grafts downward to expose the lower part of grafts. The grafts are held very gently with the second forester after pushing the skin downward around the grafts (Fig. 9.2).
- The force is applied by the straight forester to pull the grafts in the direction of hair growth, while the gentle grip of the second forester guides the grafts helps in preventing decapitation of the tight grafts. Holding the grafts tightly by second forester may crush the grafts (Fig. 9.3).
- During the extraction process continuous spray of saline is essential to prevent desiccation of grafts.
- Secondly continuous spray also prevents adherence of blood clots on the graft and prevents cohesion of multiple grafts. Insufficient saline spray would lead to increased manipulation by assistants to separate these grafts while loading the grafts into implanters.

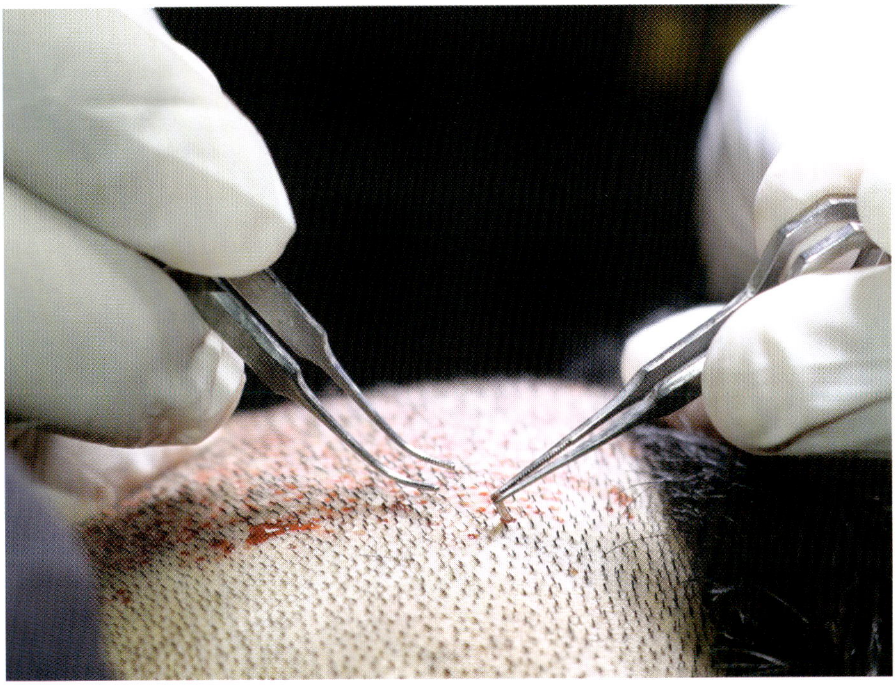

Figure 9.1

Graft is held firmly from the tip with a straight forester.

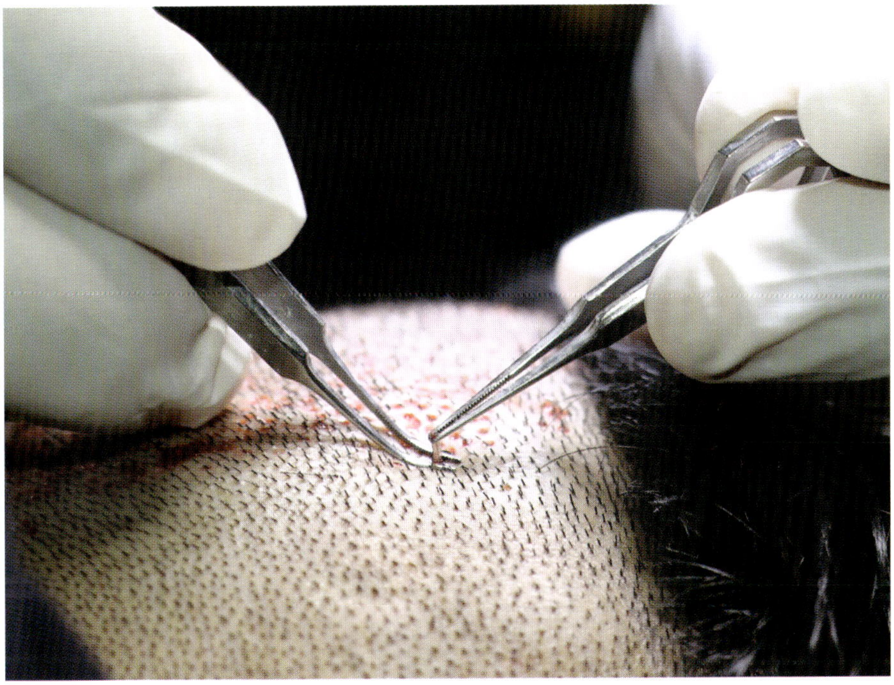

Figure 9.2

The curved forester with a grip is used to push the surrounding skin around the graft downward to expose the lower part of grafts.

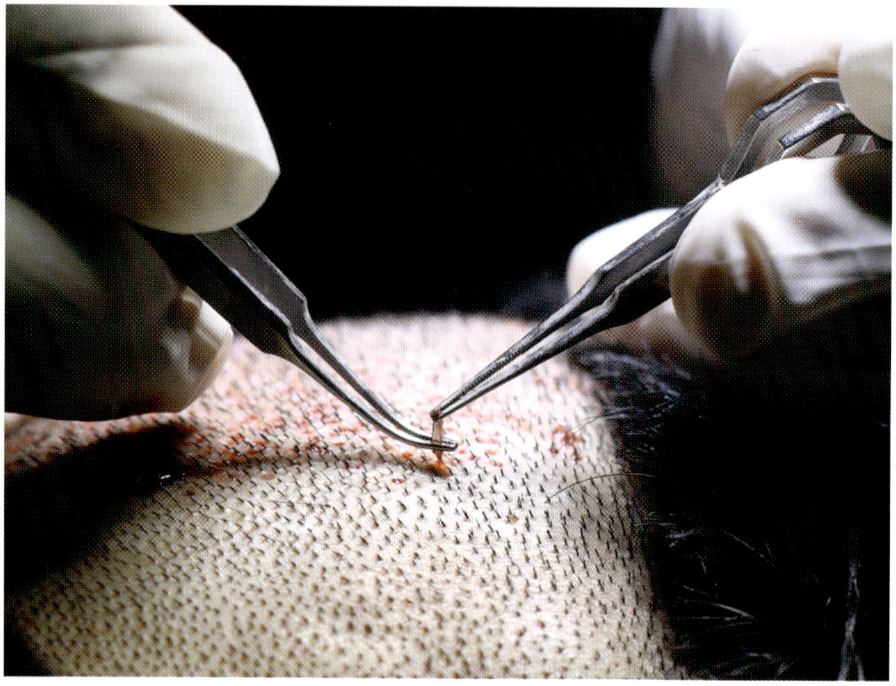

Figure 9.3

The force is applied by the straight forester to pull the grafts in the direction of hair growth.

GRAFT STORAGE

After the extraction of grafts, the grafts are kept in chilled saline (0.9% NaCl) at 4–8° or ringer lactate or in hypothermosol with liposomal adenosine triphosphate (ATP).

We illustrate the various types of grafts which are extracted during the extraction process (Figs. 9.4A to C).

The grafts should be held with forceps at the epidermal end. The authors follow "no root touch policy" where the bulb of hair from the point of extraction to implantation are never touched by either forceps, forester or manipulated in any way. Multiple follicle grafts are never split into individual follicles. This ensures minimum possible damage to the grafts.

Grafts can be damaged during the extraction process especially the single follicle grafts. They can be extracted without the fat with intact roots (Fig. 9.4D).

One can encounter grafts which are bent near the roots. These roots are damaged and will probably not survive after transplantation (Fig. 9.4E).

One can also encounter partially transected or completely transected grafts. A graft can be totally transected with all its follicles cut transversely or partially transected with one or more of its follicles cut. The International Society of Hair Restoration Surgery Terminology Committee officially defines transection to reflect *any microscopically visible breakage of a follicle anywhere along its entire length.* These grafts get transected due to wrong punch size, the excessive curl of the grafts, flaying of grafts or wrongly aligned motorized or manual FUE punch (Fig. 9.4F).

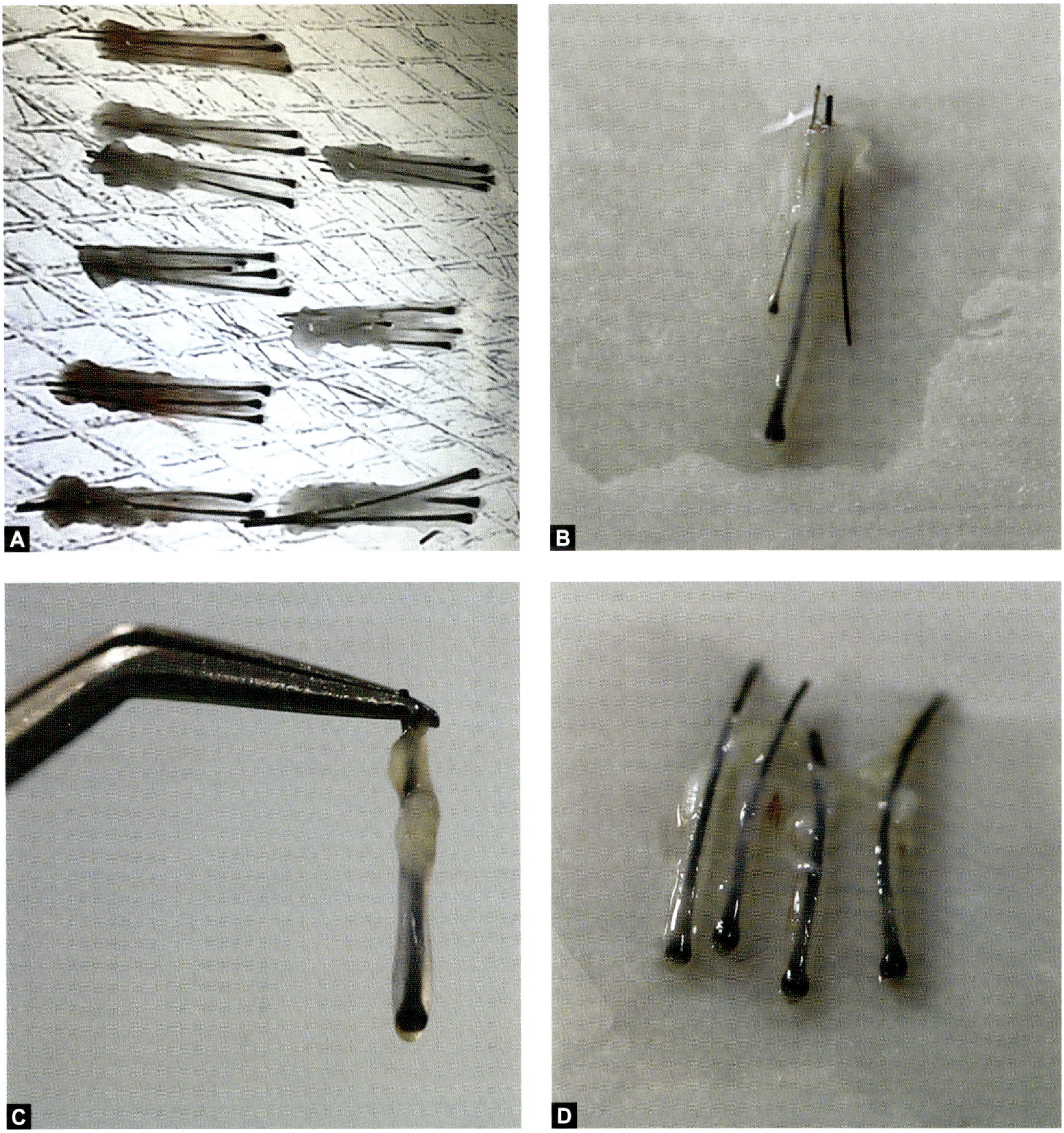

Figures 9.4A to D

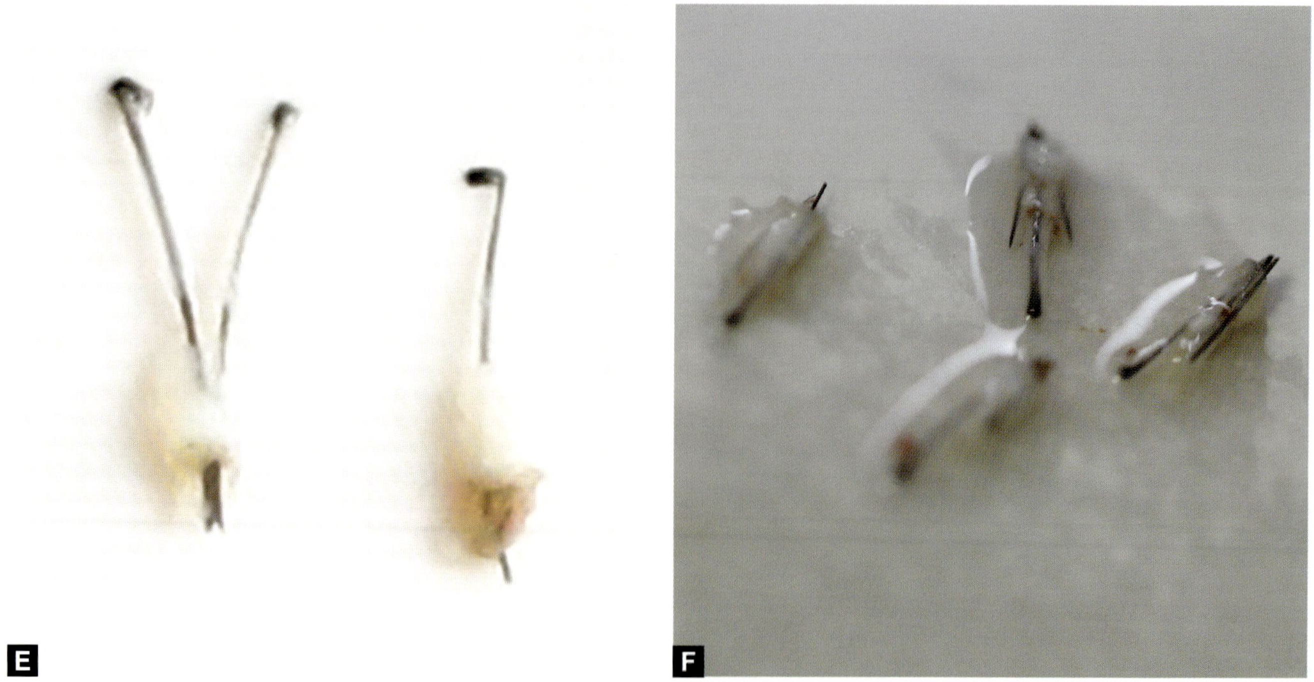

Figures 9.4E and F

Figures 9.4A to F

(A) Double and triple grafts. These grafts have been extracted with a sharp serrated 1.0 mm punch. These grafts are straight and do not flay or curl; (B) A three follicle graft with one telogen hair, one transected hair root and one intact hair root of anagen hair. The telogen hair is often missed by naked eye. They are considered single hair grafts and implanted in the hairline transition zone by mistake; (C) Holding of grafts at the tip; (D) Grafts with intact roots but devoid of the surrounding tissue. Such grafts are alive but should be implanted immediately with the help of implanters without touching the roots; (E) Depicts the bent hair roots which signify damage during the extraction and graft handling; (F) Long, curved and splayed grafts which have high transection rates. Such grafts need to be scored less deep and preferably with large punch size of 1.0 mm or 1.05 mm or trumpet punch. Such grafts may protrude out of the implanter due to splaying and curvature. Correct loading of grafts to minimize graft handling is essential.
Courtesy: Dr Chiara Insalaco (Fig. A).

LOADING OF GRAFTS INTO IMPLANTER

Since we are following the no root touch policy, we prefer the implanter for implantation of grafts.

Steps of loading the grafts into the implanter:

1. The dull needle implanter is held in one hand in the way as shown in Figure 9.5.
2. The graft is held from the epidermal end as depicted Figure 9.6.
3. The graft is pushed from behind through the channel as depicted Figure 9.7.
4. The graft is pushed till the root reaches the middle of the bevel, ensuring that graft does not protrude out or bend in the channel. Always use correct size of implanter depending on the number of follicles in the graft. The forcep in Figure 9.8 points to the level at which grafts have to reach the implanter for

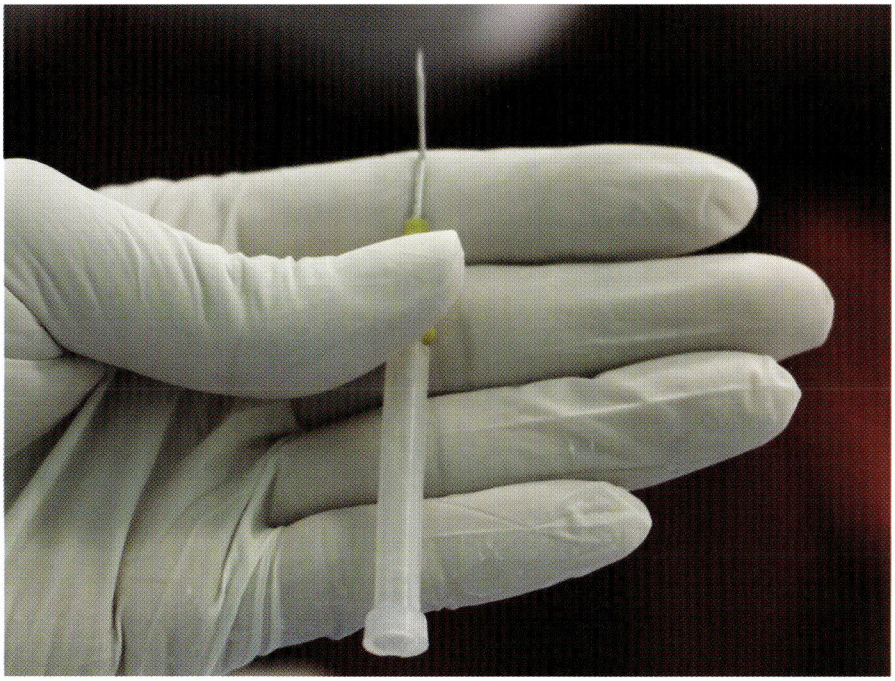

Figure 9.5

SAVA™ (dull needle) implanter is held in one hand.

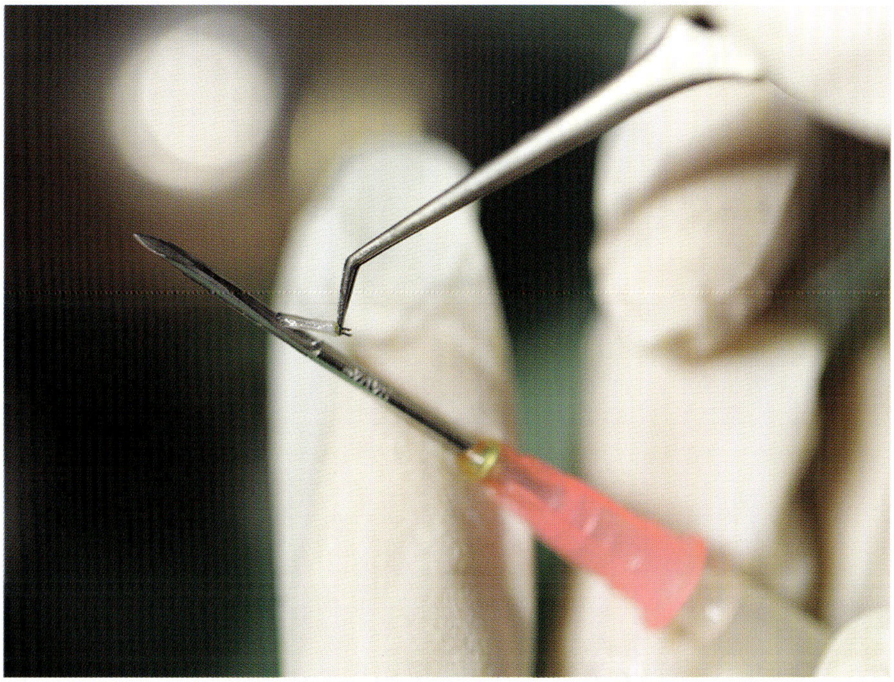

Figure 9.6

Graft is held from the epidermal end.

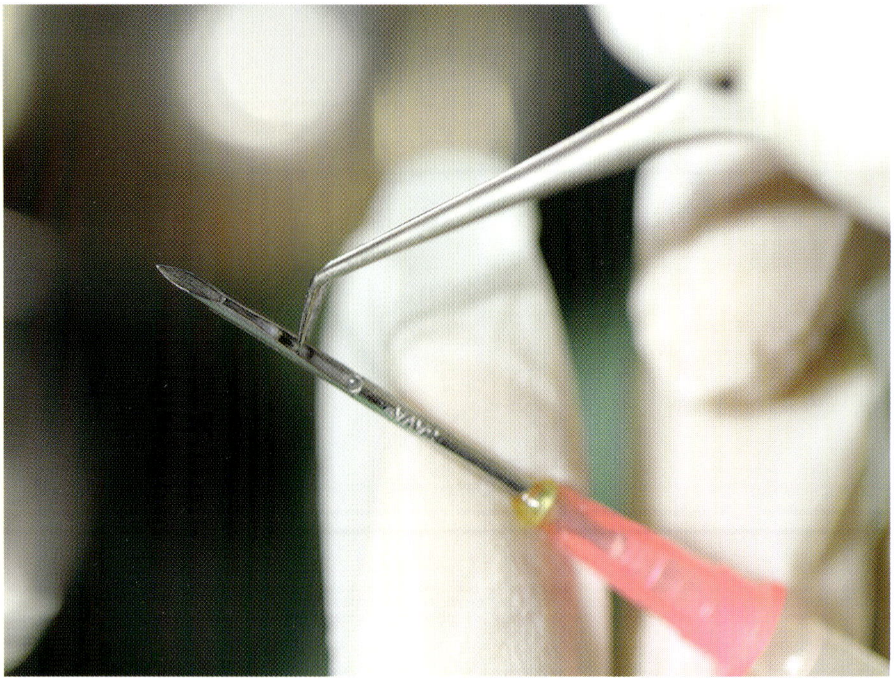

Figure 9.7

Graft is pushed from behind through the channel.

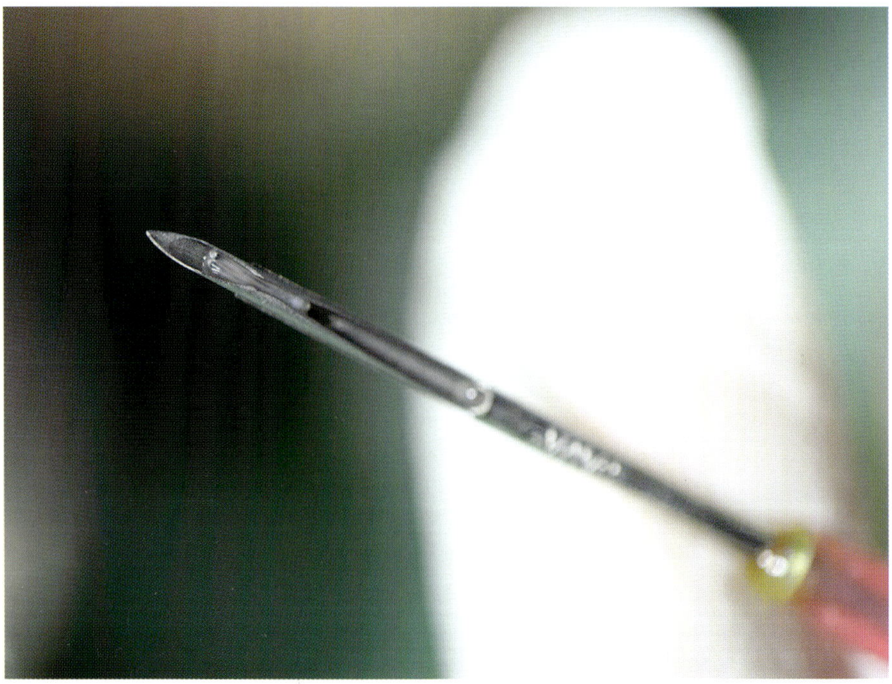

Figure 9.8

The graft has to reach the mid-point of the bevel for correct unloading during implantation.

correct unloading during implantation. However, one can face issues in cases of splayed grafts, curved grafts, or grafts with excessive tissue and fat where one or more follicle may protrude out of the implanter. It is important to increase the implanter size in such cases. Taking out test grafts before making slits helps in overcoming such situation.

IMPLANTATION OF GRAFTS

We demonstrate implantation of grafts in sagittal slits with the use of SAVA™ dull needle implanters. These implanters are blunt implanters which do not increase the size of slits during implantation into the premade slits. Other ways of implantation is using forceps which helps in dilating the slits and grafts are inserted into the dilated slits.

1. The first step is pushing the needle of dull needle implanters into the premade slits. In Figure 9.9, sagittal slits have been made. The implanters are inserted in alignment with the slits. The angle of implanter's entry should match the surgeon's angle during slit making, thus technicians should be aware about the direction and angles during slit creation.
2. After inserting the implanter fully, the implanter is rotated 90° to dilate the slits as shown in Figure 9.10.

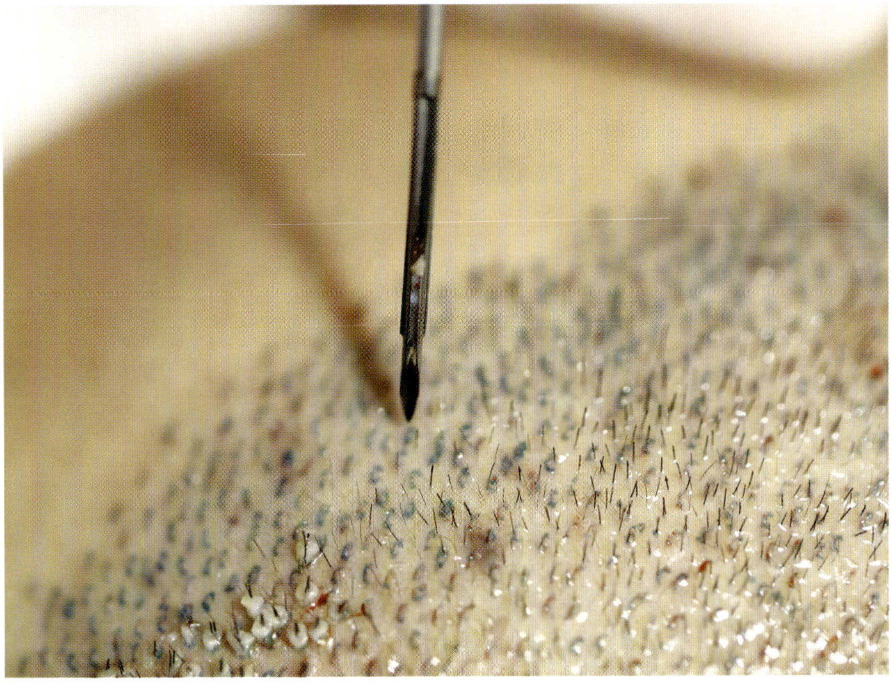

Figure 9.9

The implanters are inserted in alignment with sagittal slits.

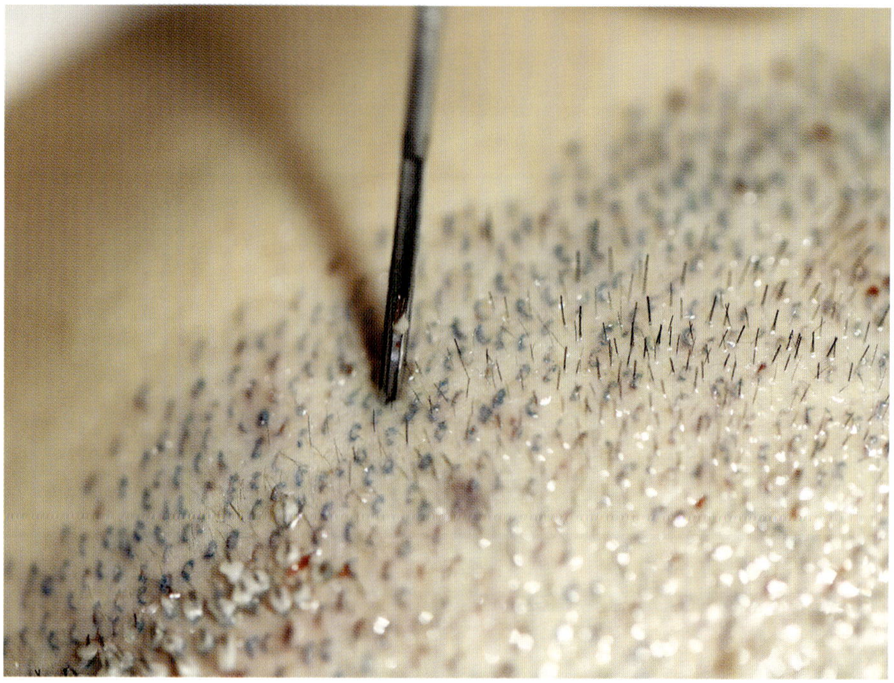

Figure 9.10

After inserting the implanter fully, the implanter is rotated by 90° to dilate the slits.

3. The graft is pushed with forcep from the top till the graft is inserted with just the epidermal portion protruding out. When the insertion of grafts is almost complete, the implanter is pulled out with the forcep preventing the implanted grafts from sliding out along with the implanter during this process as shown in Figure 9.11.
4. After the completion of unloading process, the implanter is withdrawn and given to the loader for further loading. Notice the orientation of bevel during the insertion and the exit from the slits (Figs. 9.12A and B).

CONCLUDING THOUGHTS

Graft handling is equally important part of hair transplantation. An excellent surgeon with poorly trained technicians cannot deliver results since the staff may damage the grafts during the extraction and implantation process. However, an average surgeon with good technicians can still deliver acceptable results.

Comments by Dr Chiara Insalaco

In order to get a great hair restoration result many steps have to be performed in a correct way. Of course harvesting good grafts, with no transection or damage is mandatory. But it is not enough. Immediately after the extraction phase, the grafts have to be kept at a constant and low temperature inside a storage solution.

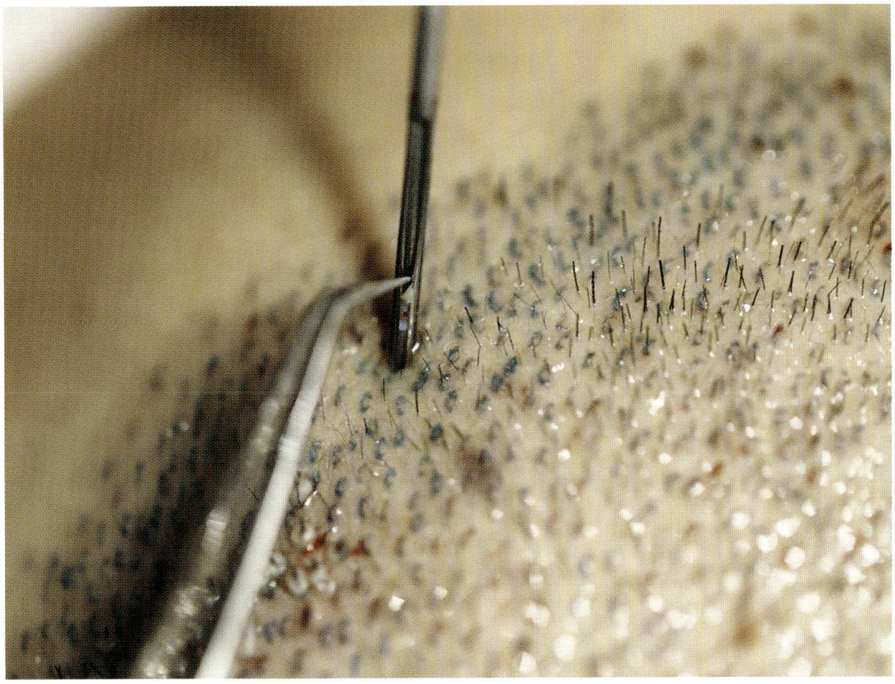

Figure 9.11

The graft is pushed with forcep from the top till graft is inserted with just the epidermal portion protruding out.

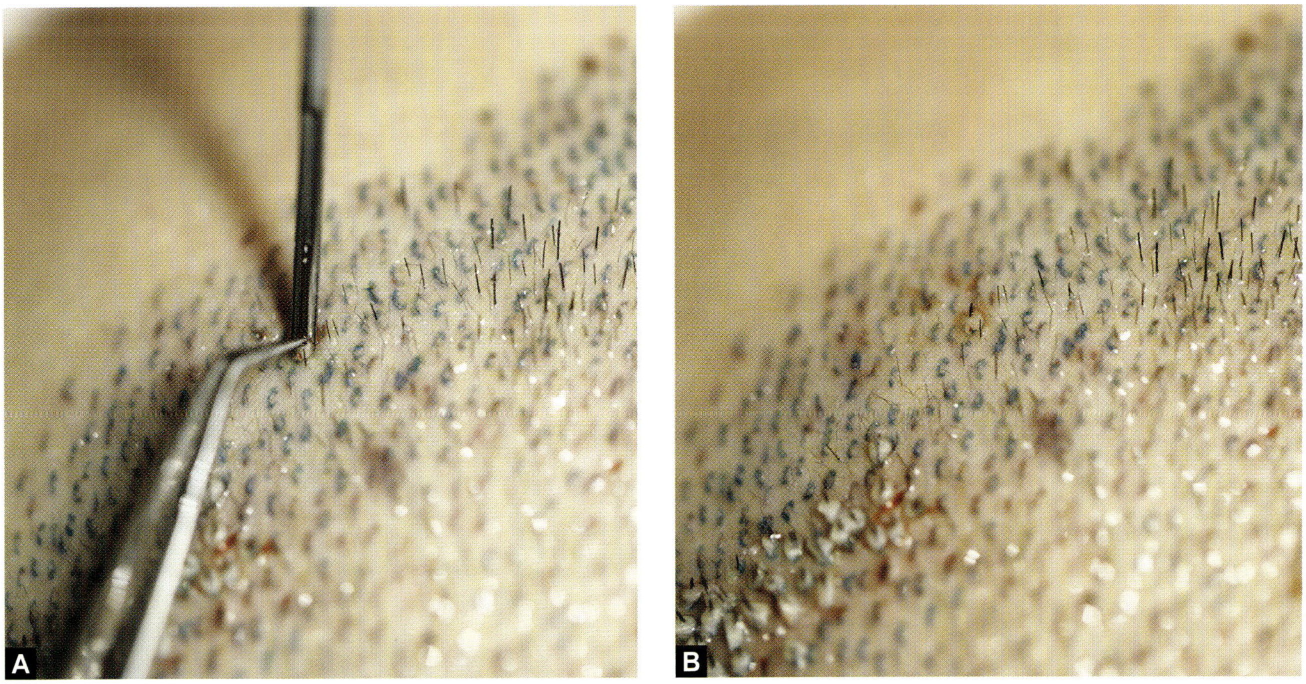

Figures 9.12A and B

The graft is pushed inside the slits. The epidermal portion of the grafts remain protruded out. Note the orientation of bevel during the exit of implanter from the slit.

It can be a simple saline solution, Ringer lactate or much better the more advanced hypothermosol. This last one improves and extends preservation of the follicles. We do not know yet how long the grafts are able to stay outside the body before they start to degenerate. For this reason, it would be better to place them inside the recipient sites as soon as possible. The second step is to create recipient sites using different size of blade or needle based on the punch size used during the harvesting. The average length of the hair follicle is 4 mm, but it can vary from a patient to another patient and from an ethnicity to another one. It is important to measure with a ruler the length of the graft in order to create sites with the perfect depth to welcome the follicular units. The grafts implantation can be done using implanter or the traditional forceps, straight or 45° angled. The main goal is to manipulate as less as possible the graft, that is a very delicate organ. The dedicated person has to be well-trained and with a long placing experience. The follicle unit is full of stem cells in all sheath length, inside the bulge and the bulb area. It means that in order to get a good yield we need to follow all these steps in the right way, always paying attention to the grafts. It is not important how fast we are but how gentle and precise we are with the follicles.

SUMMARY

- No root touch policy is to be followed throughout from extraction to implantation.
- Multiple grafts are never to be split into individual follicles.
- Dull needle implanters are used; which are full needles hence do not increase the size of pre-made slits.

CHAPTER 10

Complications: A Rare Thing in Trained Hands

Sarita Sanke, Arika Bansal, Abhinav Kumar

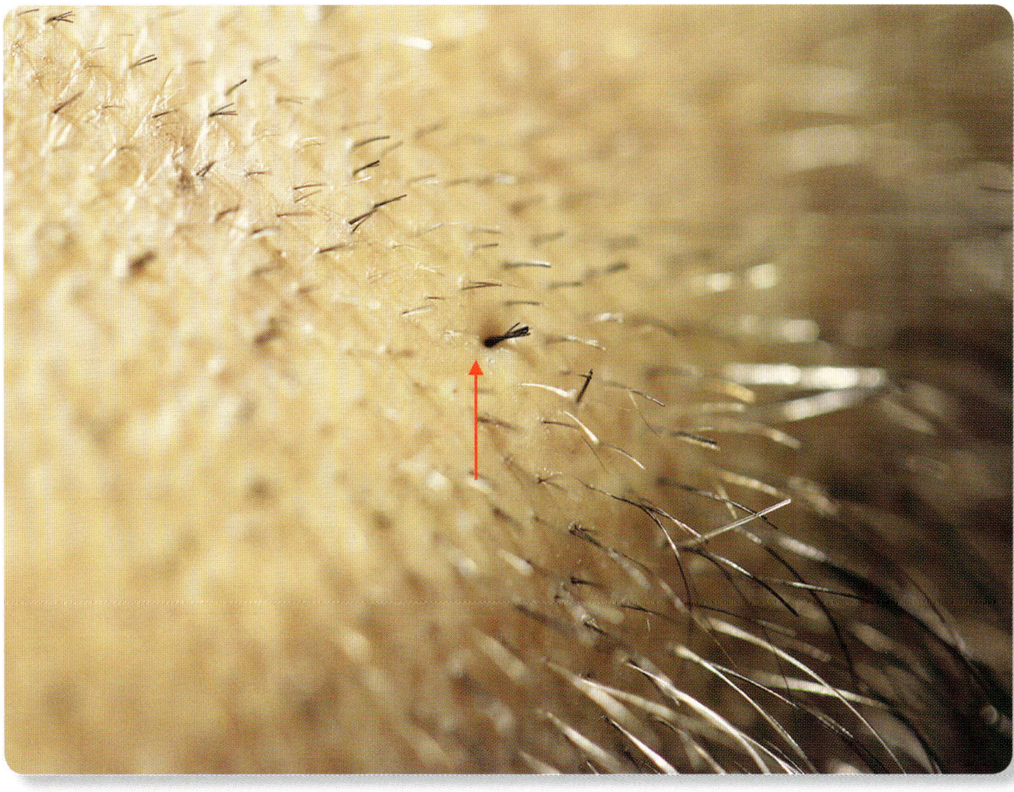

Pitting of grafts.

Complication is something which is unforeseen, unexpected and unwanted. A diligent, experienced team with academic, ethical, compassionate and one pointed focus can obviate many complications.

INTRODUCTION

Complications in hair restoration surgery are usually few and temporary. It can occur either at donor site or recipient site.

Complications can be divided into medical complications and aesthetic complications (Table 10.1).

PAIN-RELATED COMPLICATIONS

Pain during the surgery is the most common complication and also the easiest to manage. Adequate anesthesia, analgesics and anxiolytics will help in reducing the pain. Few patients complain of numbness, hypoesthesia or hyperesthesia or postoperative pain in the donor or recipient area. This usually disappears in few months. Neuralgic pain or sharp shooting pain may occur rarely. It occurs due to nerve injury during the surgery.

BLEEDING

Minimal bleeding is the norm in hair restoration surgery. However, excessive bleeding is uncommon. The patients should be asked to stop medicines like aspirin, nonsteroidal anti-inflammatory drugs (NSAIDs), vitamin E at least 2 weeks before the surgery. Routine investigations like complete hemogram with platelet count, bleeding time, clotting time, prothrombin time and viral markers should be done in all patients. Alcohol intake a day before surgery and high blood pressure can also lead to increased bleeding. This can be countered with tumescent injections of adrenaline and bupivacaine. Increased bleeding hamper the operating field and can make graft extraction inefficient. Constant pressure for 10–15 minutes with a gauze piece will stop the bleeding. We have been giving tablet alprazolam and oral tranexamic acid tablet to patients who are hypertensive to control bleeding

Table 10.1: Medical and aesthetic complications.

Medical complications	*Aesthetic complications*
Pain, hypoesthesia, hyperesthesia, neuralgic pain	Temporary hair loss and permanent hair loss
Bleeding	Unnatural hair line, poor density, unnatural crown and temple
Infections	Poor growth of transplanted hair
Edema	Pitting
Scars [follicular unit transplantation (FUT) scar, follicular unit excision (FUE) scar], keloids	Tenting
Donor and recipient necrosis	Poor donor aesthetics
	Absence of growth

during surgery. Similarly few patients may experience postoperative bleeding in next 24–36 hours following surgery which is a normal finding.

INFECTION

Localized infections can occur both at the donor as well as the recipient site; however, the risk of serious infection is extremely rare. Papulopustular lesion or folliculitis is the most common form of infections and can occur within 2 weeks to 4 months (Fig. 10.1). The chances of infections are increased if there is improper removal of the crusts from the donor site, improper cleaning of the recipient site at frequent intervals with normal saline, or if the patient is diabetic. Localized infections can be easily taken care of with oral antibiotics. Medical literature does not support the routine use of prophylactic antibiotic in skin surgery. The primary treatment for infections is debridement and then antibiotics. In the age of methicillin-resistant *Staphylococcus aureus* (MRSA), culture should be done routinely in the presence of infection and initial antibiotics should cover MRSA before the culture results arrive. Considering the Indian scenario we prescribe a 7-day course of systemic antibiotic after the procedure. Moist compresses and regular gentle shampooing should be advised after 7 days.

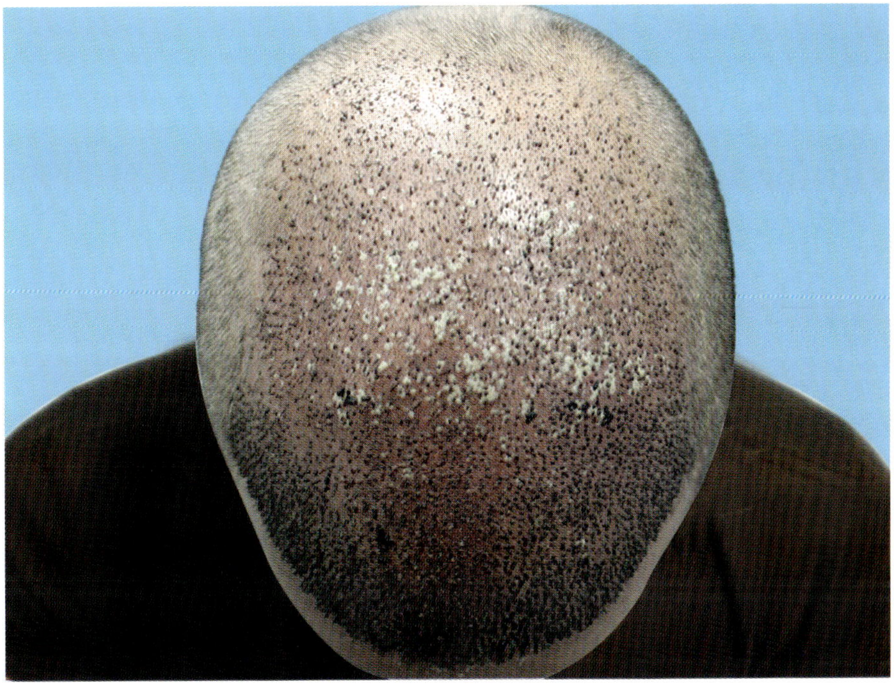

Figure 10.1

Folliculitis in the recipient region on day 3 of surgery. We changed the antibiotic immediately and sent it for culture sensitivity and it healed within 3 days.

EDEMA

Postoperative edema is another common complication which can occur either due to the anesthetic and tumescent fluids or due to venolymphatic congestion. The edema is maximum on days 2–4. We put a dynaplast on the forehead and ask the patient to massage from the center towards the periphery carefully in front of the mirror (Fig. 10.2). A short course of oral steroids can also be helpful.

SCARS, KELOIDS, HYPERTROPHIC SCAR

Keloids and hypertrophic scar are uncommon in a patient with no prior history. In case of any doubt, a small patch of test grafting can be done in an area of scalp which can be easily camouflaged. They can be managed with intralesional injection of triamcinolone acetonide 40 mg/ml. However, wide scars, cross-hatch scars, multiple large scars are rarely seen with follicular unit excision (FUE) (Figs. 10.3 to 10.6).

TEMPORARY HAIR LOSS AFTER SURGERY

Hair loss can occur both at the donor area as well as the recipient area. Hair loss at donor area occurs due to local vascular compromise; inflammation and edema postsurgery and is a temporary phenomenon (Fig. 10.7). It recovers within 3–4 months.

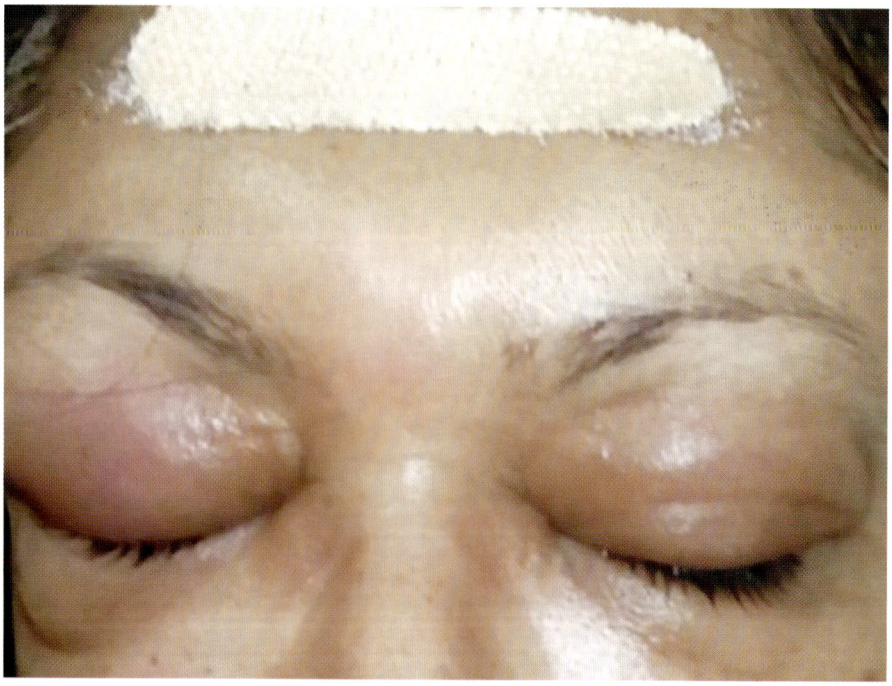

Figure 10.2

Massive periorbital swelling which developed on third day following female hair transplantation.

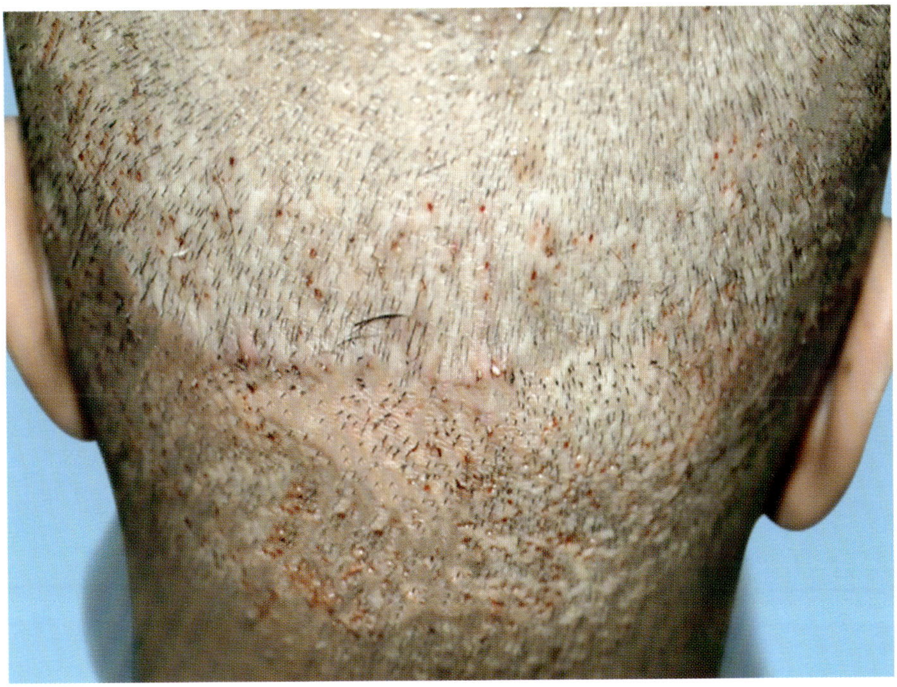

Figure 10.3

Presence of hypertrophic follicular unit transplantation scar. In this patient even the follicular unit excision (FUE) scars, earlier made with blunt 1.0–1.2 mm punch were mildly hypertrophic. We still did FUE in this patient after two failed surgeries and managed to plant 1,500 grafts from the scalp and 2,500 grafts from the beard.

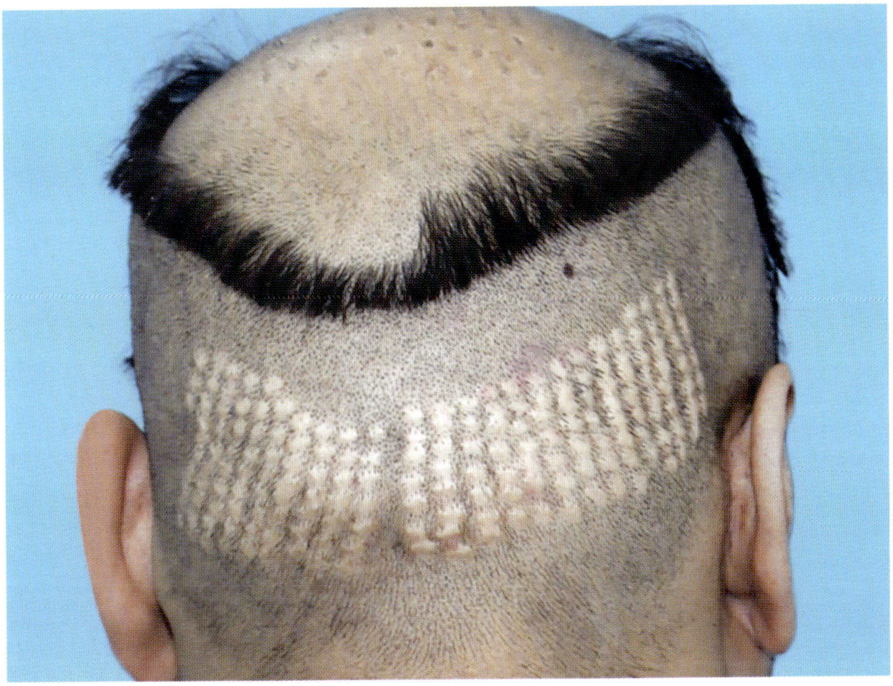

Figure 10.4

Depiction of hypertrophic scars of punch harvesting which was practiced earlier years.

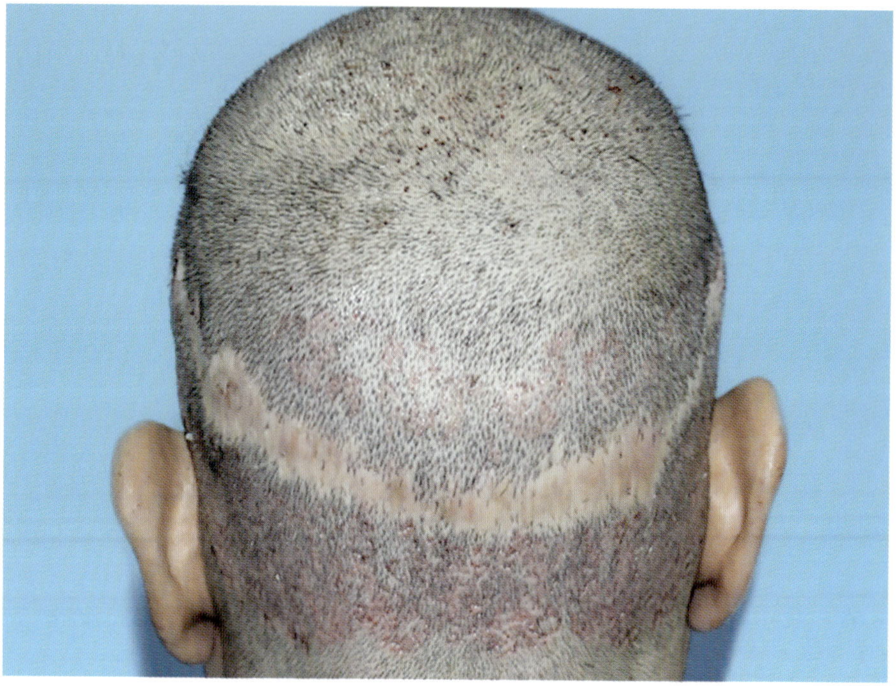

Figure 10.5

A bad follicular unit transplantation (FUT) scar.

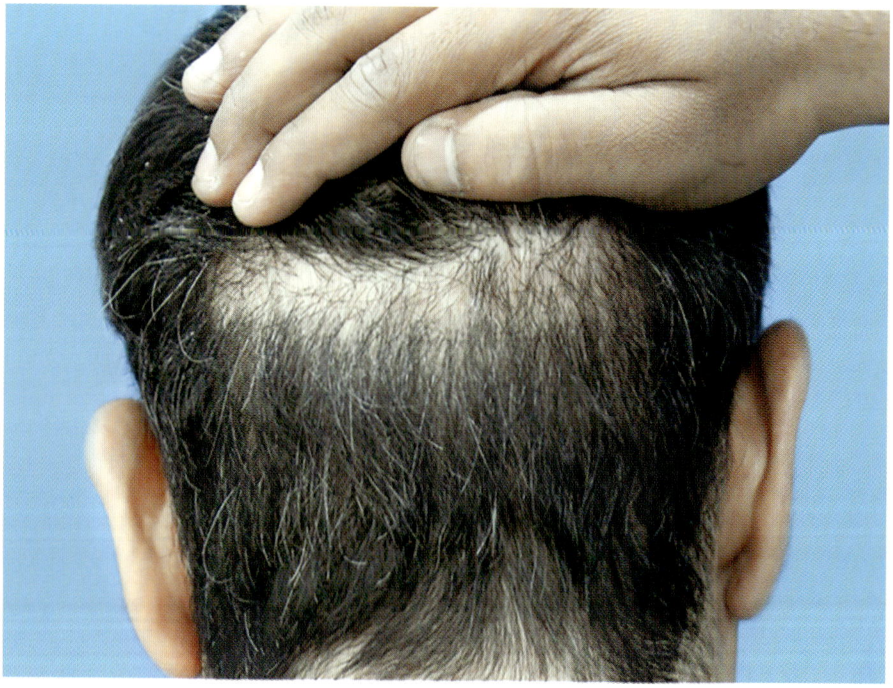

Figure 10.6

Further improvement is expected as it is photographed at 6th month following surgery.

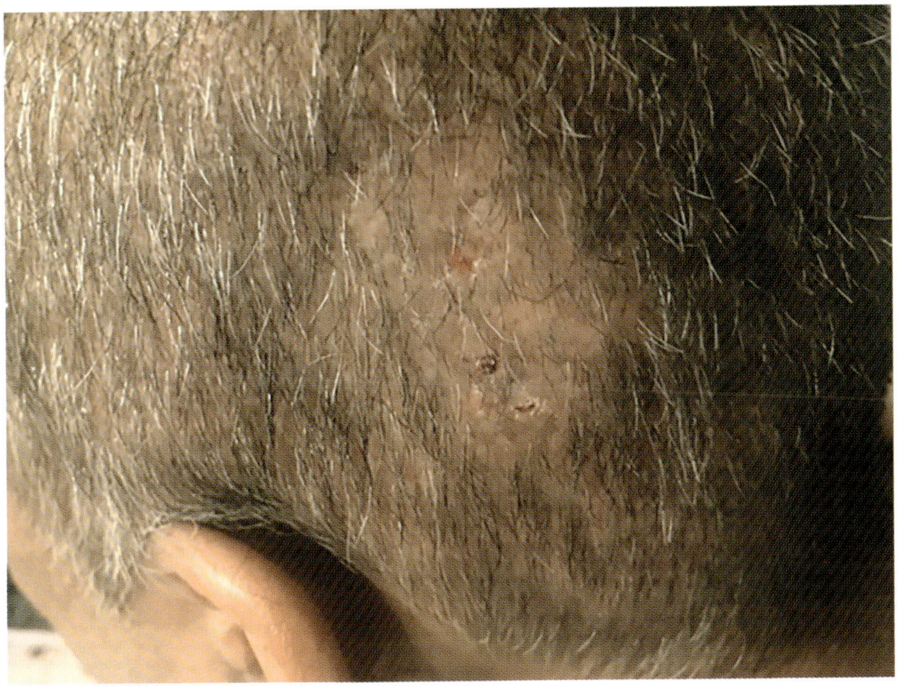

Figure 10.7

Donor region shock loss which recovered in 3 months. Shock loss in donor region is a rare phenomenon.

Hair loss can occur in recipient area when transplanting between native hair. It is an inevitable and normal process rather than a complication; occurring due to poor circulation associated with capillary damage after multiple needle insertions. It is the duty of doctor to counsel the patients that while this hair loss is usually temporary. Some of the hair may not regrow. Native hair that are miniaturized are most vulnerable to both shedding and failure to regrow. Daily intake of finasteride 1 mg along with micronutrient support, high protein diet and minoxidil may help in preserving those pre-existing hair.

NECROSIS

It happens in the donor region due to deep or too close punching during FUE surgery (Fig. 10.8). It can even happen in the recipient area during slit making when the needle or the CTS blade goes very deep and damages the blood vessels underneath it.

UNNATURAL HAIRLINE

Creating a natural hairline is an art to master and comes with experience. Certain mistakes like implanting 2 or 3 follicle grafts instead of 1 follicle graft on the anterior hairline and not breaking the hairline by creating the micro- and macroirregularities can give an unnatural appearance to the hairline (Figs. 10.9 to 10.11).

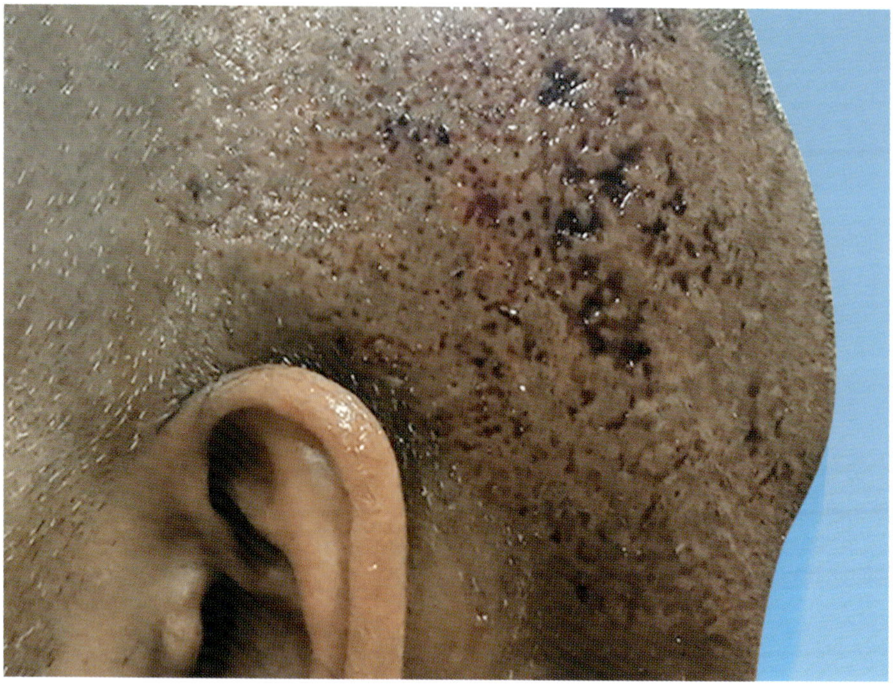

Figure 10.8

Donor necrosis at the punched site due to very close and deep punching.

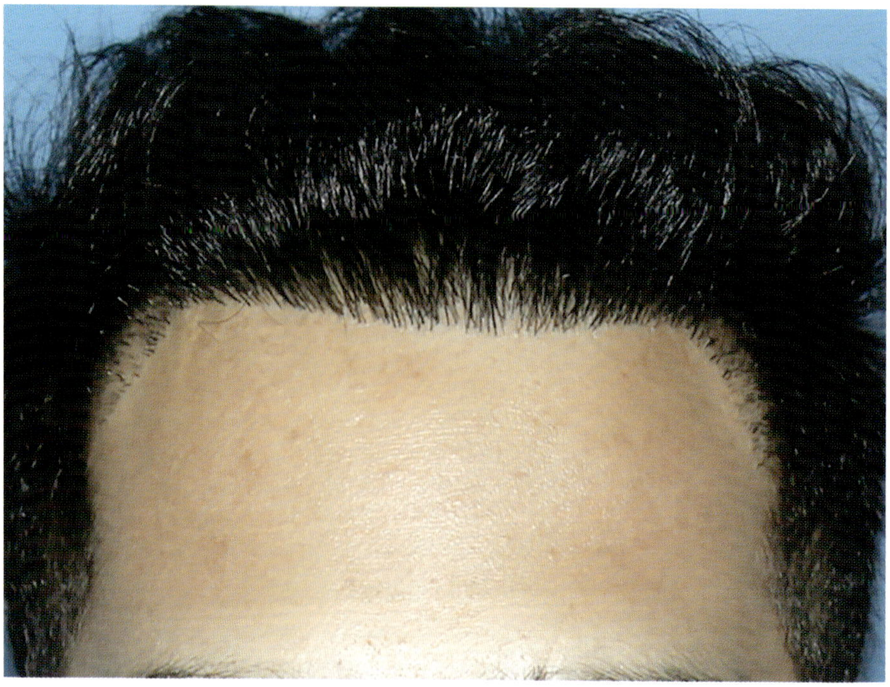

Figure 10.9

The hairline is absolutely sharp, totally symmetrical, with filled frontotemporal angles. There are no microirregularities. One should never create a hairline like this.

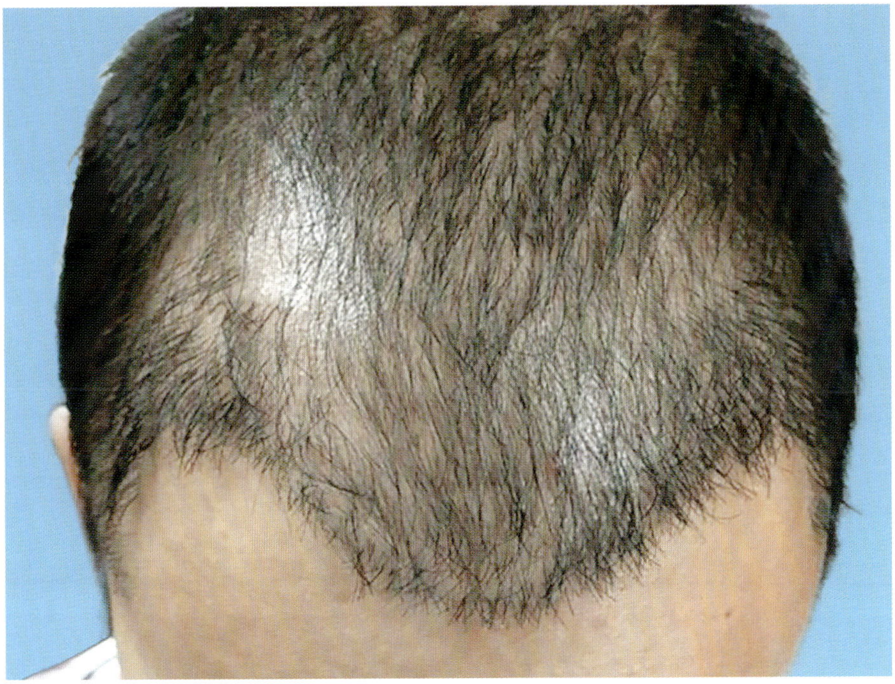

Figure 10.10

In this patient, surgeon planted hair in the hairline and extended the hairline by 1 cm. No effort was made to plant behind the hairline zone. The hairline which was created was not dense, does not merge with the surrounding hair, has wrong direction. The fronto-temporal angles were filled by the surgeon.

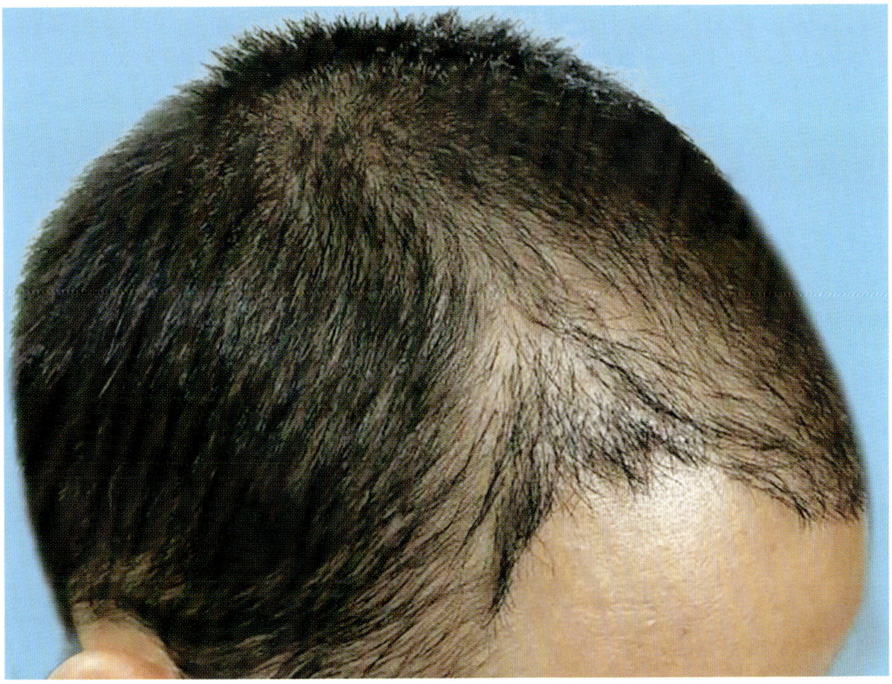

Figure 10.11

Filled frontotemporal angles making it a female hairline. The transplanted hair stand out and has not merged with the pre-existing hair.

POOR GROWTH OF THE TRANSPLANTED HAIR

The transplanted hair sometimes do not survive due to various reasons like: transection, over manipulation, oxygen deprivation, desiccation, etc. These problems can be corrected by doing the surgery with corneal loupes of high magnification to avoid mal-handling of the grafts and by following the direct hair transplantation (DHT) technique to ensure better survival of grafts.

In the upcoming example shown in Figures 10.12 and 10.13, there was hardly any growth after the failed follicular unit transplantation (FUT). We corrected his hairline as shown in Figure 10.13. The hair at frontotemporal angles still need to be removed by laser or through FUE.

PITTING

Pitting is defined as the depressed appearance of the grafts. It occurs if the grafts are placed too deep or if the slits are bigger than the grafts (Fig. 10.14).

TENTING

Tenting is defined as the elevated appearance of the grafts and occurs due to superficial placement of the grafts.

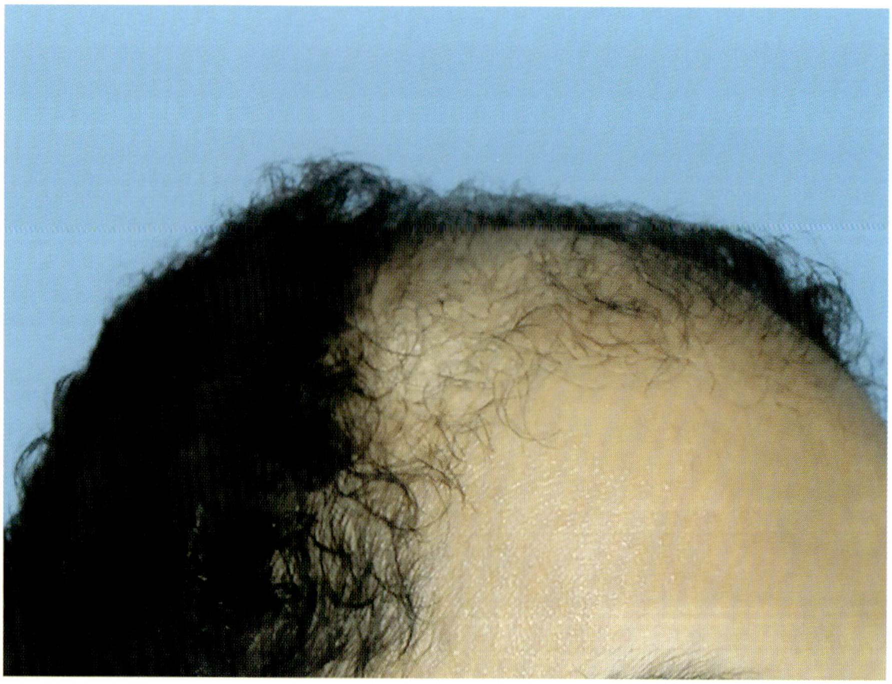

Figure 10.12

Virtually no growth after first hair restoration surgery.

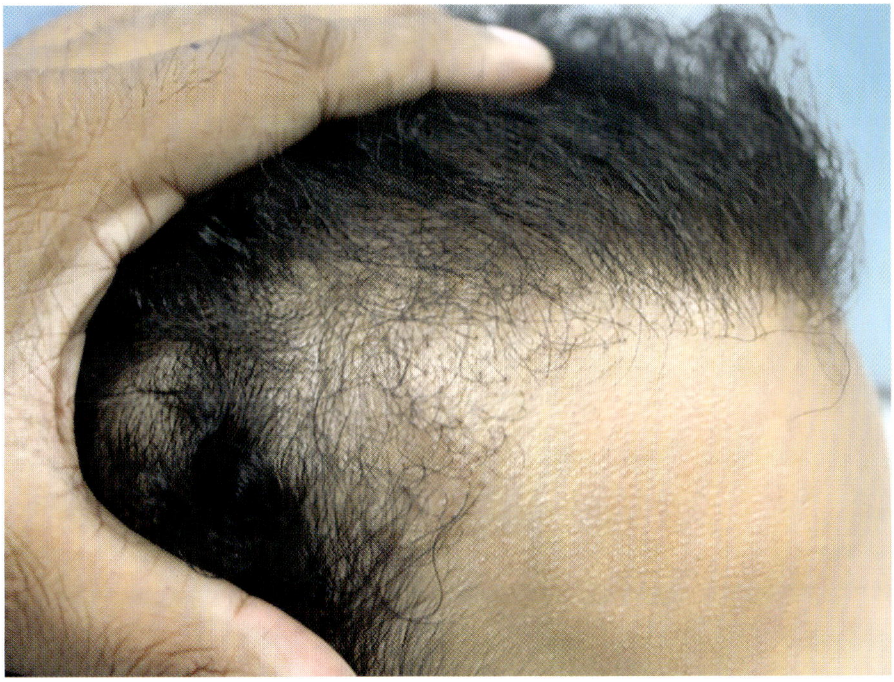

Figure 10.13

We used the hair of the failed restoration surgery in the hairline as sentinel hair to provide naturalness to the hairline. The hair in frontotemporal angles need to be removed by laser or FUE by a 0.8 mm sharp surrounded punch to thus ensuring minimum possible scar.

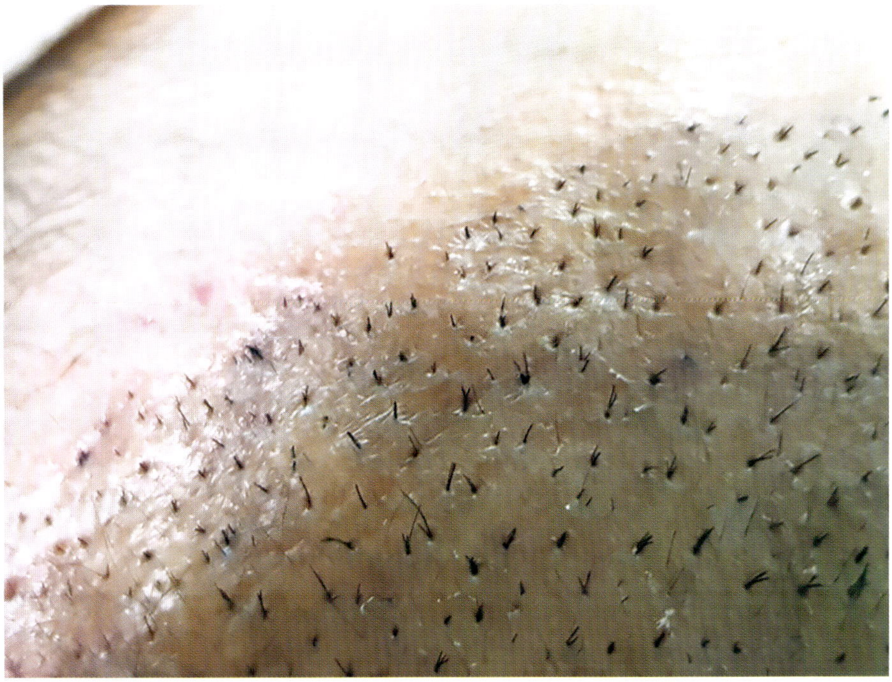

Figure 10.14

Pitting of grafts.

POOR DONOR AESTHETICS

Uneven extraction from the donor region can lead to visible difference in density of different region of scalp. During extraction of graft by FUE, the surgeon should keep in mind about the presence of FUT scar, any traumatic scar, presence of reverse thinning, presence of coronet, difference in donor density at temporal region and occipital region (Fig. 10.15).

HALO

A rim of hairless zone usually forms in patient who does not take finasteride after hair transplant (Fig. 10.16).

ABSENCE OF GROWTH OF HAIR OF ONE TYPE

We have observed in rare cases that beard grafts have failed to grow in a patient but scalp grafts have grown (Figs. 10.17 and 10.18).

CONCLUDING THOUGHTS

Complications can be predictable as well as nonpredictable. One should take the maximum possible precaution to avoid the possible complication but fear of complications should not tie a surgeon's hand.

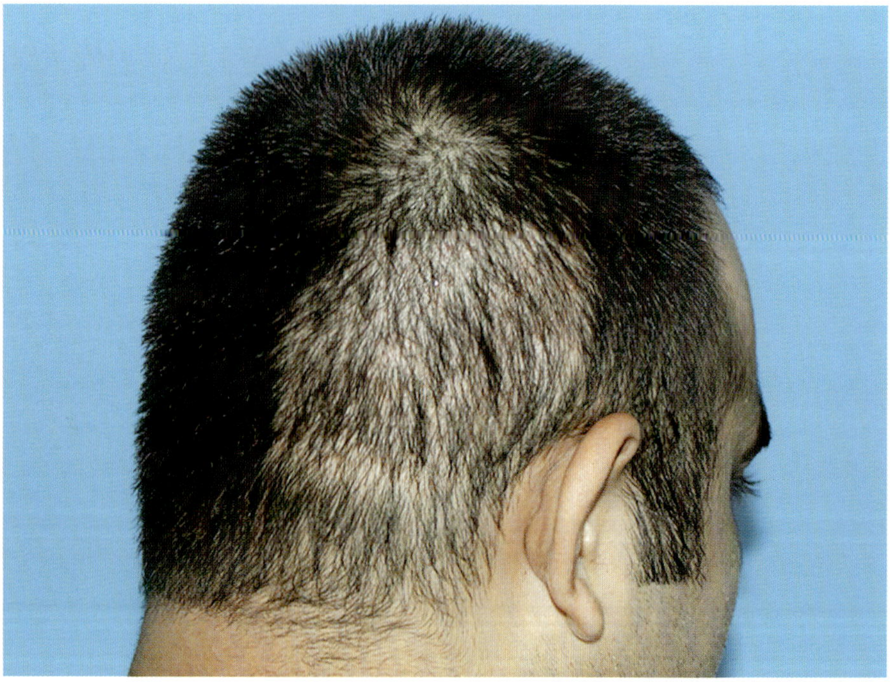

Figure 10.15

Moth eaten appearance due to excessive extraction from the one region of the scalp.

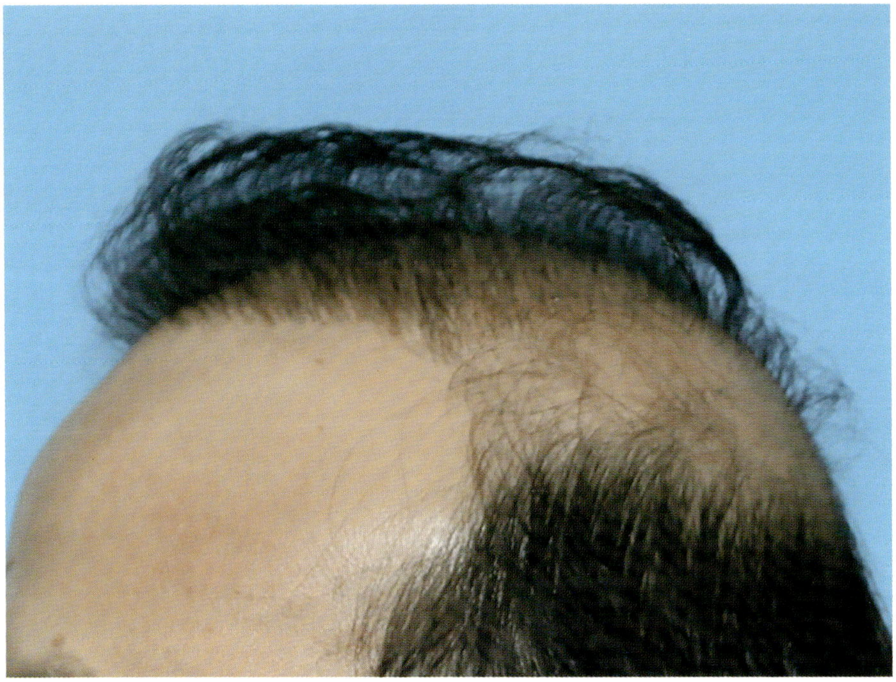

Figure 10.16

Note the recession of hair in the temporal region as baldness progressed from Norwood grade VI to Norwood grade VII. This created an island of hairless zone around the transplanted hair. Patients are advised to take finasteride lifelong to decrease the risk of progression of baldness.

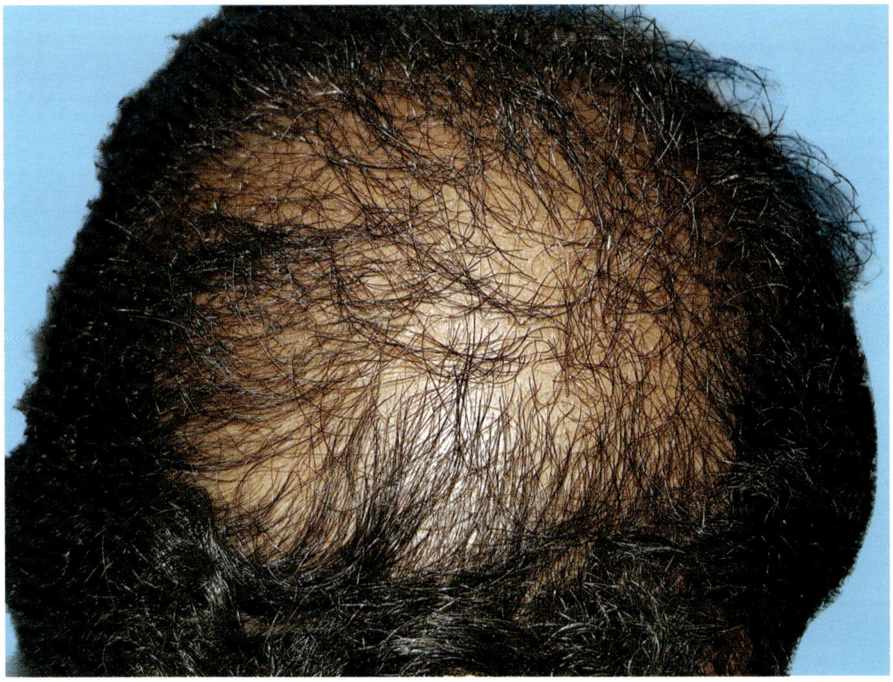

Figure 10.17

From the mid-scalp till the vertex transition point, we had planted beard grafts. The hairline and the crown were reconstructed with scalp grafts. The grafts at the hairline zone grew but most of the beard grafts failed to grow as seen in this picture. Probably it had to do with scoring with 0.75 mm punch resulting in grafts with minimal fat, trauma during extraction as they were more fragile compared to beard grafts in other patients and our poor graft handling of these beard grafts.

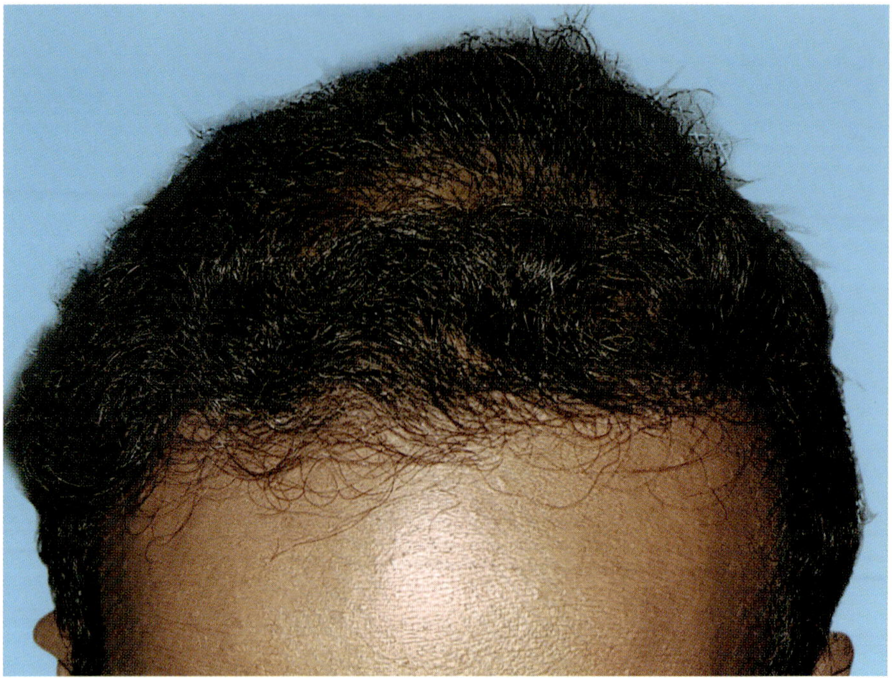

Figure 10.18

The same patient, in whom the beard grafts failed to grow in mid-scalp but as the hairline was made with scalp grafts, they grew perfectly in the most aesthetic way.

Comments by Dr Piero Tesauro

The iconography of this chapter is impressive. If someone had thought of this kind of surgery as an operation with little to no complications, he would have been disappointed.

"My grandfather was a peasant from the countryside. He owned corn fields in the middle of Italy. A part of which had been strenuously taken away by the slopes of the mountain. The land changed in that area and as the ascent began, stones of various sizes filled the harsh surfaces surrounded by the roots of the trees.

Every crop in that area was a gamble.

My grandfather spent weeks preparing and farming the land. He ploughed the fields carefully and hand planted every seed carefully at the same distance one after the other. Then he waited.

At the beginning of spring, when the first crops started to come out, he would run out every morning before coffee, to make sure they had all survived the cold night.

Some years he would just plough the land without planting any crops, he knew it was not ready yet, it needed time to rest.

My grandfather achieved many good harvests over the years, but despite his commitment and the care he put in each one, he still had some less fruitful years."

I think that hair restoration surgery has many similarities with my grandfather's story. A good and dedicated surgeon can achieve many good results, but this does not make him immune from bad outcomes. For this reason, every experienced surgeon knows better than to say "transplanted follicles will last forever" because their destiny is not always the same (Table 10.2).

Many of the complications highlighted in the chapter can worry a surgeon who is just beginning, but at the same time it is very clear what to avoid and how to deal with many of the problems shown.

Year after year, they will become more cautious, growing confident in their technical skills they will realize that the most frequent complications today are due to two main factors, that have surprisingly very little to do with the technique itself.

1. The first and most striking one is related to poor consultation. It has already been said in Chapter 1 that we must take into account the patient's history of hair loss and yet this is often overlooked. Since a picture is worth more than thousand words here is an example for you to judge (Figs. 10.19 to 10.21).
   In this specific case, the patient came back to my practice worried about the aggressive operation he had undergone. This over-harvested donor area in fact, leaves him without many possibilities to face his progressive hair loss in the future.
2. The second reason of many complications and bad results is related to some common pitfalls in communication that I tried to group briefly in Table 10.3. "What goes around comes around" "as you sow, so shall you reap is the meaning of this chapter. So far remember, the basic law of cause and effect works in hair transplantation like in any other field.
   A personal thank you to my friend and colleague Dr Pradeep Sethi for requesting my comment in this book.

Table 10.2: Transplanted follicles destiny.

Stable	Transplanted follicles will grow old following the natural aging of the donor area
Stable + therapy	Transplanted follicles tend to miniaturize earlier without therapy
Unstable	Transplanted follicles miniaturize over time

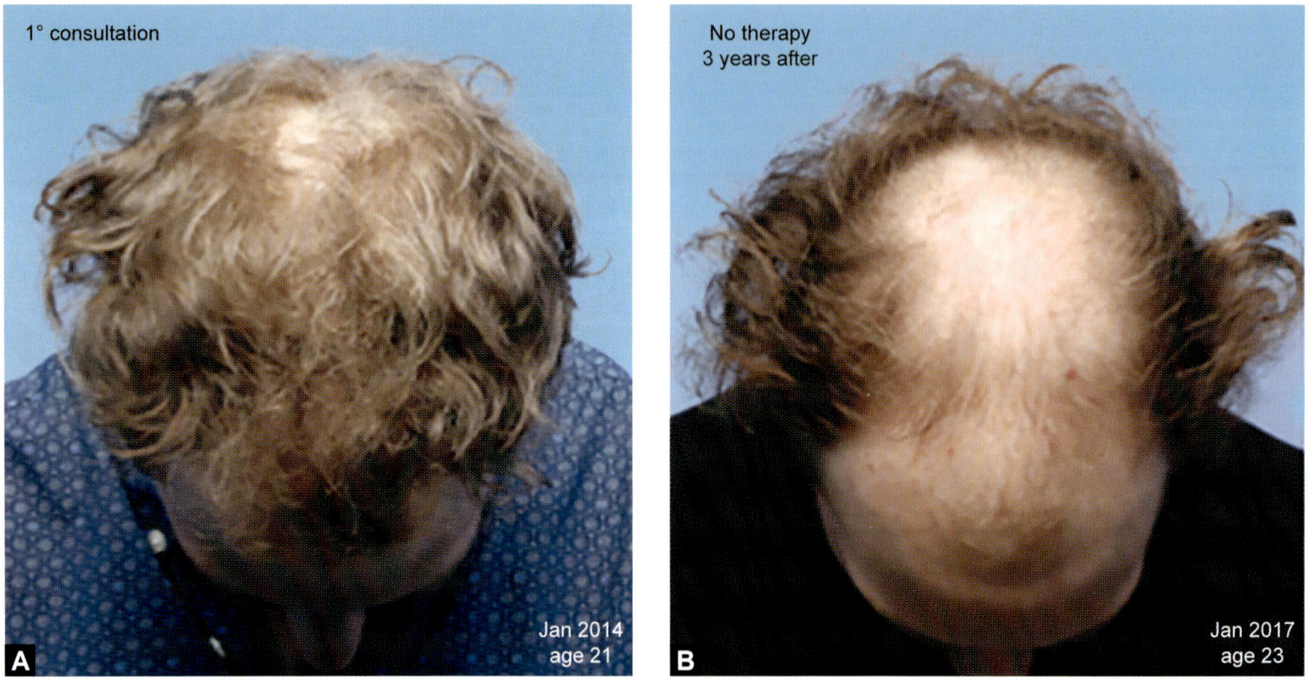

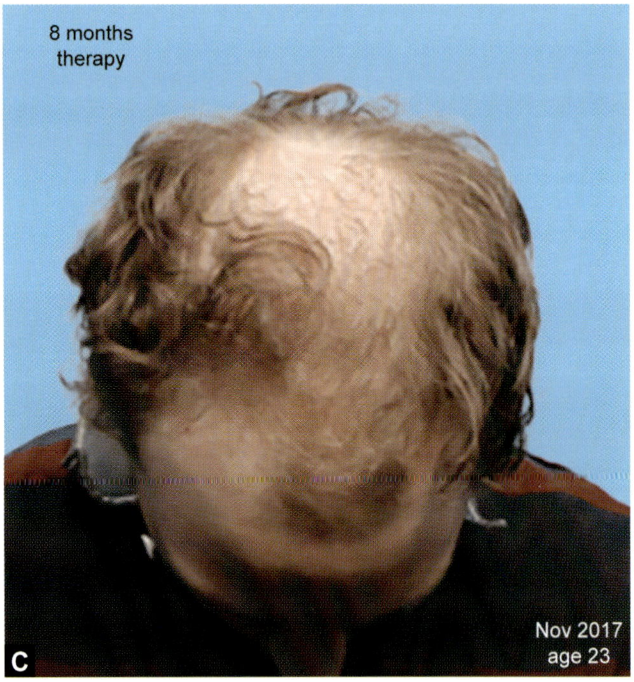

Figures 10.19A to C

My plan was to wait more years, then make a clear evaluation of therapy stabilization, and then consider whether to perform a conservative hair transplantation.

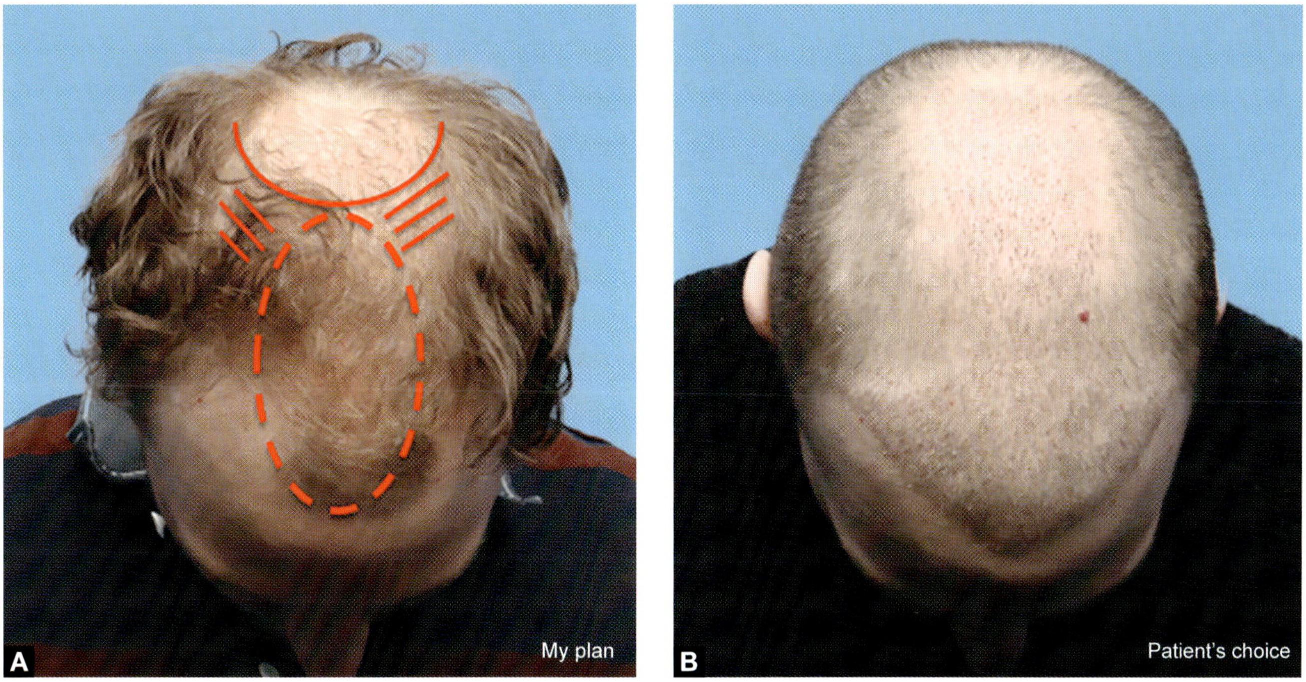

Figures 10.20A and B

(A) My plan has gone unheard; (B) The patient decided not to wait and he did 3,300 follicular units (FUs) in another clinic with no prior consultation.

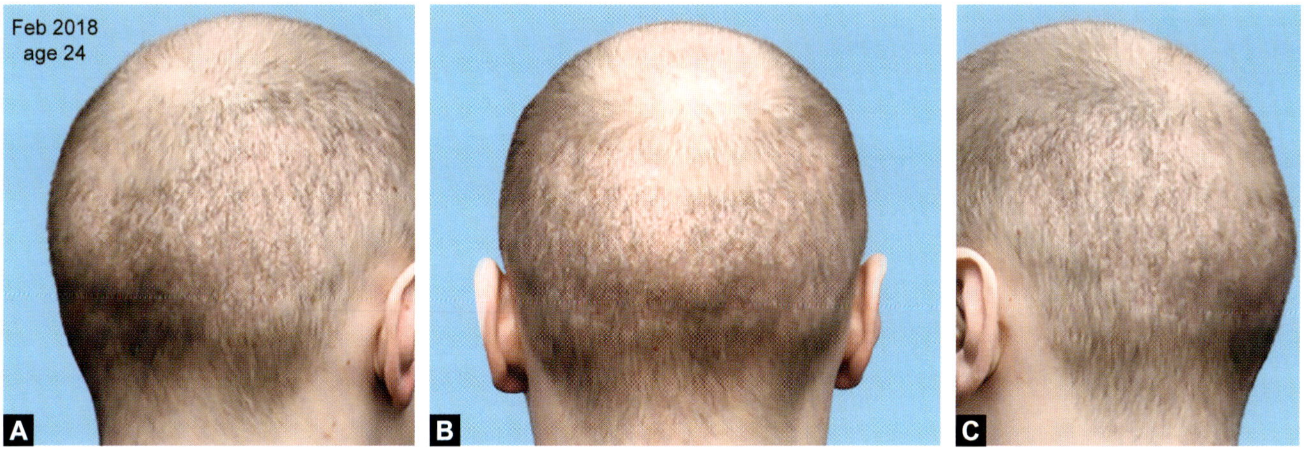

Figures 10.21A to C

Will this patient be happy in the future? How much donor still exists?

Table 10.3: Communication pitfalls.

Social media-Doctor Social media-Patient	The influence of social media must be frequently disempowered because it heightens the expectations and encourages aggressive plans
Doctor-Patient	A good result will be obtained when both the doctor and the patient, clearly understand their own responsibilities
Doctor-Surgical team Surgical team-One another	Appropriate knowledge, intense training, structured communication and clear understanding of each others' responsibilities make the perfect staff

SUMMARY

- Complications though rare can happen to the best of the surgeons but they are often always avoidable with proper precautions as well as patient education.
- Both medical as well as aesthetic complications are to be taken care of seriously whether or not it affects the final outcome.

CHAPTER 11

Corrective Hair Transplant

Pradeep Sethi, Arika Bansal, Abhinav Kumar

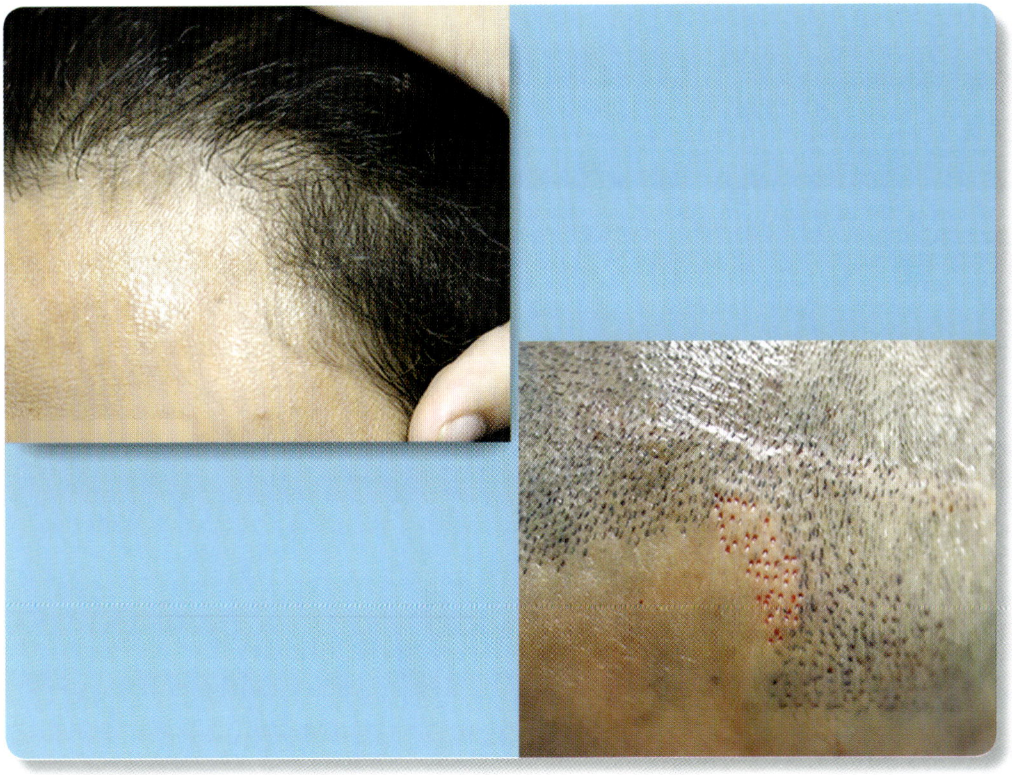

Correction of frontotemporal angle (FTA) and temple.
Top image: Pre-existing angles.
Bottom image: Pre-made slits for correcting FTA and temple. The holes depict the extracted grafts.
"Do no harm", the first principle of medical science! Once the hair is grown it is permanent! Wrongly positioned and grown hair give unaesthetic looks as well as more mental agony! It takes a mammoth task and sometimes not possible to correct the wrongly done procedure. Do it once, do it right!

INTRODUCTION

With the rising popularity of hair restoration surgery in India, a large number of people are undergoing hair restoration surgery. The numbers of trained surgeons who can perform quality hair transplant are limited but due to its huge demand, a number of clinics and hospitals are seeking professionals who have some experience in hair transplantation. Designing the hairline and transplanting hair by such inexperienced doctors often lead to poor results. Such patients who are unsatisfied by their prior hair transplant then seek experienced professionals for corrective surgery.

There are several issues in patients who need corrective hair transplant. Firstly, the donor area is compromised excessively as a result of first surgery. Over extraction is usually done from the scalp as role of beard is never taken into consideration by inexperienced hair transplant surgeons. There may be a previous surgery follicular unit transplantation (FUT) scar, restricting the area immediately above the FUT scar for extraction in view of the scar becoming visible. There is pulling of the neighboring hair due to the fibrosis which occurs secondary to punching. In the recipient area, the grafts could have been placed at wrong sites which results in a very low mid-frontal point and a flat hairline. The frontotemporal angle may be obliterated and might need correction. The angle and direction of the transplanted hair may be wrong. There may be hypertrophic FUT scar or multiple FUT scar and rounded punch scars by the previous surgery. Also, there can be scarring and fibrosis in recipient zone due to previous failed implantation. Virtually no growth at recipient sites may be possible in inexperienced hands. Lastly, a patient may refuse to take oral finasteride resulting in progression of baldness thus needing corrective surgery after few years. Some patients may not be able to achieve transformation through hair transplantation alone, scalp micropigmentation offers meaningful additional technique to normalize the appearance.

We present a series of cases where corrective hair transplant has been done.

CASE 1

Issues

He was a 26-year-old male with Norwood grade VI baldness, with a dolichocephalic like head and a dense donor area. He underwent a hair transplant surgery of 3,000 grafts, however resulted in virtually growth of only 500 donor hair (Figs. 11.1 and 11.2). He approached us for corrective surgery. He now had a compromised donor area but was lucky to have good and dense beard, however they were curly. He was also willing to take finasteride (Figs. 11.3 to 11.6).

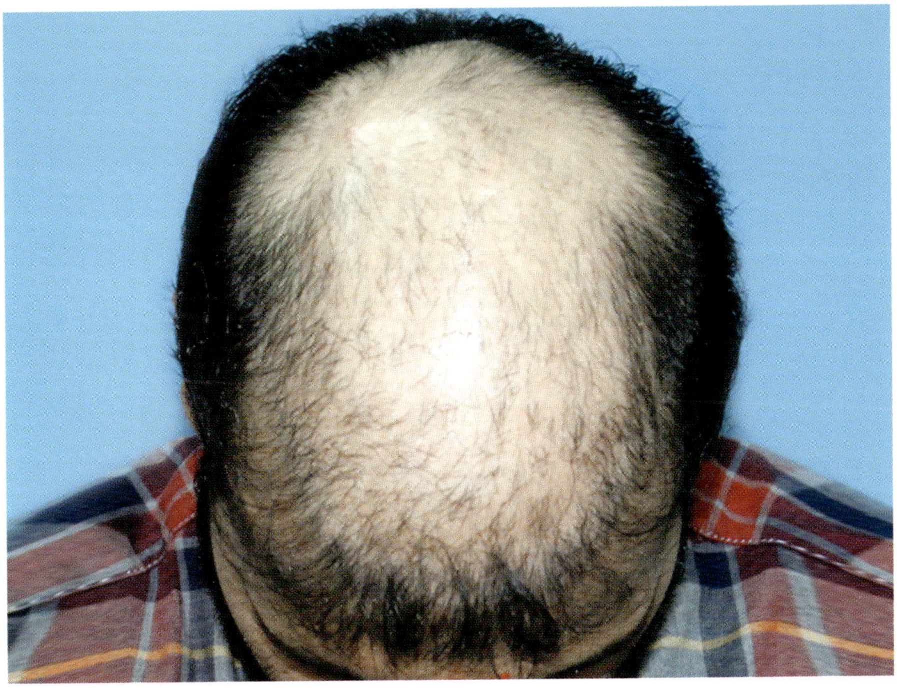

Figure 11.1

Depicting the failed previous hair transplant surgery showing the growth of not more than 500 grafts out of 2000 grafts in the front. This patient came to us for corrective surgery.

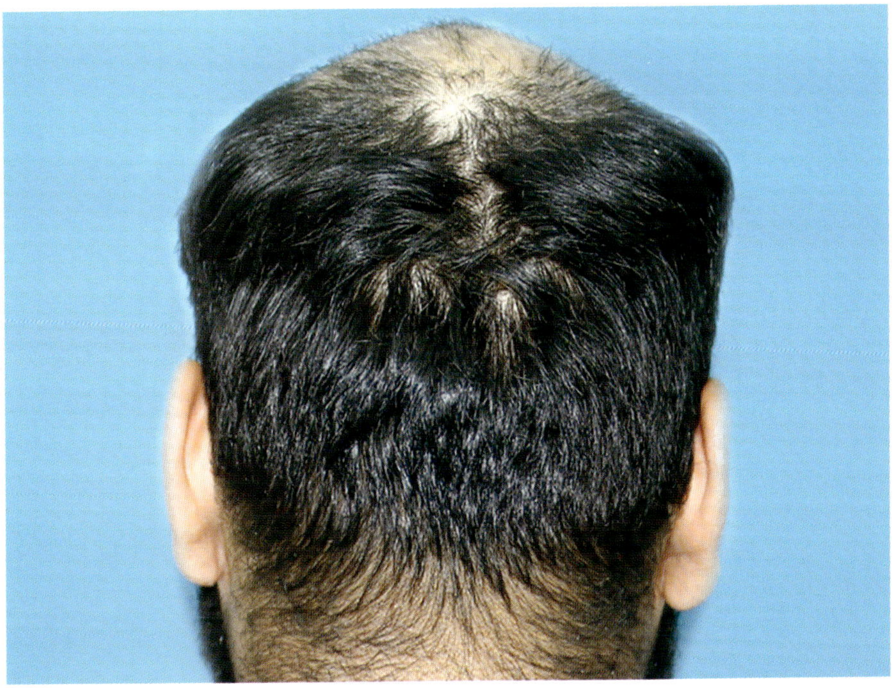

Figure 11.2

Note the reverse thinning at the lower part of occipital region. Donor hair should not be extracted from such site.

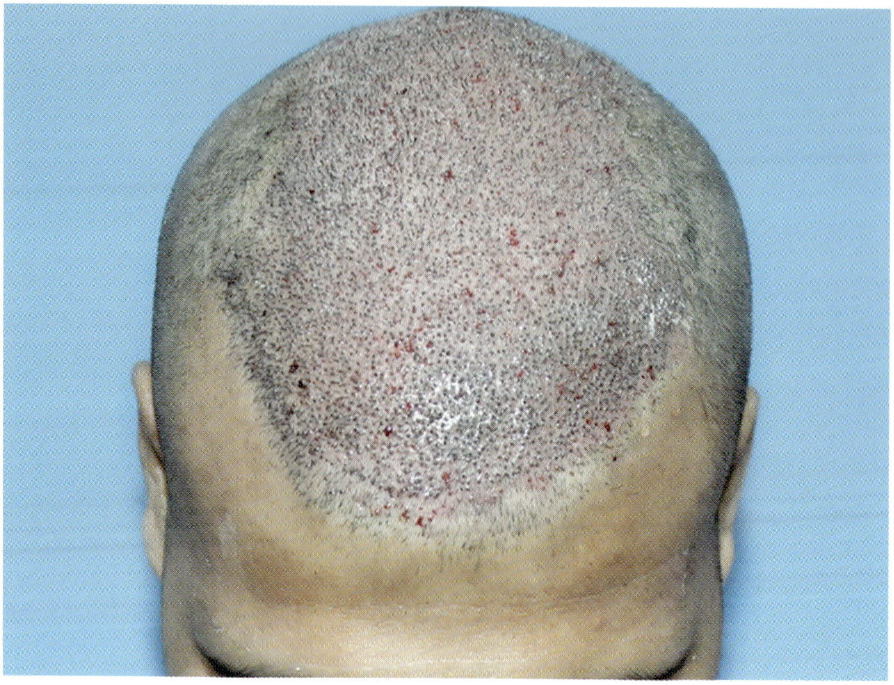

Figure 11.3

Corrective hair transplant was performed with 5,100 grafts (2,500 scalp grafts plus 2,600 beard grafts). We used the scalp grafts to improve the hairline by making a rectangular hairline which fits his face. We filled the scalp with beard grafts, leaving a small part of the crown.

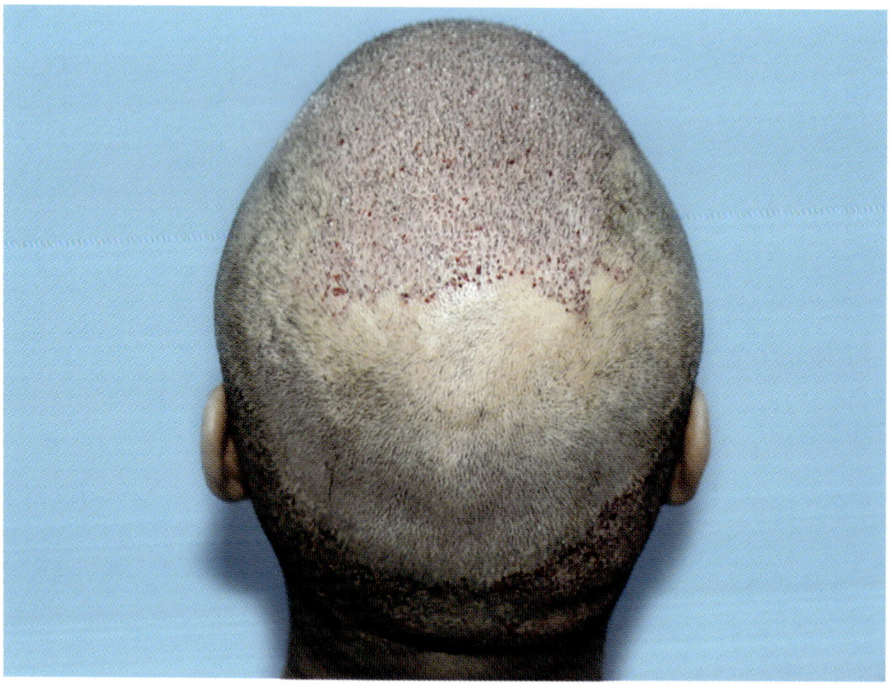

Figure 11.4

A part of crown was left untouched since it needs purely scalp hair and not beard hair. After extracting 3,000 grafts from a dolichocephalic head thus having a compromised donor, no further extraction was possible from safe donor region.

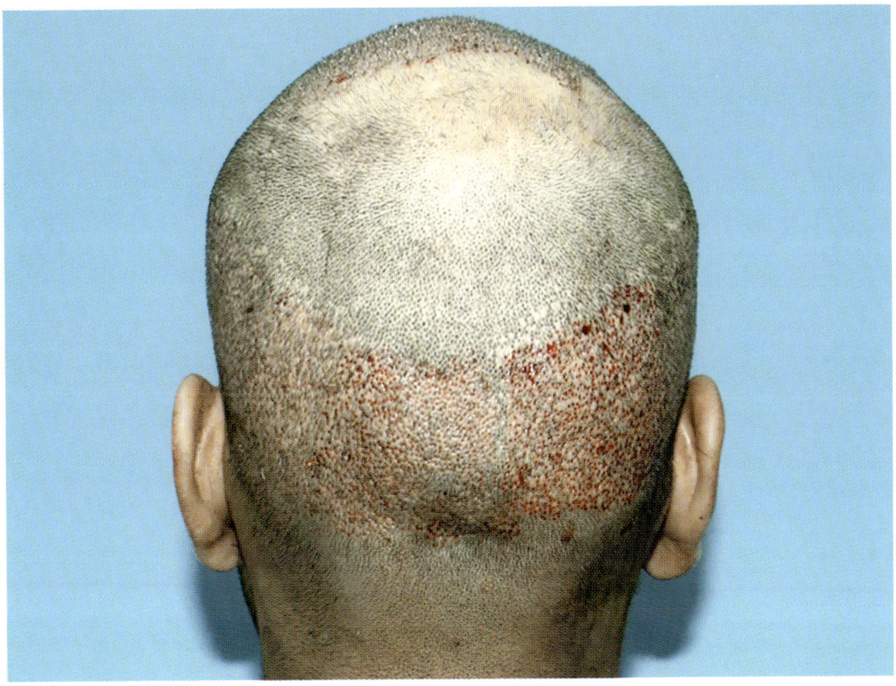

Figure 11.5

The appearance of scalp immediately after extraction. Note no extraction has been done from the region of reverse thinning. Sharp serrounded 0.9 mm follicular unit excision (FUE) punch was used for extraction. Note the pre-existing FUE scars.

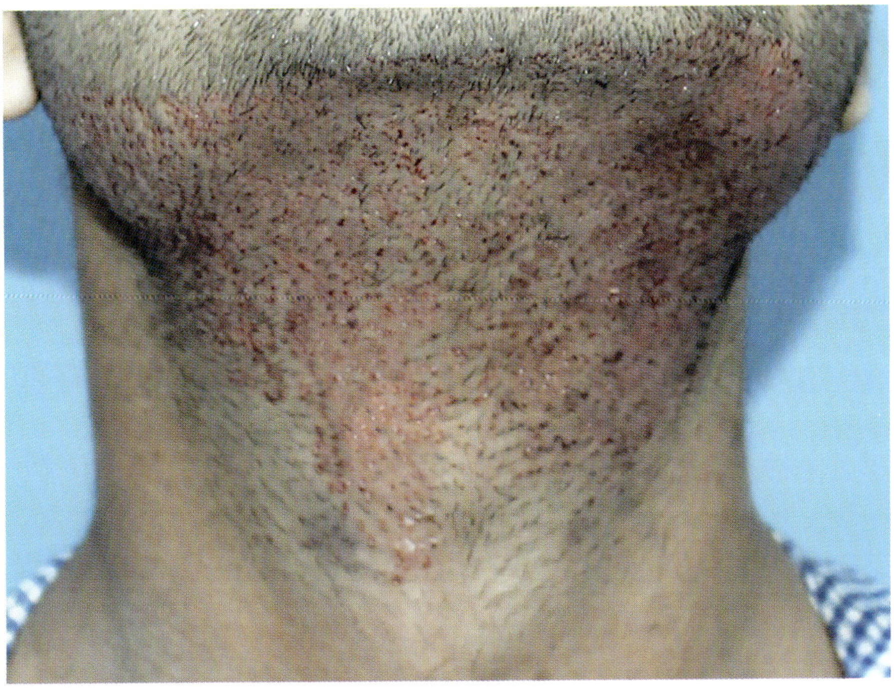

Figure 11.6

The appearance of beard area after extraction of 2,600 grafts. We used 0.8 mm sharp serrounded punch. Extraction was done from the shadow region of the face and extended the extraction up to the jaw line.

Results (Figs. 11.7 and 11.8)

After just 4 months, significant growth was visible which dramatically changed the patient's look. Further improvement of density by up to 30% is still expected.

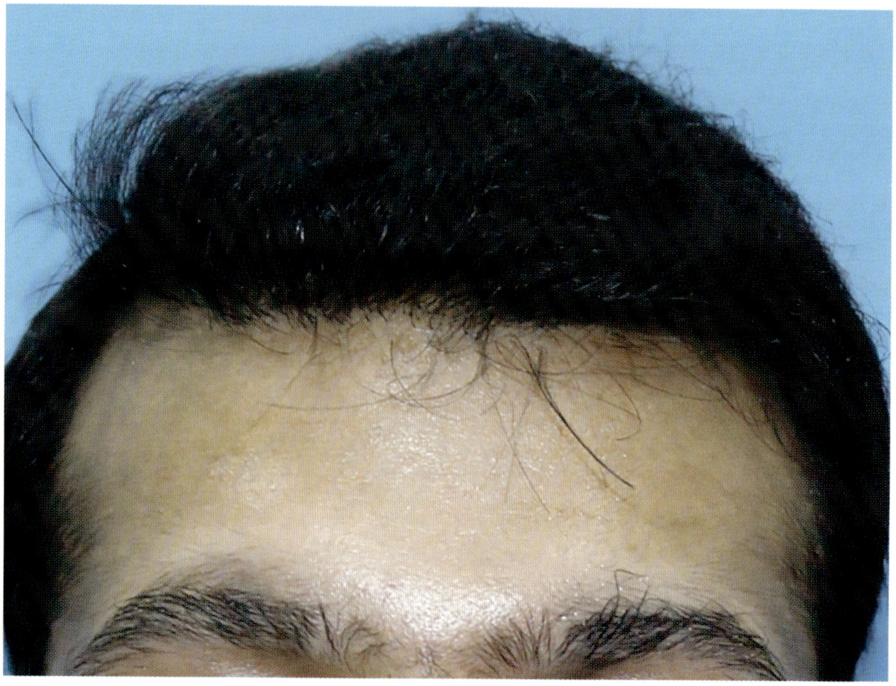

Figure 11.7

Note the improve aesthetics of hairline. The hairline is dense, fits the face. The hairline is nonsharp and shows micro-irregularities and has natural fall.

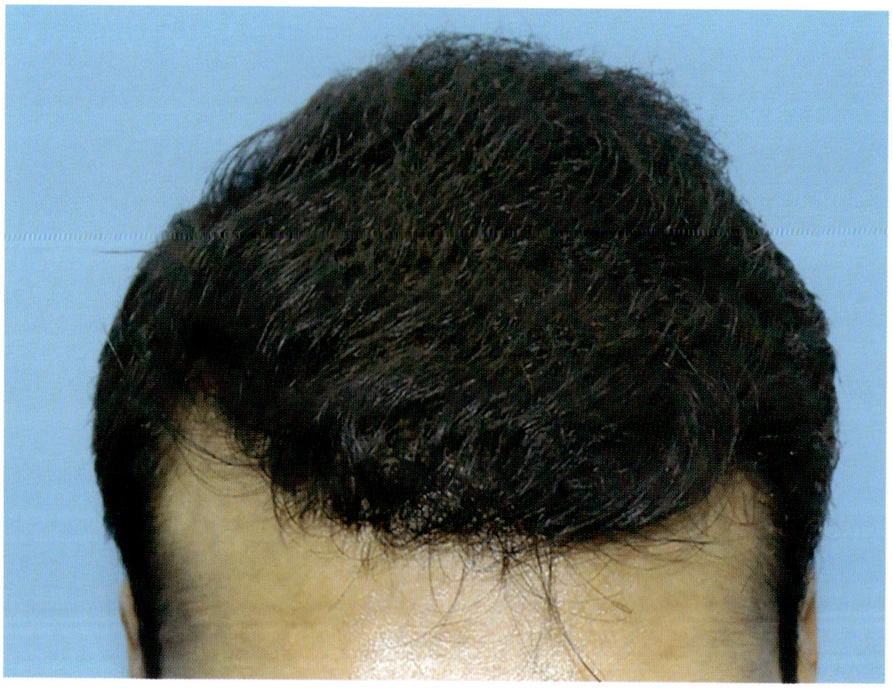

Figure 11.8

Six-month postoperative picture. The central part of the scalp was implanted with beard grafts while the frontal zone and a part of crown were filled with scalp grafts. The beard, despite being curly did not look out of place since it was placed in mid-scalp over a small area.

CASE 2

Issues

A middle aged man with Norwood grade VI baldness and a brachycephalic like head had undergone punch grafting for hair restoration leading to severely compromised scalp donor. He now demanded an aggressive hairline with good hair density. He had a good beard as donor area (Figs. 11.9 to 11.14).

Results

The results have been shown in Figures 11.15 to 11.17.

CASE 3

Issues

A 30-year-old male with dolichocephalic like head, had got hair transplant done by FUT method. He had a wrong hairline (Figs. 11.18 to 11.23).

Results

The results after 9 months have been shown in Figures 11.24 to 11.27.

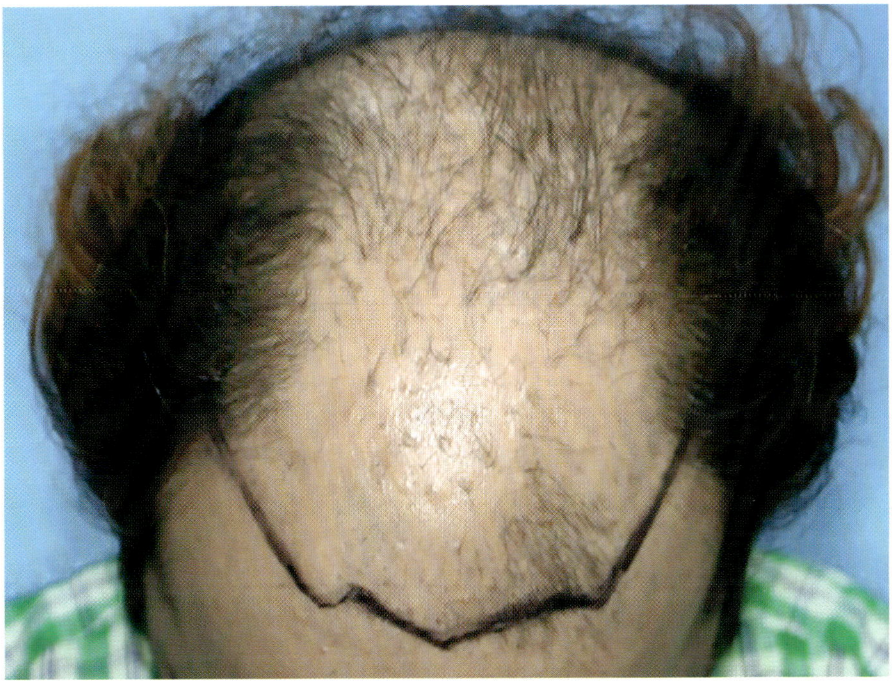

Figure 11.9

A 40-year-old man with previous scars of punch grafting at donor as well as recipient sites, having Norwood grade VI baldness presented to us. We drew a semi-aggressive three peaked rectangular hairline which matched his facial structure. The hairline was 7.5 cm from the glabella. The patient's donor density was good in spite of terrible looking punch scars.

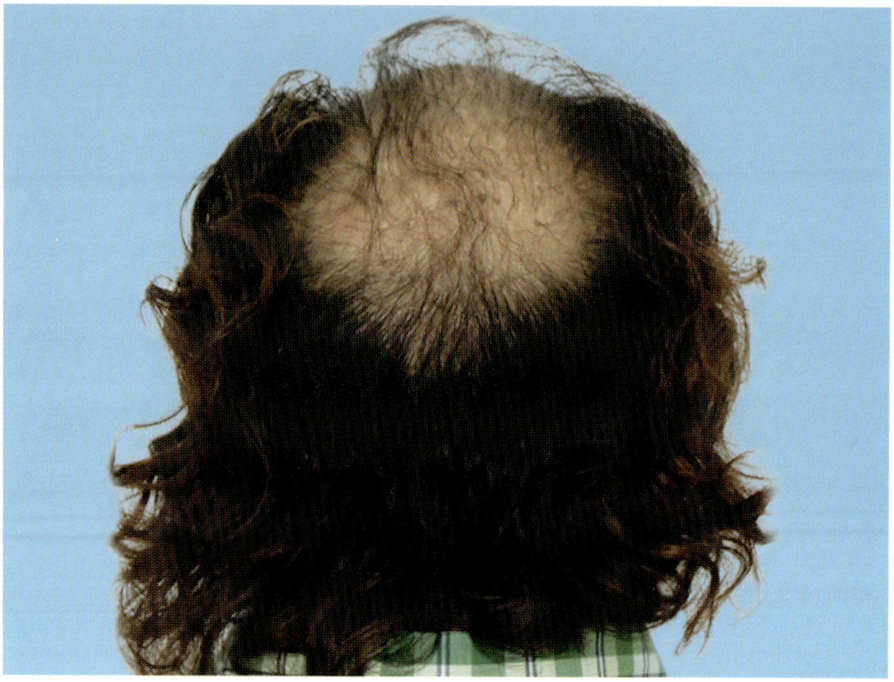

Figure 11.10

The donor region seemed fine until we trimmed those long hair. Crown was sparse and visible.

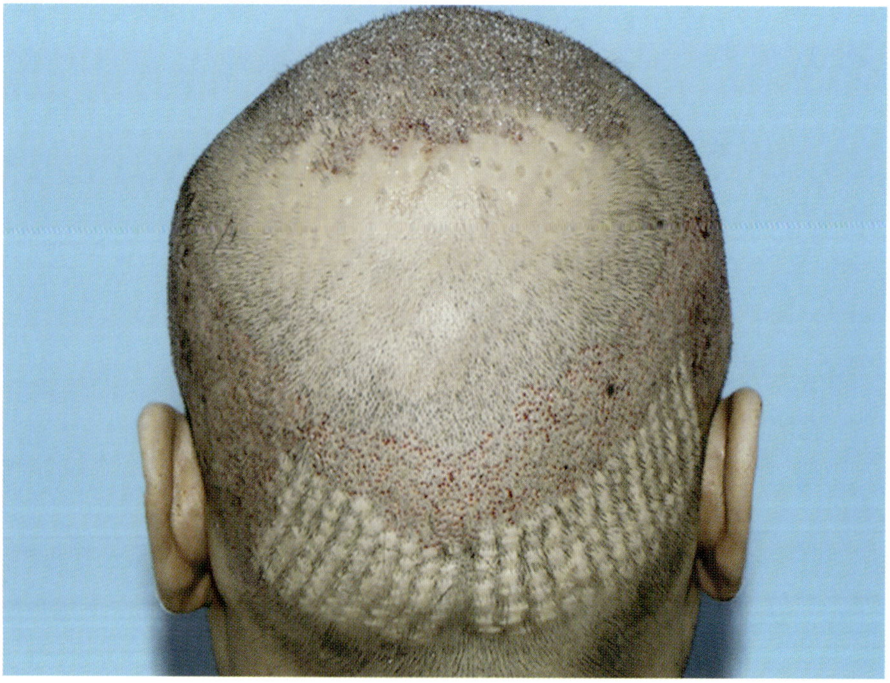

Figure 11.11

Since massive scars of previous punch grafting were present, extraction was only possible from the temporal region and the region above scars. The region below the punched scars showed reverse thinning, hence they were spared. No extraction was done in between those punched scars. There was a risk of breaching the safe donor zone if we went above the punched scars but patient promised to take finasteride lifelong and the family history of extreme baldness was absent. We extracted around 1,800 grafts from the back with sharp serrated 0.9 mm punch.

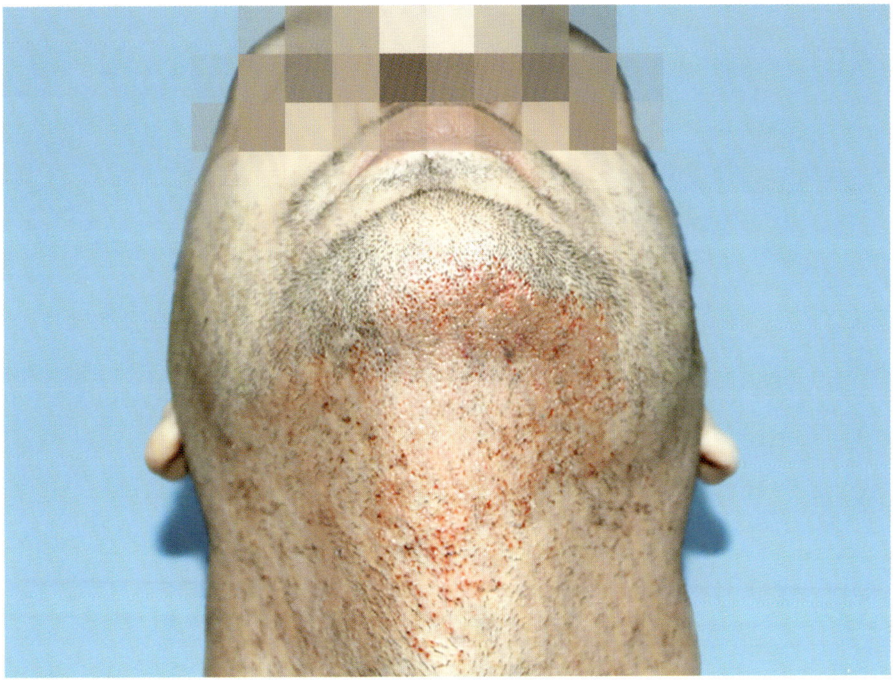

Figure 11.12

We almost took his entire beard from the shadow region of the face below the jaw line. Patient never desired to have the beard. Total number of grafts extracted from beard were 2,800.

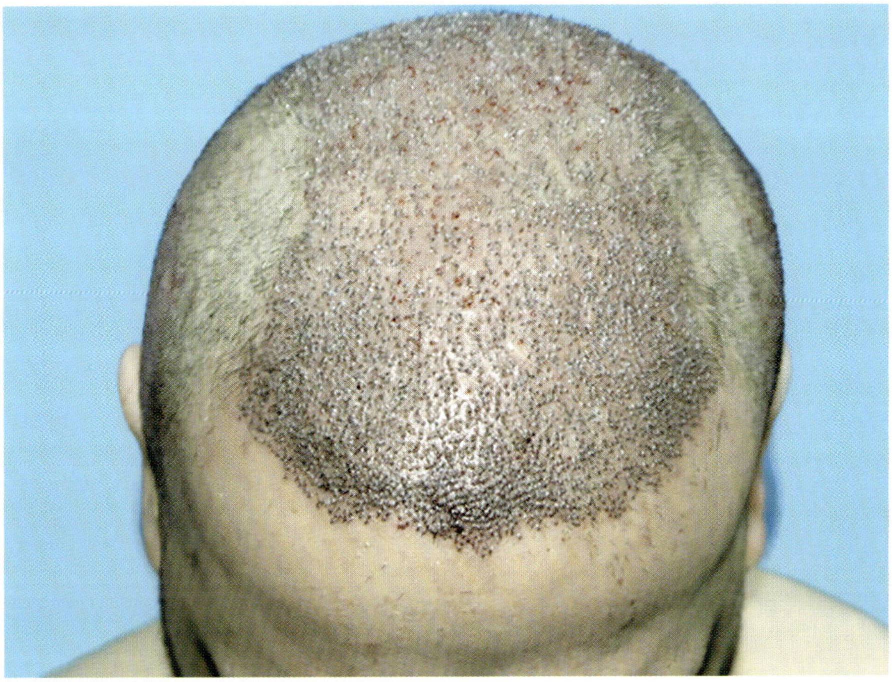

Figure 11.13

A total of around 4,300 grafts were implanted having maximum density at the hairline zone and graded decrease in density as one proceeded toward the crown. Beard was implanted in mid-scalp.

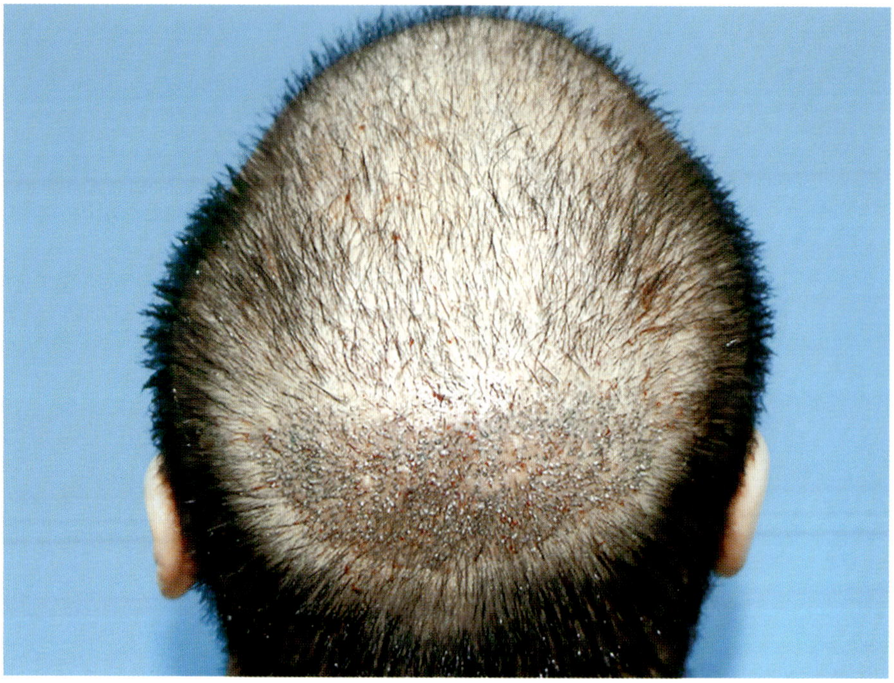

Figure 11.14

After 2 months, another session of around 1,000 grafts was performed to partially cover the crown.

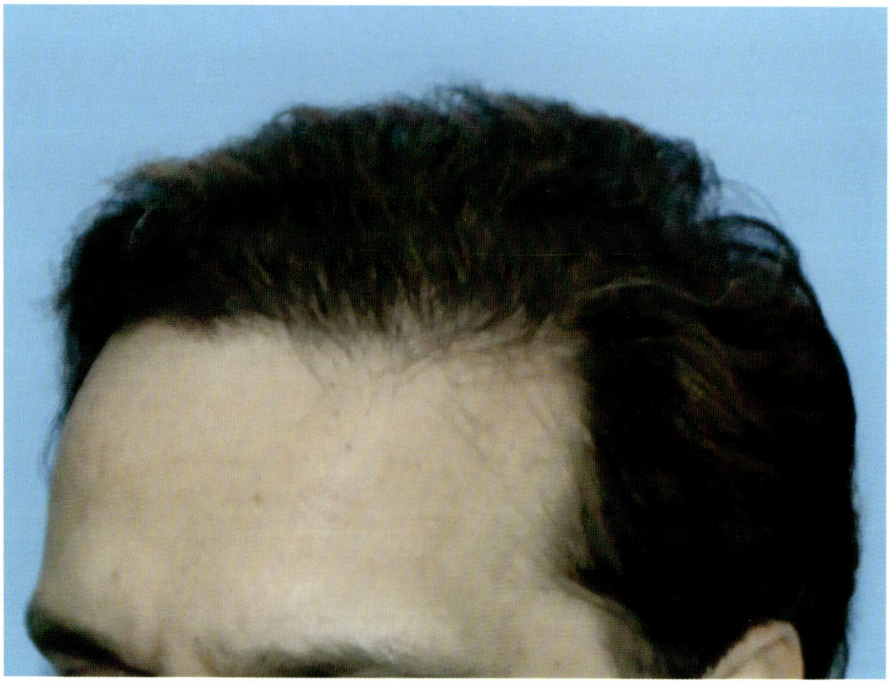

Figure 11.15

After 7 months, one can see an aesthetically designed hairline with no see through effect.

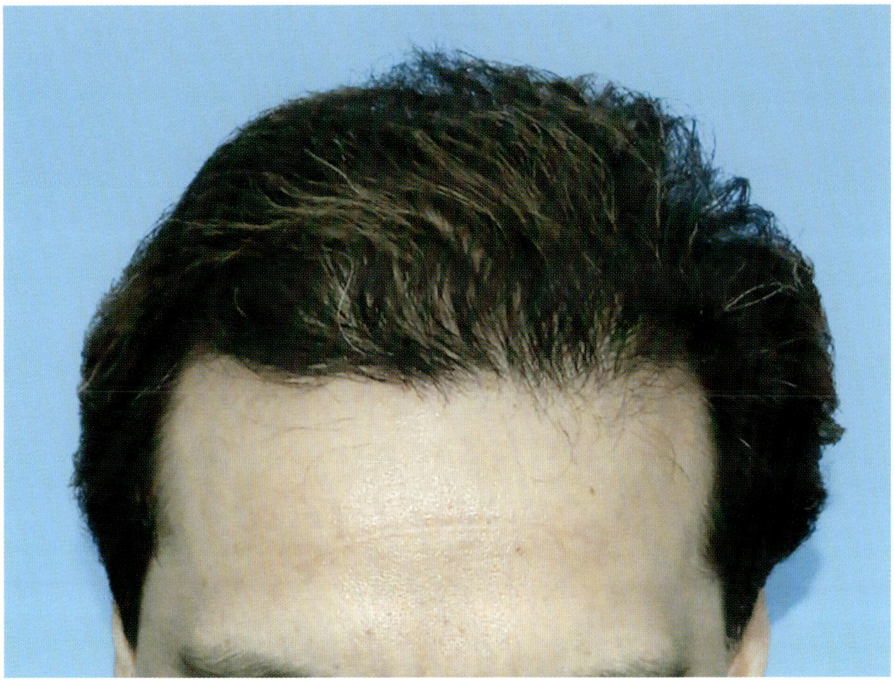

Figure 11.16

The density in the mid-scalp is equally good. The hairline is asymmetrically designed as seen from the sketched hairline, has three peaks, has micro- as well as macroirregularities.

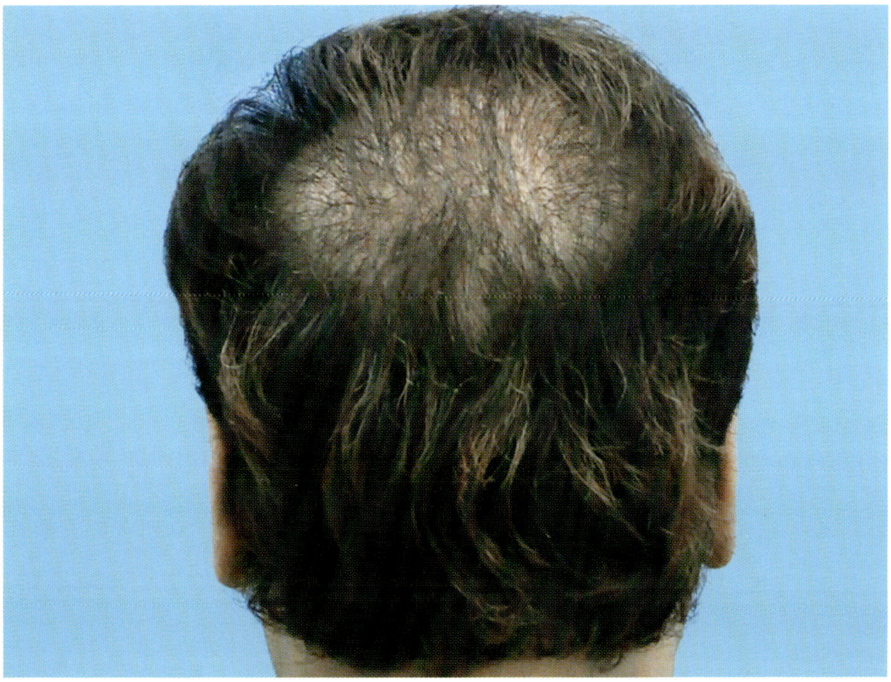

Figure 11.17

Donor aesthetics is preserved after extraction. We have fanned the thousand grafts over the crown to minimize the "see through" effect.

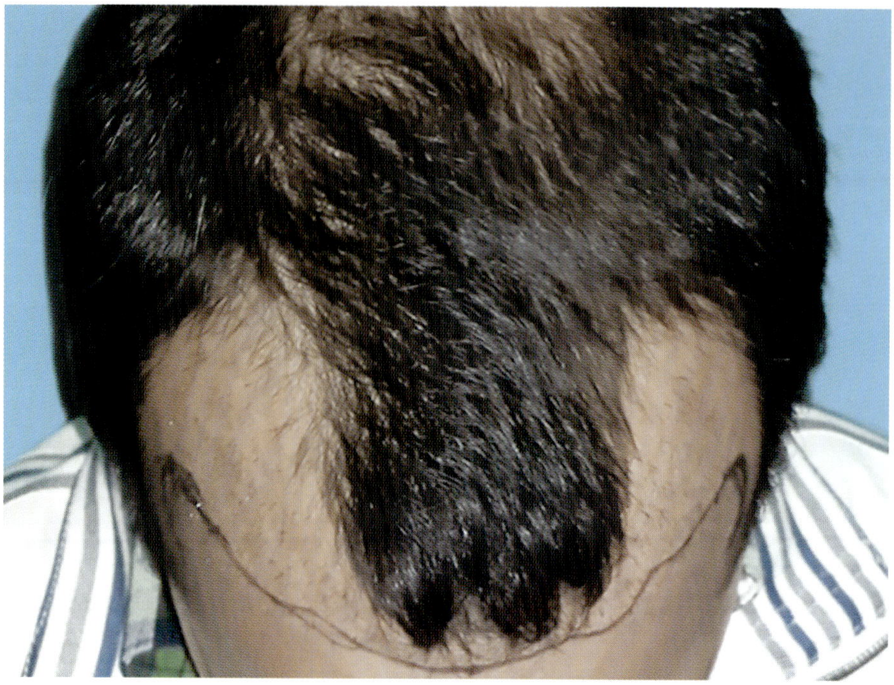

Figure 11.18

Patient got follicular unit transplantation (FUT) done for hairline restoration with poor growth of the transplanted hair.

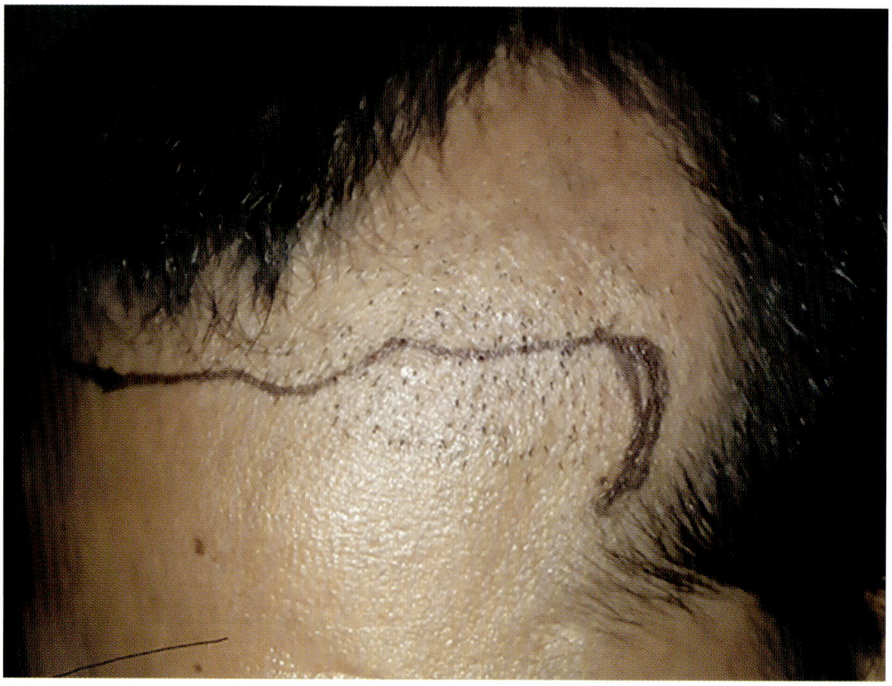

Figure 11.19

We redesigned the hairline. Note the poor growth of the previous transplanted hair, obliteration of frontotemporal angle and sparse growth behind the hairline zone. Patient was so unsatisfied with the results that he kept those hair shaved.

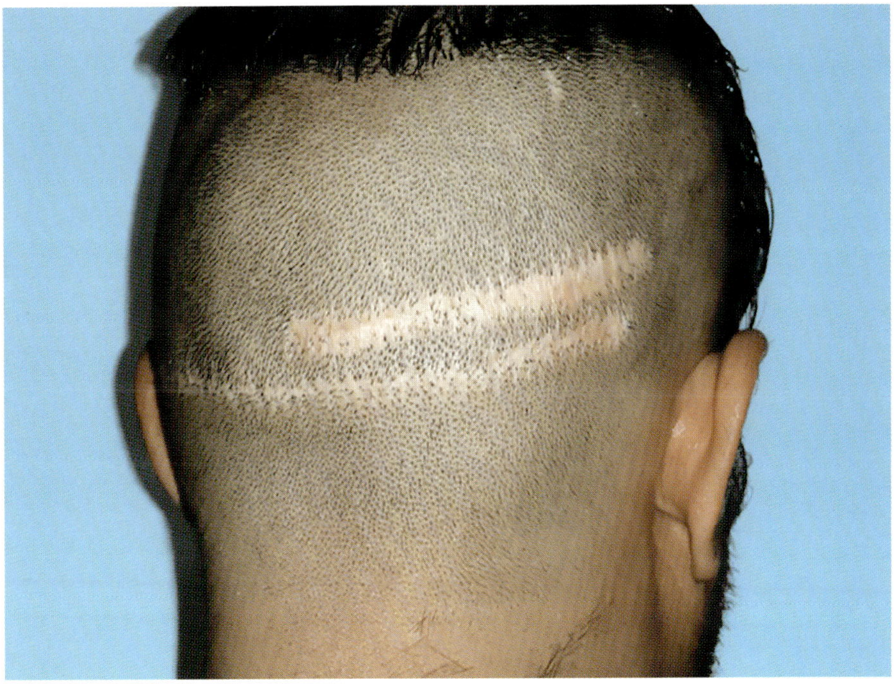

Figure 11.20

He had two follicular unit transplantation (FUT) scars as well. Note the width of the upper FUT scar.

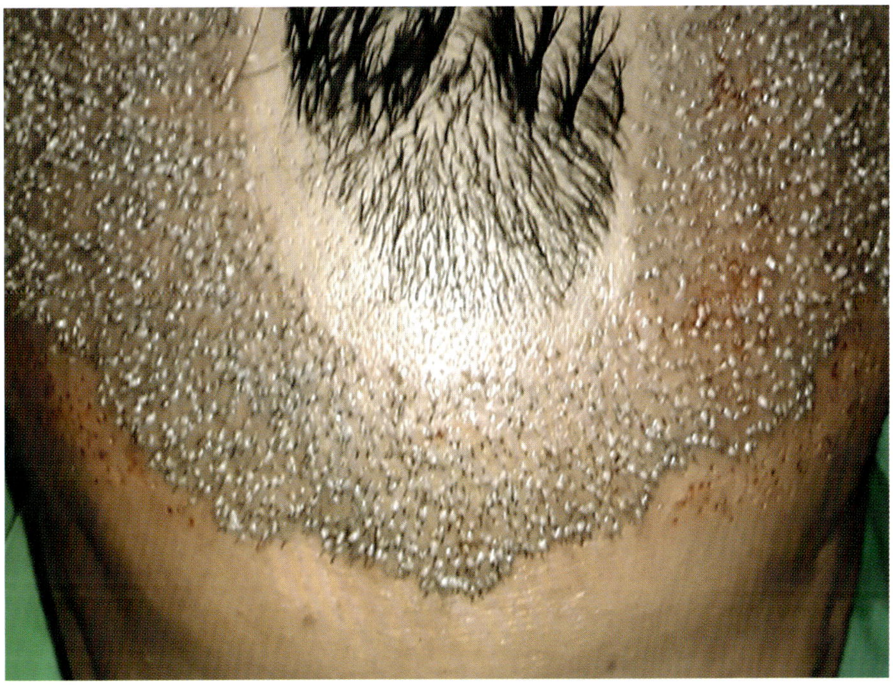

Figure 11.21

We redesigned the hairline. Note the macroirregularities and the wavy nature of the hairline. We implanted 3,000 grafts by direct hair transplantation (DHT) method.

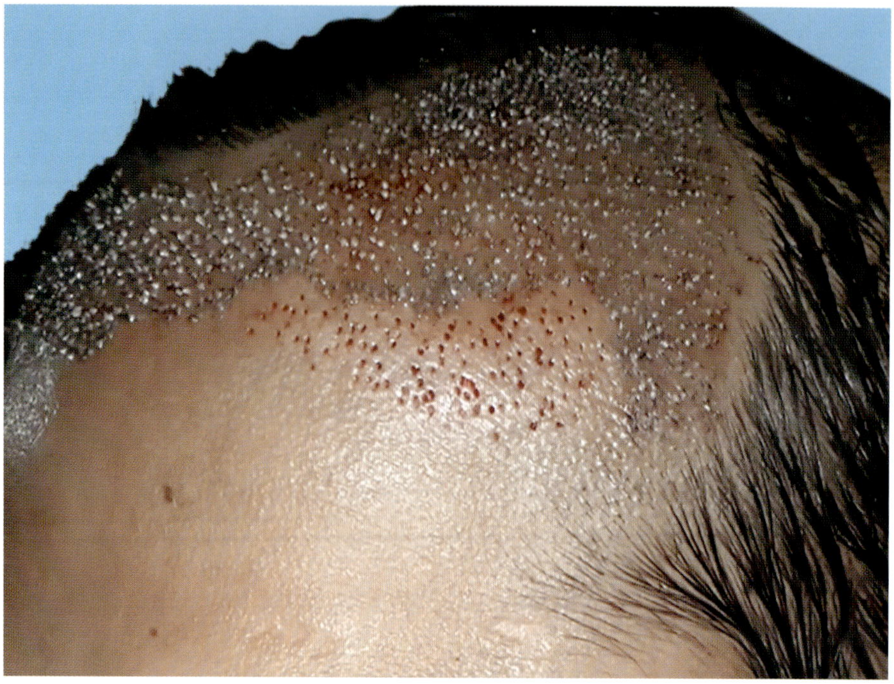

Figure 11.22

We extracted the wrongly implanted grafts and put it back at right places.

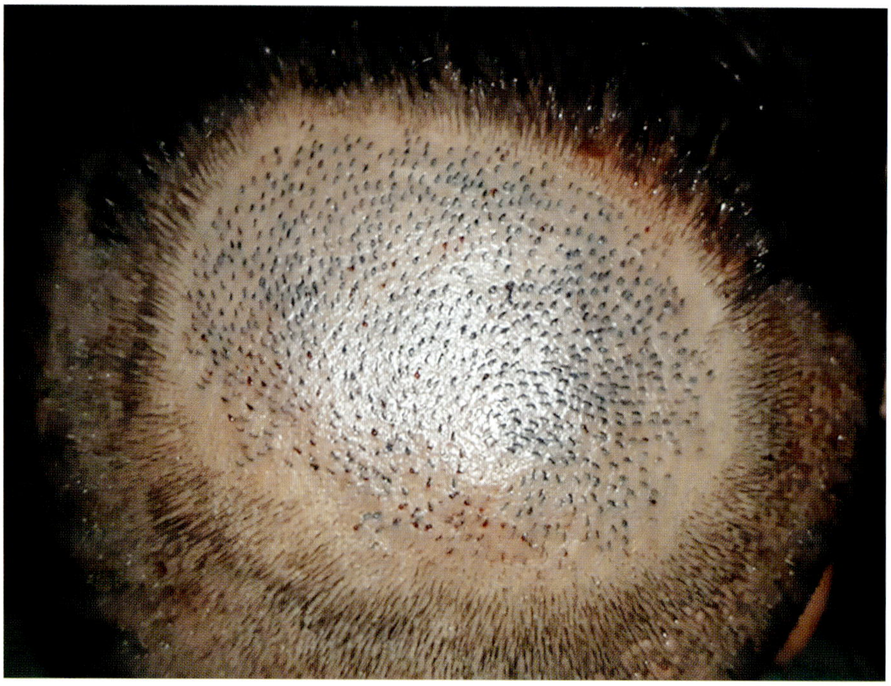

Figure 11.23

We restored his crown as well. Note the beautifully designed whorl which radiates outward and merges with the surrounding hair.

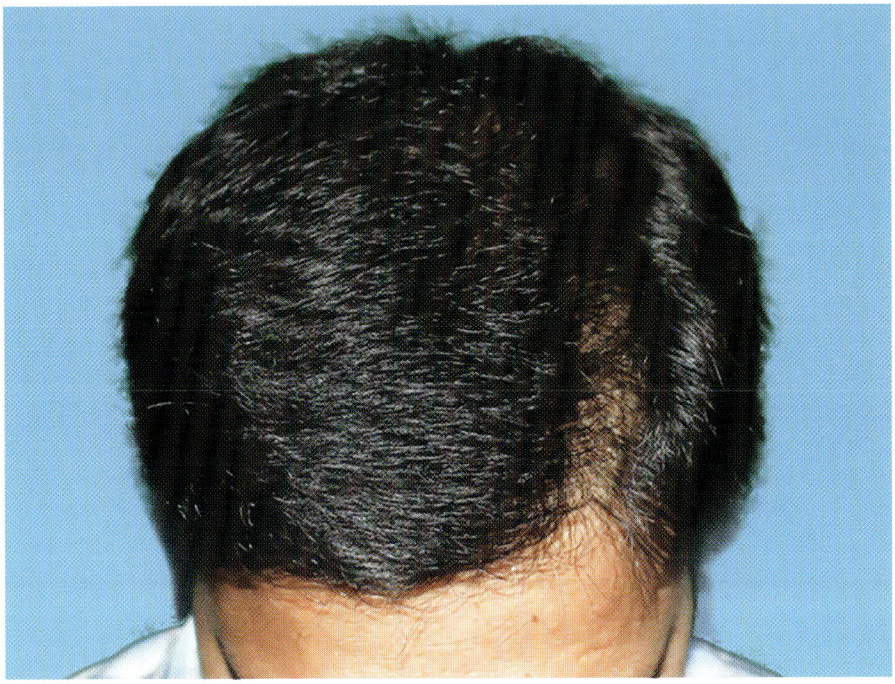

Figure 11.24

Note the restored hairline, its naturalness and correct frontotemporal angles. Visual density of transplanted hair matches with the pre-existing hair.

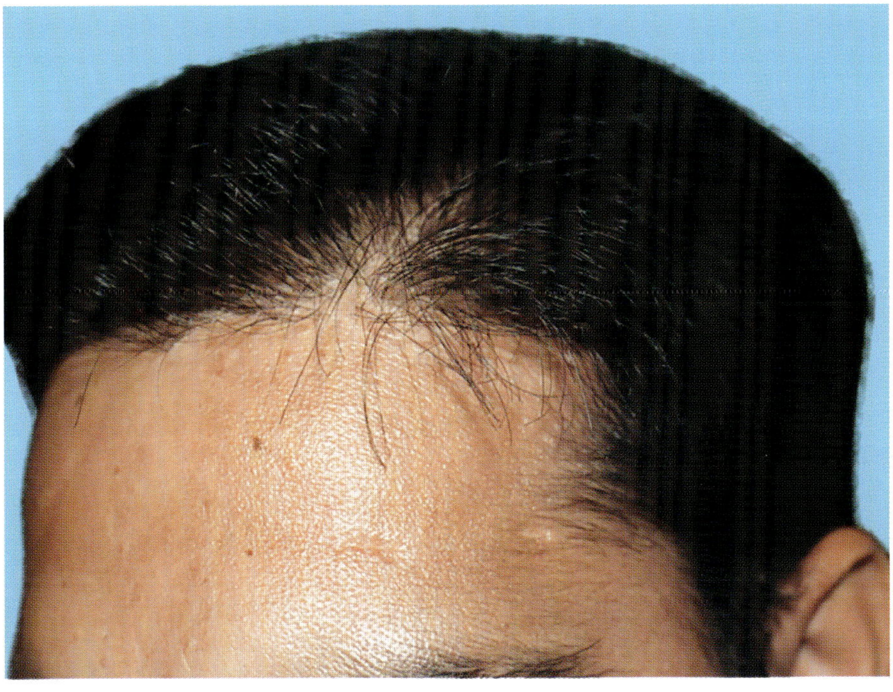

Figure 11.25

Note the absence of any visible scars, irregularity of the hairline, correct frontotemporal angles.

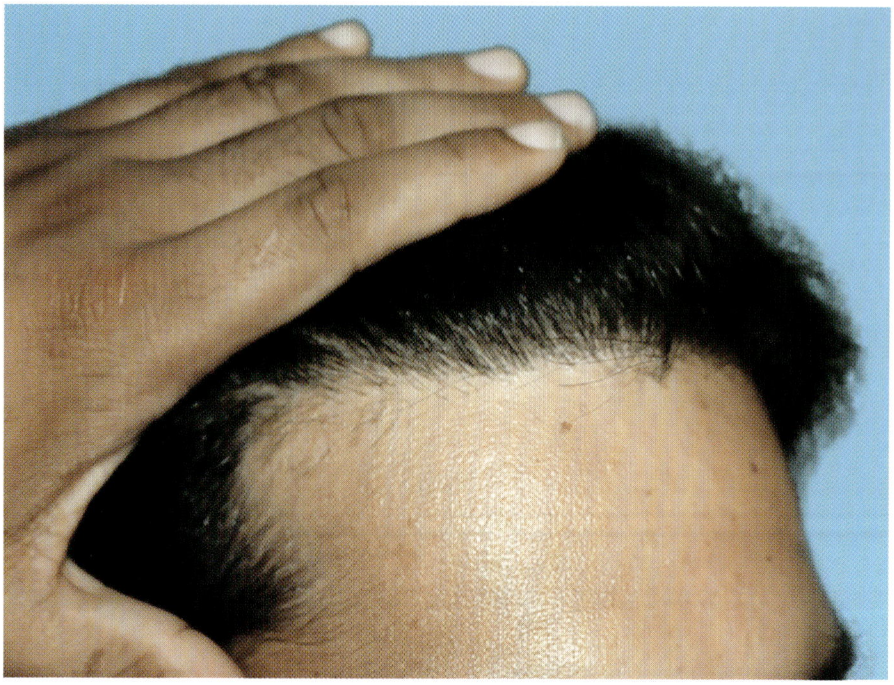

Figure 11.26

Close view of the hairline. No visible FUE scars on the right side of the forehead as well. Note the hairline naturalness.

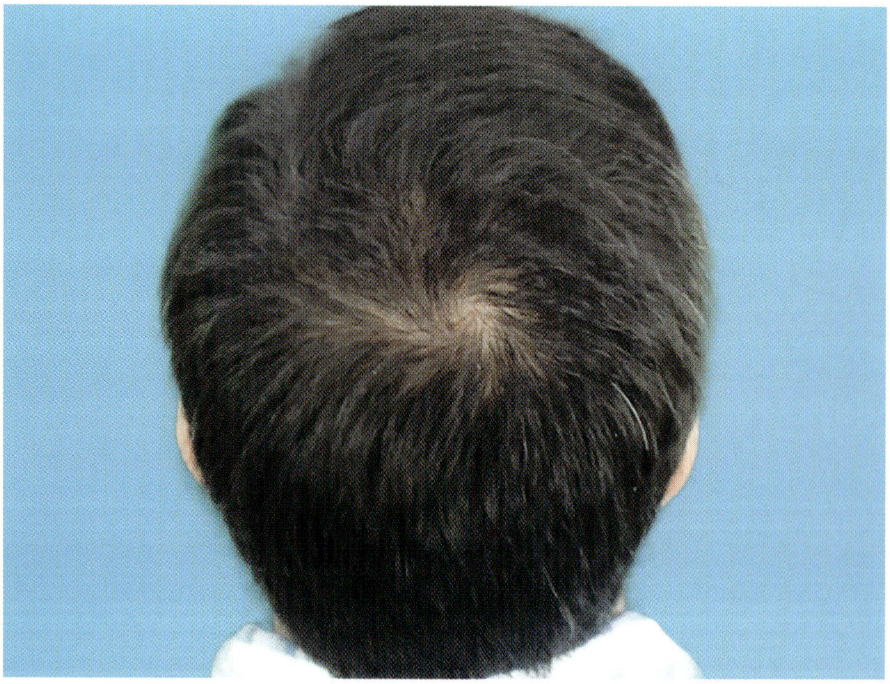

Figure 11.27

Reconstructed crown. Note the direction of transplanted hair in the recreated crown matches with the directions of the pre-existing hair.

CASE 4

We decided to present one of the dramatic cases of corrective hair transplant done by Dr Arvind Poswal here.

Issues

Massive scars on the scalp were present. there was virtually no scalp donor to cover his massive scalp. A total of 10,509 grafts procedure was done using FUSE technique in different sessions, over a period of 3 days each time (Figs. 11.28 to 11.31). The grafts details are as follows:

- *First session*: A total of 5,183 FUSE grafts procedure was done using 2,043 scalp, 2,586 beard and 554 chest hair.
- *Second session*: A total of 4,037 FUSE grafts procedure was done using 1,299 scalp, 1,931 beard and 807 chest hair.
- *Third session*: A total of 1,289 FUSE grafts procedure was done using 361 scalp and 928 beard hair.

Comments by Dr Arvind Poswal

Over the years, I have shared with the author and he also agrees now, that there is no need to reinvent the wheel.

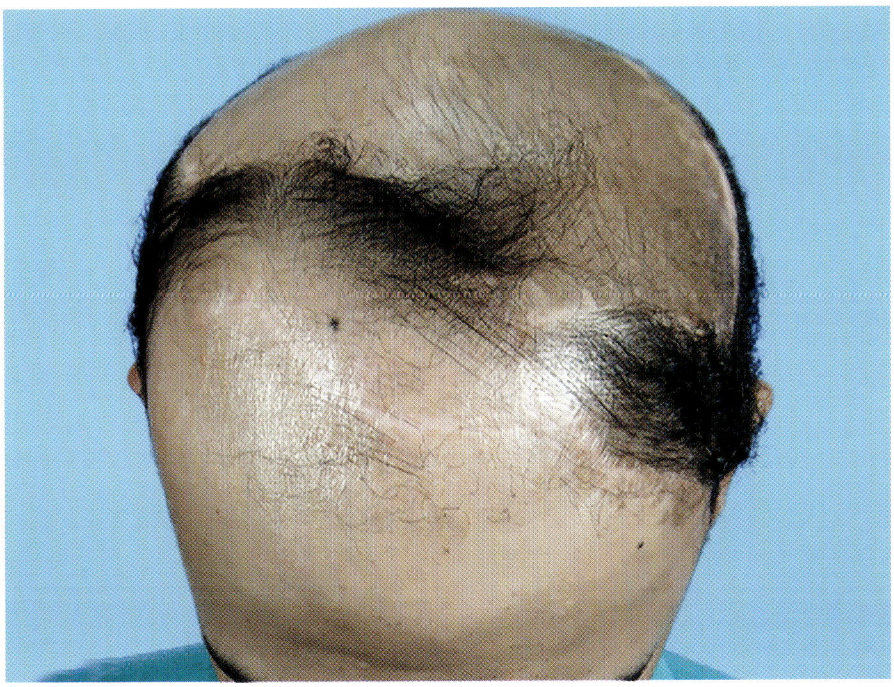

Figure 11.28

The top view of the patient showing the massive head size.

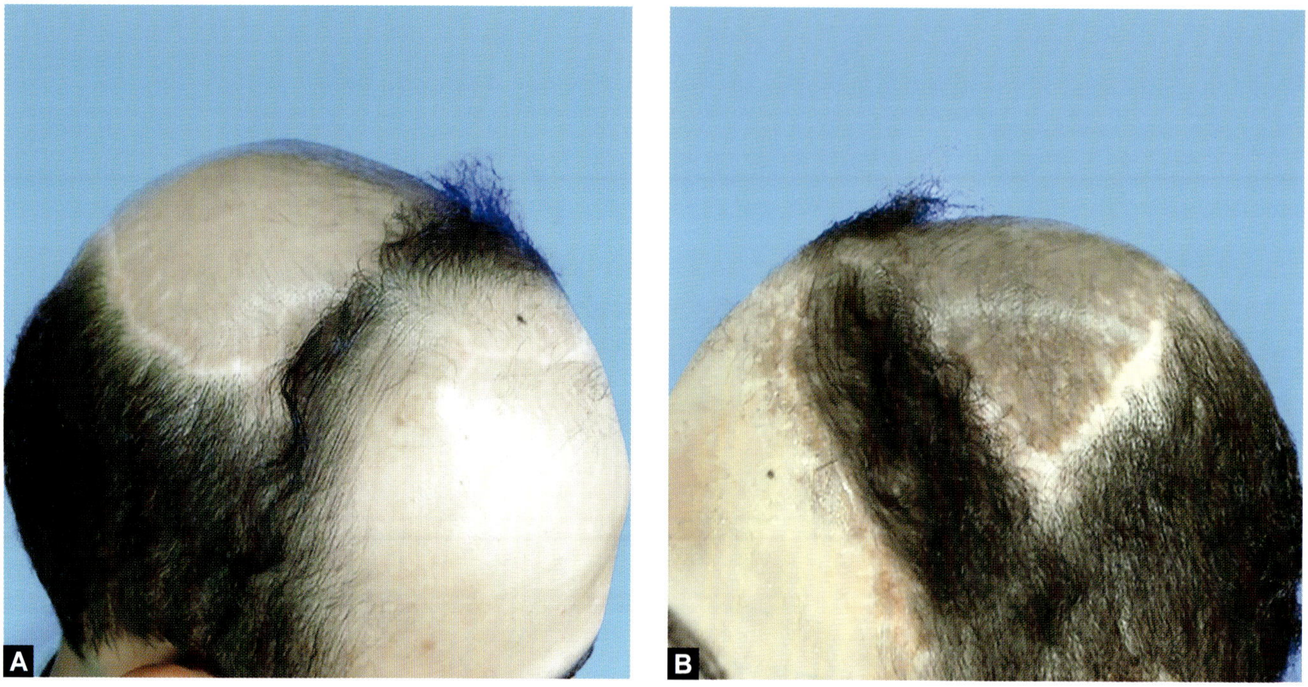

Figures 11.29A and B

The set of photographs shows the extent of coverage needed and the donor available for the same patient on the scalp.

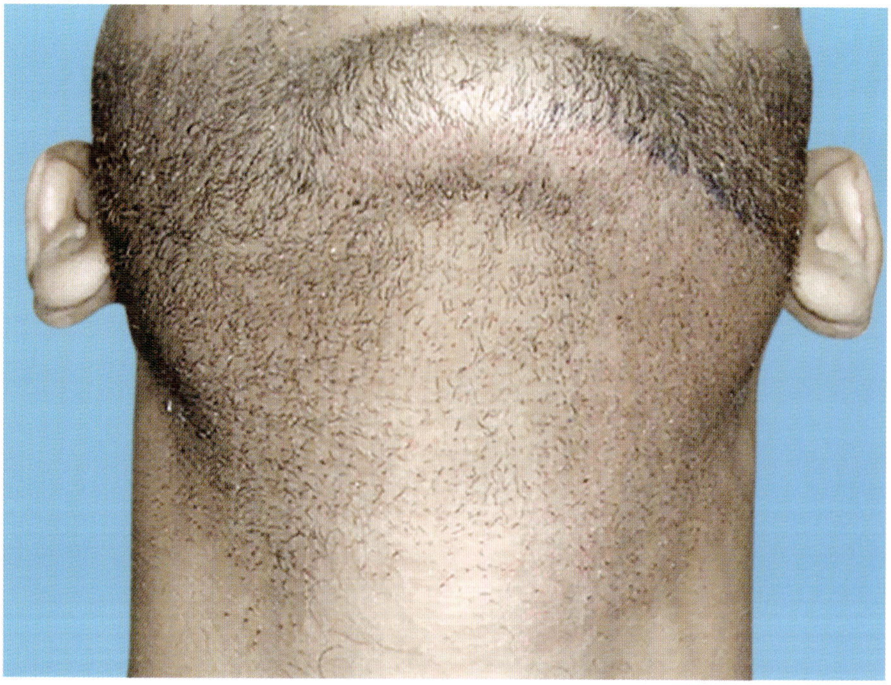

Figure 11.30

Beard grafts were the major contributor to the coverage.

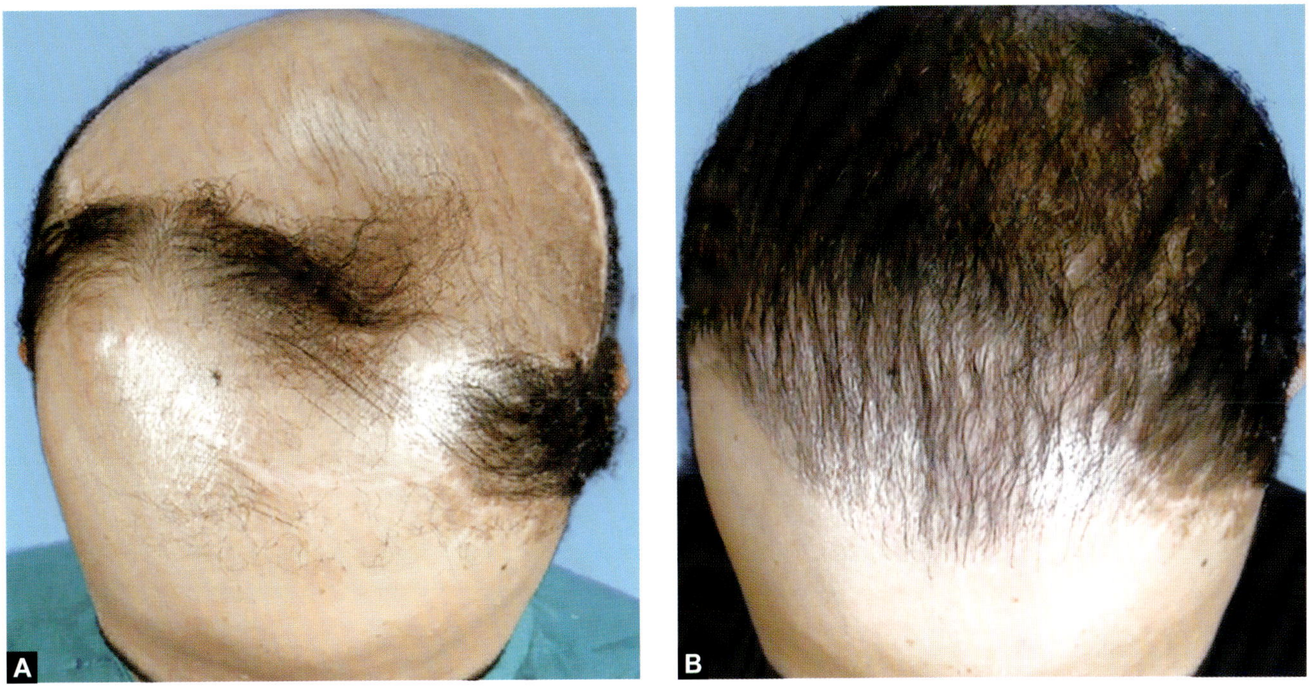

Figures 11.31A and B

(A) Before and (B) after photographs. A total of 10,509 grafts were implanted by Dr Arvind Poswal and his team over three sessions with each session of 3 days (total 9 days).

It is not possible to learn the art of hair transplant from short workshops or YouTube videos just like any other surgery, it needs to be taught in the following manner:

Observing the surgery, then assisting the teacher/professor in surgery, then performing the surgery under supervision of the teacher.

This is all doctors know is the correct way of learning hair transplants instead of depleting precious donor area. The links here show contribution of author in the field of corrective hair transplant.

- http://fusehair.com/portfolio-posts/sub-gallery-a80/
- http://fusehair.com/portfolio-posts/zayden-3/.

SUMMARY

- Corrective surgery is commonly sought nowadays due to rise in HT clinics run by semi-skilled doctors and surgical assistants all over the world who unknowingly mess up the surgery.
- There is gross compromise of donor area in terms of number of grafts that can be scored. This happens mostly with scalp donor as beard remains untouched by amateur surgeons.
- Most common corrections needed are flat hairlines, filled up frontotemporal angles, wrong angles of implanted hair, big FUT scars, sparsh growth in the transplanted region.
- Corrective surgery requires good understanding of the mistakes committed and proper planning before proceeding ahead with the correction.

CHAPTER 12

Megasession or Gigasession

Arika Bansal, Pradeep Sethi, Abhinav Kumar

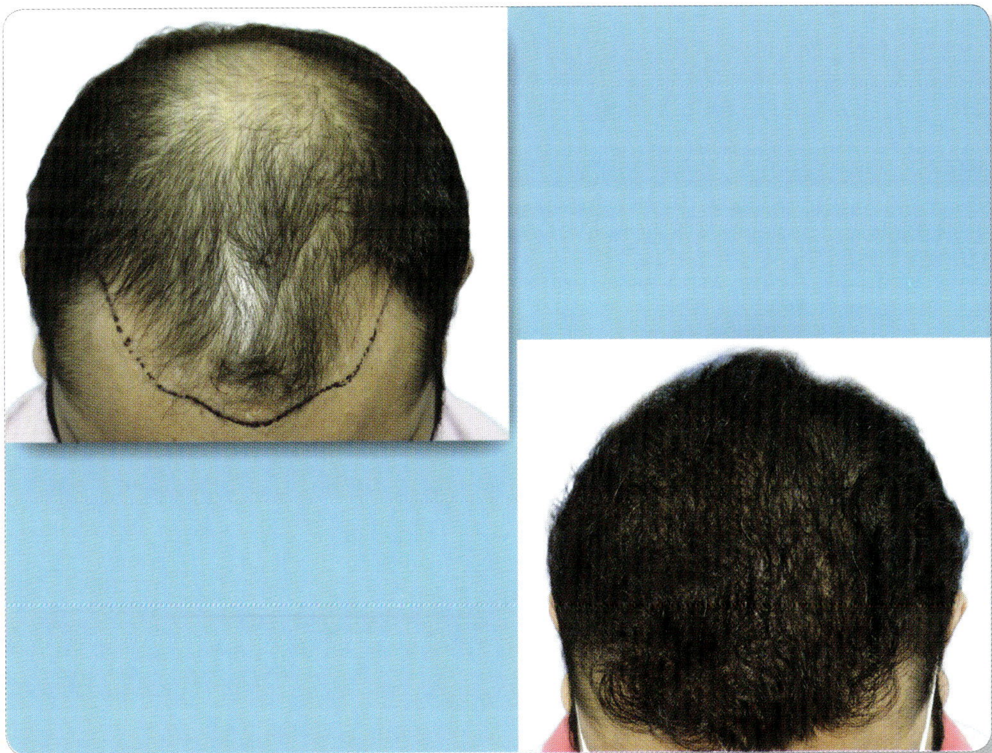

Megasession of 6400 grafts.

Hair restoration science is constantly challenged to cover the total bald area with adequate density. This requires a minimum of 50% of number of hair of the pre-bald density! Which in most cases is not possible considering the finite number of grafts available on the donor scalp. The next sources of hair are beard and rest of the body areas like chest. (According to the experience of the authors the body hair other than beard are not always trustworthy for growth and long-term sustenance! With more than 2000 odd patients where beard grafts are also used, the authors also does not pin their faith upon the beard grafts as they would for the scalp grafts).

INTRODUCTION

Megasession is a term used in the field of hair restoration surgery, when a single surgical session involves transplantation of more than 2,500 grafts.[1] A session means a single visit to the hair transplant surgeon where surgery is performed in continuation on 1–3 consecutive days. Since the term was coined a long time back, now almost every hair transplant comes under megasession. It would be better to call them "gigasession" as we were doing more than 6,000–7,000 grafts in a single session on a regular basis. Such sessions were the need of the hour as patients with Norwood grade VI and Norwood grade VII baldness visited us and wanted complete transformation in a single visit to the surgeon. We were initially sceptical of doing more than 5,000 grafts in a single session with direct hair transplantation (DHT) but after seeing successful results in hundreds of patients where we had performed gigasessions, we decided to share our experience with rest of the world.

We feel that our gigasessions are yielding good results because of two reasons:

1. We do DHT[2] where premade slits and minimum "out of body" time of the grafts leads to superior results.
2. We use dull needle implanters to implement our "No root touch "policy, where only epidermal end and gentle handling of the shaft of the hair is involved in extraction, loading and unloading of the grafts.

Gigasession is a tiring procedure for surgeons, assistants and the patients as well since it involves 2–3 continuous days of rigorous surgery involving 3,000–3,500 grafts being implanted per day. We recommend that if patient is from outstation, he should not travel immediately after the surgery and should stay at the place for at least 2 postoperative days to ensure proper care of the grafts and avoid any lapses in postoperative care due to tiredness.

PATIENT EVALUATION

Donor Density

A gigasession aimed for full scalp coverage can give fabulous results only if patient selection by the doctor is correct. A patient of gigasession with Norwood grade VI and Norwood grade VII baldness should have:

- A decent donor scalp density of at least 60–70 follicular units/cm^2, absence of reverse thinning in the scalp and good beard density with potential to donate at least 2000 beard grafts.
- A poor scalp density of less than 50 hair/cm^2 but an excellent beard density with potential to donate atleast 2500 good quality beard grafts. The scalp and the beard hair should be of similar type (curly, straight or wavy).

Head Size

We often use the "brachycephalic like" and "dolichocephalic like" mentioned here to estimate the number of grafts, though they may not be fitting the exact definition still they help us in giving a graft estimate for full coverage of scalp while conducting a gigasession (Fig. 12.1).

Normal Head

It is a rounded head with anteroposterior diameter and nearly exceeds slightly in diameter of biparietal eminences. Cephalic index is in between 76% and 81%. Such people with Norwood grade VI and Norwood grade VII needs around 6,000–7,000 grafts for full coverage.

Dolichocephalic Head (Cephalic Index of $<76\%$)

It is a condition where head is relatively long with long narrow facies. Such patients may get full coverage with around 6,000 grafts in Norwood grade VII baldness (Fig. 12.2).

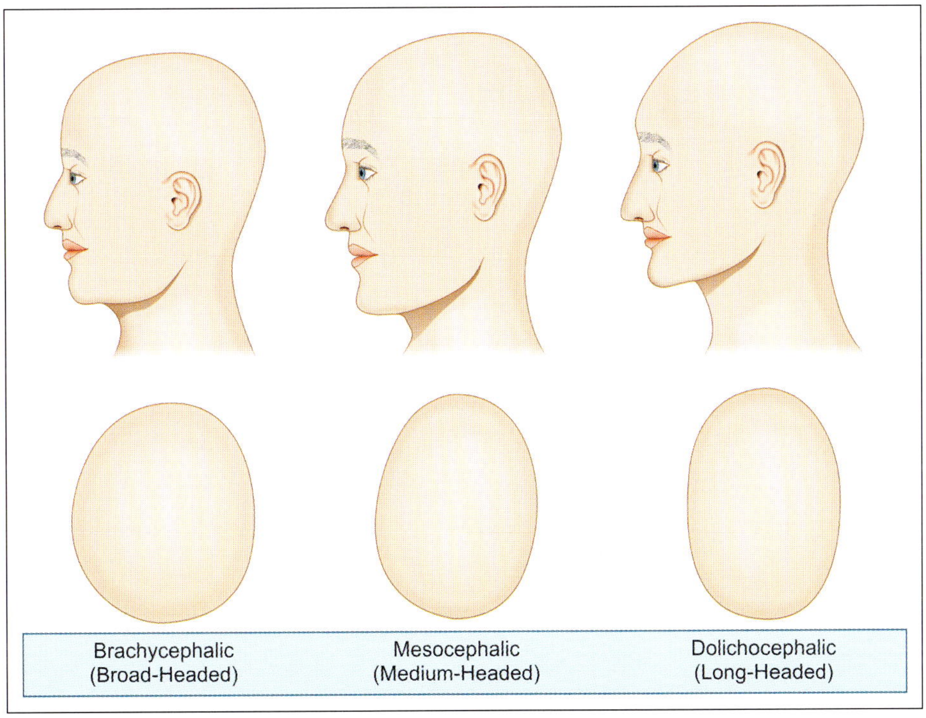

Figure 12.1
Head size.

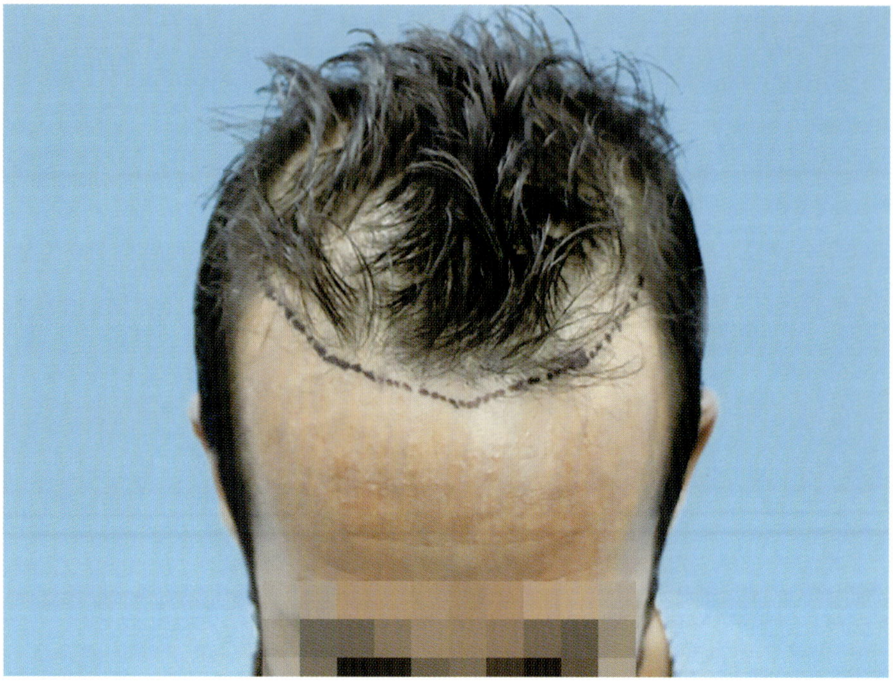

Figure 12.2

Depicts a dolichocephalic like head, which is basically a long and narrow head.

Brachycephalic Head (Cephalic Index >81%)

It is a condition where anteroposterior diameter is shorter than distance between biparietal eminences. It is a short wide head with flattened occiput. Such patients need more than 10,000 grafts for baldness of Norwood grade VII (Figs. 12.3A and B).

We will be discussing few of our cases below where we have successfully given full scalp coverage in a Norwood grade VII in a single session.

CASE 1

He was a 50-year-old man, presented to us with Norwood grade VI baldness. He wished to go for complete coverage in a single session. We counseled the patient that he would need more than 7,000 grafts for complete coverage. We also counseled him that we keep a higher hairline to give appropriate look according to his age and his crown would not be covered fully in spite of opting for a gigasession due to limitation of number of grafts which can be extracted from the scalp and the beard at one go. After mutual consensus, we went ahead with the procedure. We implanted 7,892 grafts (Figs. 12.4 to 12.9).

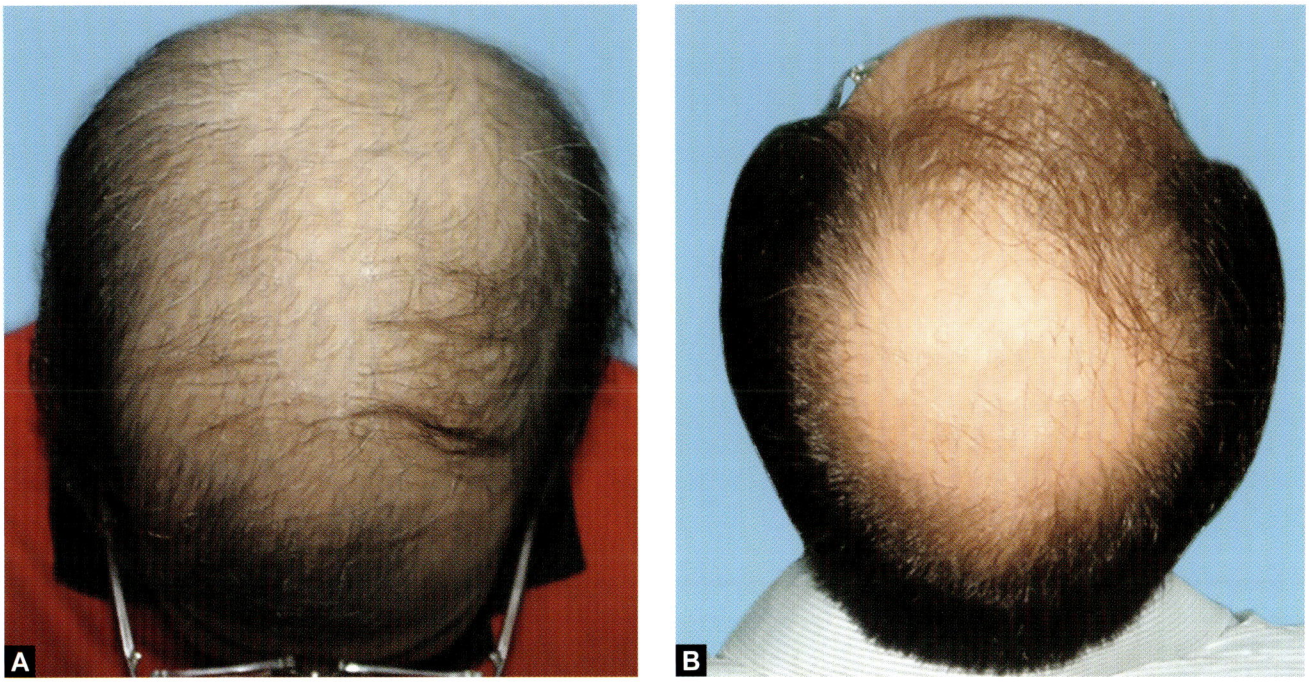

Figures 12.3A and B

Depicts a brachycephalic like head with wider biparietal eminences and big head size. Both these patients need over 10,000 grafts for complete coverage and with an average density, so going for coverage in such patients will involve two gigasessions.

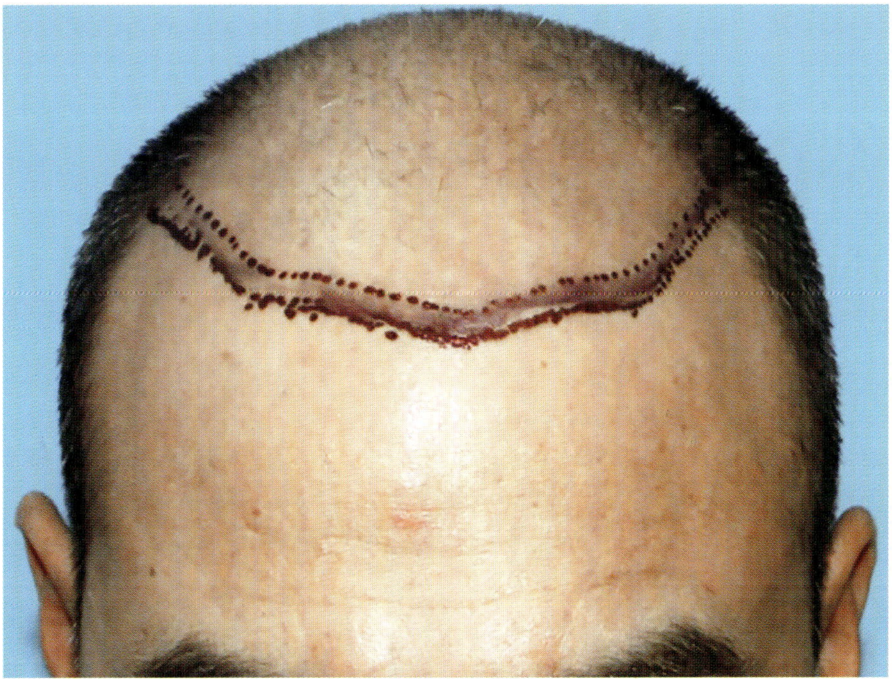

Figure 12.4

We constructed a polygonal three-peaked high hairline. The zone between the two hairlines is an area of micro-irregularity.

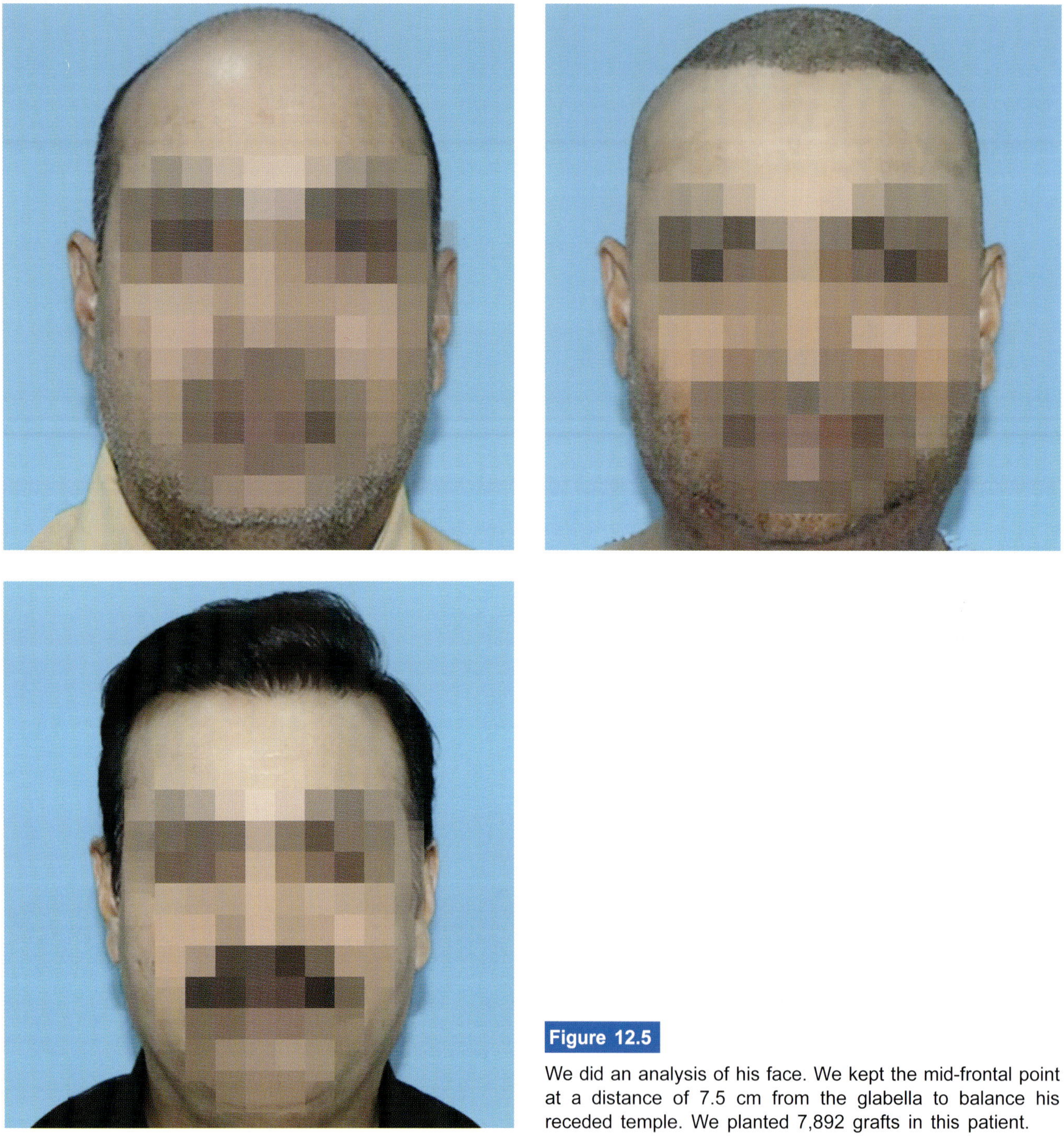

Figure 12.5

We did an analysis of his face. We kept the mid-frontal point at a distance of 7.5 cm from the glabella to balance his receded temple. We planted 7,892 grafts in this patient.

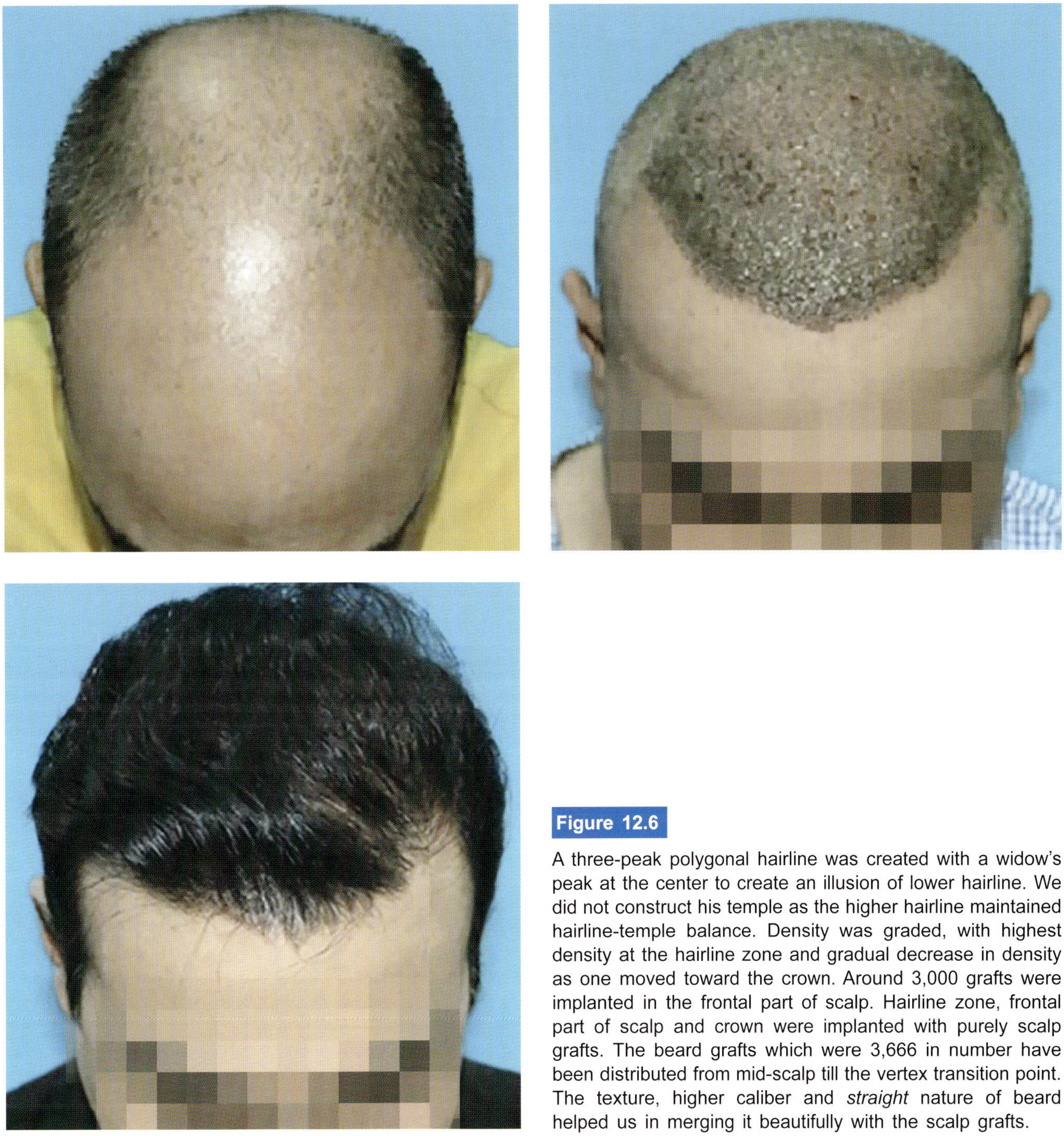

Figure 12.6

A three-peak polygonal hairline was created with a widow's peak at the center to create an illusion of lower hairline. We did not construct his temple as the higher hairline maintained hairline-temple balance. Density was graded, with highest density at the hairline zone and gradual decrease in density as one moved toward the crown. Around 3,000 grafts were implanted in the frontal part of scalp. Hairline zone, frontal part of scalp and crown were implanted with purely scalp grafts. The beard grafts which were 3,666 in number have been distributed from mid-scalp till the vertex transition point. The texture, higher caliber and *straight* nature of beard helped us in merging it beautifully with the scalp grafts.

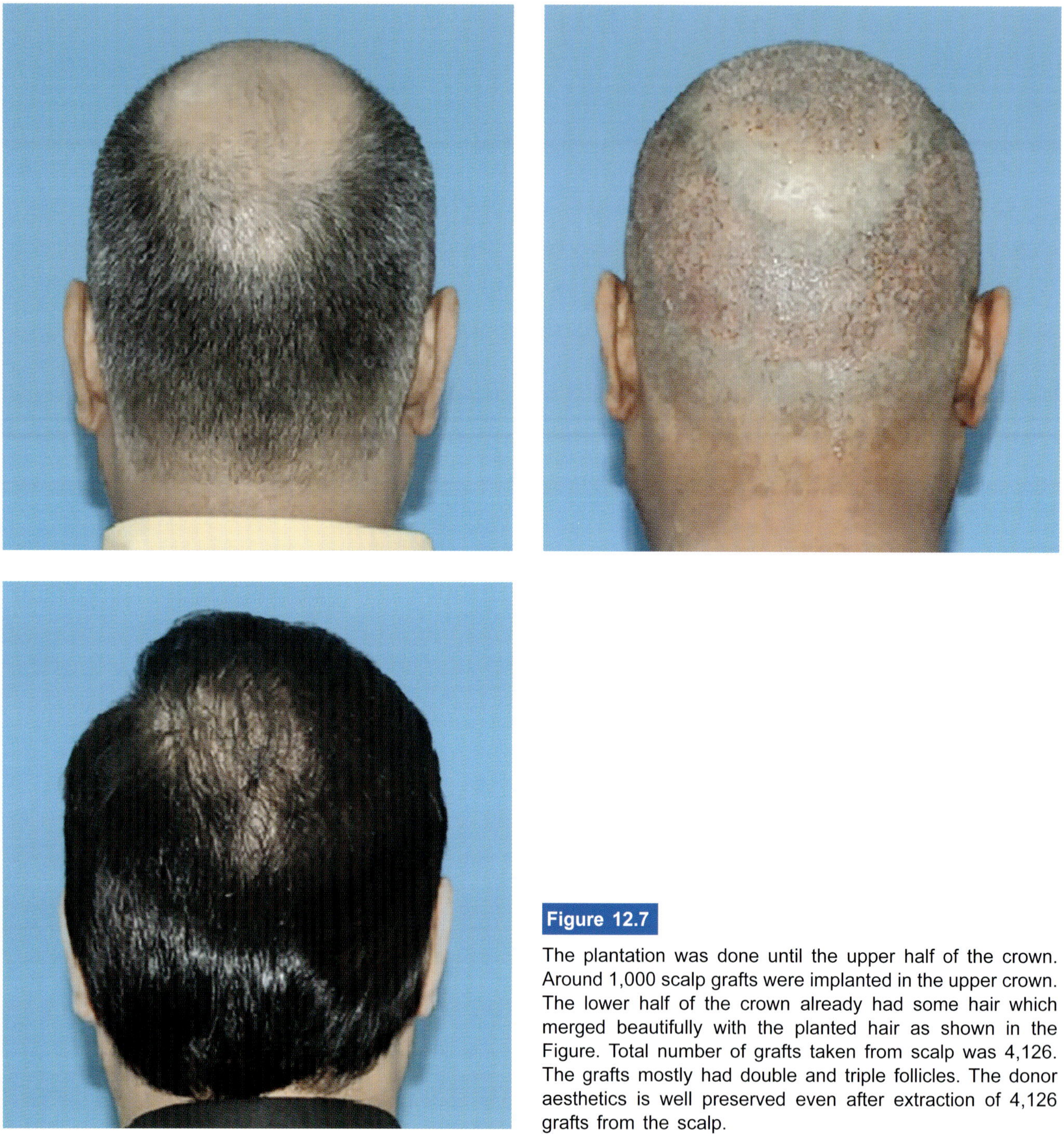

Figure 12.7

The plantation was done until the upper half of the crown. Around 1,000 scalp grafts were implanted in the upper crown. The lower half of the crown already had some hair which merged beautifully with the planted hair as shown in the Figure. Total number of grafts taken from scalp was 4,126. The grafts mostly had double and triple follicles. The donor aesthetics is well preserved even after extraction of 4,126 grafts from the scalp.

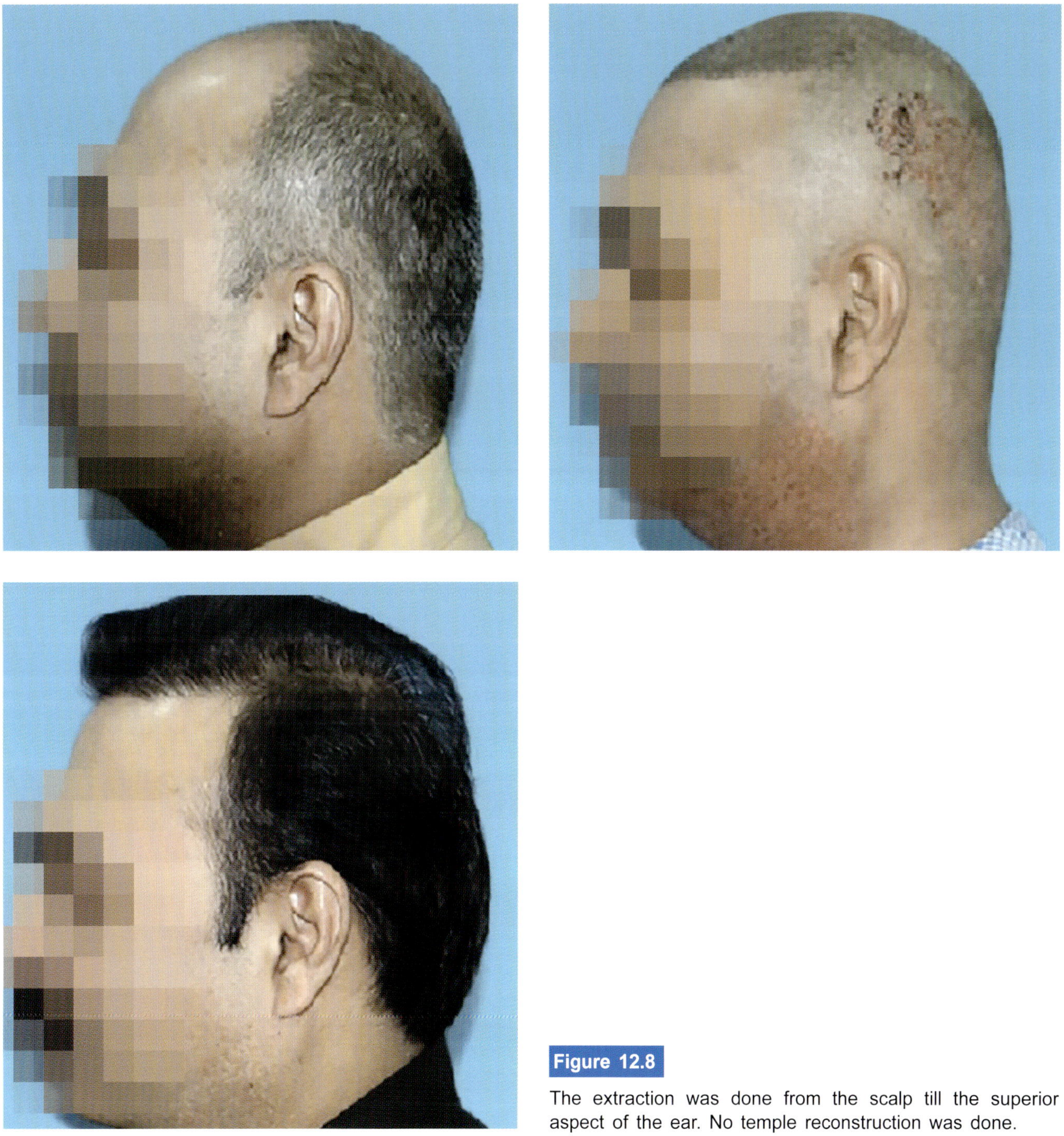

Figure 12.8

The extraction was done from the scalp till the superior aspect of the ear. No temple reconstruction was done.

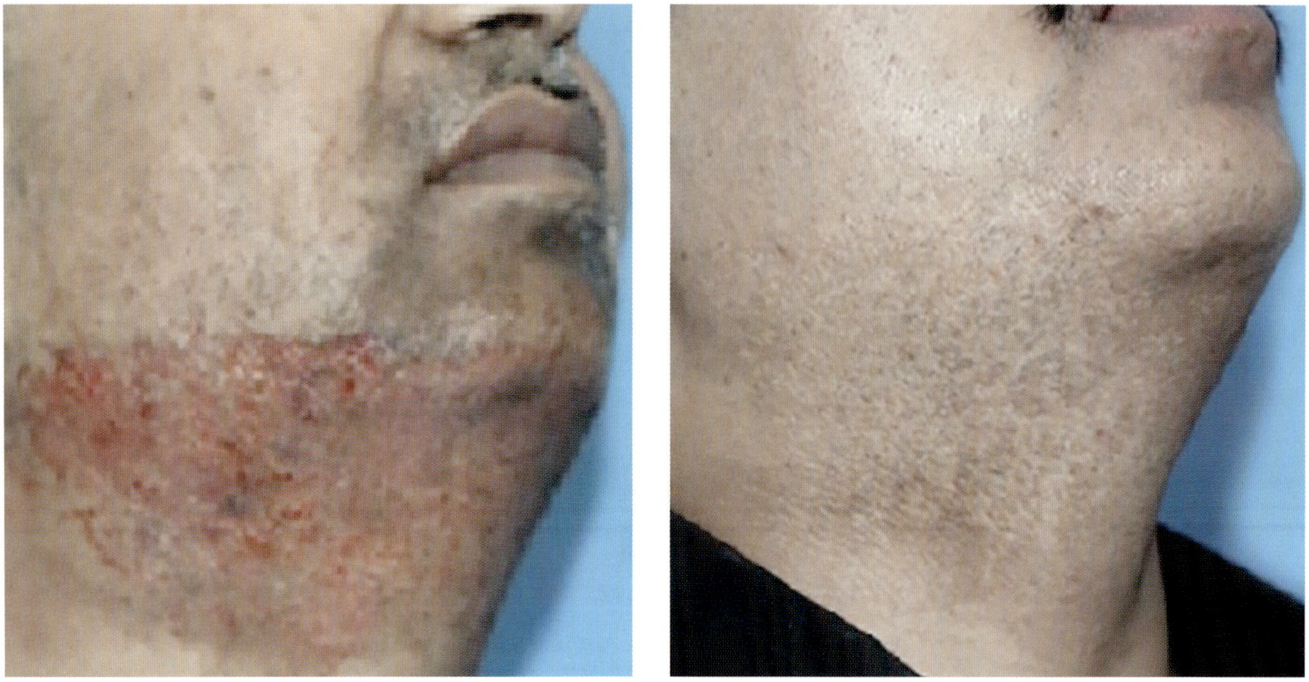

Figure 12.9

Immediate postoperative photographs, 8 months later postoperative photographs of beard after extraction of 3,666 beard grafts in a single sitting.

CASE 2

A 35-year-old male with Norwood grade VI presented to us for hair transplantation. He had a scalp donor with average density but dense beard. He had a brachycephalic head. We gave him a graft estimate of 10,000 grafts. We went ahead with the gigasession and were able to give him full coverage in two surgical visits (Figs. 12.10 to 12.14).

CASE 3

A 40-year-old man with Norwood grade VI baldness presented to us for hair transplant. He had a "Normal sized" head which needed around 6000 grafts for complete coverage. We planned his surgery in single visit. We extracted 6346 grafts over period of two days (3300 scalp, 200 side locks and 2846 from beard). We made the mid-frontal point at 7.5 cm from glabella and made a round hairline. The results are shown in Figures 12.15A to C.

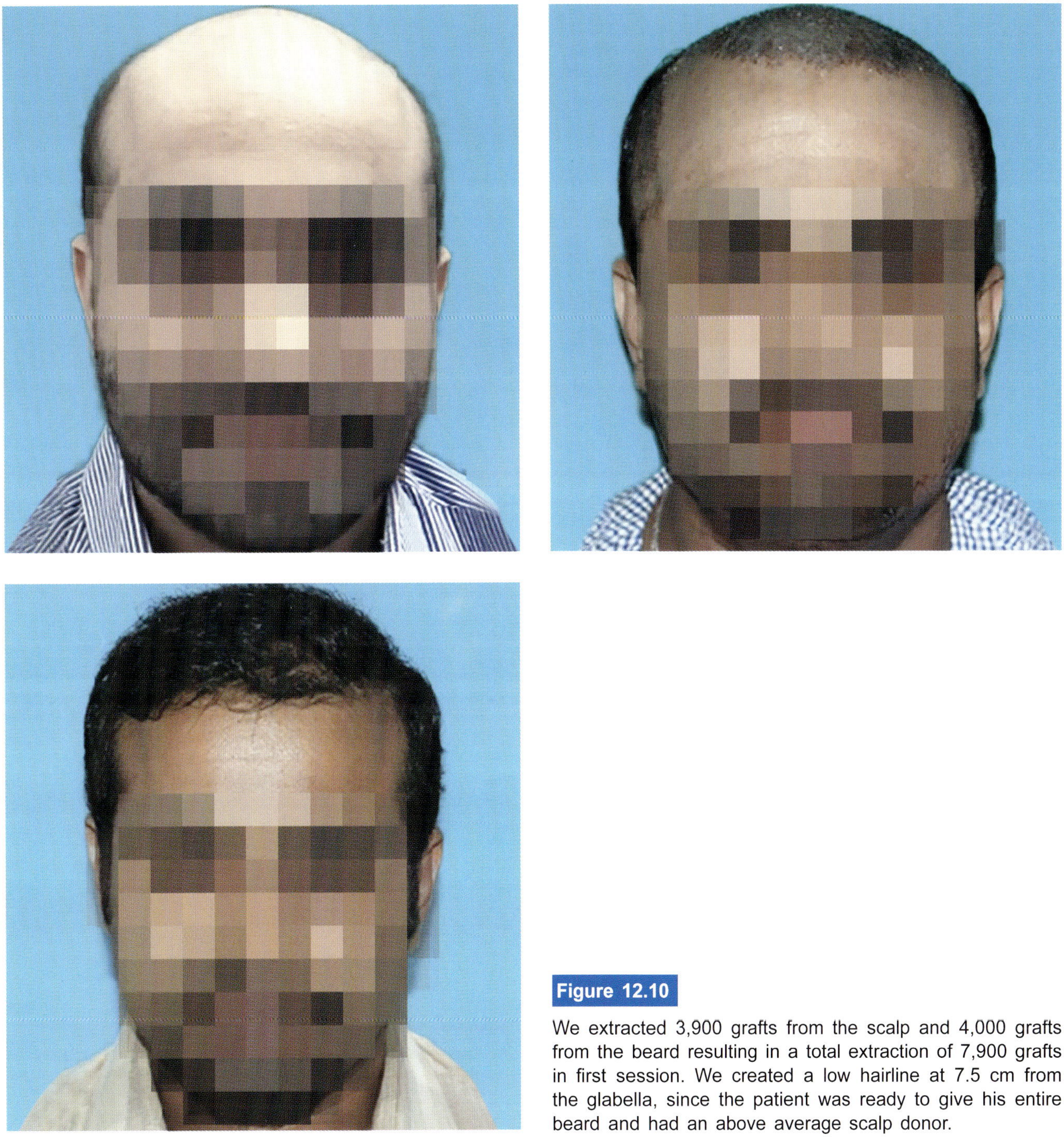

Figure 12.10

We extracted 3,900 grafts from the scalp and 4,000 grafts from the beard resulting in a total extraction of 7,900 grafts in first session. We created a low hairline at 7.5 cm from the glabella, since the patient was ready to give his entire beard and had an above average scalp donor.

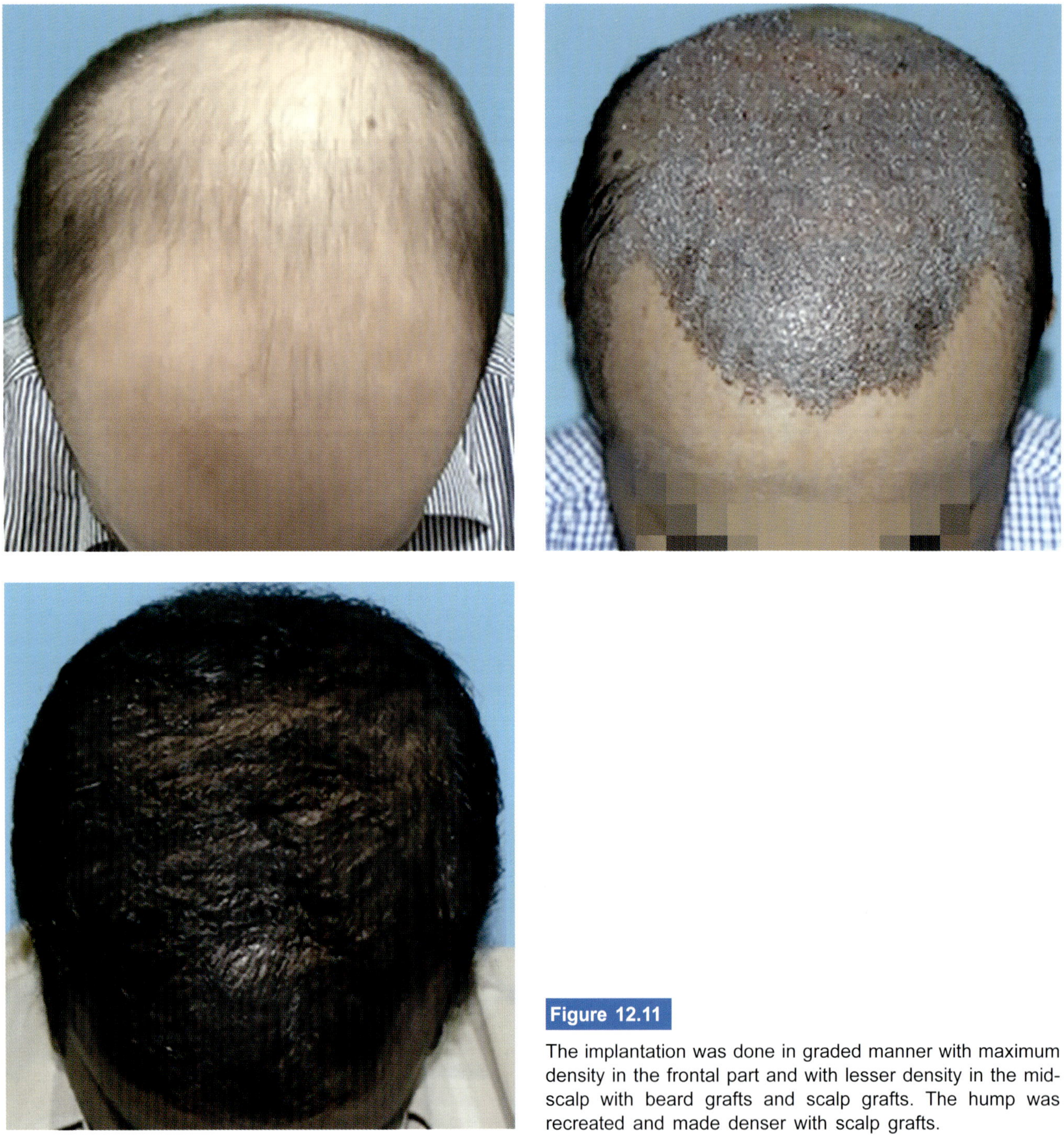

Figure 12.11

The implantation was done in graded manner with maximum density in the frontal part and with lesser density in the mid-scalp with beard grafts and scalp grafts. The hump was recreated and made denser with scalp grafts.

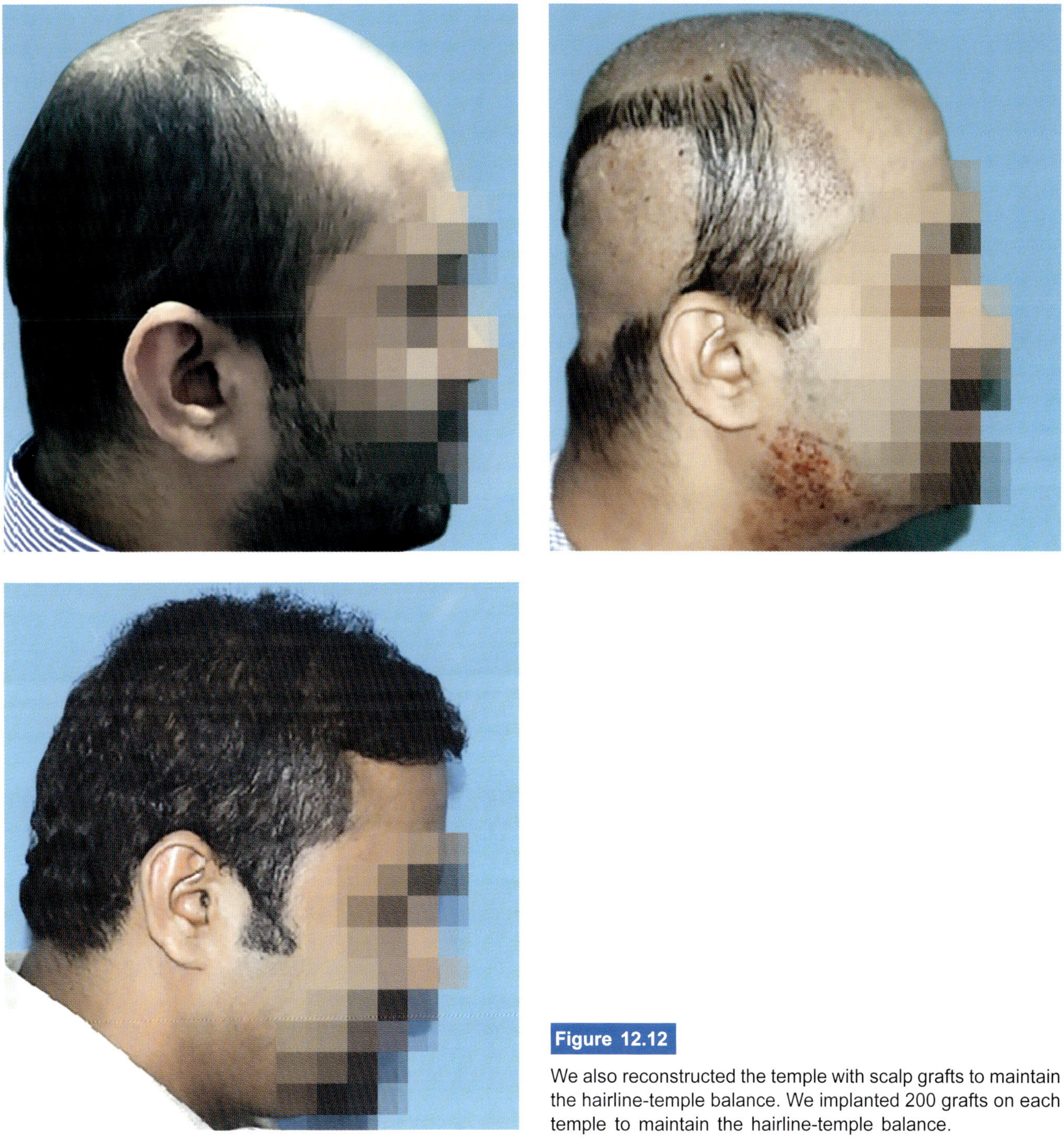

Figure 12.12

We also reconstructed the temple with scalp grafts to maintain the hairline-temple balance. We implanted 200 grafts on each temple to maintain the hairline-temple balance.

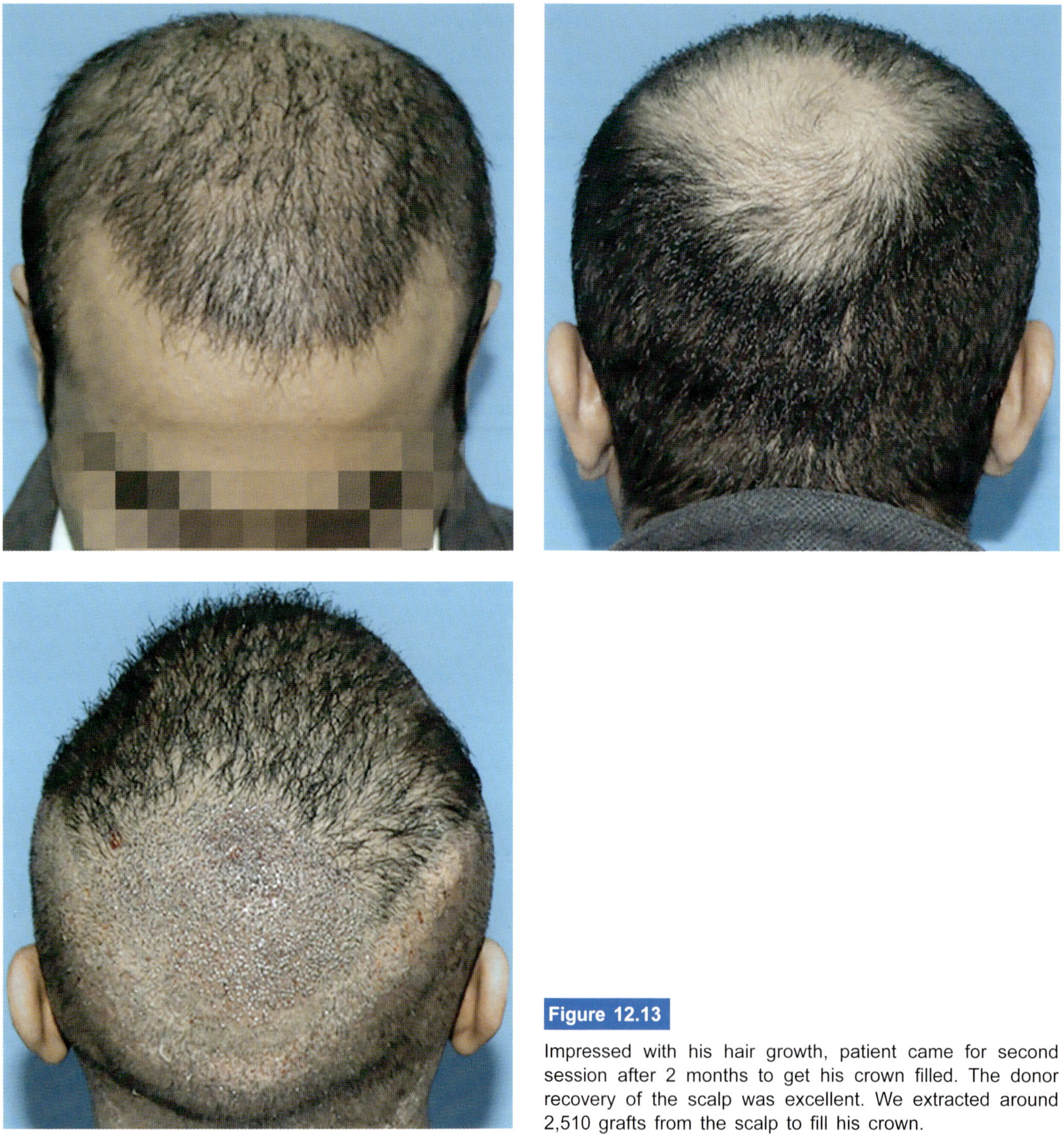

Figure 12.13

Impressed with his hair growth, patient came for second session after 2 months to get his crown filled. The donor recovery of the scalp was excellent. We extracted around 2,510 grafts from the scalp to fill his crown.

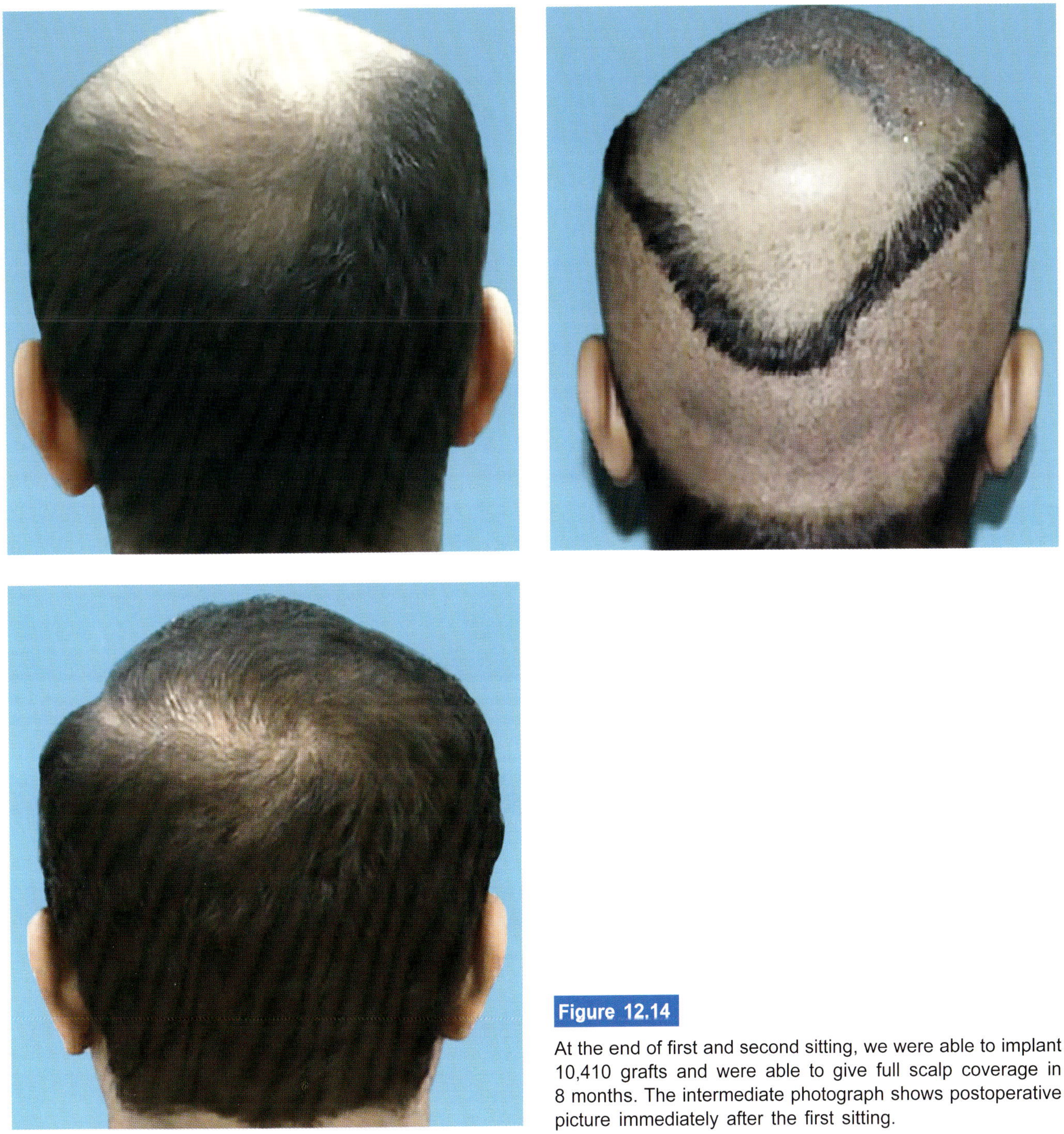

Figure 12.14

At the end of first and second sitting, we were able to implant 10,410 grafts and were able to give full scalp coverage in 8 months. The intermediate photograph shows postoperative picture immediately after the first sitting.

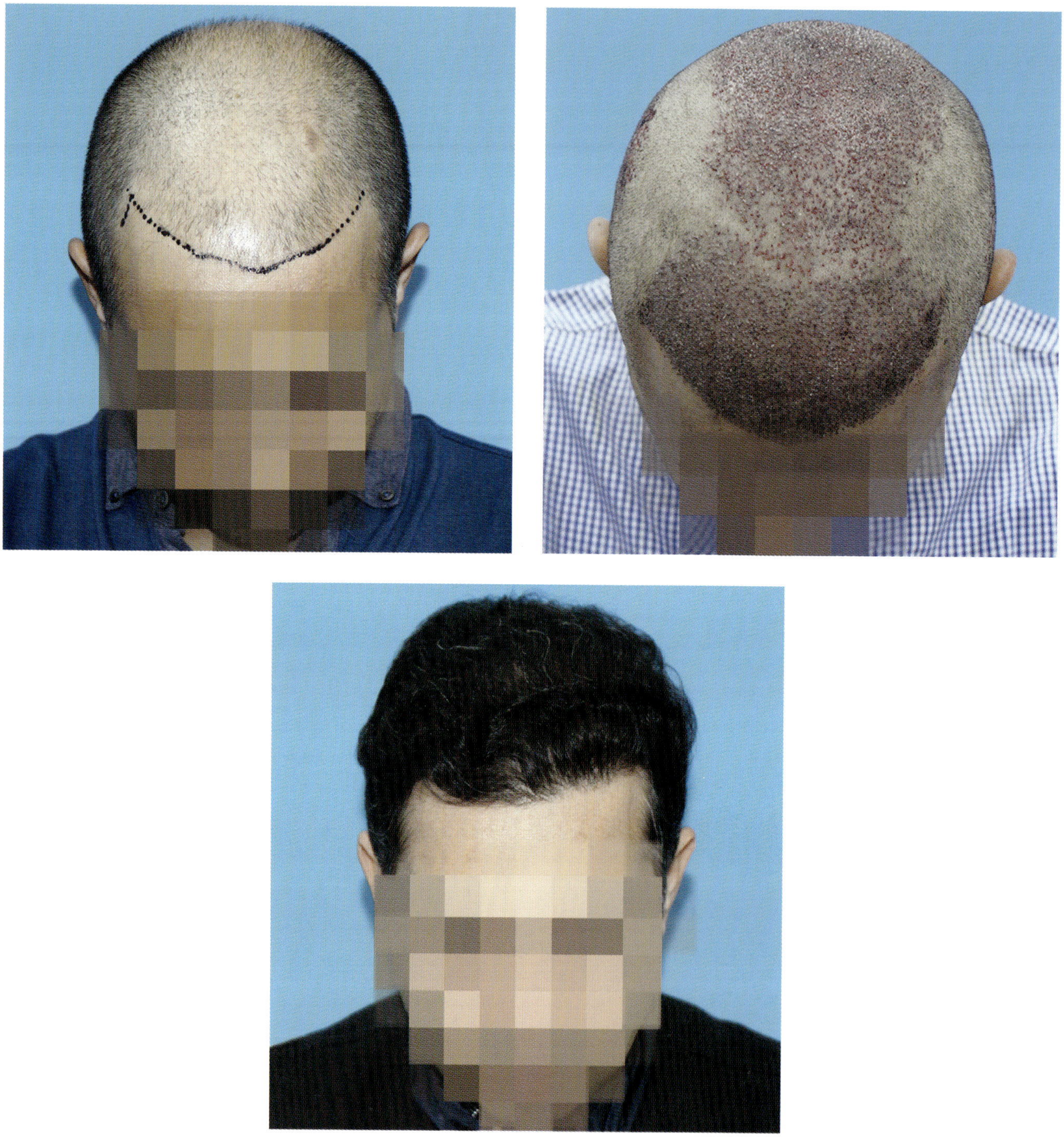

Figure 12.15A

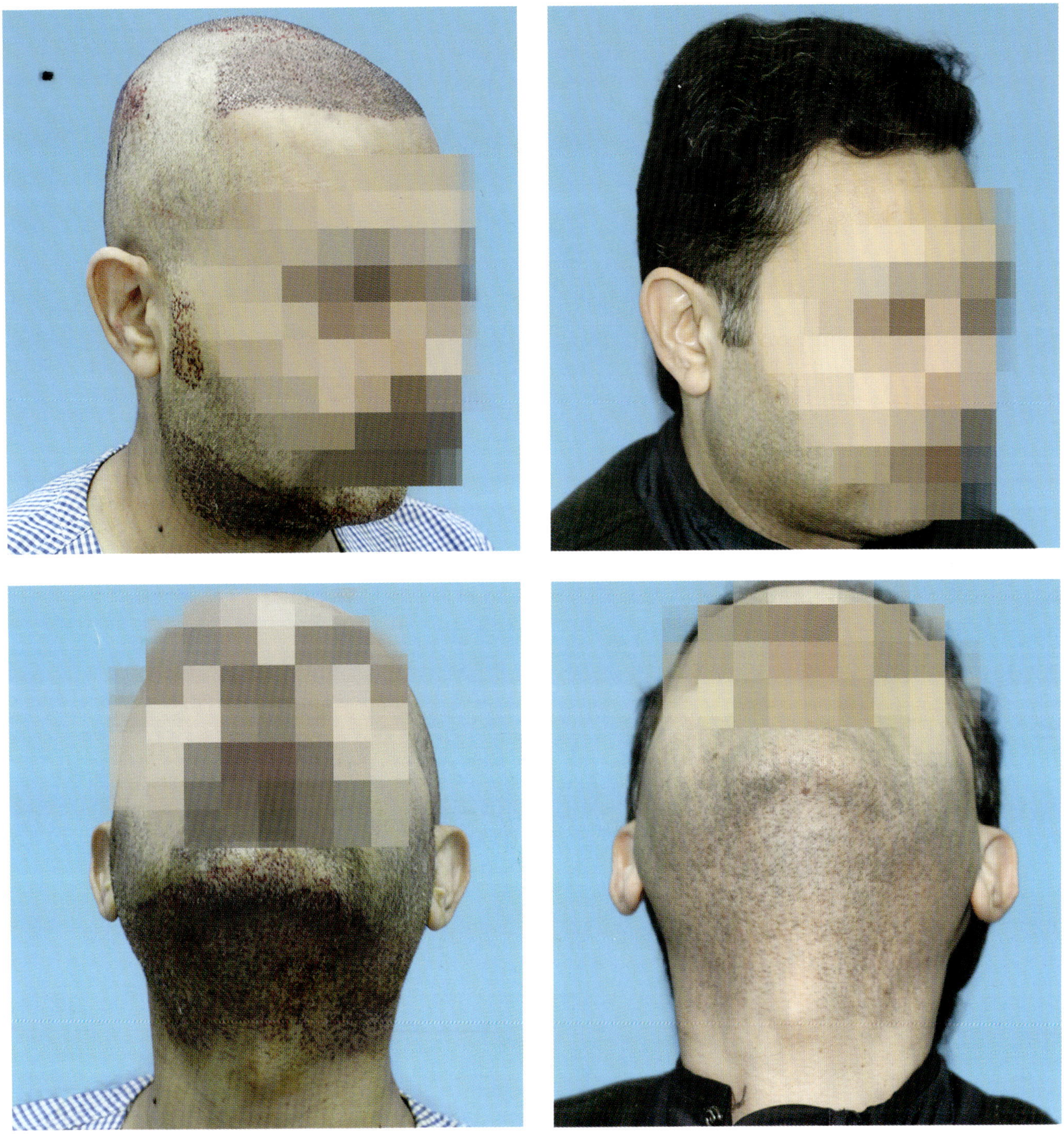

Figure 12.15B

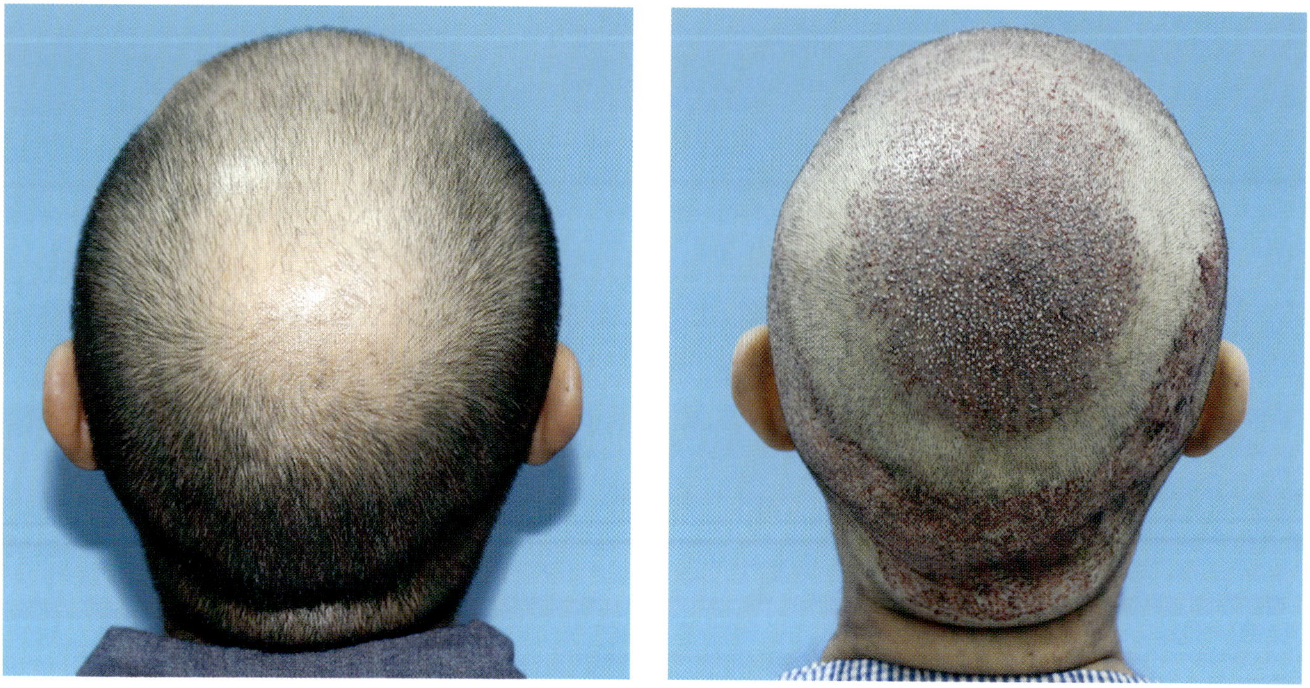

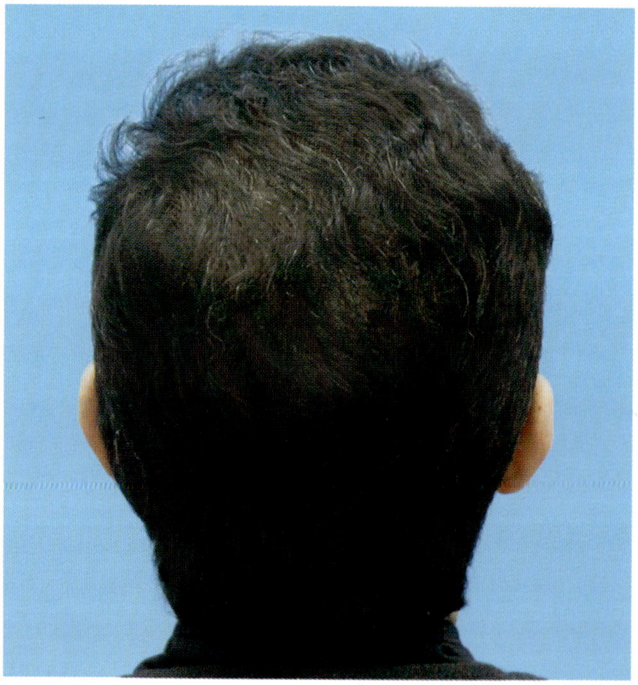

Figure 12.15C

Figures 12.15A to C

Presurgery, postoperative and 8 months later photographs of a patient. Total number of grafts implanted was 7,930.

CASE 4

A 45-year-old male with Norwood grade VII baldness presented to us for hair restoration. He had a "brachycephalic like" head which needed at least 10,000 grafts for complete coverage. We planned to cover the full head in two sittings. We made the hairline at 8 cm from the glabella and created a widow's peak to give an illusion of lower hairline. Hump and hairline were exclusively implanted with scalp grafts. The density from front to back was graded with maximum density at the hairline. We adopted the fanning technique in the crown and implanted nearly 3,000 grafts in a whorl-like fashion. A total of 10,300 grafts were implanted in two surgical visits (Figs. 12.16A and B).

CASE 5

A 55-year-old male with Norwood grade VI baldness presented to us for hair transplant. He had a "brachycephalic like" head. He needed around 10,000 grafts for complete coverage considering his large head size. We did his transplant in three surgical sessions (Figs. 12.17 to 12.21).

TECHNICAL DIFFICULTIES IN CONDUCTING GIGASESSION

Conducting gigasession is technically more challenging in many ways. One has to estimate patient's scalp grafts and beard grafts at the beginning of surgery. Such surgery usually requires more than 2,500 grafts from the beard and more than 3,000 grafts from the scalp. Bigger the head size, higher the number of grafts required. Such patients may require one gigasession or one gigasession and one small session. Sometimes due to retrograde thinning, one is more dependent on beard grafts or rarely on chest grafts than on scalp grafts for full coverage. In our DHT technique, presence of five to six assistants is always required at any point in the surgery. In DHT, either all the three processes: (1) scoring, (2) extraction and (3) implantation is happening together or two assistants are implanting the grafts after the completion of extraction, which may need two technicians for quick loading of grafts into implanters and two technicians for supplying the grafts. Doing all the three steps of surgery together helps us in implanting at least 3,500 grafts in 8 hours leaving the rest for the next day as doctor and technician fatigue also needs to be taken into account (Figs. 12.22 and 12.23). The beard grafts are usually taken on the first day of surgery after restoring the hairline as they need to be implanted on the mid-scalp and mixed intelligently with scalp grafts. We usually use the grafts on the back of the head for the hairline as they are of best quality and those on the sides for the mid-scalp and crown. Crown is implanted with either scalp grafts alone if they are sufficient or mixed with the beard grafts in the periphery of the crown. Hump and temple are always implanted with scalp grafts alone.

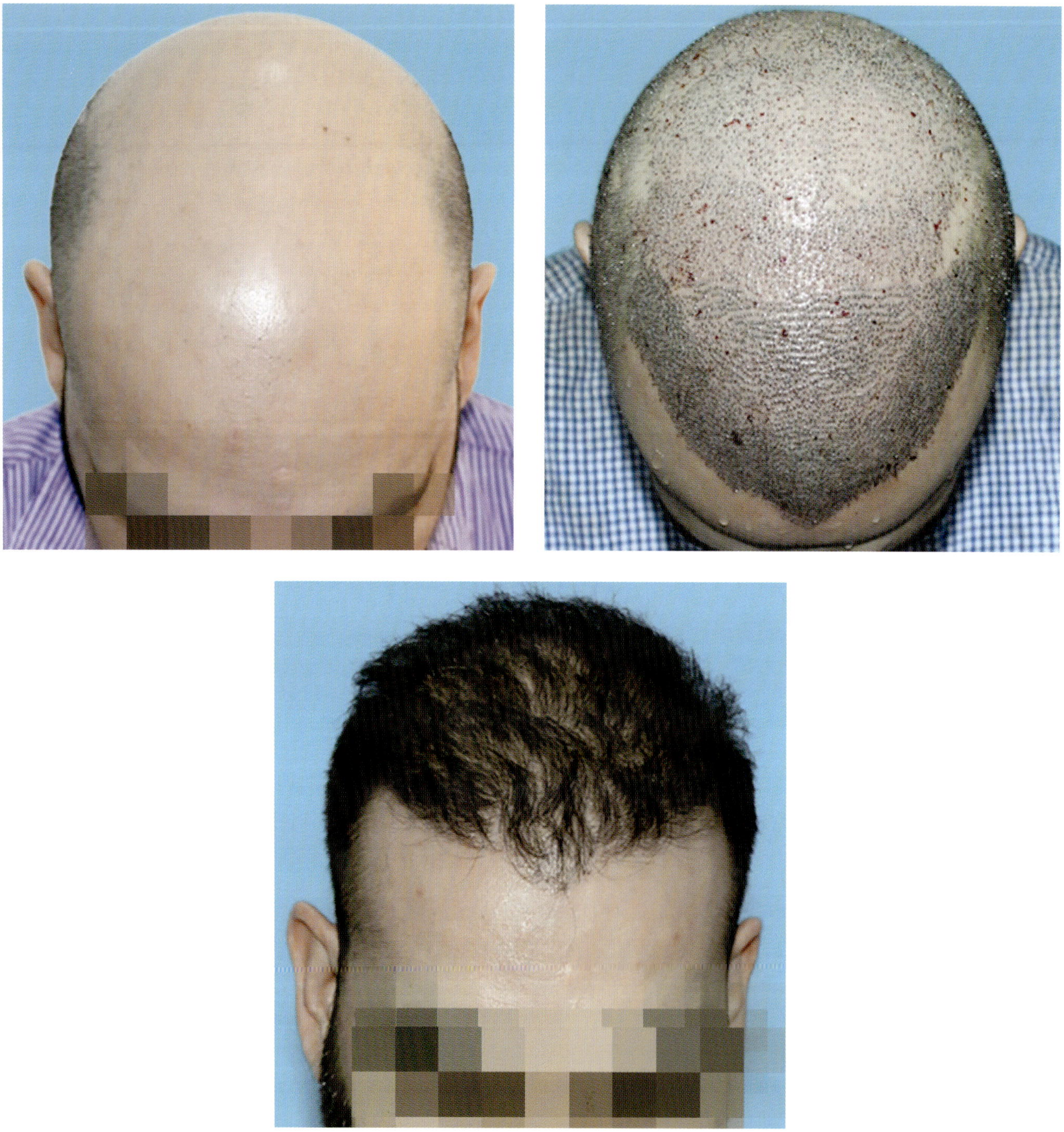

Figure 12.16A

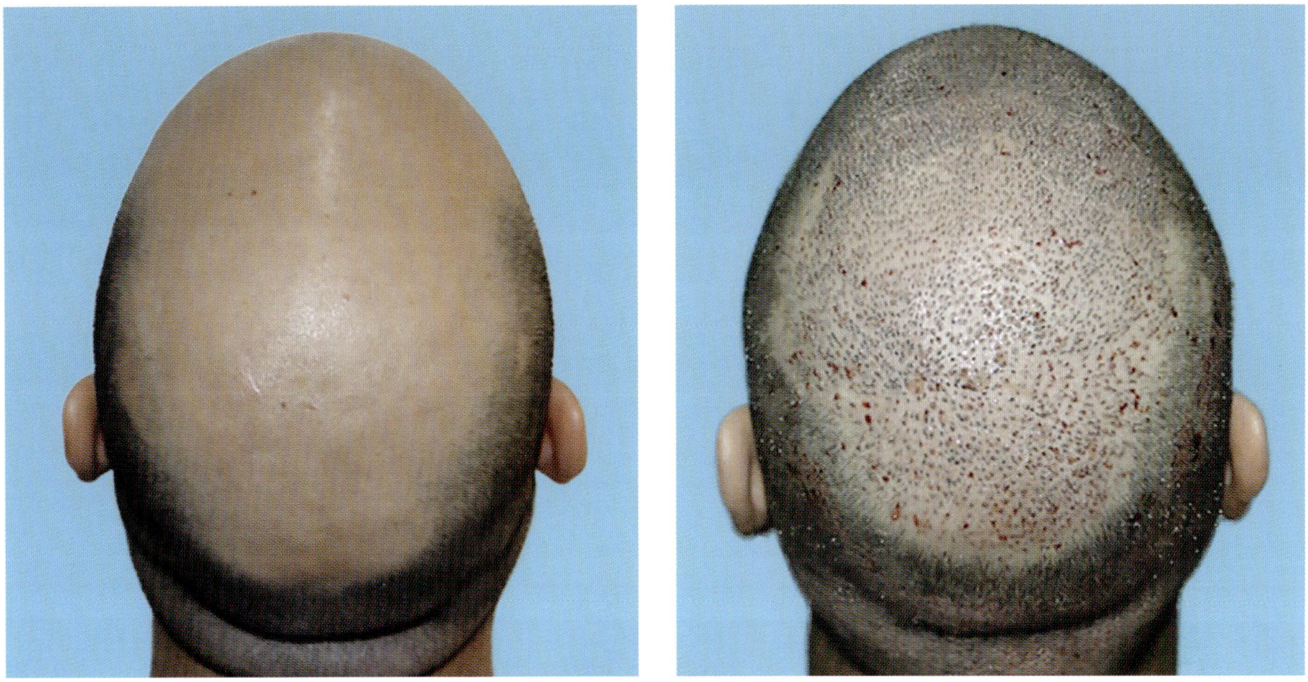

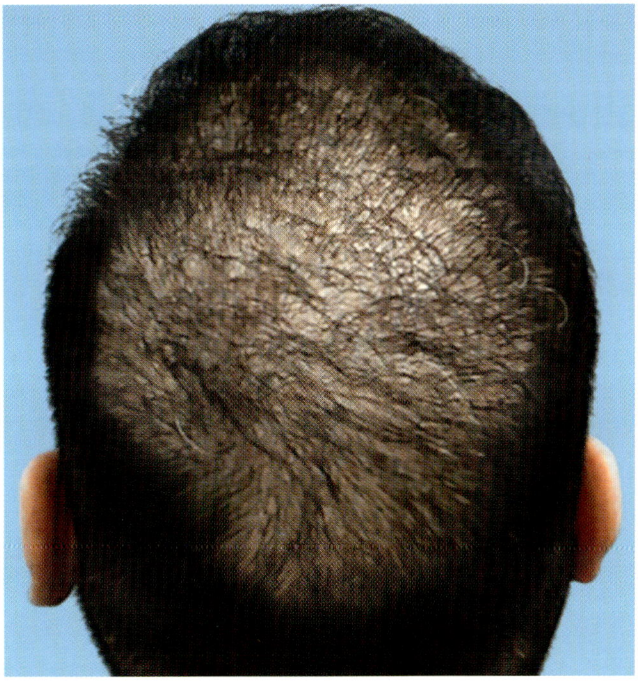

Figure 12.16B

Figures 12.16A and B

The set of photographs shows the preoperative, immediate postoperative photographs, 10 months postoperative photographs of the patient who had undergone transplantation of 10,300 grafts in two surgical visits. We implanted 50 grafts/cm^2 in frontal 2/3rd but the density we got in the front was less than optimum. This was due to the vascular compromise due to overtly dense implantation of grafts. A caution against going overboard with density in patient of high scalp-hair colour contrast.

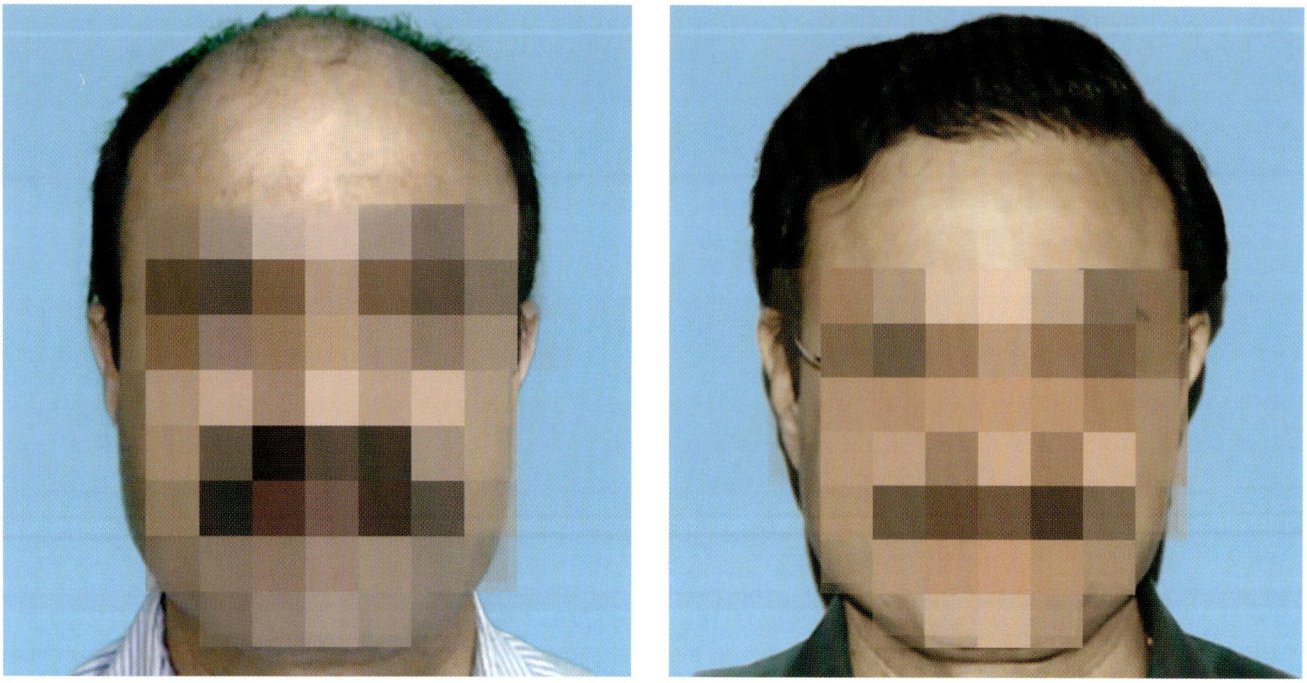

Figure 12.17

We made a rounded hairline which suited his head size and his head.

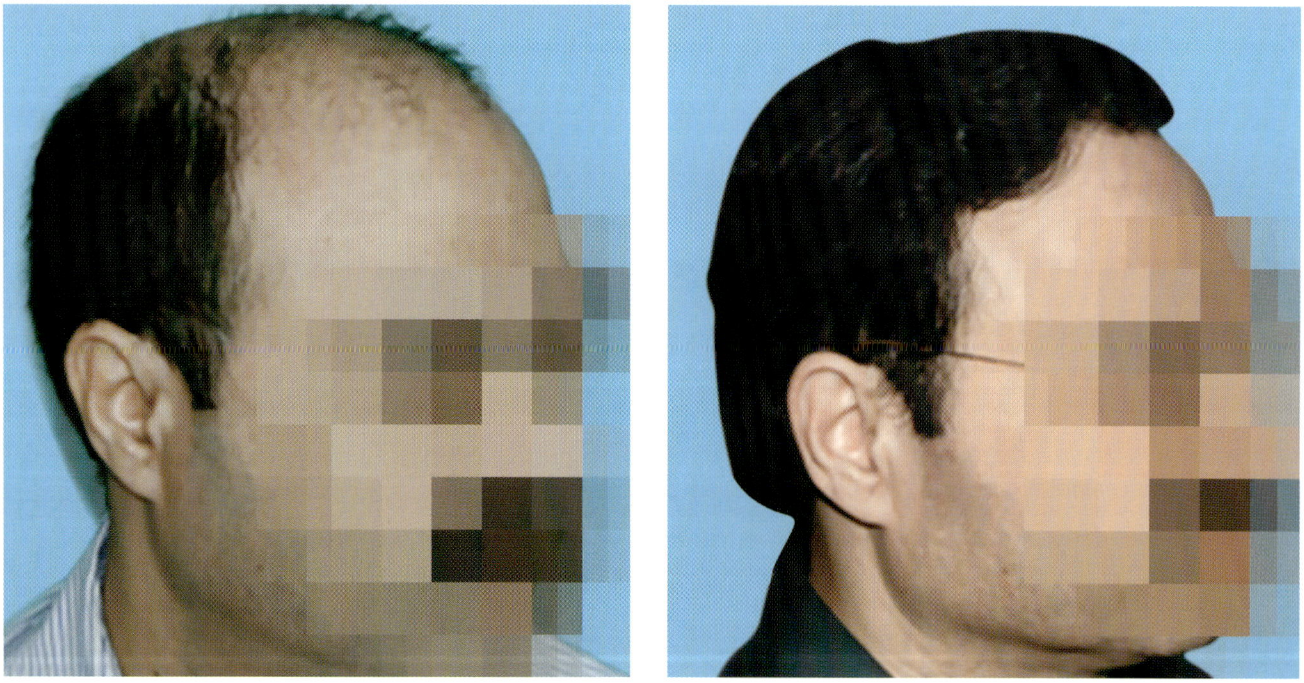

Figure 12.18

The right oblique view of the patient. We did not reconstruct the temple. The hairline-temple balance was maintained by creating a higher hairline.

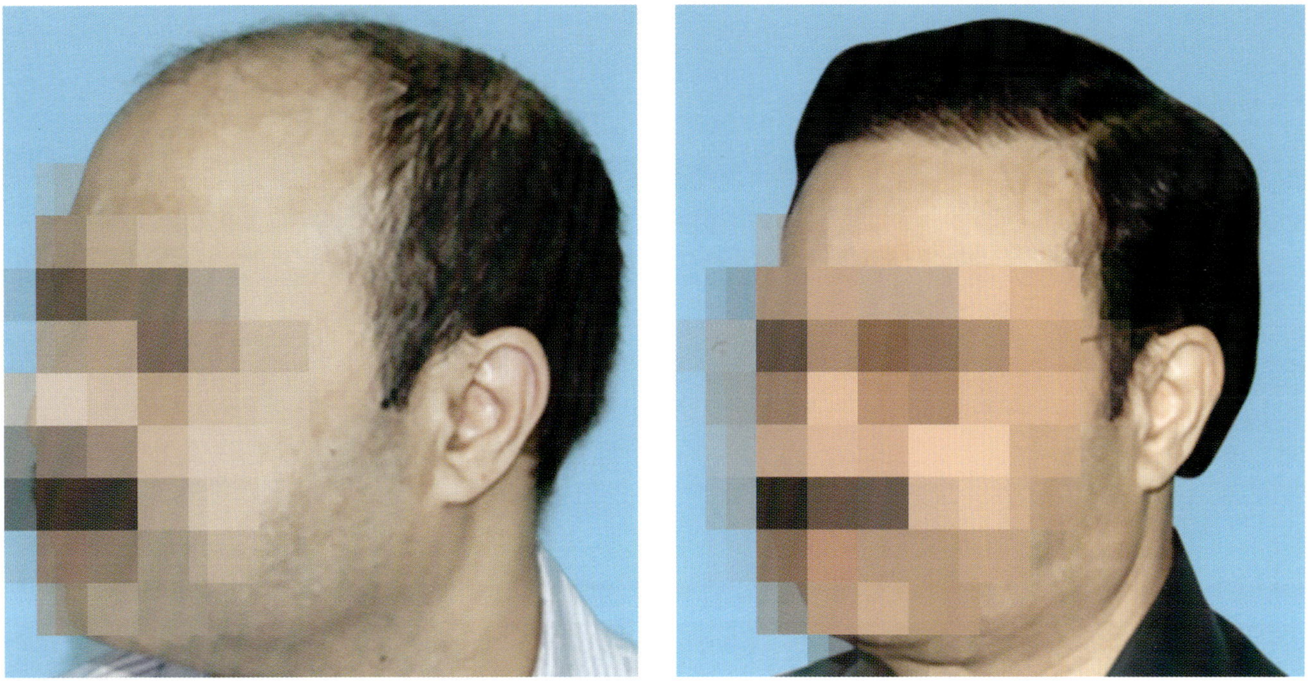

Figure 12.19

The frontotemporal angle is visible in the set of photographs. We created the crown on left side, since he parts his hair from the left side.

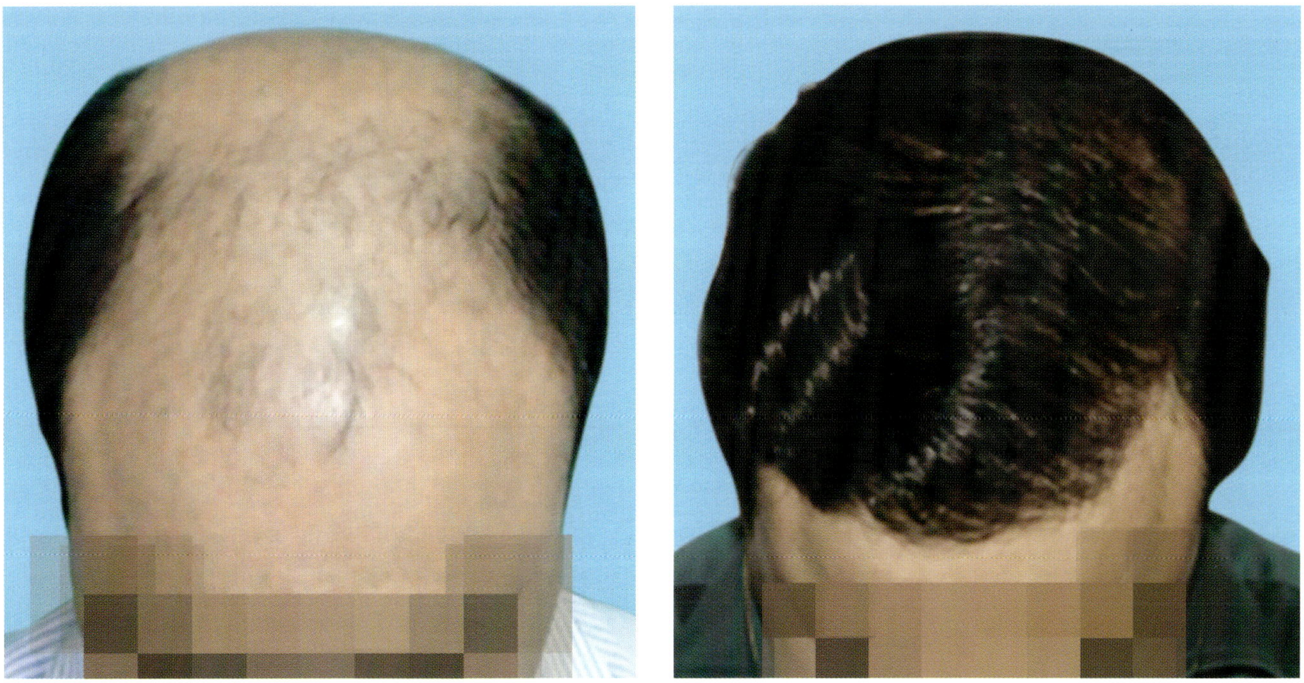

Figure 12.20

The “front bend” view showing the extent of coverage, the graded decrease in density and merging of the transplanted hair with the hair in the temporal region.

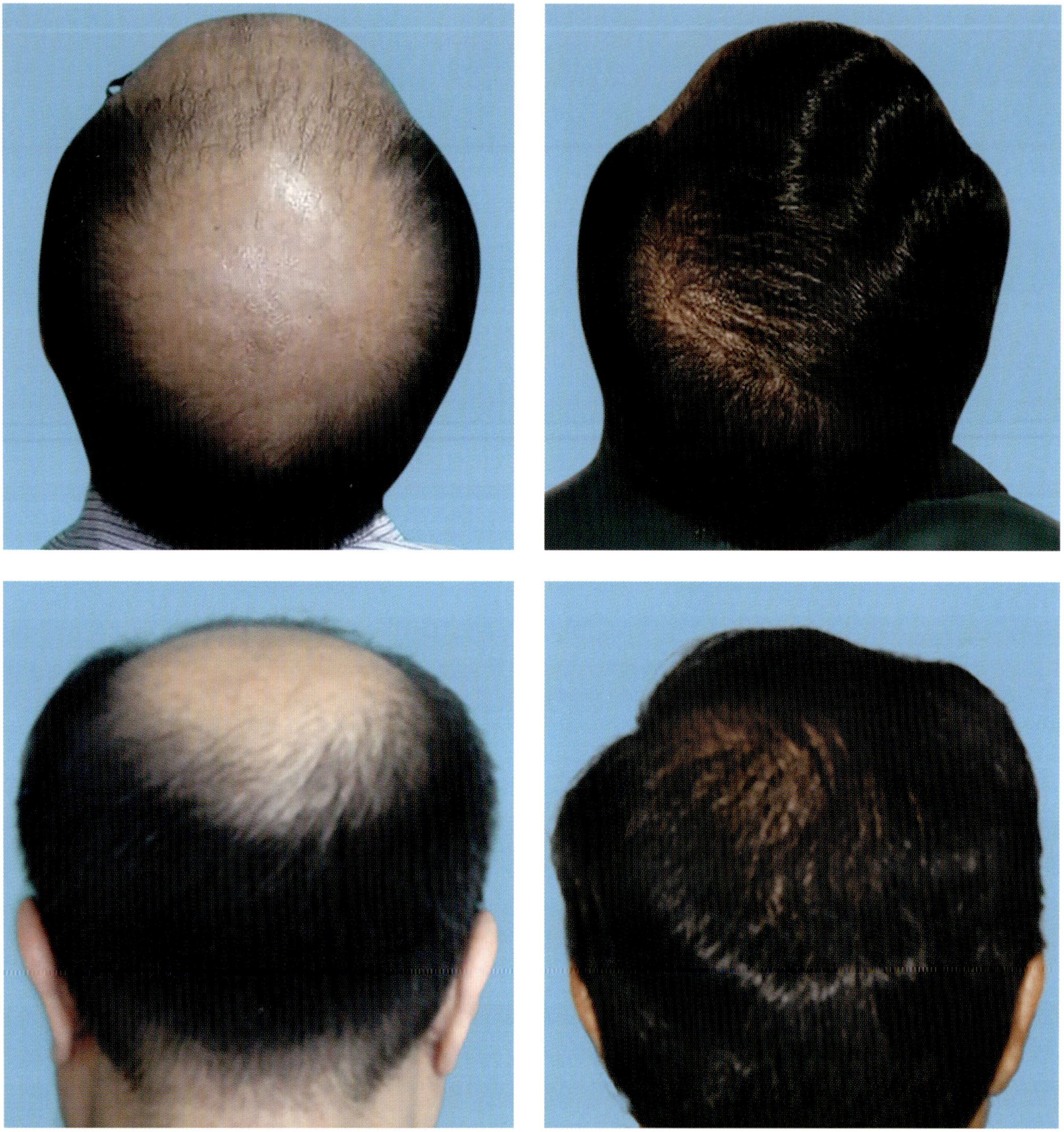

Figure 12.21

We created a left sided, clockwise crown. We implanted 5,000 grafts from the vertex transition point till superior edge of the occipital hair.

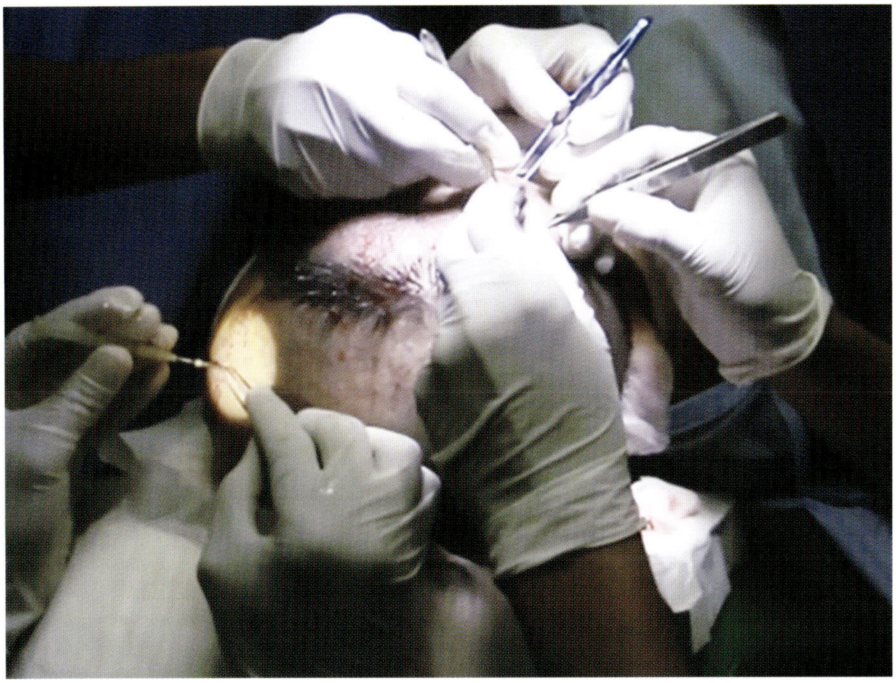

Figure 12.22

After scoring of grafts is completed by the doctor, two technicians quickly extract the grafts as seen in this photograph while one assistant continues with the plantation of grafts.

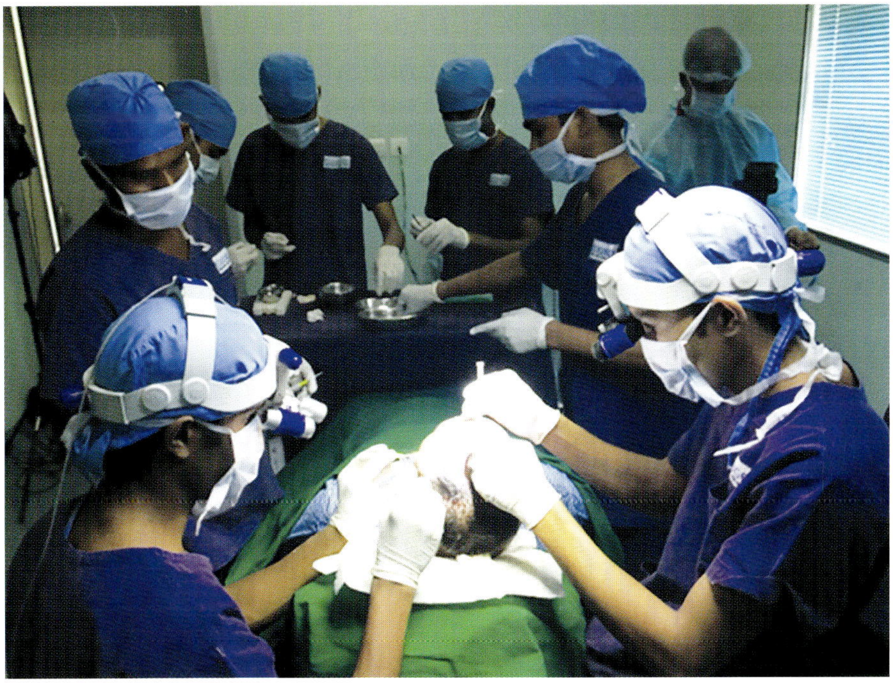

Figure 12.23

Simultaneous implantation by two doctors, loading of grafts by three technicians and transfer of grafts by two assistants.

CONCLUDING THOUGHTS

We have an experience conducting gigasession in over 500 patients now. We have implanted over 5,000 grafts in single sitting of surgery. We feel that our

DHT technique has helped us greatly in going ahead with such megasurgeries. DHT is quicker than follicular unit extraction with minimum out of body time. This ensures graft survival in gigasessions, still we want to caution the surgeons about proper assessment of patient when one conducts gigasession. These patients have extreme grade of baldness but want a youthful hairline. Their donor evaluation includes scalp and beard donor and one should have an estimate of number of grafts which can be extracted together from these areas. Breaching the safe donor area (SDA) may be a concern in such cases among few surgeons. We have been successfully able to extract 1 out 3 noncontinuous grafts from the scalp and 1 out of 2 noncontinuous grafts in beard to get optimum yield and without damaging donor aesthetics. Use of Cole punch ranging from 0.8 mm to 1.0 mm and Trumpet punch of 1.0 mm has helped us in conducting such mega surgeries in patients with even thin grafts but sufficient donor number. We remain within the safe donor region but do not hesitate to extract densely from scalp and unusual sites like side locks and beard.

Comments by Dr Hyun-Wook Baik

What an amazing review about megasession and gigasession. This review will give a big impact to hair transplant surgeons who were too worried about donor depletion, resulting in under correction of recipient area. I agree that the number of the grafts that we can transplant in one session is much bigger that what doctors are usually doing these days.

SUMMARY

- Larger sessions consisting of more than 2500 grafts are called megasession.
- It is done more often now as patients prefer to cover their scalps as much as possible in one surgical visit.
- Good donor ensures such a possibility; with a scalp donor density of atleast 60–70 FU/cm^2, absence of reverse thinning in scalp and good beard density with potential to donate 2000 plus grafts.
- A "normal" head with Norwood grade 7 requires 6000–7000 grafts.
- "Dolichocephalic like" head with Norwood grade 7 requires 6000 grafts.
- "Brachycephalic like" head with Norwood grade 7 requires 10,000 grafts.

REFERENCES

1. Thomas N. Megasessions, Lateral Slits and Dense Packing. Hair Transplant Operative 360, 2nd edn. New Delhi: Jaypee Brothers Medical Publishers (P) Ltd.; 2016. 134.
2. Sethi P, Bansal A. Direct hair transplantation: a modified follicular unit extraction technique. J Cuta Aesthet Surg. 2013;6(2):100-5.

CHAPTER 13

Female Hair Transplantation

Arika Bansal, Sarita Sanke, Pradeep Sethi

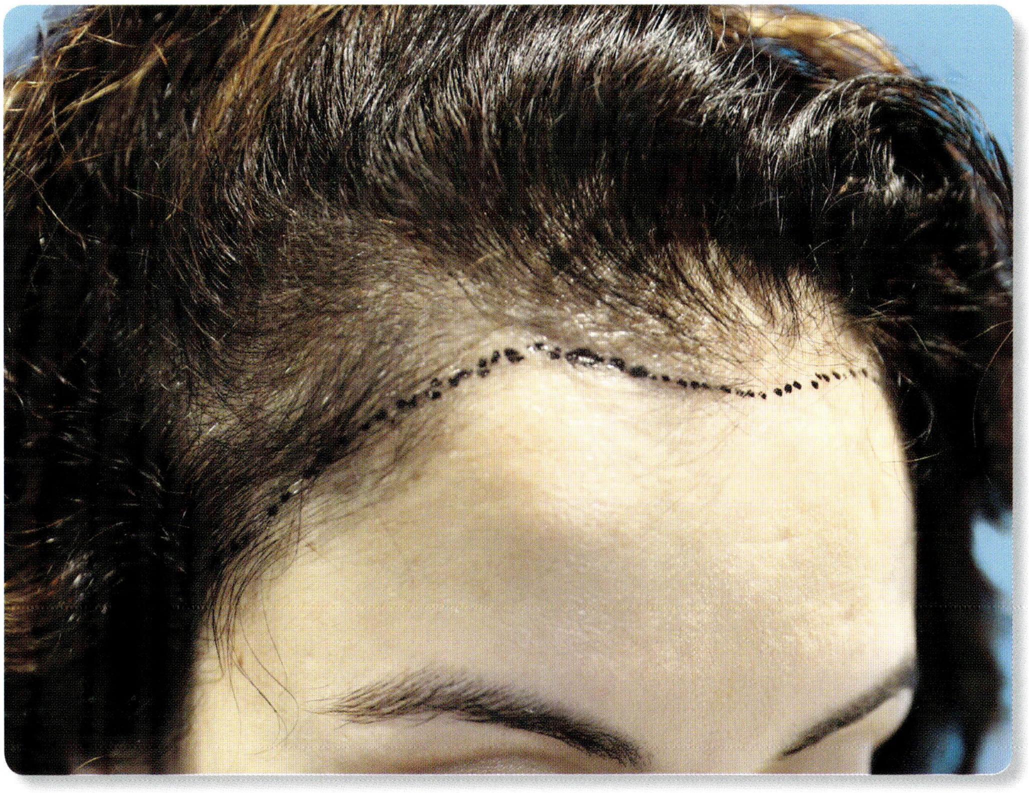

Female hairline.

The beauty of the female face lies in the proportionate positioning of the hairline and a short forehead. With evolution of human body and hair biology females are experiencing more and more receding hairline as well as pattern hair loss.

INTRODUCTION

Hair loss in females has a severe negative impact in their social life. Depending on the cause of hair loss, various treatment options are available. Hair loss in females could be either due to telogen effluvium, alopecia areata, cicatricial alopecia or female pattern hair loss. Medical treatment could be the treatment option in all the four causes; however, hair transplantation is especially indicated in female pattern hair loss.

FEMALE PATTERN HAIR LOSS

Female pattern hair loss could be of three types:[1] (1) Ludwig pattern, (2) Norwood-Hamilton pattern, and (3) Christmas tree pattern.

Ludwig Pattern

Where there is diffuse central sparsening of hair with retention of the frontal hair line (Fig. 13.1). It is the most common type, especially seen in postmenopausal women. Here, our main goal should be to increase the density of hair at the center without damaging the existing hair. The transplant density should be at least 25–30 follicular units (FUs)/cm^2. 21G needles can be used instead of the mini-blades for making the slit, to minimize the damage to the existing hair and to minimize the possibility of shock loss. Premade slits could be difficult to find in

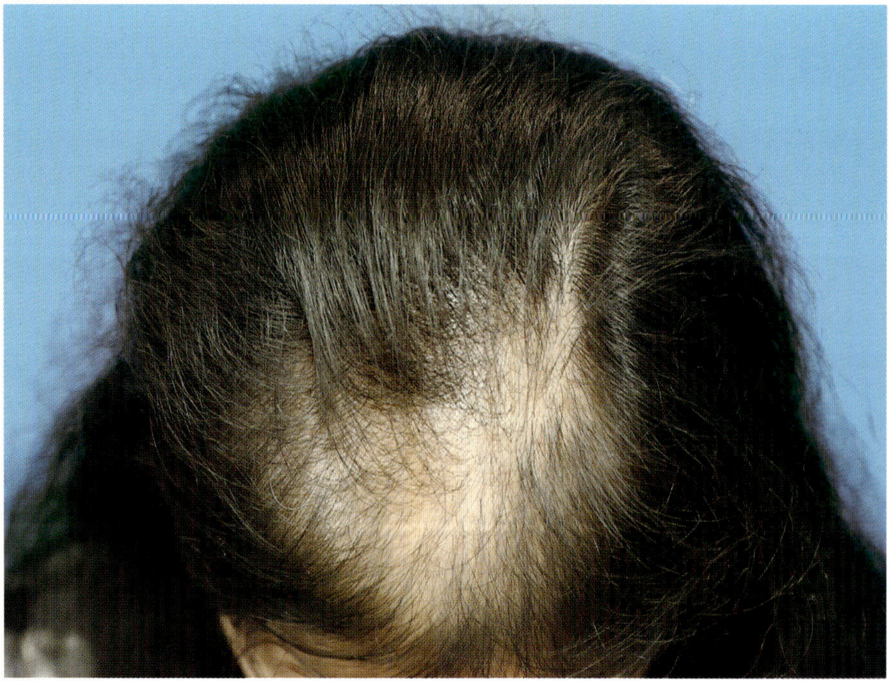

Figure 13.1

Ludwig pattern of hair loss with sparsening of hair at the center.

nontrimmed donor, so it is advisable to use high magnification loupes of 4X to 5X during implantation.

Norwood-Hamilton Pattern

This pattern of hair loss is less commonly seen. Loss of frontotemporal hair causing recession is the most common Norwood-Hamilton pattern seen in females. Here, there is more sparsening in the temples as compared to that in the center. The frontotemporal area is constructed in a manner similar to that in the males, with micro- and macroirregularities. The density should be in the range of 30–40 FUs/cm^2.

Christmas Tree Pattern

Here, there is broad frontal accentuation of hair loss tapering posteriorly.

SCARRING ALOPECIA

Scarring alopecia could be the result of either burns, or any dermatological disease like lichen planopilaris, lupus erythematosus or pseudopelade. Transplantation should be considered only in patients in whom the disease is inactive for few years. The density of hair follicles in the cicatricial areas should be around 15–20 FUs/cm^2. The patients should also be counseled about the poor results in these areas due to inadequate blood supply as compared to that of noncicatricial areas. Slits should be made with 18G or 19G needle and extraction should be done with 1.0 mm punch to ensure adequate grafts and proper survival in the slits, as coverage rather than density is the prime concern.[2]

WHEN SHOULD A FEMALE OPT FOR FEMALE HAIR TRANSPLANT?

The response to medications is slow in females; however, the pathology is same as in males. They should be given minoxidil 5% at least once daily. If they have completed their family, patient can be prescribed finasteride after proper counseling in a dose of 2.5–5 mg. Finasteride is still not the Food and Drug Administration (FDA)-approved for female pattern hair loss. Other androgen inhibitors like spironolactone, etc. can also be tried or combined with finasteride in case of poor response. Mild herbal dihydrotestosterone (DHT) inhibitors like saw palmetto, green tea extract, etc. can also be added. Topical peptides have also shown some promise, although concrete studies showing their efficacy are yet to come. Doctors should always rule out other causes of female pattern hair loss like polycystic ovarian syndrome, adrenal hyperplasia, etc. Patient should be advised minoxidil, oral finasteride or spironolactone for at least 6–8 months before considering hair transplant in early cases. However, in severe cases where results are not expected with medications, one can opt for early hair transplant as well.

Hair transplantation in a female is basically for camouflaging the existing baldness. Achieving full density and coverage is ideally not practical as females never agree for complete trimming of the scalp. Thus, placement of grafts at right position in the scalp is of paramount importance for the surgeon to appreciate a significant change in his patients, look.

HAIRLINE DESIGN AND SELECTION OF SITES FOR SLIT MAKING

In female hair transplant, the sites which need to be transplanted are straight forward as depicted in the Figure 13.2 and Figure 13.3 showing frontotemporal recession hairline recession respectively. The sites of transplantation can be tricky in certain cases like Figure 13.4 where one has to choose the sites depending on the parting style which can give maximum coverage in spite of implanting few grafts in a small area. However, the artistry involved to give naturalness should never be missed.[3]

Slits should be made at relevant sites. When we are making slits in female, we prefer a needle of 21G over 20G and use 0.9 mm sharp surrounded punch

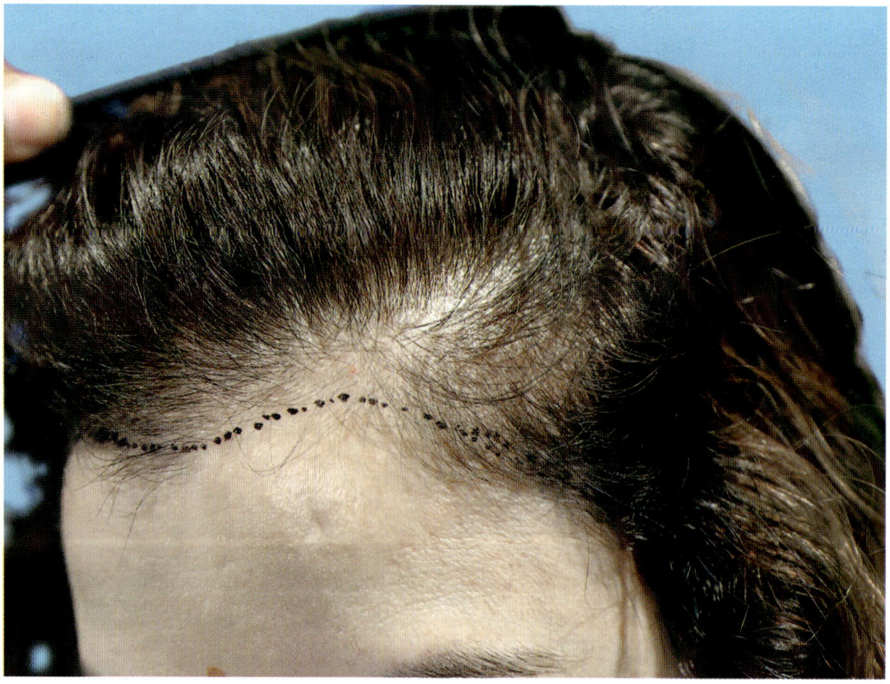

Figure 13.2

Female with frontotemporal recession (Norwood-Hamilton pattern of baldness).

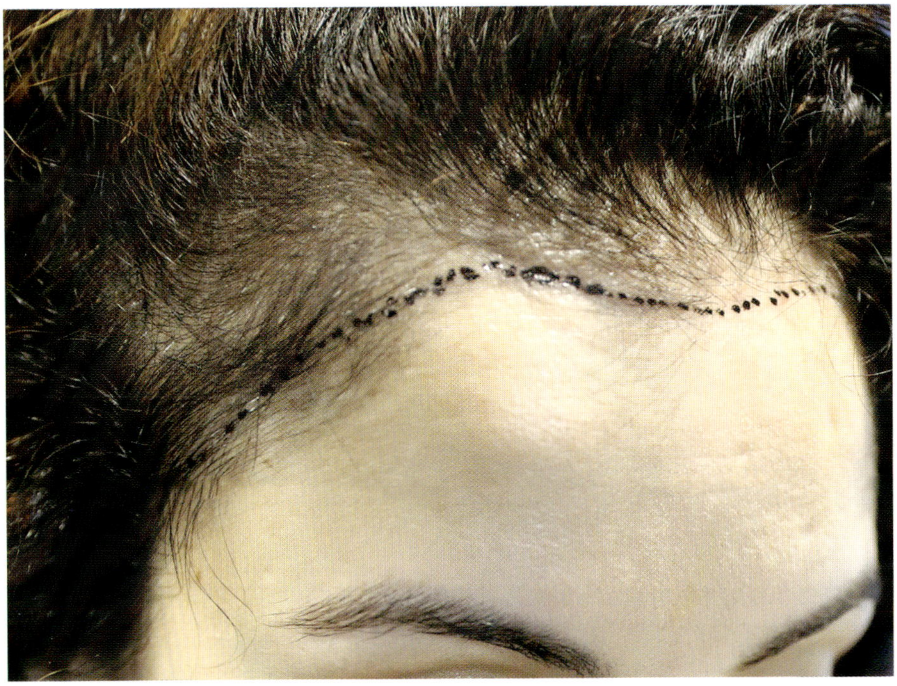

Figure 13.3

Recession of overall female hairline.

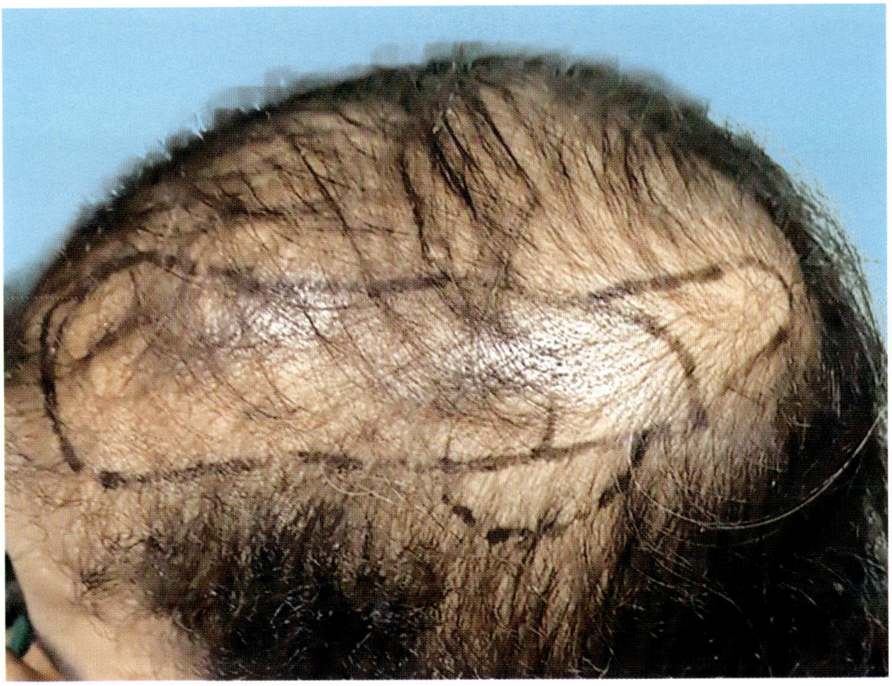

Figure 13.4

An unconventional approach where a huge area of the scalp needs to be filled in this female which is not possible considering the Indian scenario, where complete trimming is not possible. So keeping this in mind, the authors decided to make a triangular zone with a broad base at the hairline and tapering peaks at the vertex with side convex, which merges with temporal hair and the other side concave to conserve the grafts. These hair will grow long and cover the rest of the scalp.

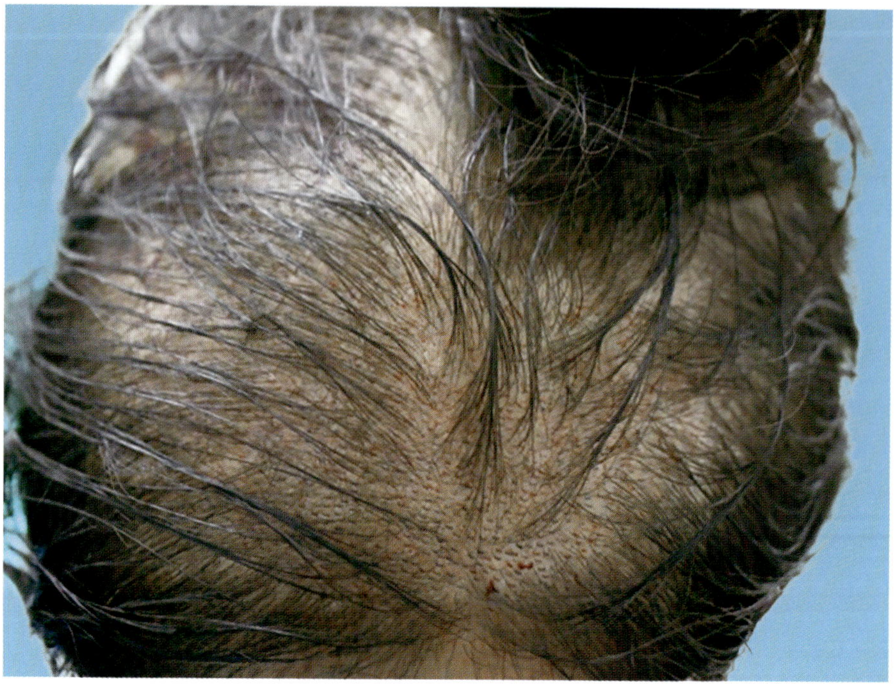

Figure 13.5

Slits have been made strategically in the forelock to improve the density at the partition and improve the frontal look.

for extraction. This modification has been done to minimize shock loss of the pre-existing hair in females. In Figure 13.5, we have not redrawn the hairline. Slits have been made in the frontal forelock which will make the frontal area appear dense and reduce the partition width.

TRIMMING

While doing the window trimming one should carefully decide the length and width of the window depending on the donor density and the type of grafts (Fig. 13.6). It is preferable to extend the window or create new window. Extending it downward may cause exposure of the trimmed scalp.

IMPLANTATION

We prefer blunt dull needle implanters used in the premade slits. This ensures minimum graft handling and minimum resistance during insertion of implanters.

RESULTS

Results are visible over a period of 8 months to 1 year. If the patient and the surgeon are careful and lucky enough and there is no shock loss, results are evident as early as in 6 months (Figs. 13.7A and B).

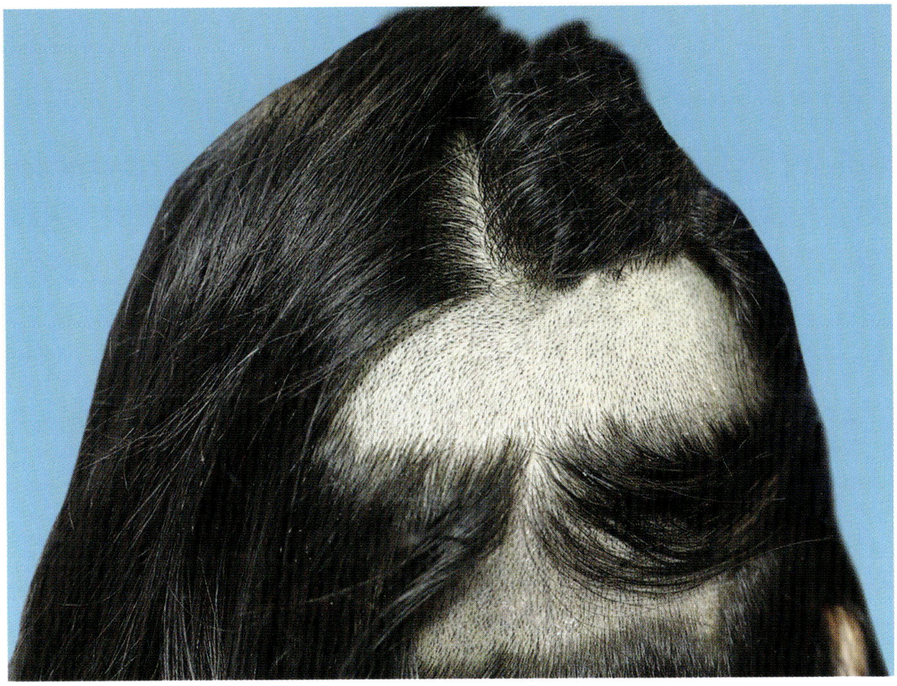

Figure 13.6

Window trimming done in a female with long hair. When she will let her upper hair down, the window area would be hidden beneath these long hair without giving her any cosmetic disadvantage. Care should be taken not to increase the height of window, as it would be difficult to camouflage it.

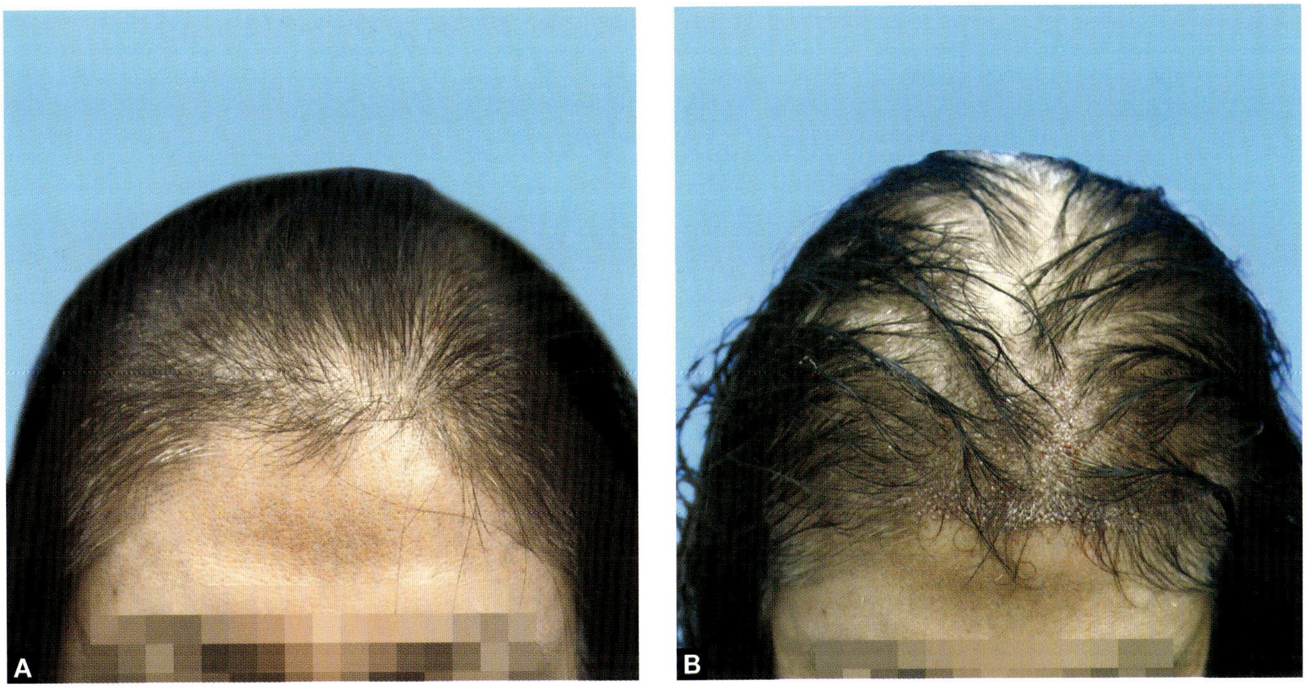

Figures 13.7A and B

The strategic graft placement.

CASE 1

A 35-year-old female with widening of partition came to us for the surgical correction. She had tried all types of medical management but with minimal improvement. We encouraged her to stick to medical management and decided to proceed with surgical correction of hairline. We placed 1066 grafts predominantly in the central forelock (Figs. 13.8A to C). She is happy with result.

CASE 2

An old female had widening of partition and thinning at the hairline zone. Only the frontal zone was implanted with 1,000 grafts for giving good frontal coverage (Figs. 13.9 to 13.11).

CASE 3

A 67-year-old female with recession of frontal hairline came to us for hair restoration (Fig. 13.12). Seeing the size of the bald areas, we were scared initially. She needed at least 2000 to 3000 grafts and was ready to trim her hair. We knew that we could not extract so many grafts from her scalp in one sitting. We promised around 2036 grafts and counseled her about expected result time of 1 year. She went ahead with the surgery. We drew the hairline as shown in Figures 13.13A and B. The slits which have been made are in graded density. We implanted 2036 grafts in those premade slits (Figs. 13.14A and B). The quality of donor hair is extremely important for survival of transplanted hair in female.

CONCLUDING THOUGHTS

Female hair transplant is a tough technique to master due to limitation of trimming. The approach of placing grafts in a concentrated area is usually followed in surgery.

Comments by Dr Nicole Rogers

Hair restoration for women can be just as successful as it is in men. Women with female pattern hair loss generally can achieve the best, most predictable results when the grafts are placed into the most cosmetically concerning areas, as opposed to scattering them all over the scalp. Examples include the part line, the frontal central scalp, or deep bitemporal recessions, which can look masculine until the hairline is rounded and lowered. Other women may benefit from transplantation into brow lift scars or facelift scars along the sideburn area.

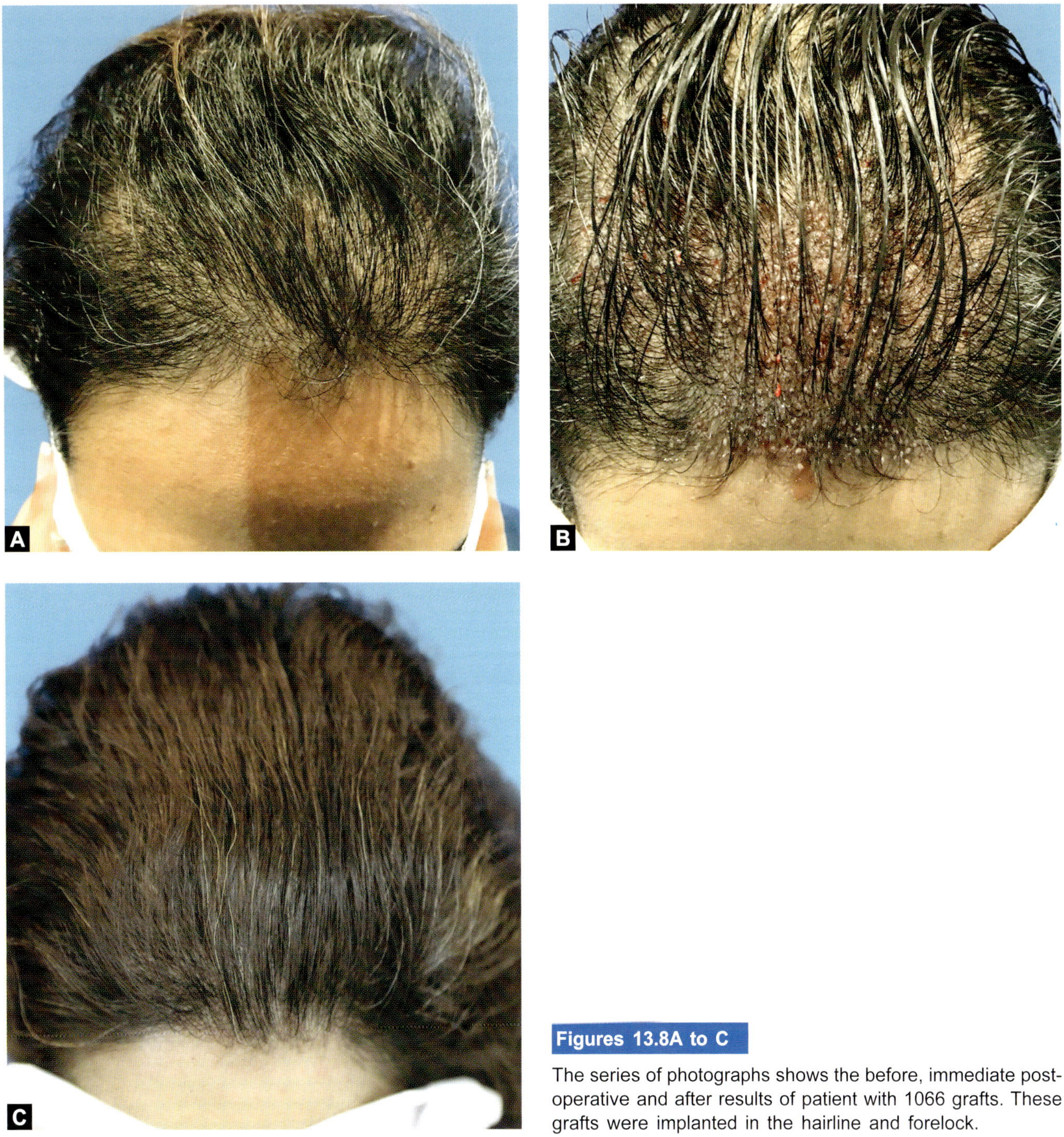

Figures 13.8A to C

The series of photographs shows the before, immediate post-operative and after results of patient with 1066 grafts. These grafts were implanted in the hairline and forelock.

Most women choose to have traditional donor ellipse [strip, or follicular unit transplantation (FUT)] harvesting so that they would not have to shave their head. Occasionally women who are concerned about the possibility of a linear scar

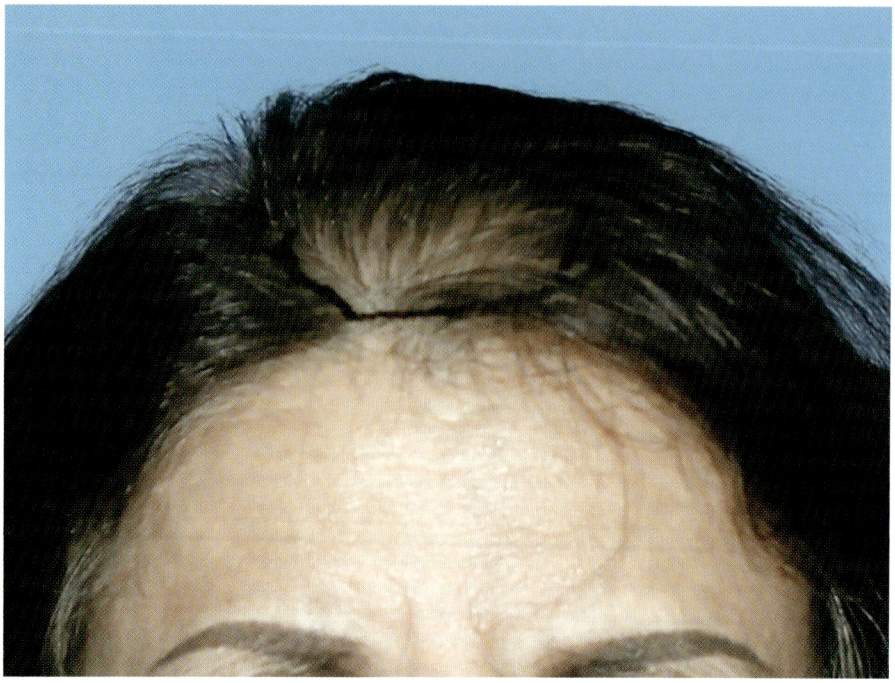

Figure 13.9

Hair loss at the partition site is evident. The area to be implanted is first marked.

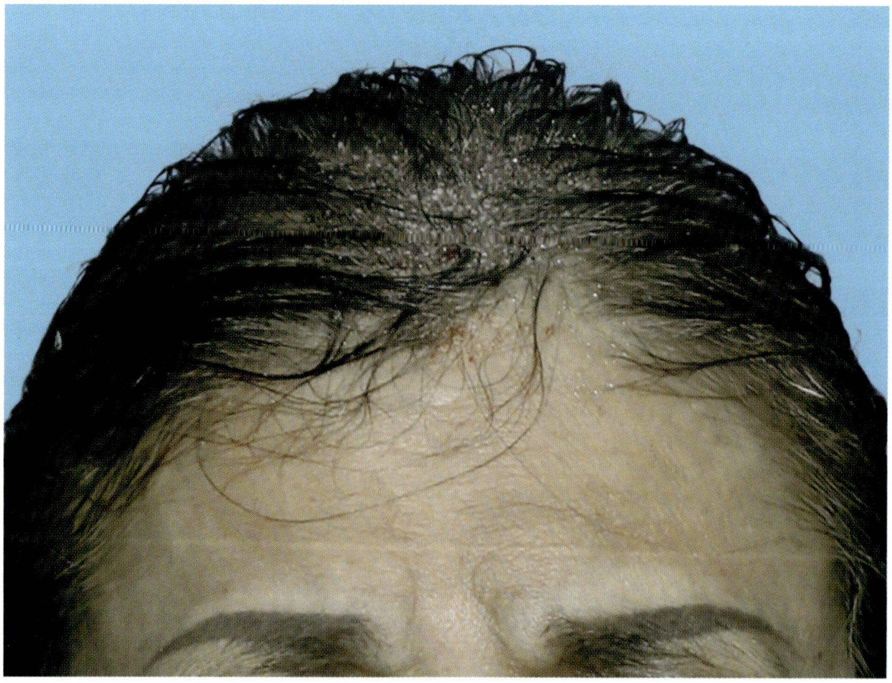

Figure 13.10

Immediate post-transplant photo showing the implanted grafts (1,000 grafts) at marked sites.

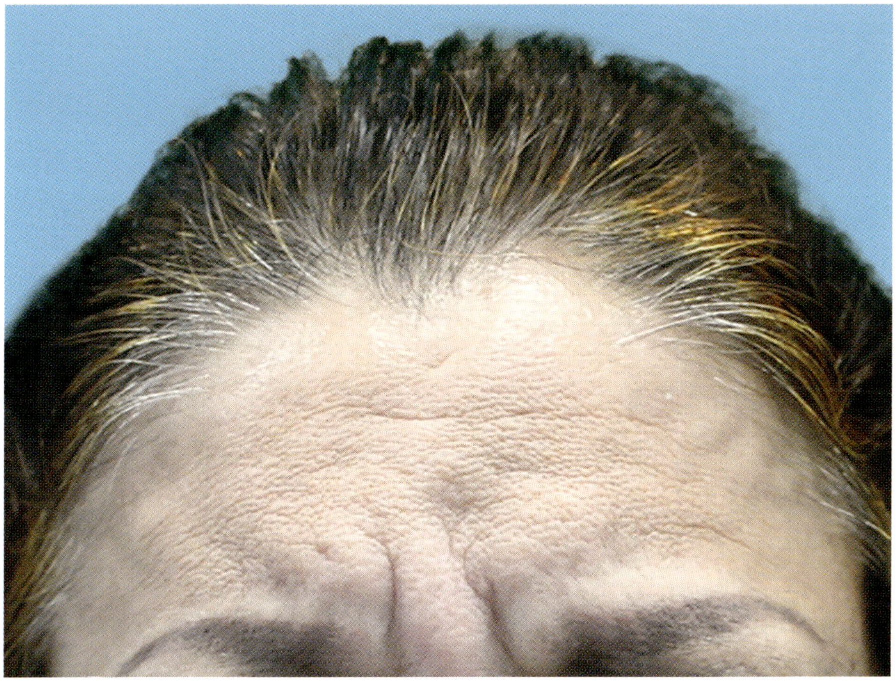

Figure 13.11

Eight months post-transplant photo showing that even fewer number of grafts implanted at the right sites can give a good coverage in a female and can change the look dramatically.

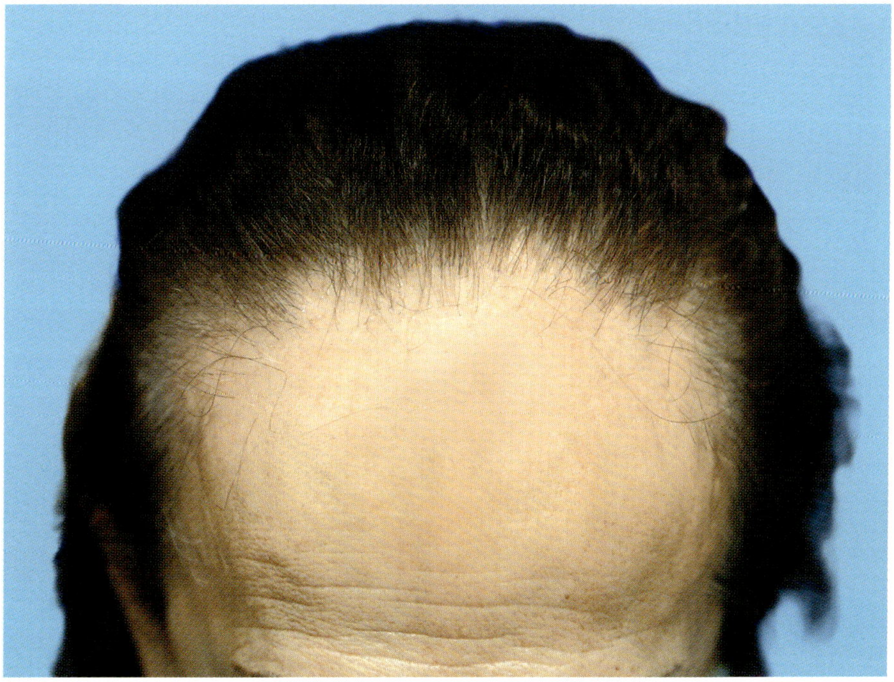

Figure 13.12

Note the pre-existing receded hairline in this patient. This was a case of male pattern baldness in female. This should not be confused with frontal fibrosing alopecia (which we thought initially). The baldness was stable since last 15 years.

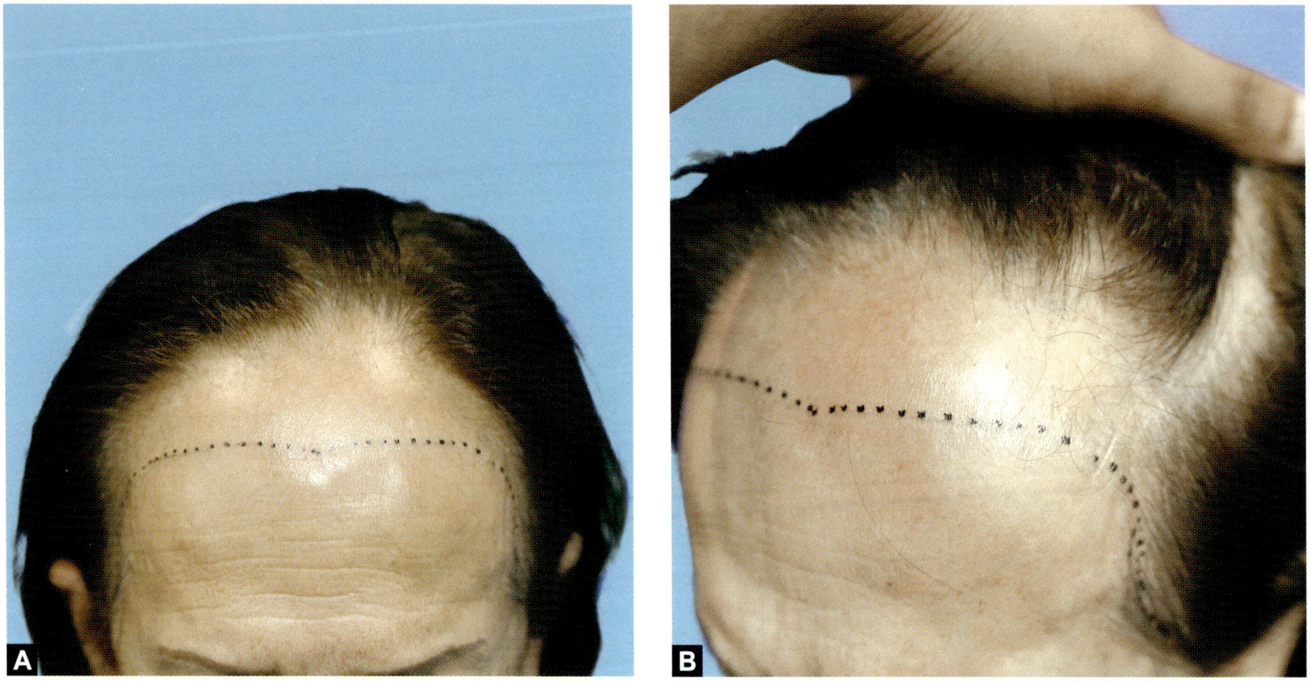

Figure 13.13A and B

The redrawn hairline with the plan to extract around 2000 grafts.

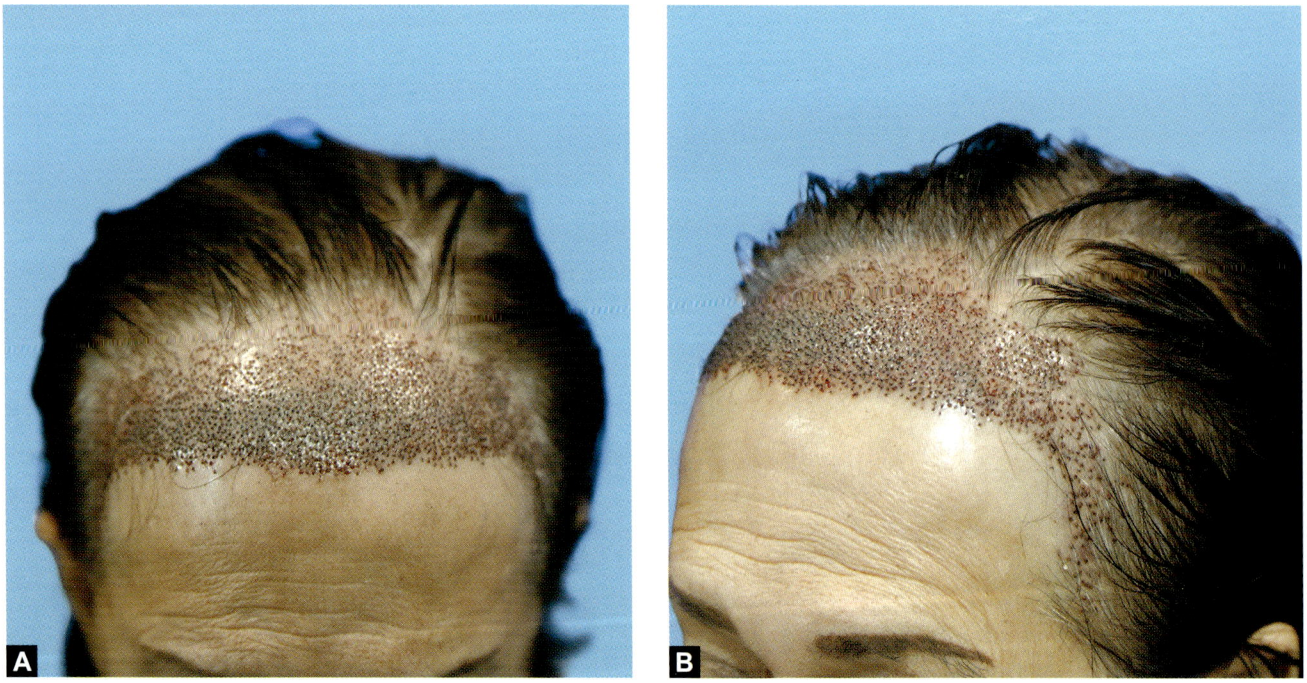

Figures 13.14A and B

We implanted 2036 grafts in this patient.

may choose follicular unit excision (FUE). A fair number of women may develop a postoperative telogen effluvium (shedding of surrounding nontransplanted hair). This usually resolves with time and the hair grow back along with the transplanted hair. Topical minoxidil, spironolactone, finasteride, LLLT, and PRP can all help to enhance surgical results and prevent future thinning.

SUMMARY

- Hair loss in female is on the rise and each day we see more of them. Much more concern and stigma is associated with it when it comes to women with baldness.
- *Reasons: Telogen effluvium, Cicatricial alopecia,* or *simply FPHL.*
- *Patterns:*
  - *Ludwig:* Diffuse central sparsening with retention of frontal hair line.
    Transplantation should be done with a density of 25–30 FU.
  - *Norwood:* Hamilton pattern—common. Sparsening at temples than at centre. Transplant density should be around 30–40 FU
  - Christmas tree pattern—broad frontal accentuation tapering posteriorly.
- *Scarring alopecia:* LPP, Lupus erythematous, Pseudopelade of Brocq. Transplanted only if diseases is burnt out.

  Transplant density around 15–20 FU. Results are variable due to decrease blood supply in Cicatricial areas. Slits to be made with 18 or 19G needles. Punch 1.0 mm.
- *When to for sure go ahead...* medical treatment to be tried before, viz. minoxidil 5%, finasteride 2.5–5 mg. Others like aldactone, saw palmetto, green tea extract, topical peptides.
- *Artistry* to give naturalness.
- Preferred needles 20G and punch 0.9 mm sharp surrounded.
- Window trimming
- Blunt SAVA implanters.
- *Points to keep in mind:*
  - *Avoid shock loss*
  - Coverage is given more importance than density
  - To rule out existing PCOD, adrenal hyperplasia.

REFERENCES

1. Jung JH, Rah DK, Yun IS. Classification of the female hairline and refined hairline correction techniques for Asian women. Dermatol Surg. 2011;37:495-500.
2. Shapiro R. Principles and techniques used to create a natural hairline in surgical hair restoration. Facial Plast Surg Clin North Am. 2004;12:201-17.
3. Wong J. Planning for ultra-refined follicular unit transplantation and the hairline design. In: Pathomva D, Imagawa K (Eds). Hair Restoration Surgery in Asians. Tokyo; London: Springer; 2010. 37-9.

CHAPTER 14

Eyebrow and Eyelash Transplantation

Sarita Sanke, Manas Chatterjee, Pradeep Sethi

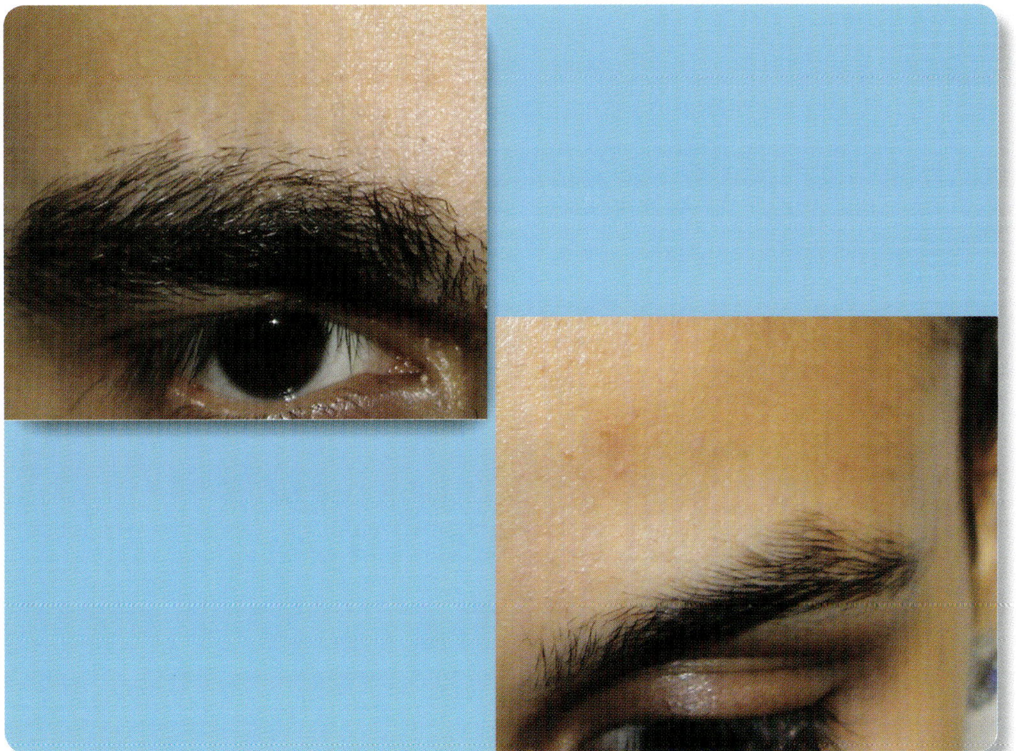

The hair in the eyebrows are placed differently with different angles and graded thicknesses along the total brow. The patients need to be educated enough about the requirement of regular trimming and grooming of the grown hair to keep them short enough to just be at the length of the normal eyebrow hair. This does not take away the responsibility of the physician to chose the right kind of hair which are having optimum pigment, slow growing with long anagen phase. Wrongly planted eyelashes can give regular trichiasis and do more harm to the eyes!

INTRODUCTION

Eyebrows play an important role in making a person look beautiful, especially in Asians.[1] They form an integral part of the face. Eyebrows can be lost as a part of cicatricial alopecia in diseases like lichen planopilaris, discoid lupus erythematosus or it could be secondary to burns, chemotherapy or radiotherapy or due to congenital inability to grow hair.

For reconstructing an eyebrow, a surgeon must have an idea about the natural appearance of the eyebrows in both males and females. A female will like her eyebrows to have an arch at the junction of medial two-thirds and lateral one-third (Figs. 14.1A and B). The density of hair should be more in the center, widening in the medial portion, becoming narrow and dense in the lateral part. A slight feathering at the upper and lower border would please the female. In contrast, the eyebrows in a male are uniformly thick and dense throughout with no arch (Fig. 14.2).

An important thing to know for a surgeon is that the eyebrow hair, unlike the scalp hair are fine, soft and thin. The hair of the hairline at the periphery of scalp are said to be fine with thinner caliber simulating the eyebrow hair. Hence, an area of scalp near the periauricular area or nape of the neck close to hairline margins is chosen as the donor area for eyebrow transplantation.[1] There should not be any evidence of retrograde thinning while choosing hair from those regions.

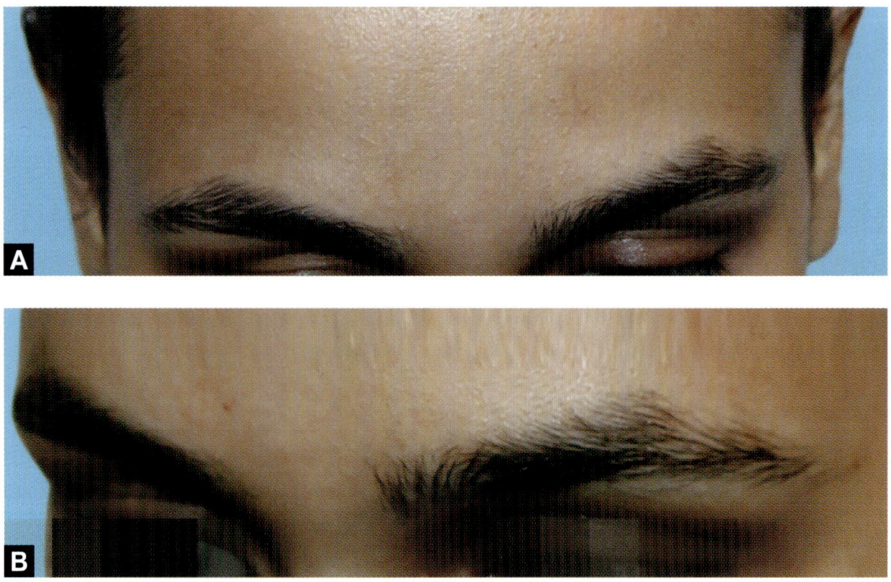

Figures 14.1A and B

An ideal female eyebrow. Note the arched appearance, widening at the junction of medial two-thirds and lateral one-third. There is feathering at the upper border.

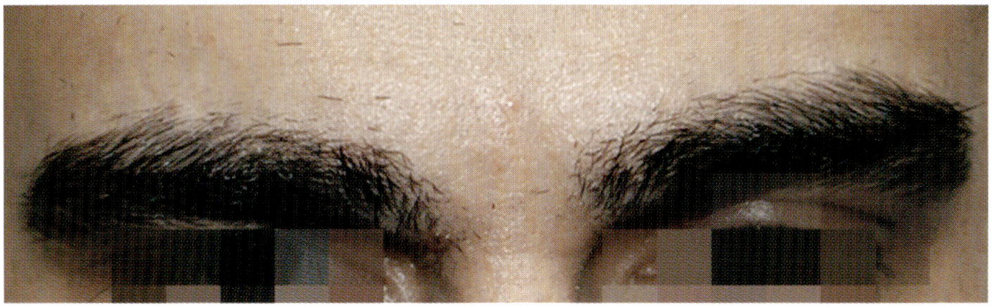

Figure 14.2

Male eyebrow. Note the uniform thickness and absence of arch.

PROCEDURE

An outline of the eyebrow must always be drawn beforehand and reviews of the patient himself must always be taken regarding the shape and design desired (Fig. 14.3).

The donor region should be trimmed but hair are kept slightly longer to know the curl of the hair in the donor region so that the transplanted eyebrows stick to the skin surface.

The donor area as well as the eyebrow area is anesthetized with 1% lidocaine and epinephrine. An area not more than 1×6 cm^2 is usually needed to reconstruct the eyebrows. The grafts should be harvested using a smaller diameter punch usually of 0.8 mm or 0.9 mm punch by the follicular unit extraction (FUE) method.[2] One should deliberately make follicular transections in case of multiple grafts or extract only single hair grafts. In case of multiple grafts, manual dissection of the grafts should be done. It is important to harvest single follicle grafts only for eyebrows.

The grafts in eyebrow construction are usually pointed in three different directions as shown in Figure 14.4. The bulb of the medial, most grafts should be pointed downward (red arrows), the bulb of the upper grafts in lateral area should be pointed medially and downward (blue arrows), while the lower lateral grafts should be pointed medially and upward (green arrows). Also, a good surgeon must always consider the color and caliber of the grafts to be transplanted to achieve fantastic results. The hair at the medial end are lighter in color with smaller caliber, becoming darker and thicker as we proceed laterally in the middle. Again, in the lateral end, the hair are of smaller caliber.

On an average at least 100–250 single hair grafts are needed on each side depending on the area involved.

We create the slits first with a 20G needle to create the space for the placement of grafts. The slits should be made keeping the hair directions and angulations in mind (Fig. 14.5).

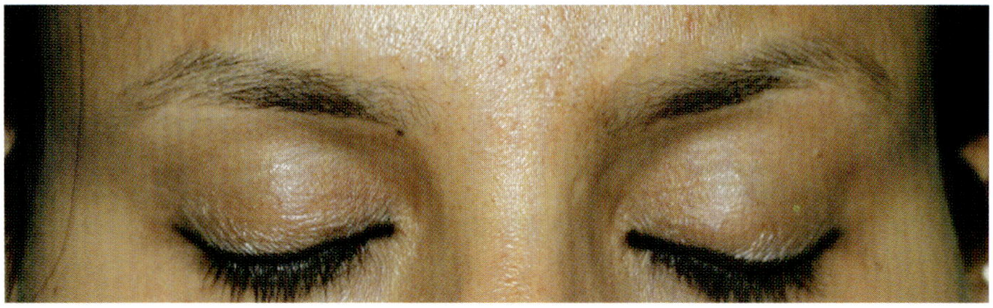

Figure 14.3

Designing and marking the eyebrow with a skin marker should always be done before the surgery. Asking the patients opinion about the design and incorporating any inputs makes them feel satisfied.

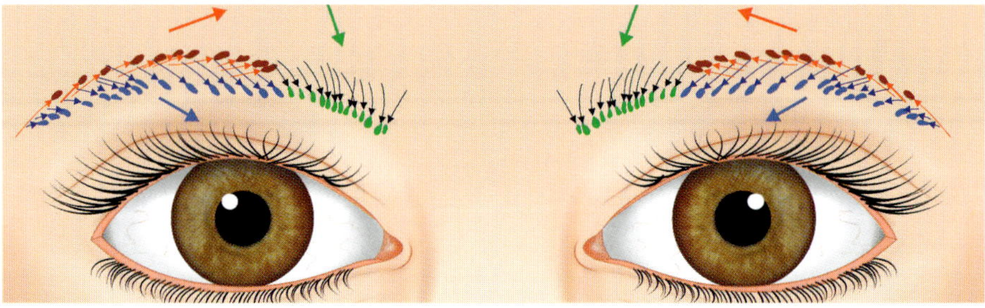

Figure 14.4

Note the orientation of the bulb at various sites of eyebrow. The density of hair also varies at various sites.

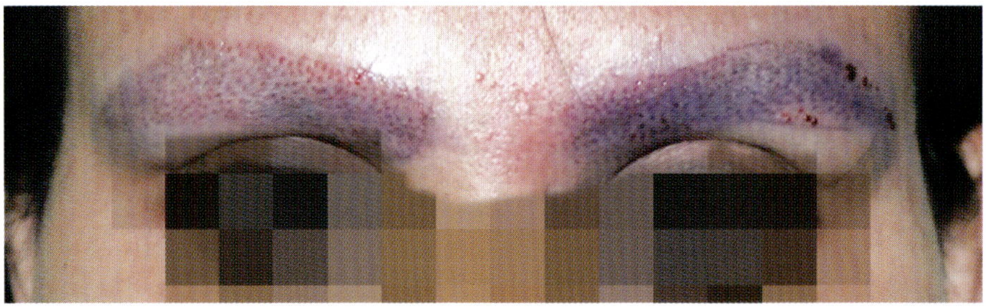

Figure 14.5

Note the premade slits created in this patient. The direction and angulation of slits is critical in this patient. Even a slight change in direction of the slits may lead to bad results.

The direction and angle of the hair to be inserted should be in accordance to a natural eyebrow. We use SAVA™ implanters to insert the grafts in the premade slits. The most experienced technician or the surgeon himself should insert the grafts in the premade slits since orientation of the grafts is critical to ensure quality result (Fig. 14.6). The curl of the hair needs to be kept in mind so that hair kisses the skin when it starts growing.

After the complete procedure is done, the patient should always be asked to examine the grafts and the eyebrow shape that has come out, and any adjustments if required should be done immediately.

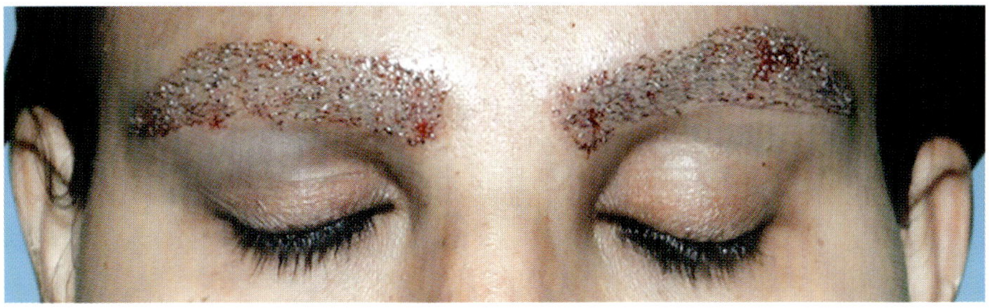

Figure 14.6

Grafts are inserted keeping the directions of the premade slits in mind.

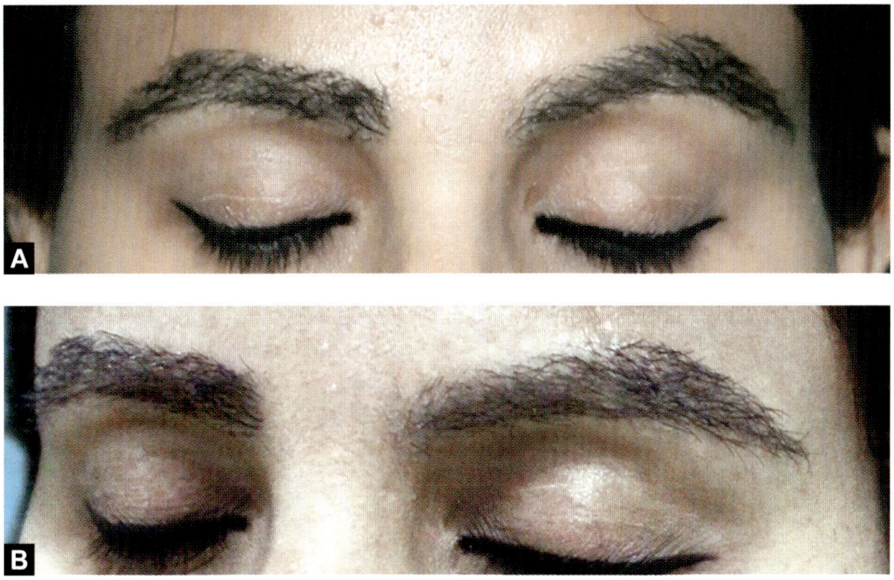

Figures 14.7A and B

Considerable growth of eyebrow hair after 8 months of transplantation. Note the arch and the direction of hair. Also note that the caliber of the hair is slightly thicker as compared to normal eyebrow hair. Hence choosing a right donor area with fine hair is important.

The patient should be asked to follow-up after 5 days. If we find any hair growing in any abnormal direction, it has to be extracted immediately. The growth of hair takes about 6-8 months, achieving the final result by 1 year (Figs. 14.7A and B).

The shortcomings in eyebrow transplantation include a few hair growing out of alignment, giving an unnatural appearance. This is especially common in patients with curly grafts. Mimicking the medial most part of eyebrow to give a natural look is very difficult and comes with expertise.

EYELASH TRANSPLANT BY DR MANAS CHATTERJEE

Eyelash transplantation is a procedure in which hair follicles from hair-bearing areas are transplanted in eyelashes. It has been used as a therapeutic option for loss of eyelash resulting from diverse etiology like trauma or trichotillomania and vitiligo. Eyelash transplantation can be performed by various methods. It can be done using pluck and sew technique as described by Caputy GG et al.[3] It can also be done using single hair transplant with Choi hair transplanter or by strip composite eyebrow graft as described by Kasai K.[4]

Procedure[5]

Mild sedation is ensured by using tablet diazepam 10 mg per oral half an hour prior to starting of procedure. Corneal eye shield applied after topical anesthesia with lignocaine. Local anesthesia is administered in donor and recipient site with 2% lignocaine with adrenaline. Temporal area is prepared by clipping of hair and single hair follicle is harvested using 0.8 mm punch with FUE motor. The involved eyelashes are removed with a 20G needle similar to creation of chambers for hair transplantation of the scalp. Black hair obtained from the temporal scalp of the patient was harvested as in hair transplant surgery and single hair grafted onto the chambers created, using fine jeweller's forcep or implanter. About 15–20 hair per eyelash is transplanted in one sitting. Donor lash is trimmed to size of other lashes. Thereafter, a pad and bandage is applied to the affected eye for a week (Figs. 14.8A to D).

Postoperative Evaluation

After procedure, eye pad is applied and treated eye is kept covered for 7 days. There is formation of scab around transplanted follicle and transplanted hair falls off by 2–3 weeks and regrowth of eyelashes is first noticed by 8–10 weeks. Surgery is usually free from major complications and most common complications noticed are bruising and swelling of eyelids. Patient should be instructed and told to use curling devices to give direction to eyelashes. Scalp hair grow faster and hence required trimming of these lashes by patient at regular intervals (Figs. 14.9A and B).

CONCLUDING THOUGHTS

We believe that we still have to improve in eyebrow and eyelash reconstruction. The caliber of hair of scalp and placement of thinner caliber grafts at medial end and lateral end are critical in providing naturalness. Probably taking body hair and mixing with scalp hair will provide better alternative to taking only scalp hair at these sites. Choosing the right donor region and orienting the grafts correctly are critical in these cases. The eyebrow hair should kiss the skin, so it is essential to examine the curl before implanting the graft. Similarly in eyelash transplant, the eyelash should grow away from the eyeball which is only possible if the curl of the transplanted eyelash is correct.

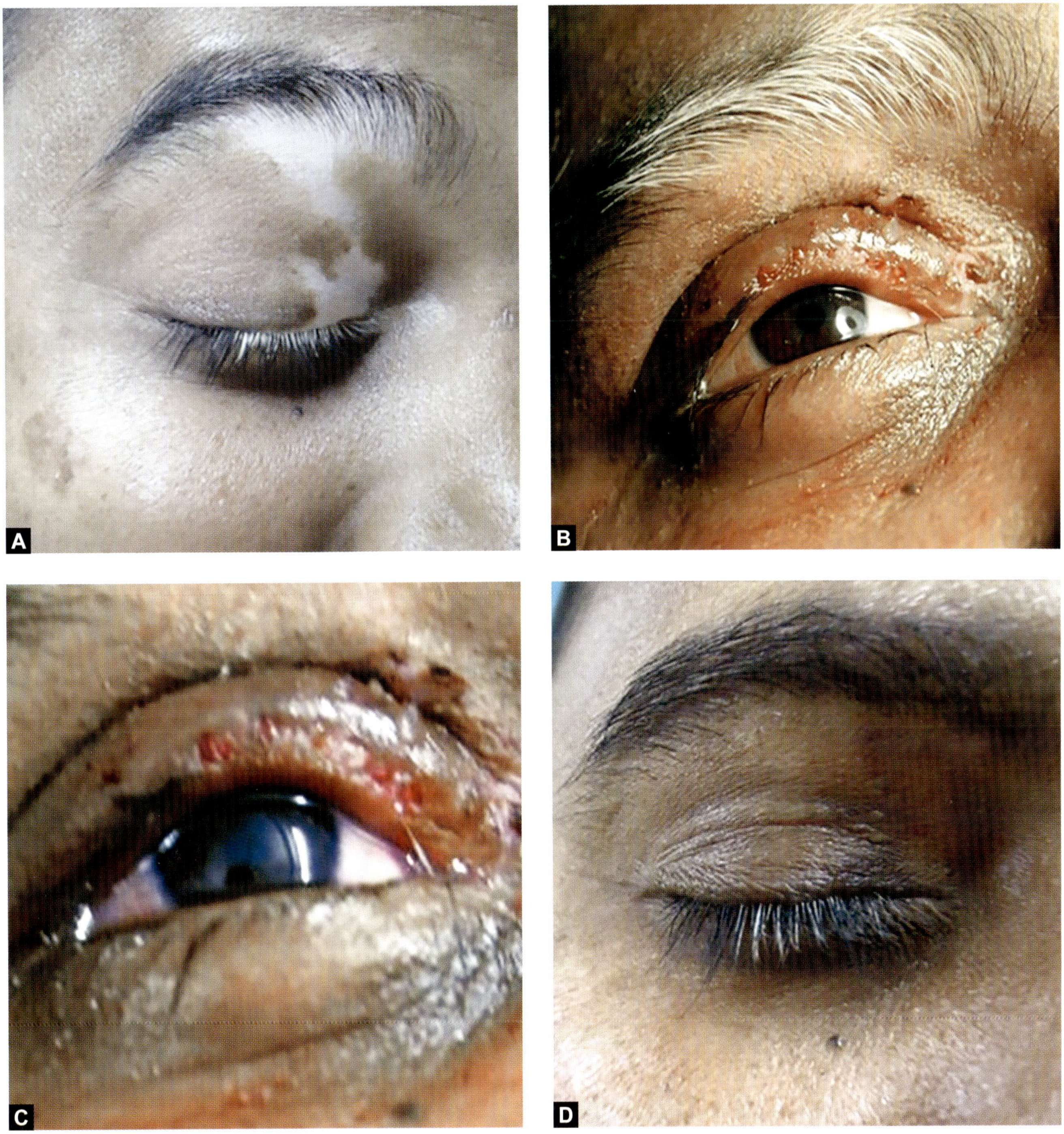

Figures 14.8A to D

Eyelash transplantation was in this for vitiligo with eyelash leukotrichia. Swelling is seen immediately after transplant as shown in Figure 8C. Figure 8D shows growth of pigmented eyelash and eyelid after 3 months.
Courtesy: Dr Manas Chatterjee.

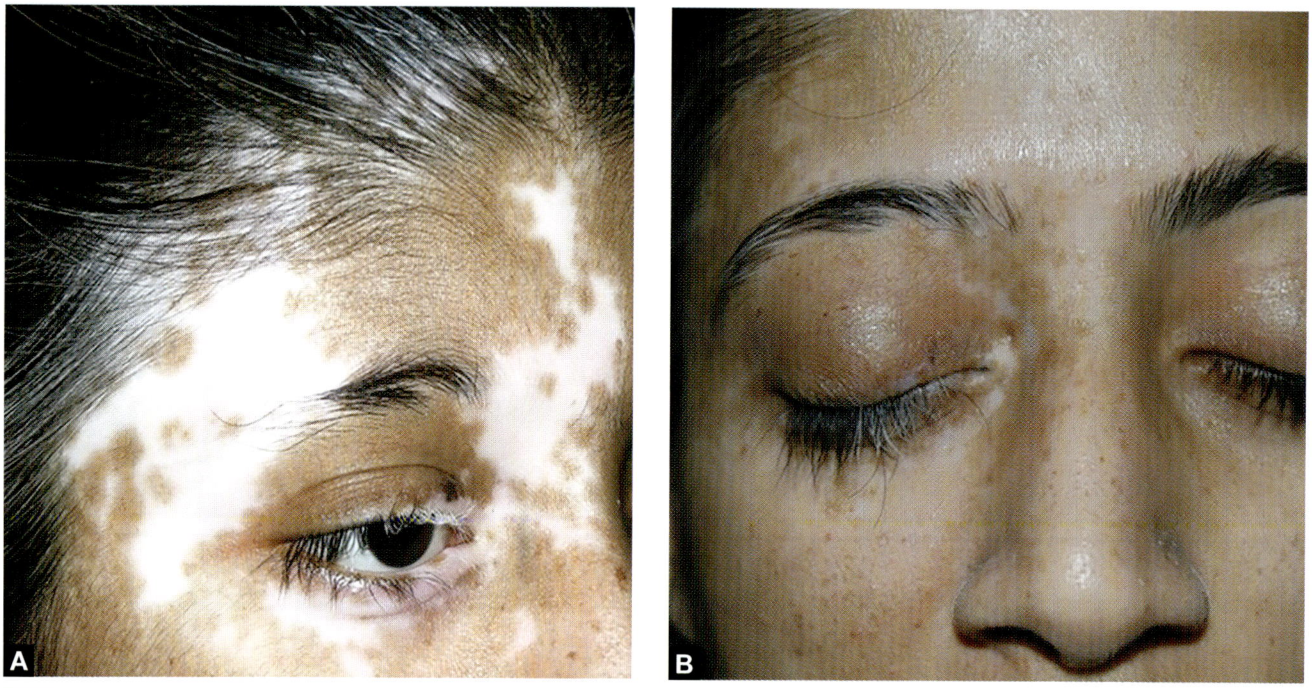

Figures 14.9A and B

The relatively longer transplanted eyelash which needs to be cut every 2 weeks. The transplanted eyelash ensured pigmentation of the depigmented eyelid margin.
Courtesy: Dr Manas Chatterjee.

Comments by Dr Nicole Rogers

Eyebrow restoration can be one of the most challenging and rewarding aspects of hair surgery. Eyebrows have an anagen (growth) phase lasting just 3 months. Patients must understand the most obvious difference, which is the longer growth phase of transplanted follicles. As a result, hair taken from the scalp must be trimmed every 2–4 weeks. Also, the hair are not naturally tapered so the distal tips can look thicker and less natural. Because of the difficulty achieving such a natural appearance, some have argued that eyebrow restoration should be limited to purely reconstructive cases of scarring or total eyebrow loss. Transplantation of eyebrows in frontal fibrosing alopecia or lichen planopilaris may grow in the short run, but it can be difficult to predict or guarantee long-term growth especially if other medications controlling the disease process are discontinued. Each case must be considered on an individual basis and with the informed consent of the patient.

SUMMARY

- Female eyebrow demands an arch at the junction of medial two-thirds and lateral one-third; with density more in center, widening in medial portion, becoming narrow and light laterally.
- Male eyebrows are uniformly thick and dense throughout without arch.
- Only single follicle grafts are implanted and punched out with 0.8 or 0.9 mm size punch.
- Orientation and curl of graft is extremely critical to ensure quality result in eyebrow and eyelash transplant.

REFERENCES

1. Laorwong K, Pathomvanich D, Bunagan K. Eyebrow transplantation in Asians. Dermatol Surg. 2009;35(3):496-503.
2. Tomc CM, Malouf PJ. Eyebrow restoration: the approach, considerations, and technique in follicular unit transplantation. J Cosmet Dermatol. 2015;14:310-4.
3. Caputy GG, Flowers RS. The "pluck and sew" technique of individual hair follicle placement. Plast Reconstr Surg. 1994;93(3):615-20.
4. Kasai K. Eyelash reconstruction with strip composite eyebrow graft. Ann Plast Surg. 2008;60(6):649-51.
5. Chatterjee M, Neema S, Vasudevan B, et al. Eyelash transplantation for the treatment of vitiligo associated eyelash leucotrichia. 2016;9(2):97-100.

CHAPTER 15

Hair Transplantation in Cicatricial Alopecia

Sarita Sanke, Pradeep Sethi, Priyadarshini Das, Abhinav Kumar

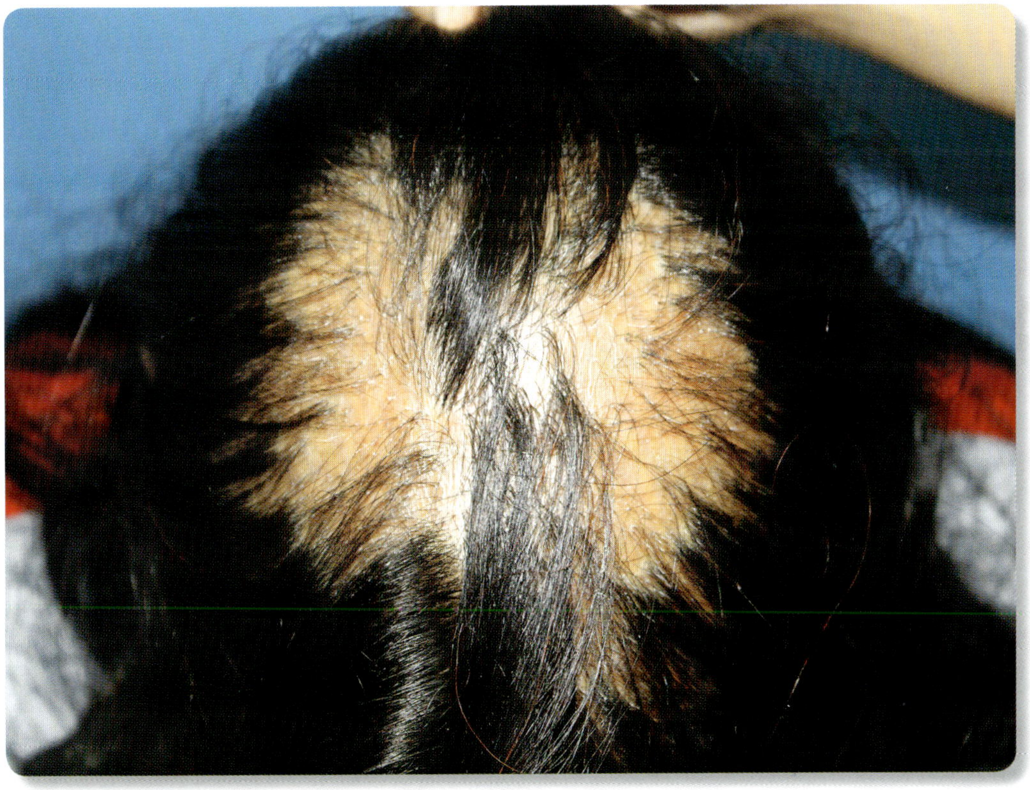

Lichen planopilaris.

The scars on body are always difficult to manage. But most scars on the hair-bearing areas can be managed to great extents if the physician is experienced enough with the behavior of the scar tissue with hair transplantation. The gratification achieved is much more when a scarred eyebrow or scalp grows hair to cover it than grown hair upon normal bald area.

INTRODUCTION

Cicatricial alopecia is a condition wherein the hair follicle is the primary target and is permanently destroyed and replaced by fibrous tissue. Cicatricial alopecia leads to permanent damage of the stem cells in the hair follicle bulge. It can either be primary (lichen planopilaris, discoid lupus erythematosus, folliculitis decalvans, etc.) or secondary (to burns, radiation, trauma, etc.).

Pharmacological treatment in these cases can halt the progression of disease, but it cannot cause regrowth of the hair thus, effecting the self-esteem and self-image of the patient. This is where, hair restoration surgery (HRS) comes as a boon to restore the aesthetic look of the patient.

CHALLENGES FACED DURING HAIR RESTORATION SURGERY IN CICATRICIAL ALOPECIA

- Graft survival is an issue
- Compromised vascular supply of the scarred area
- May lead to koebnerization, if the disease is active
- Donor area itself, may be compromised by the disease
- May need multiple sessions
- Higher rate of complications
- Low blood flow can cause infection, tissue ischemia, and necrosis after surgery
- Unpredictable results
- Close monitoring after surgery for any signs of relapse of the disease.

PREREQUISITES FOR HAIR RESTORATION SURGERY IN CICATRICIAL ALOPECIA

- The disease should be stable/nonprogressive (at least 1 year of quiescence).[1]
- A good donor area should be available.

HAIR RESTORATION SURGERY IN CICATRICIAL ALOPECIA

Follicular unit excision (FUE) is definitely better than other procedures for HRS in cicatricial alopecia. It also gives the added advantage of using body/beard hair for transplant when donor area in the scalp is inadequate. A scarred tissue has poor blood supply and scalp oxygenation which is of utmost importance for a good uptake of the grafts. The depth of slit making also varies in the scarred tissue. If the scar is hypertrophic, the slits should be made deeper than normal, and if the scar is atrophic, the slits need to be less deep. The graft survival also depends on the number of grafts/cm^2. It is better if this number does not exceed 30 grafts/cm^2

when performing hair transplant in cicatricial alopecia.[1] More number of grafts may hamper the uptake due to poor blood supply.

Adrenalin should be avoided during local anesthesia injection, so that the areas of poor vascular supply can be assessed by the surgeon. In such relatively avascular areas, the number of graft implantation should be restricted to 15–20 grafts/cm^2. Minoxidil can be used to induce vasodilation in the period preceding and/or following surgery to improve oxygenation of the grafts. Pentoxifylline 400 mg three times a day with meals, for 2 weeks before surgery, can be another alternative method for increasing oxygenation of the scalp tissue.

The institution of pharmacological therapy for the primary disease immediately postsurgery is questionable. We recommend starting therapy to protect the newly implanted grafts as well as the uninvolved grafts from the inflammatory process of the primary disease and to halt disease progression/koebnerization.

Test Patch

Ideally, in cicatricial alopecia cases, the HRS should first be done in a small patch of the affected area to look for the results and to ensure if uptake of the grafts is sufficient to give visible results.[2] Once evident results of hair growth are seen, the rest of the areas can be taken up for grafting. In cases, where extensive areas need to be covered, the surgery can be done in sessions. The second session should be done after 10–12 months of the first one. In the second session, we can also increase the density and give an aesthetically better look, reducing the see-through effect.

COMPLICATIONS IN HAIR RESTORATION SURGERY IN CICATRICIAL ALOPECIA

The chances of certain complications like tissue necrosis, ischemia, and infection are more in cicatricial alopecia cases due to the decreased perfusion of tissue. In case necrosis occurs, the area should be debrided and left to heal with secondary intention.

CASE SCENARIO 1 (FIGS. 15.1 TO 15.4)

Female patient aged 32 years, presented to us with cicatricial alopecia of 17 years duration, secondary to lichen planopilaris.

As we could see, the recipient area was very large. Hence, we first did the test patch of the grafts to look for the uptake and growth. A small area was chosen in the center of the scarred area and FUE was done. A good growth of the hair was noted after 6 months, signaling a good uptake. The rest of the scarred area was

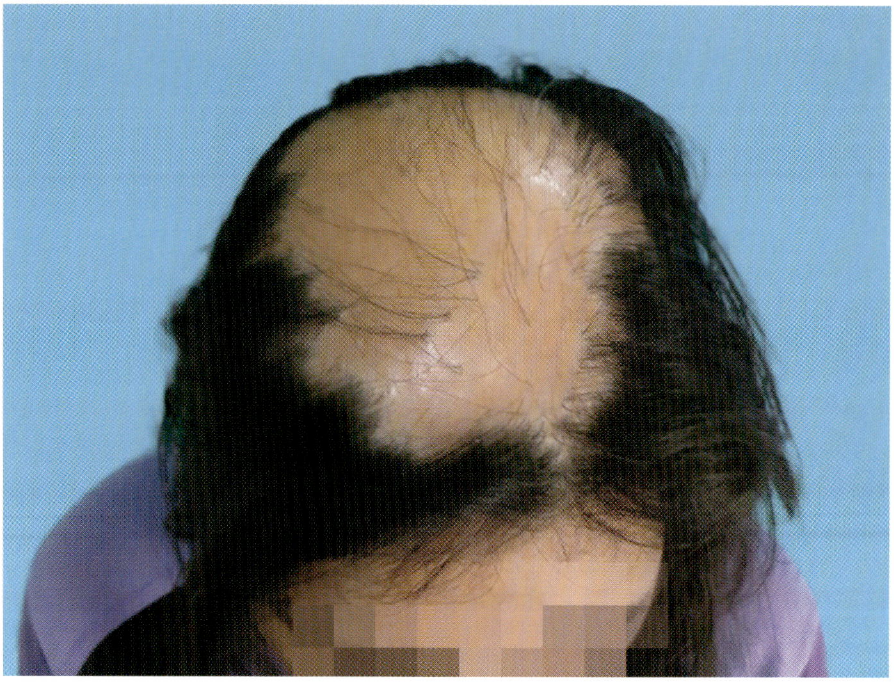

Figure 15.1

Extensive area of cicatricial alopecia, secondary to lichen planopilaris, extending from the frontal area to the vertex.

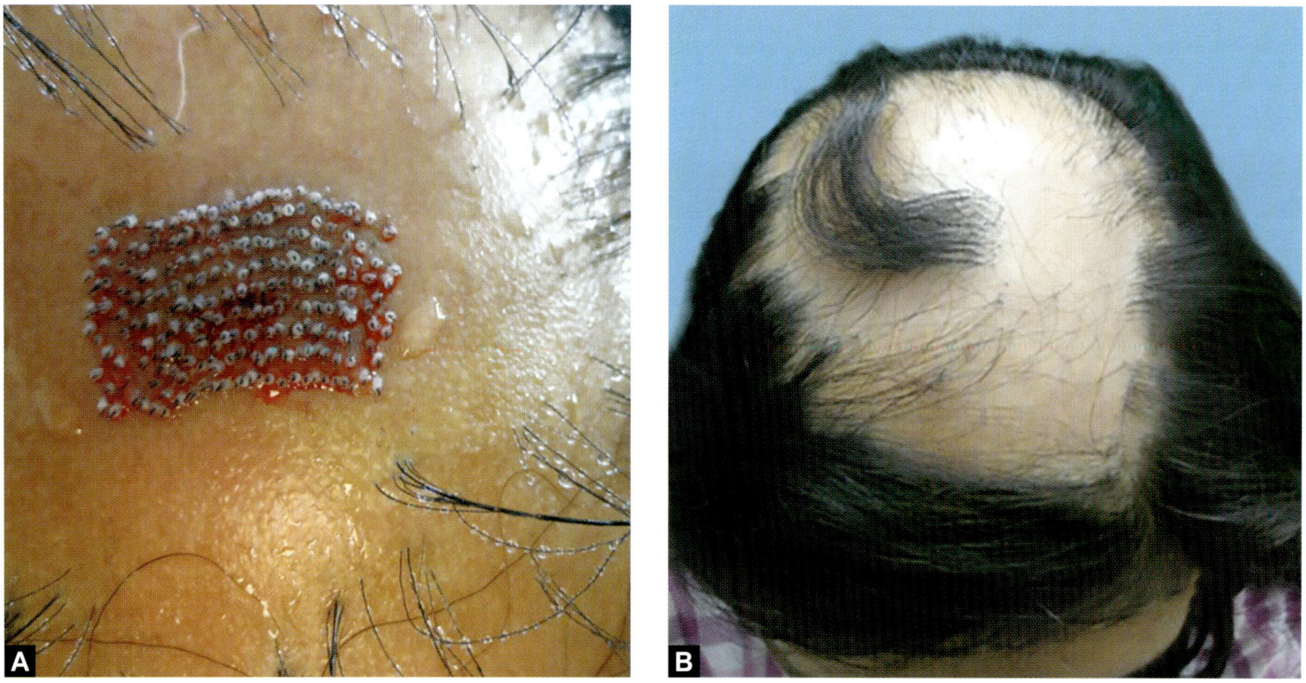

Figures 15.2A and B

(A) A small area "Test patch" is initially tested for the uptake of the grafts and hair growth; (B) Grown test graft after 6 months.

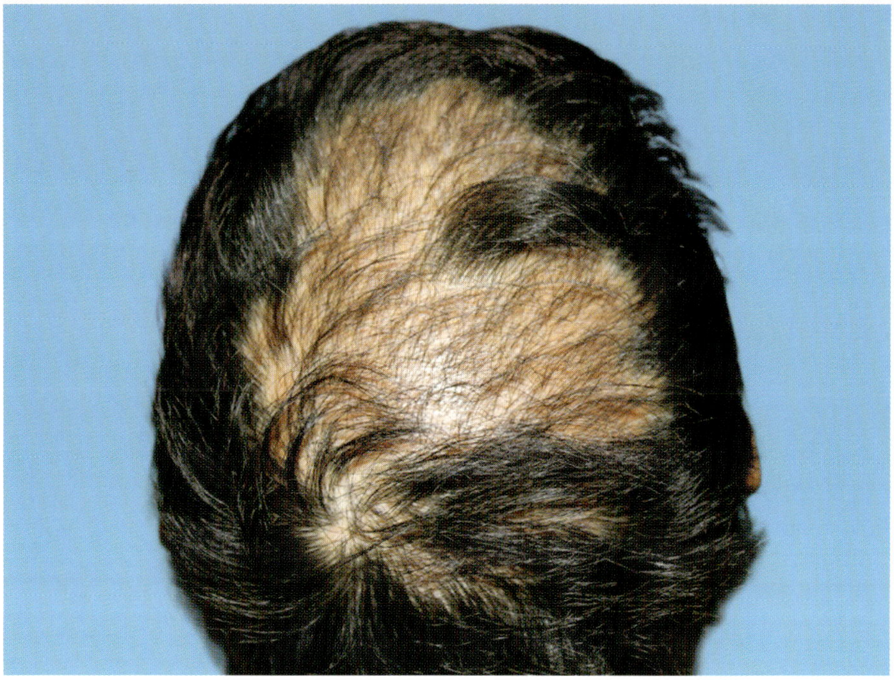

Figure 15.3

Once, the test patch showed the growth of hair (as seen by a bunch of long hair in scarred zone). We transplanted the remaining area. The transplanted hair can be seen growing 4 months after the transplant in this image.

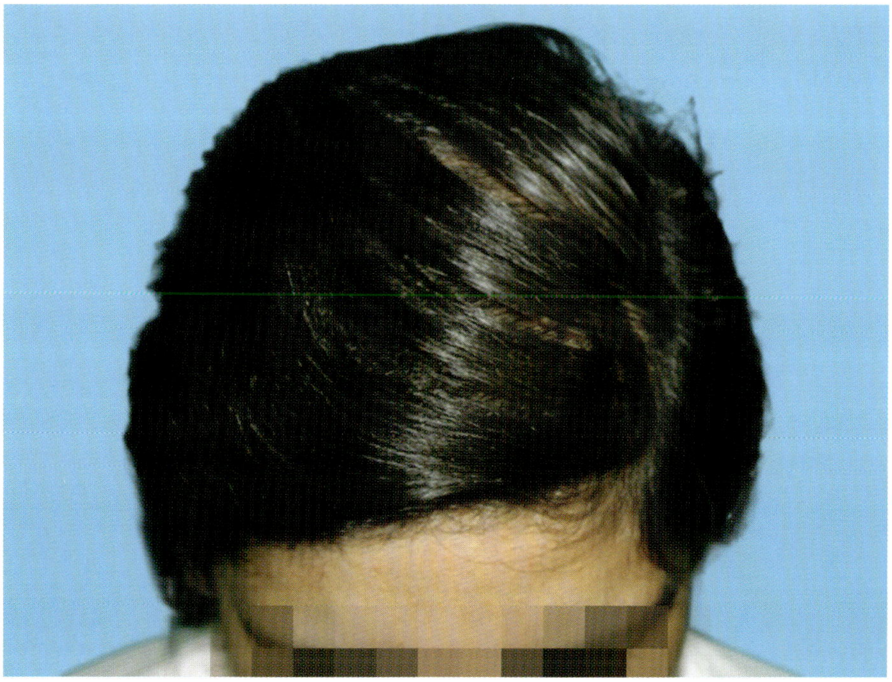

Figure 15.4

Excellent growth of hair seen after 15 months over the entire scarred area. There was no disease recurrence in the follow-up period.

then transplanted. Approximately, 2,000 grafts were implanted keeping the density of grafts to 25 grafts/cm^2. Successful growth of the hair was seen after 1 year.

CONCLUSION

Hair restoration surgery in cicatricial alopecia cases is difficult but not impossible. Appropriate selection of the candidates and meticulous planning of the surgery will definitely yield good results.

SUMMARY

- Lichen planopilaris is the most common cause of primary cicatricial alopecia.
- The major challenges are compromised vascular supply, reactivation of disease after surgery and compromised and diseased donor region.
- Prognosis is relatively better in secondary causes of cicatricial alopecia like burns, trauma, etc.

REFERENCES

1. Unger W, Unger R, Wesley C. The surgical treatment of cicatricial alopecia. Dermatol Ther. 2008;21:295-311.
2. Dahdah M, Lorizzo M. The role of hair restoration surgery in primary cicatricial alopecia. Skin Appendage Disord. 2016;2:57-60.

CHAPTER 16

Setting Up a Hair Transplant Center

Pradeep Sethi, Abhinav Kumar, Sarita Sanke

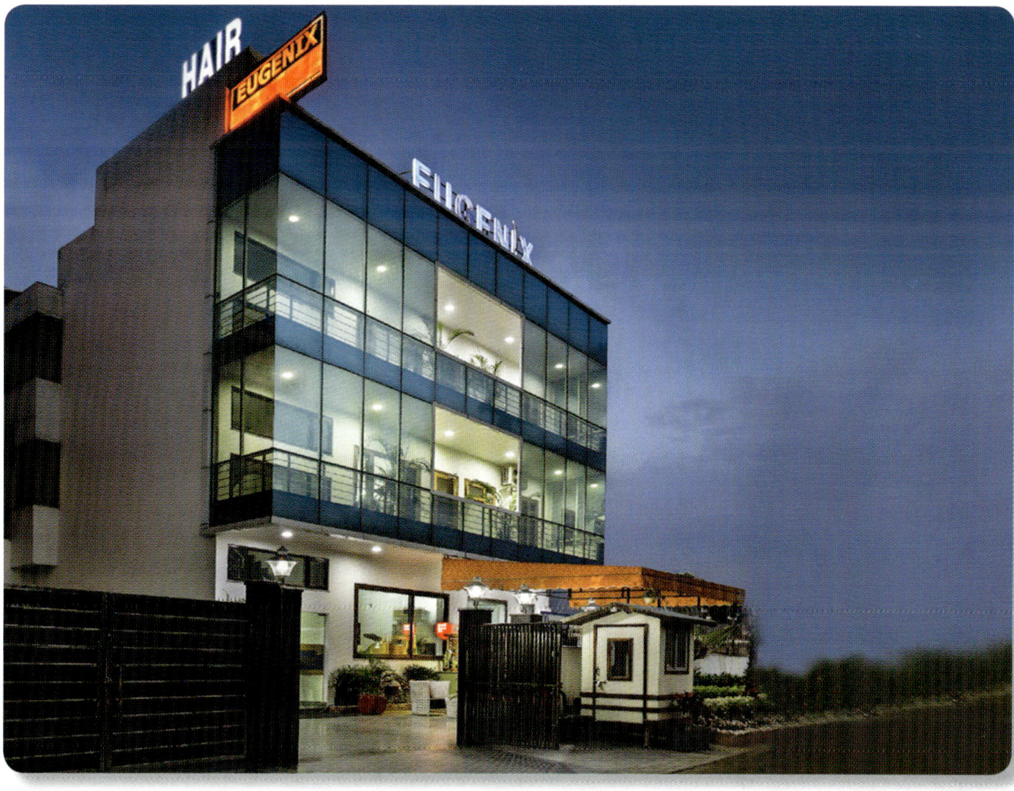

Without a dedicated, well thought setup, the ultimate results would not be the best that would have happened in the hands of the surgeon. For the best results, the team should be doing only hair restoration, focusing upon the flow of the workup and the procedure the setup should be designed to ensure sterilization and comfort of the team members and patients. The facility shows the amount of passion the physician has for the procedure and the ultimate results!

INTRODUCTION

The focus of this chapter is emphasizing the importance of setting up a good hair transplant center.

Hair transplant is conducted under local anesthesia. Patient is awake and is often relaxed during this procedure. He is neither hungry since there is no requirement of being empty stomach and also gets break when he is fatigued and can have snacks at that time. As a result, doctors or directors of hair transplant center believe that this surgery can be conducted in any setup. The only requirement is a room, instruments and proper lighting and sterilized environment. In India, hair transplant is being done illegally at even salons resulting in bad results and post-transplant complications. We will try to highlight the salient features of a dedicated hair transplant setup. Young doctors who aim to become hair transplant surgeons should invest their time and energy in solely learning hair transplant at a proper facility for at least 1 year before trying to open their own setup. Knowing the importance of a setup is critical for a young hair transplant surgeon and it can be gained only if he works in a good and scientifically designed hair transplant center.

LOCATION

The clinic should be located on a prominent road of the city or town to gain maximum visibility (Fig. 16.1).

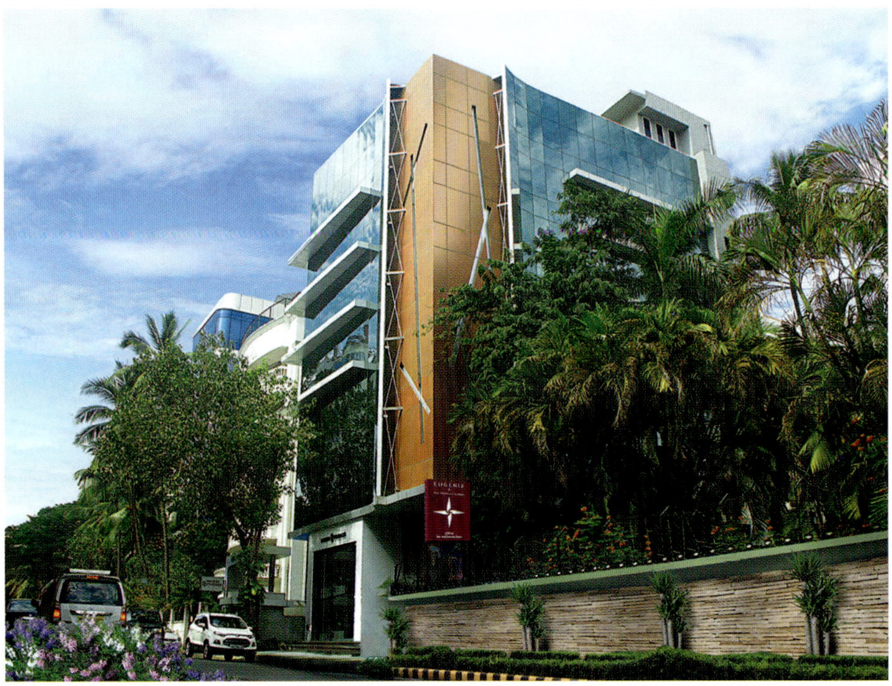

Figure 16.1

The center should be on a wide road, with ample parking space. The entrance of the center should be properly illuminated.

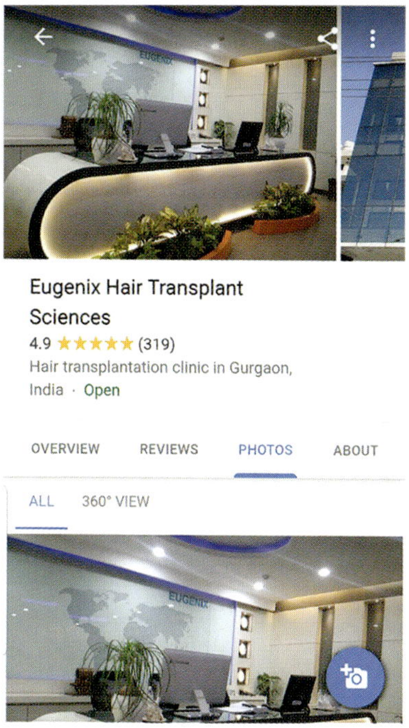

Figure 16.2 The center should be listed on Google Business and Google Maps for easy reach. The information about opening timings, closing hours should be listed there.

There are a lot of walk in patients in hair transplant industry. The location should be available on Google Maps and Google Business for easy search (Fig. 16.2).

The clinic should have a large board preferably which illuminates at night and should prominently highlight the facility you have at the center. Displaying doctor's name is optional and depends upon how you want to project the center.

RECEPTION AREA

The reception area should be pleasant. The reception staff should have a soothing personality who greets the patient, offers them a seat and politely note down all the details. The front desk staff should be able to handle and manage new/old appointments, answer all the queries of the patients, provide the basic details to the patients and should have a sound knowledge about computers (Excel sheet) to be able to maintain the records of the patients (Fig. 16.3).

CONSULTATION ROOM

This is the room where the patient will interact with the doctor. This room should be spacious, well illuminated and equipped with a handy mirror and a skin marker so that the patient can see himself in the mirror and show the problematic areas to the doctor (Fig. 16.4). It gives a good impression to have a trichoscope and a hand lens to examine the scalp of the patient. A catalog displaying the best results

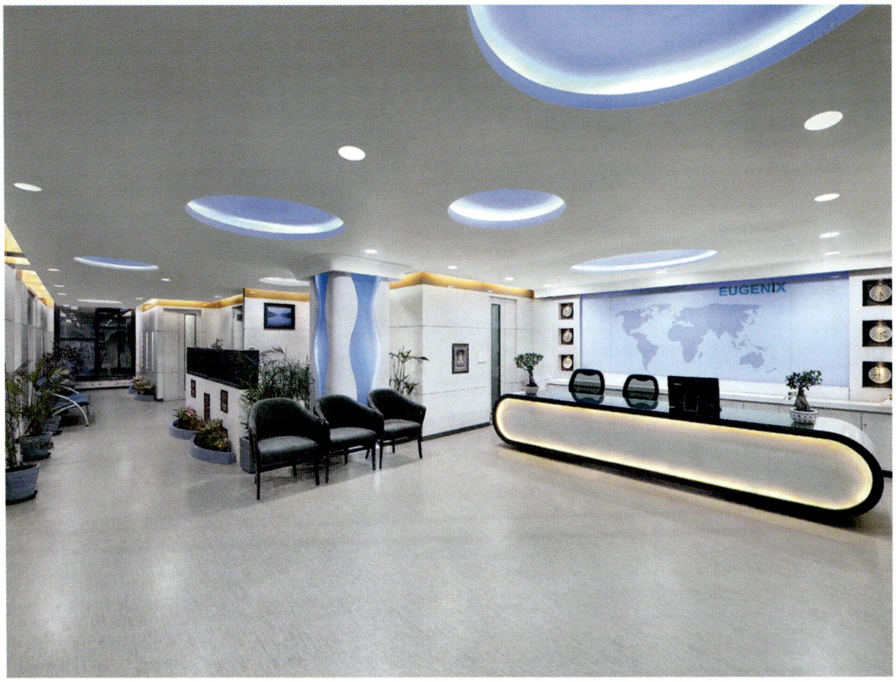

Figure 16.3

The reception area should be well-illuminated, with proper seating arrangement and pleasing staff.

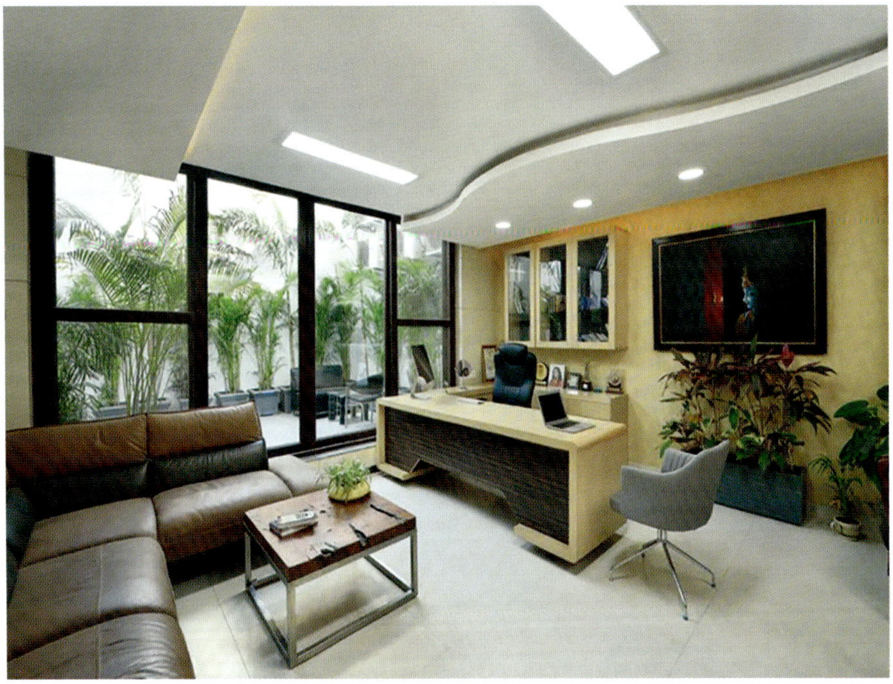

Figure 16.4

Spacious and well-illuminated consultation room.

of the doctor (pre- and postsurgery results) is essential to gain the confidence of the patient. The room should have 3–4 chairs for the accompanying person/relative. The achievements/medals/certificates of the doctor should be displayed in the room to gain the trust of the patients.

COUNSELOR

There is a huge importance of a counselor in hair transplant facility but in initial days doctor can be a counselor as well. The counselor explains the patient about the surgery, pain during surgery, the setup, shows them the results and in fact handles the pricing issues as well. The counselor handles the finer details of patient's arrival and smoothly executes his departure (Fig. 16.5).

PHOTOGRAPHY ROOM[1]

This is the second most important room for a hair transplant center after operation theater (OT) (Figs. 16.6 and 16.7). The hairline is drawn in this room. Preoperative, immediate postoperative and follow-up photographs are taken here. Effort should be made to take photographs at all scientific angles at every visit. The photography room should have digital single lens reflex (DSLR) camera of a good brand, a scale, preferably a hairline drawing instrument, a mirror, surgical marker pen hairline, spirit, gauze and a trimmer.

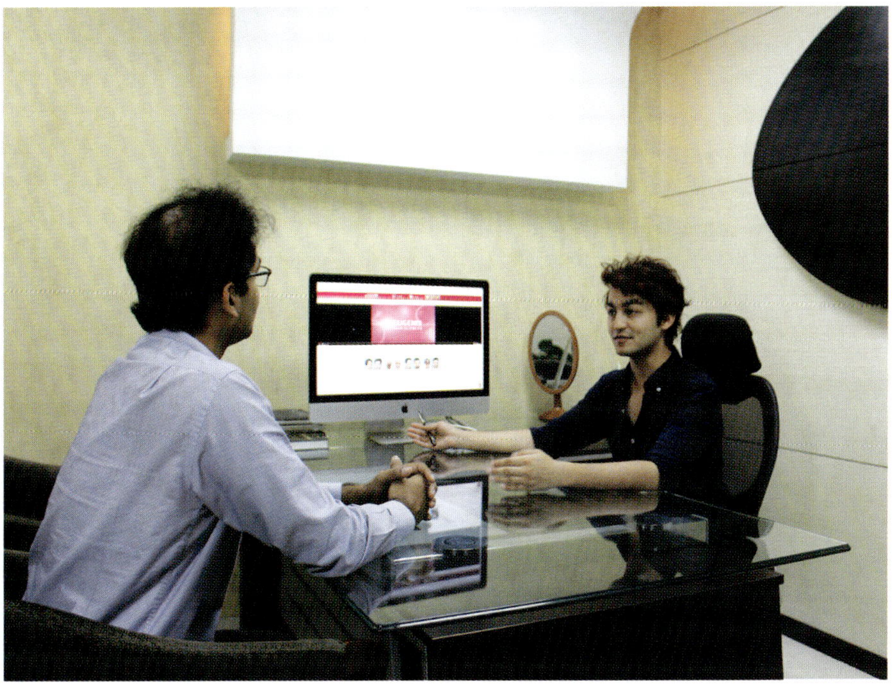

Figure 16.5

Counseling session by the counselor who explains everything about the procedure in detail.

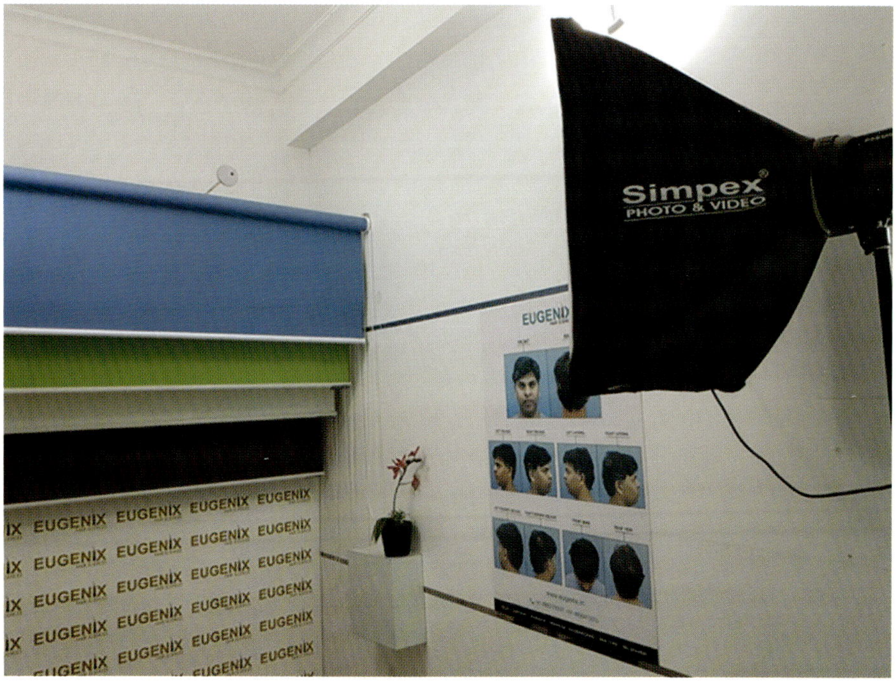

Figure 16.6

Photography room.

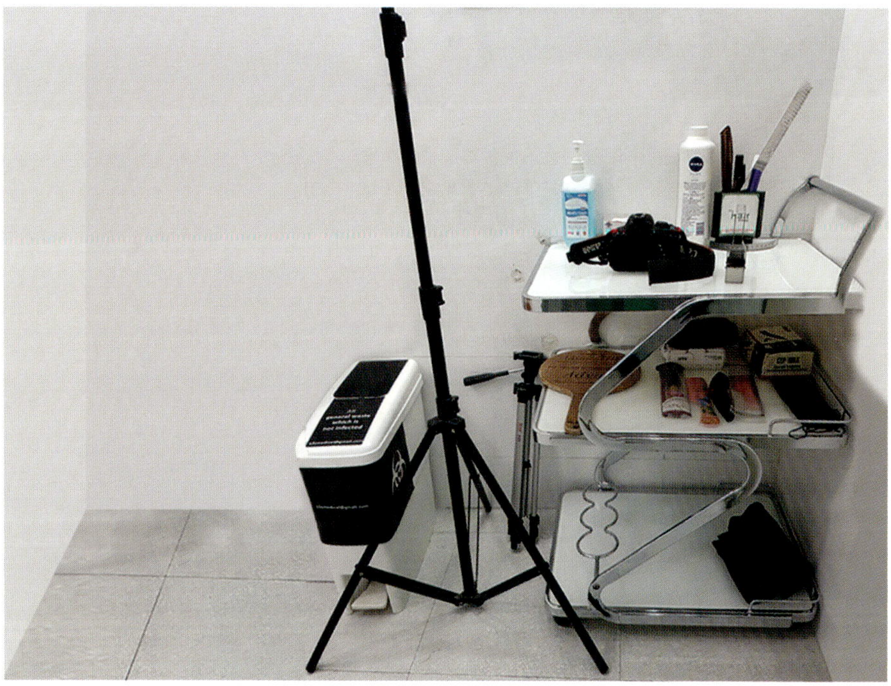

Figure 16.7

Camera room setup.

ASSISTANTS

At the end, it is the team and teamwork which matters. Well-trained assistants should be available to assist the doctor in minor works like trimming the scalp, counting the grafts, mopping the blood, dressing the donor area and for head wash 1 week post-transplant.

OPERATION THEATER SETUP[2]

1. *Sterilization*: Fumigation facility with formalin or glutaraldehyde along with chemical sterilization of the surgical instruments should be available. Other method of sterilization like use of ethylene oxide gas can also be adopted along with ultraviolet light. One cannot risk the occurrence of complications post-transplant. Hence, sterilization of OT as well as the instruments should be a priority.
2. *Hand wash facility*: Wash basin with disinfectant with a tap with nontouch panel or a long handle (Fig. 16.8).
3. *Changing room*: Provision of a room where the patient can change his clothes with a locker facility to keep their bags should be there.
4. *Hair trimming area*: A separate area should be reserved for the trimming of the patient's scalp. It should not be done on the OT bed as the minor trimmed

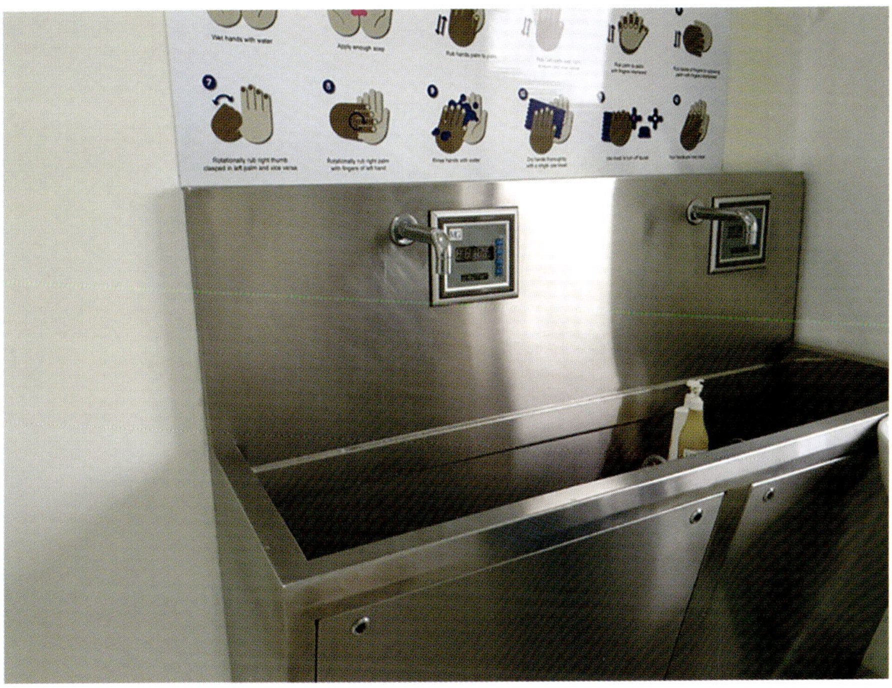

Figure 16.8

Hand wash basin with provision for scrubbing.

hair can cause irritation to the patient as well as the doctor and hinder the procedure.

5. *Operation theater*: A big OT (Fig. 16.9) which can accommodate up to eight assistants who can move around the OT easily, a light-emitting diode (LED) OT light which does not radiate heat and emits at least 120,000 lux, a motorized table is the basic minimum requirement.
   Other features of a good OT is conical roof (Fig. 16.10) and floors (Fig. 16.11) with rounded edges for easy cleaning, antibacterial walls.
6. Waste disposal should be according to standard guideline laid by the government both inside the OT and in other parts of the clinic as well.
7. Standard trolley made of stainless steel with wheels is needed to keep various instruments (Fig. 16.12).
8. Instruments needed for hair transplant are shown in Figure 16.13.
9. An illuminated loupe with attached LED light used for illumination and seeing grafts under 4X to 5X magnification (Fig. 16.14).
10. A rotating chair with adjustable height, adequate back support and foot support, and firm cushion should be available (Fig. 16.15).
11. Emergency trolley with all the necessary emergency drugs like adrenaline vial, dopamine vial, injection Avil, injection Efcorlin, oxygen support and pulse oximeter must always be handy in case of any untoward emergency. Other equipment for resuscitation like Ambu bag, airway mask and intubation pipe should also be available.

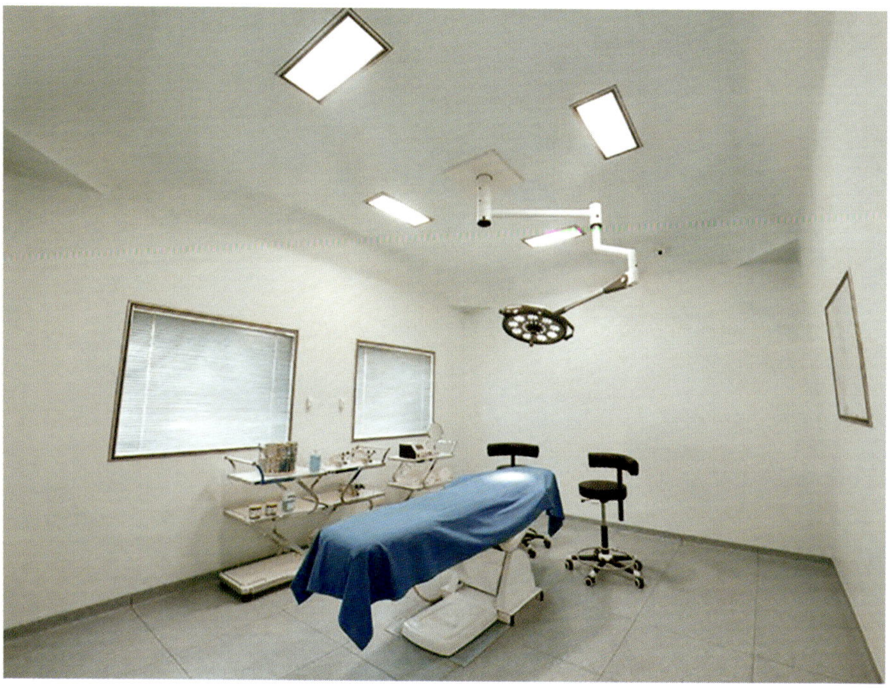

Figure 16.9

A spacious operation theater.

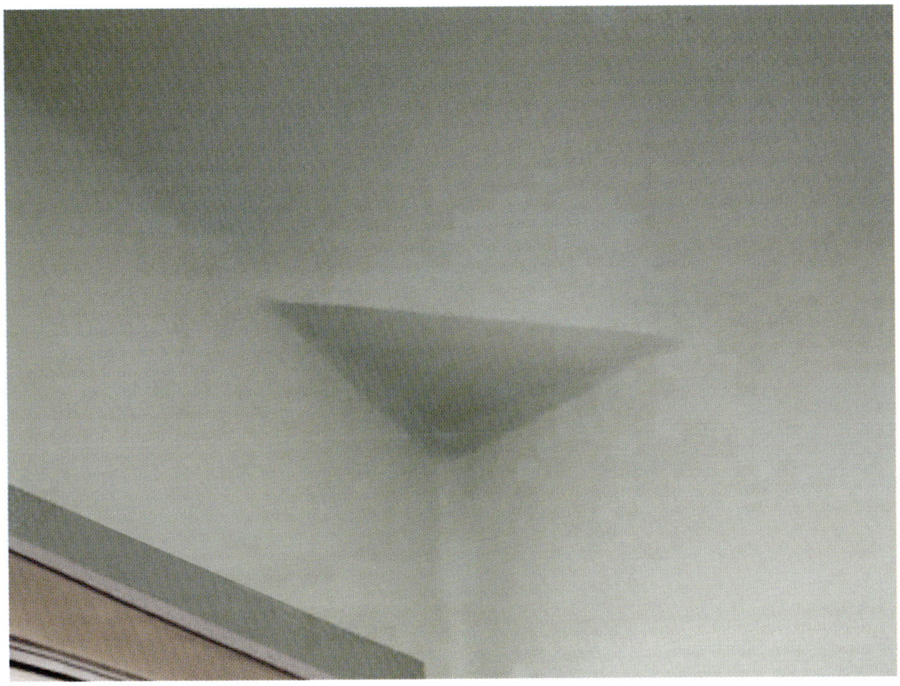

Figure 16.10

Roof with conical edges.

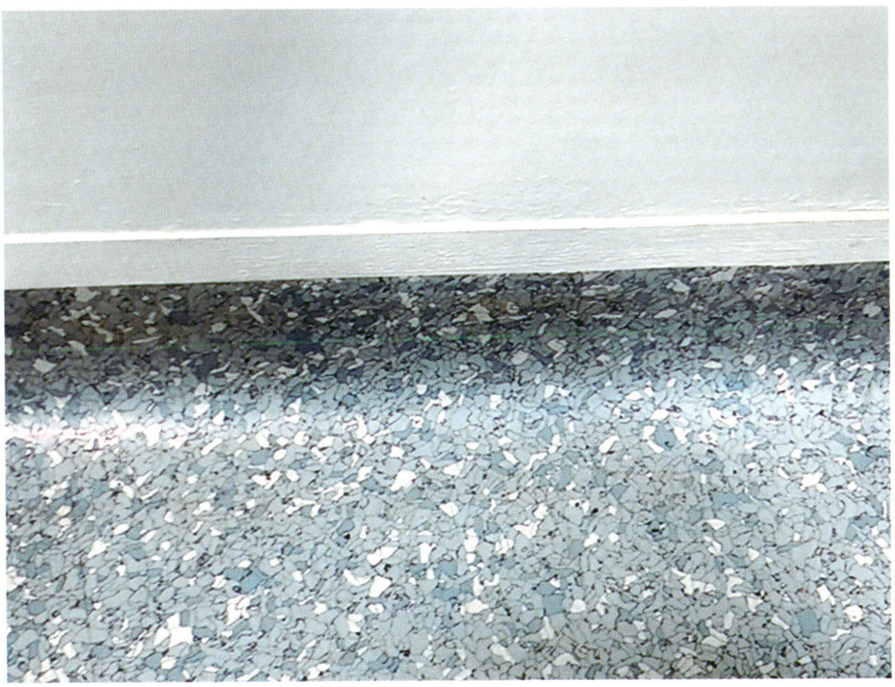

Figure 16.11

Floor with rounded edges for easy cleaning.

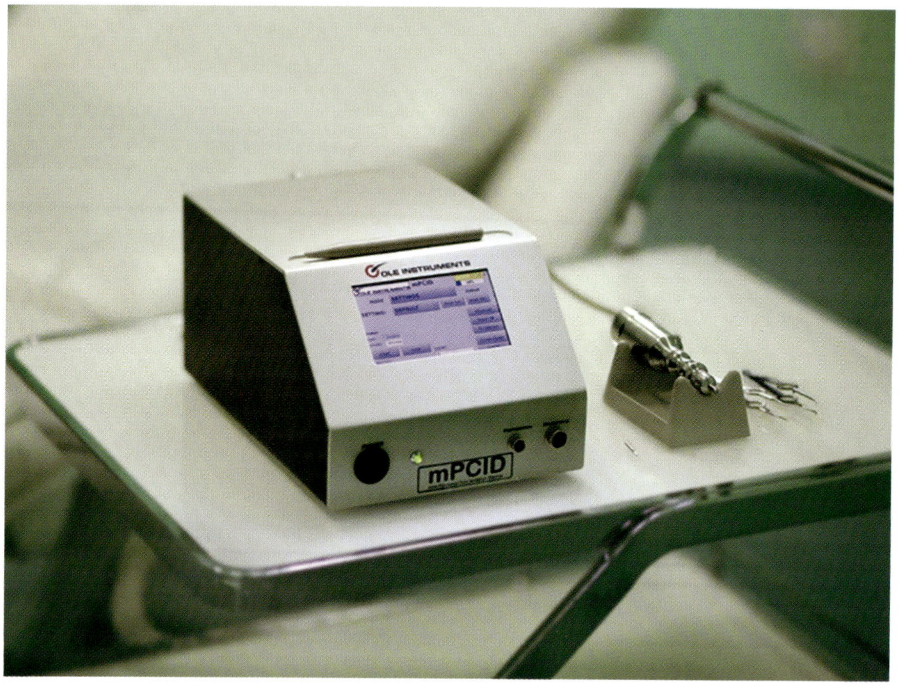

Figure 16.12

Stainless steel trolley with wheels to keep the surgical instruments.

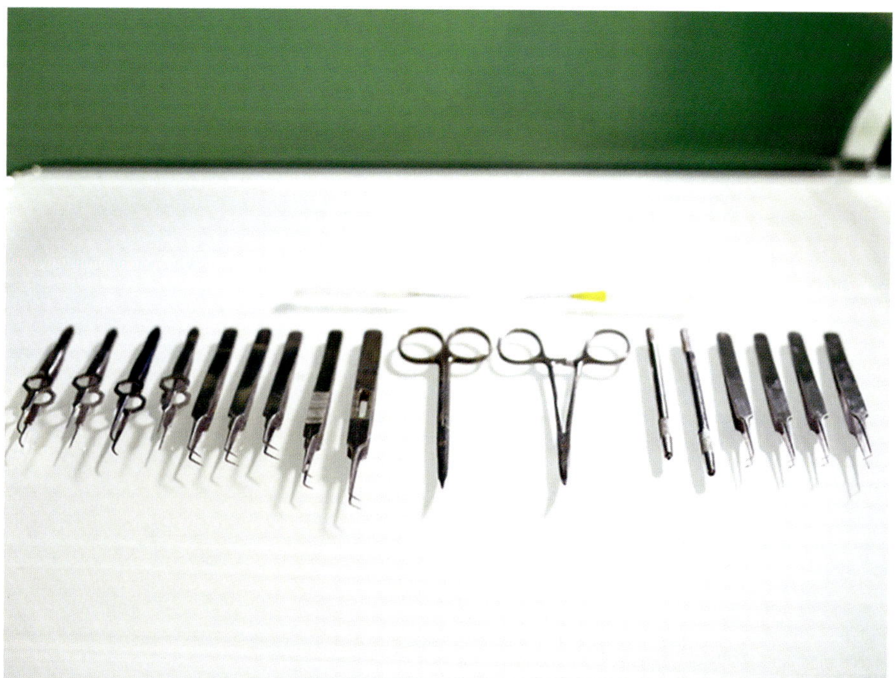

Figure 16.13

Various instruments required in hair transplant (HT) surgery.

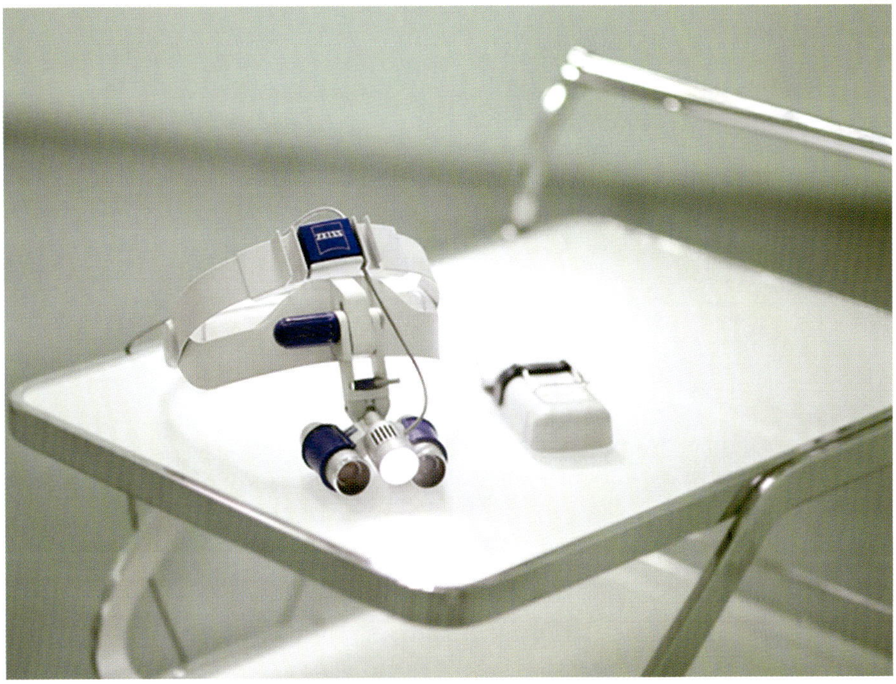

Figure 16.14

Carl Zeiss loupe with attached LED light.

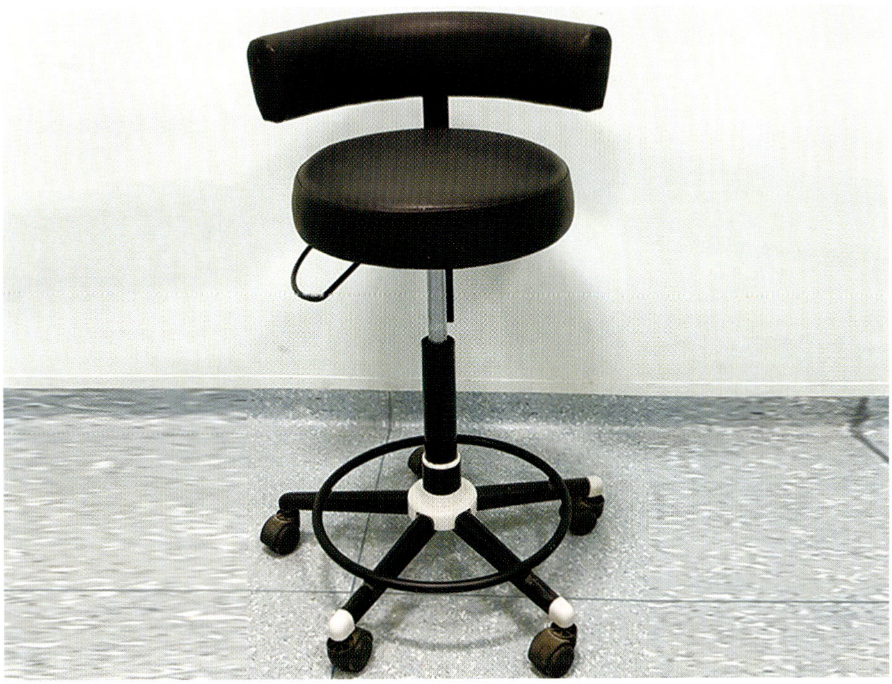

Figure 16.15

A rotating surgeon's chair.

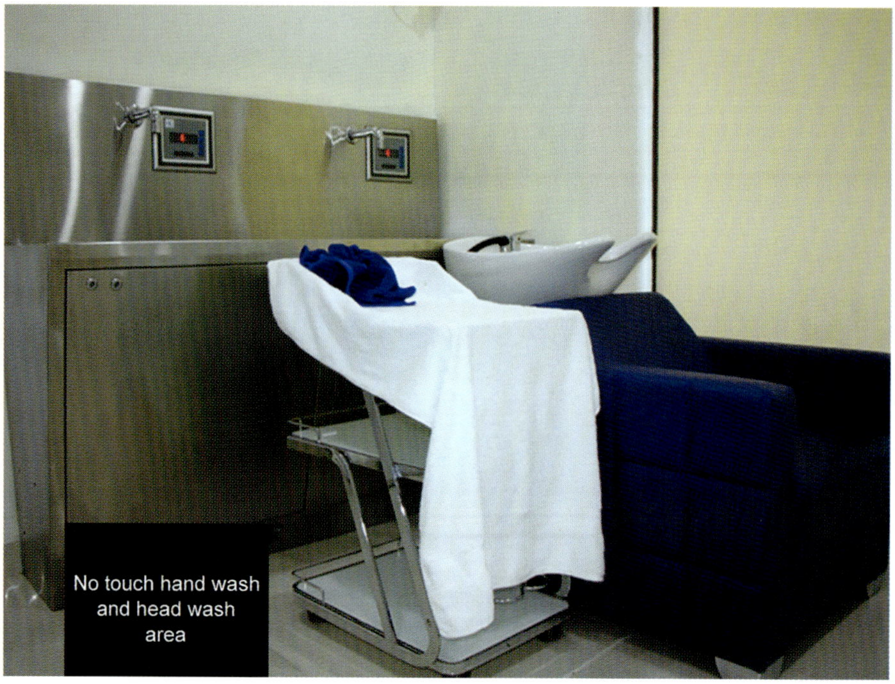

Figure 16.16

Scalp washing area needs to be comfortable with supply of warm as well as cold water in the basin.

12. *Dressing room*: A minor OT like room should be there for dressing up the scalp after surgery, and also for removal of the dressing after 1 day. The tray for the dressing should include Betadine scrub, normal saline, sterile gauze pads, scissors and mupirocin cream 2%.
13. *Head washing area*: Head needs to be washed pretransplant and 7 days after transplant (Fig. 16.16).
14. A hair transplant center should also provide facility for platelet-rich plasma (PRP) procedure in view of its potential role in hair loss. For this, a good company centrifugation machine and PRP vials with an anticoagulant should be available.

GOVERNMENT REGULATIONS FOR SETTING UP CLINIC

Registration of doctor: The doctor should always register in the particular state council in where he plans to open the clinic at.

Clinic registration: Registration of the clinic should be done and license obtained from the Indian Medical Council (IMC). Registration with the municipal authorities should also be done. Authorization should be obtained for the generation of biomedical waste.

Rules governing the employment of staff should be followed while employing any doctor, nurse or pharmacist.

The following certificates/lists should be displayed in the clinic:

- State medical council registration certificate of the doctor
- Certificate of registration of the clinic with the municipal authorities
- Charges for various procedures as per the IMC Regulations, 2002
- Opening and closing timing of the clinic.

The following documents should be available at the clinic:

- Clinic registration certificate
- Employment letters issued to the staff
- Registration certificates of the doctors/pharmacists/nurses
- Degrees of the staff
- Authorization letter of biomedical waste
- Consent forms for the various procedures
- Data/medical record of the patients.

SUMMARY

A well established clinic in a prime location with pleasant reception staff, comfortable consultation rooms, enthusiastic and smart counselors who understands the patient's point of view, a well-lit photography room, well trained assistants and lastly but most importantly fully equipped and sterilized operation theater are integral part of a successful set up.

REFERENCES

1. Witmer WK, Lebovitz PJ. Clinical photography in the dermatology practice. Semin Cutan Med Surg. 2012;31(3):191-9.
2. Rajendran SC, Omprakash HM. Standard guidelines for setting up a dermatosurgery theatre. Indian J Dermatol Venereol Leprol. 2009;75:76-82.

CHAPTER 17

Photography in Hair Transplant

Pradeep Sethi, Abhinav Kumar, Priyadarshini Das

This chapter is dedicated to Dr Bessam Farjo, the Guru in this subject and a great influence in our medical practice.

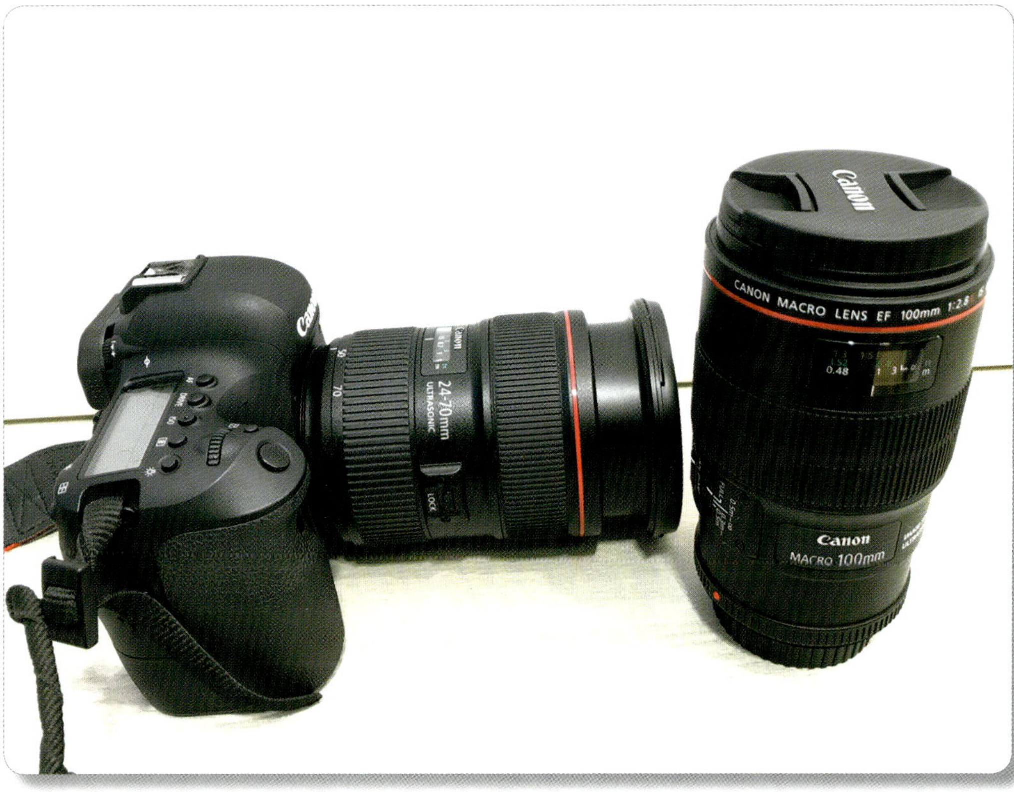

The beauty lies in the eyes of the beholder (camera/picture)! Hair restoration which is an aesthetic medicine is based primarily upon photographs, both for the patients and the physicians. The authors suggest the physicians to have some basic knowledge of the camera and the reproducible frame, angle, lighting and backgrounds for medical documentation and future references.

INTRODUCTION

Capturing a moment on lens makes it stay forever. That being true, it has much more serious implications in our lives. Any hair transplant institution which wants to work hard in making people look better every day; the camera will always play a crucial role. It helps in documenting all the finer details. The camera can point out our mistakes and also celebrate our fine work. It has almost become a person; like a constant friend who has our back. The camera sees what we see and vice versa. Knowing how to use the camera to give you that one perfect shot needs understanding and training. However, some are born photographers.

Being the authors of this book, we kept scanning the images which we took over years, many of the images which seemed perfect while taking them ultimately turned out to be imperfect when zoomed or when seen on desktop. As a result, we had to look for similar condition in other patients for including in our book.

Through this chapter, we want to share with the world, the science behind taking good images in hair transplant along with the tips and tricks of good photography so that a uniform photographic language can be spoken throughout anyone's work.

THE CAMERA

Choosing the right camera (or the right smartphone) for photography is essential especially if you are in a serious profession of hair transplantation where documentation is absolutely essential. One should always prefer a digital single lens reflex (DSLR) camera over smartphone. The benefits of using a camera over phone is ability to use various types of modes (auto, manual, AV, close up, etc.), ability to change the lens type, its durability and customization ability. Shooting with a DSLR camera brings professionalism and seriousness in the process of photography.

On the other hand, a good flagship high end smartphone may shoot one the best of image when you look at them on mobile screen, the problem arises when you see those images on desktop or send it to the publisher for using the image in the text book. Often, a part of the image which was supposed to be highlighted is not in focus. However, a flagship smartphone offers the convenience of transmitting image via mail, Google drive, and messaging applications. Secondly, it also offers instant back-up facility. Nevertheless, the image may be lost in hundreds of other images in the gallery. When you have to shoot photograph at multiple angles of one patient, this may not be the best option. There is also a risk of losing your smartphone.

Thus, we suggest surgeons to buy a good DSLR camera.

PHOTOGRAPHY ROOM

It is the real workshop for designing of the hairline, for planning of procedure, and for introduction of artistry into the procedure. Personally, the authors believe that one should spend a lot of time with the patient to understand his/her expectation. This helps in making patient understand what is practically and aesthetically doable and gives him/her realistic expectation. The patient and the doctor should be on the same page before proceeding ahead with the surgery. Spending more time in the photography room also avoids future hassles, litigations and need for future correction in the operated area.*

Creation of a photography room inside the center will create a professional environment for taking photograph (Fig. 17.1). The size of the room should be at least size 10 × 6 feet.

The things to be kept inside photography room are:

- Uniform background in photography room along with a rotating chair and bright light (Fig. 17.2).

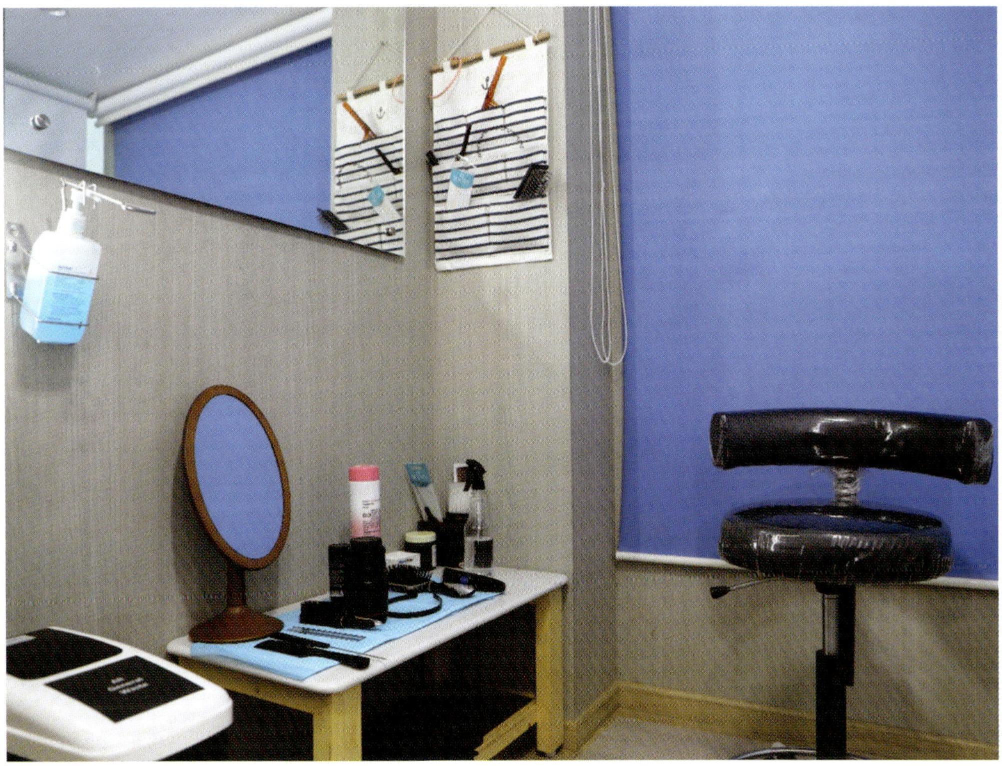

Figure 17.1
A photography room.

*No two faces on earth are similar, so no two hairlines can be same. Every face has a customized nose, eyes and lips. The ultimate creator for customization is God. The humble human being while designing the hairline, which is the gateway to the face, should take as many scientific photographs as possible in order to understand and get inside thoughts of the patient. This may ultimately help in ideation for hairline designing and planning of the overall surgery.

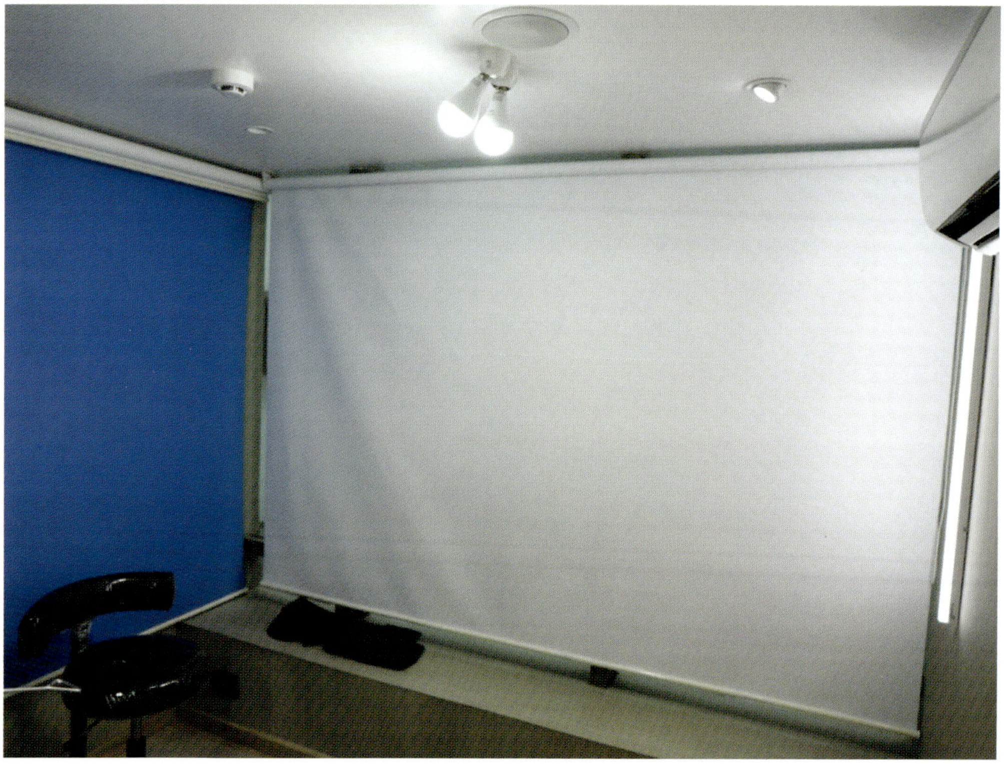

Figure 17.2

Uniform background in the photography room with a rotating chair.

- Dressing table and mirror—components of dressing table include comb, trimmer, gauze, spirit, marker pen, scale, hair band, trimming cloth, Path D laser assist hairline design device, and space for lens (Figs. 17.3A to D).
- It is important to understand that while taking photograph of patient at various angles, the photographer should bend to bring the camera lens at the level of patient's head (Fig. 17.4A). One should take picture of patient with hairline design in front of the mirror to check its symmetry (Fig. 17.4B). One should also look at the hairline from the back with neck hyper-extended and take a photograph of the hairline in that position to check the symmetry from the back as well. One should also discuss with the patient, regarding restoration of areas which are not visible to the patient in the mirror like crown (Fig. 17.4C).

Various Photographic Angles in Hair Transplant[1] (Figs. 17.5A to J)

The various photographic angles in hair transplant are as follows:

- Front and back
- Left lateral and right lateral
- Left anterior oblique and right anterior oblique
- Left posterior oblique and right posterior oblique
- Front bend and roof view.

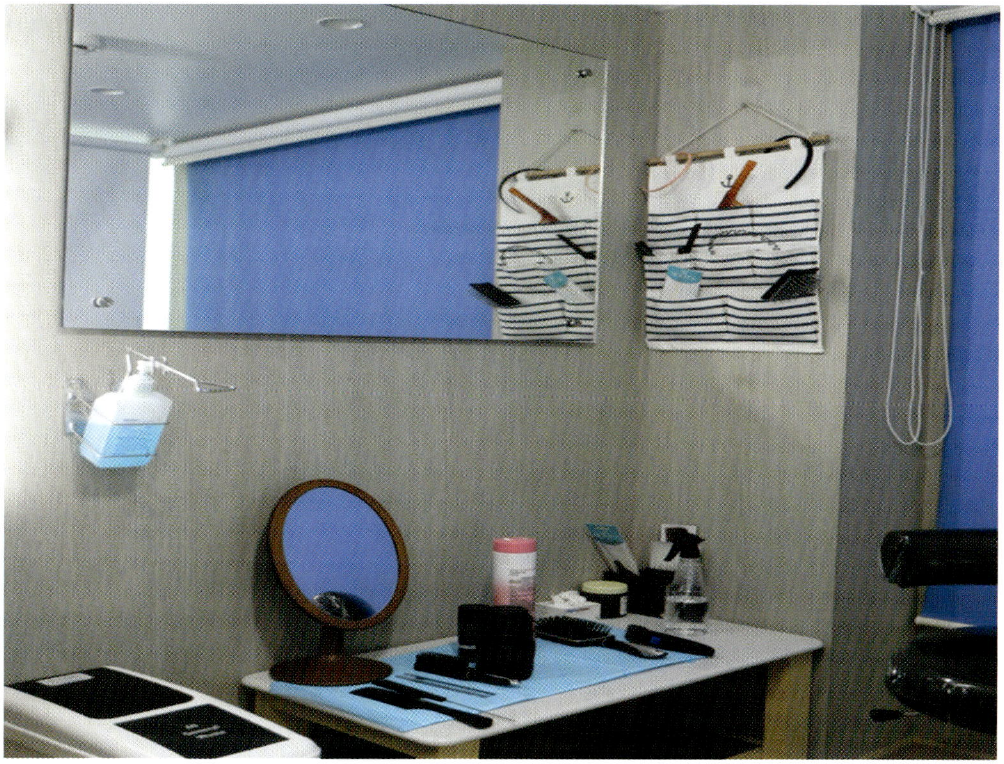

Figure 17.3A

Mirror and gadgets of photography room.

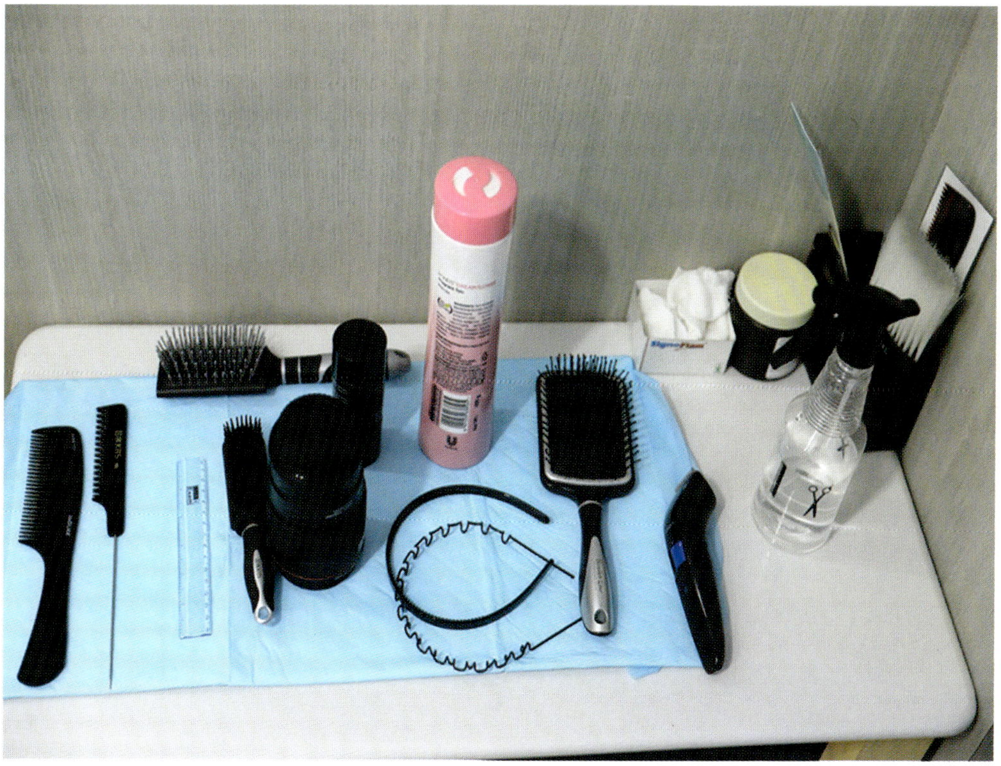

Figure 17.3B

Close-up view of the gadgets.

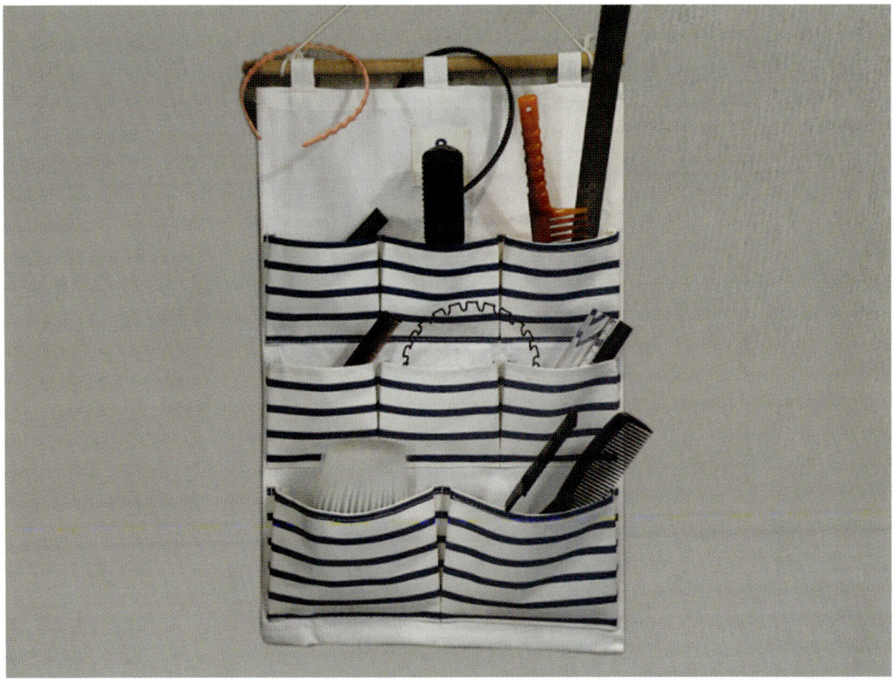

Figure 17.3C

Various types of combs to unshackle the hair and hair-band for taking photograph of the constructed hairline.

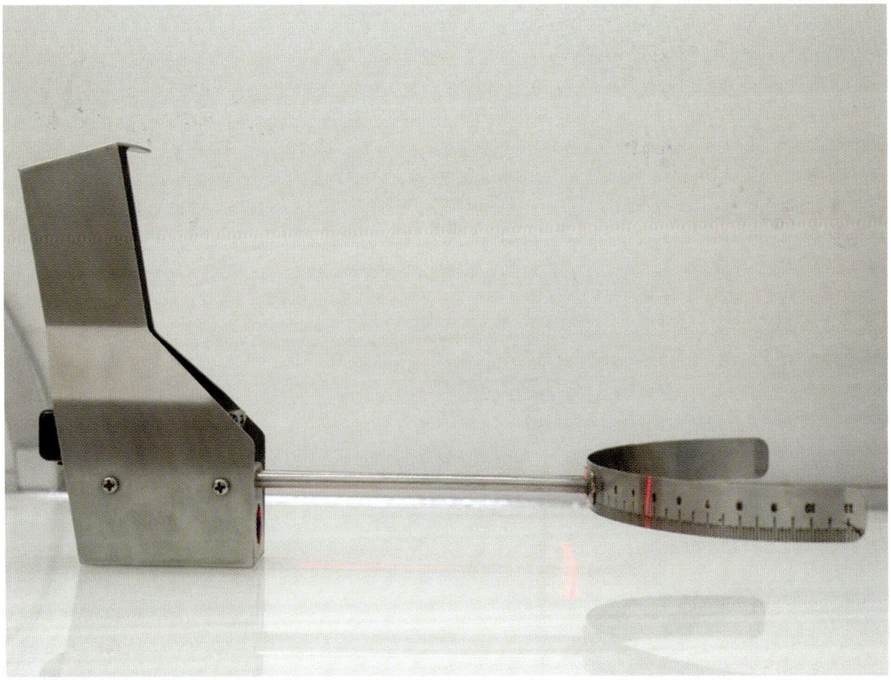

Figure 17.3D

Path D Laser Assist Hairline Design Device.

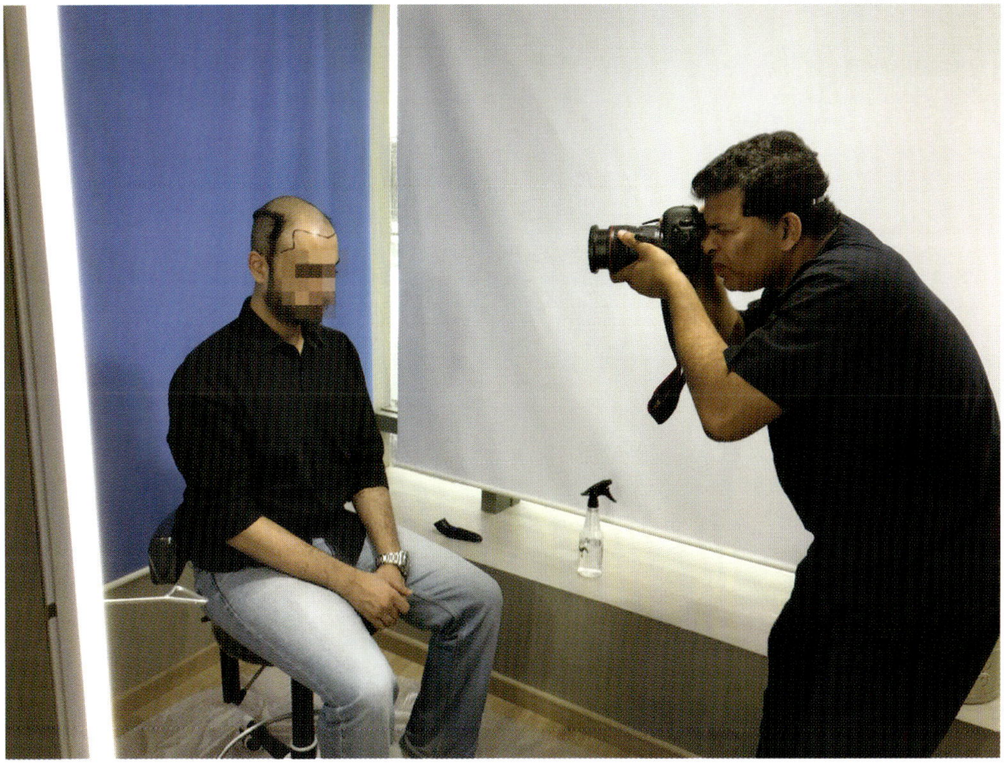

Figure 17.4A

Camera should be at the level of head of the patient.

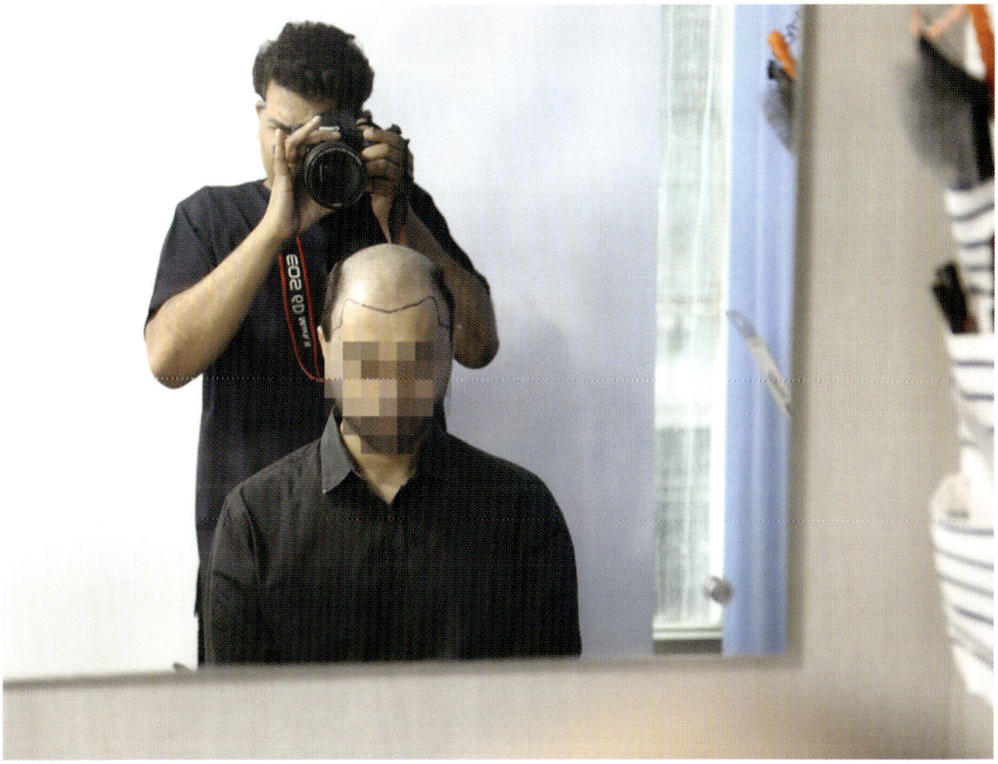

Figure 17.4B

Photograph of the patient in front of the mirror to check the symmetry of hairline from the back.

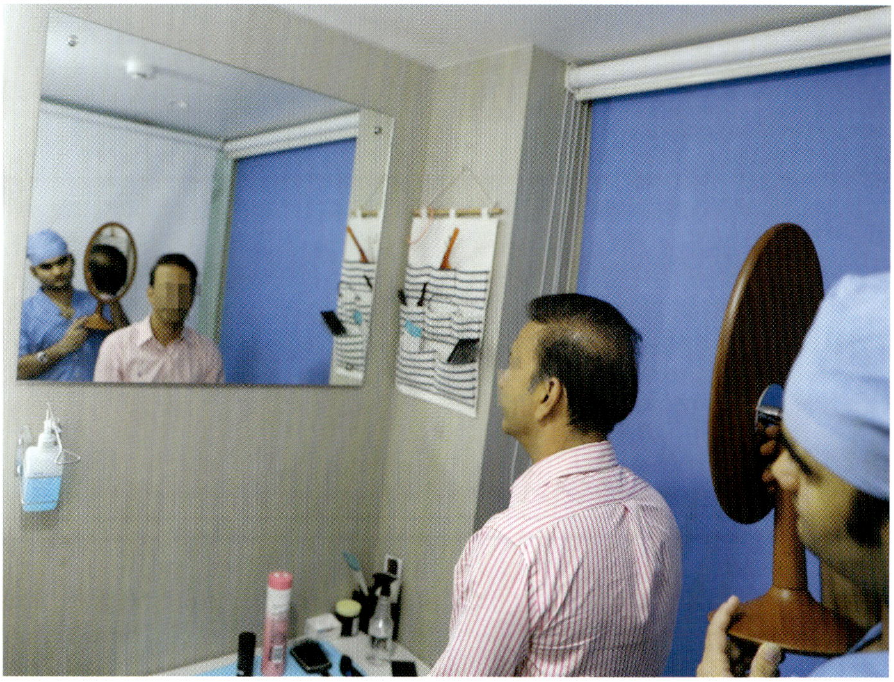

Figure 17.4C

Discussion regarding crown restoration with the patient. Unless patient visualizes the crown, he cannot point out the areas of concern. The doctor and the patient should come on the same page for correcting the areas which are not visible to the patient in front of the mirror.

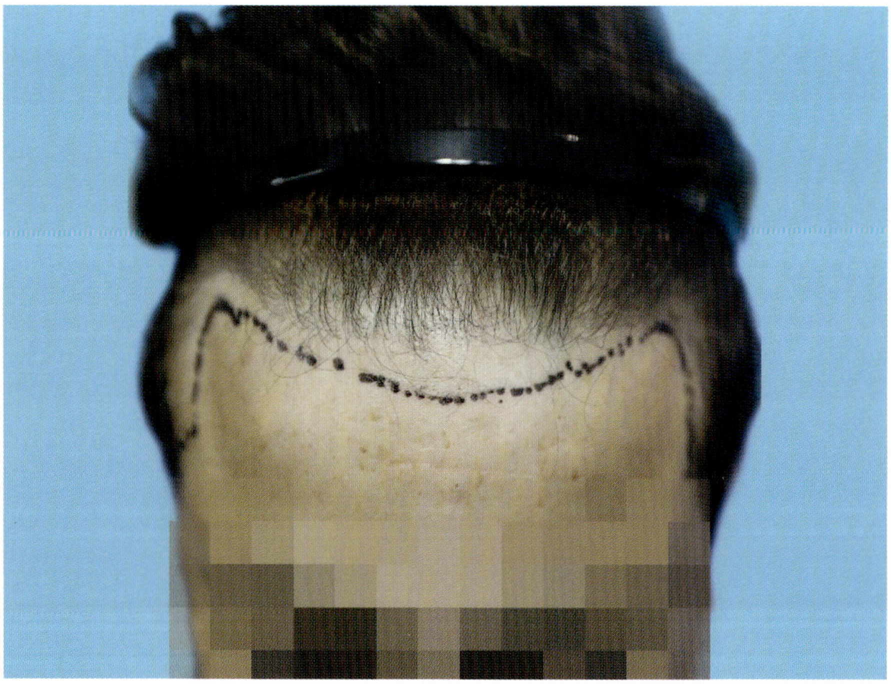

Figure 17.4D

Photographic evidence of the drawn hairline.

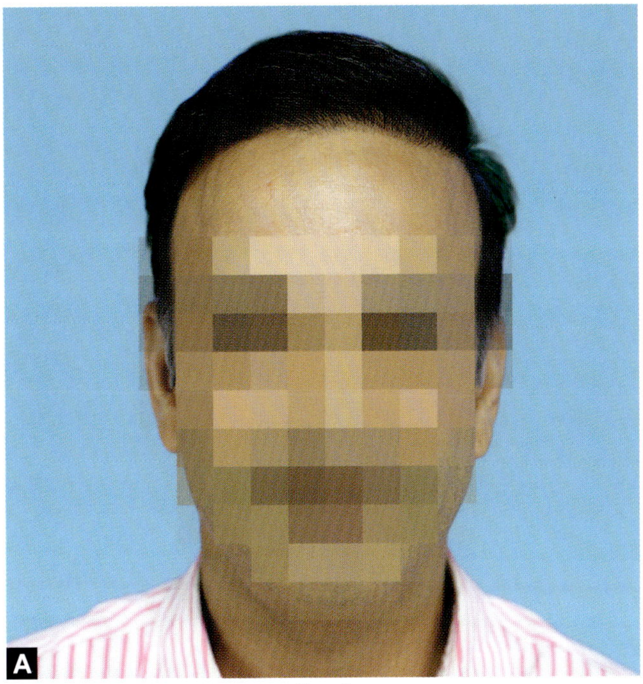

Front

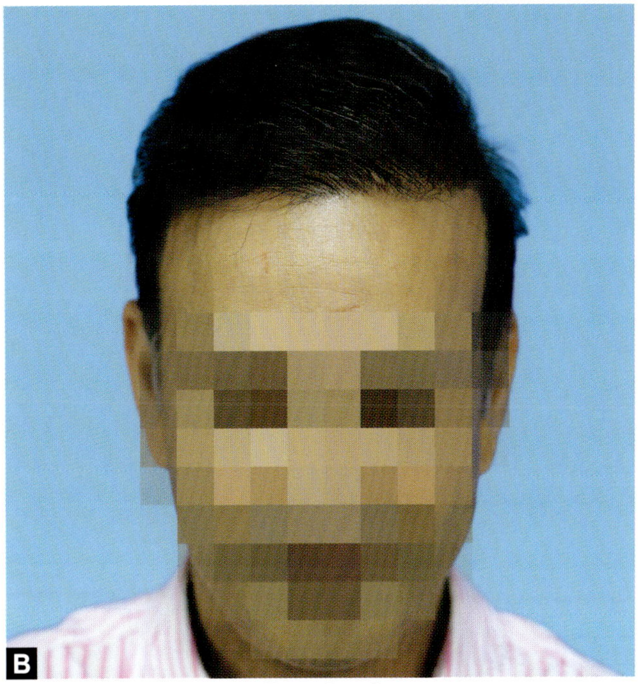

Front bend

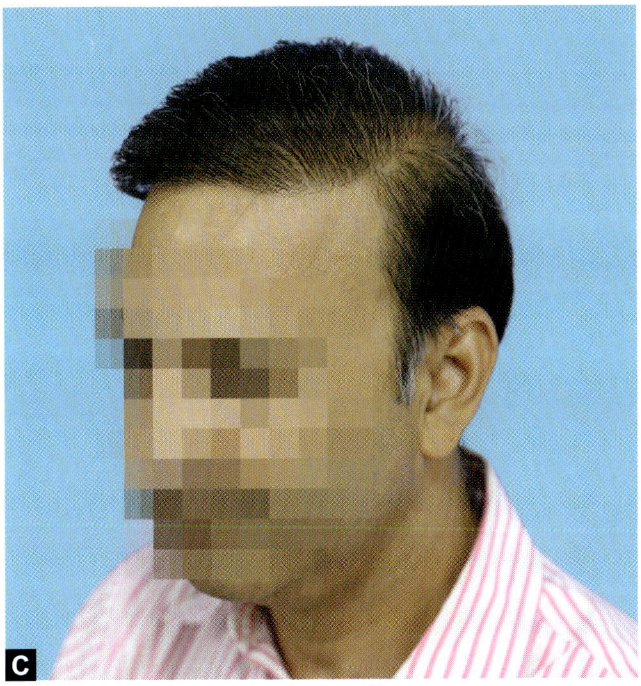

Left anterior oblique

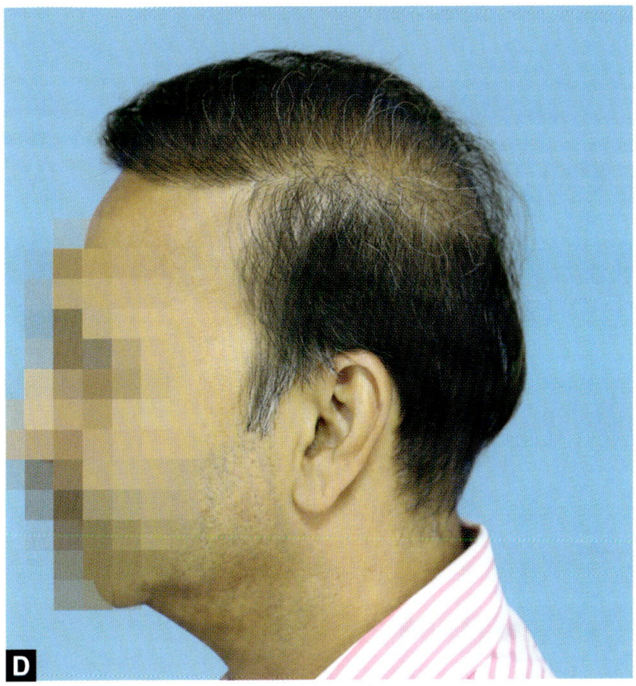

Left lateral

Figures 17.5A to D

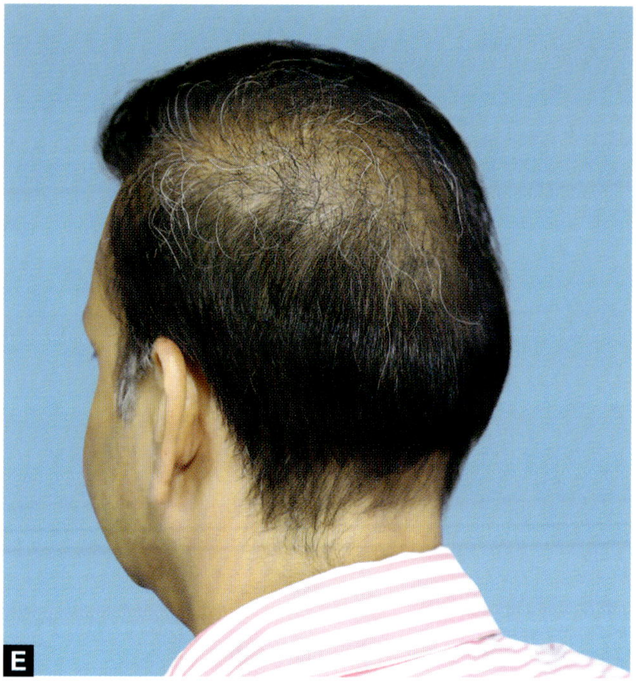

Left posterior oblique

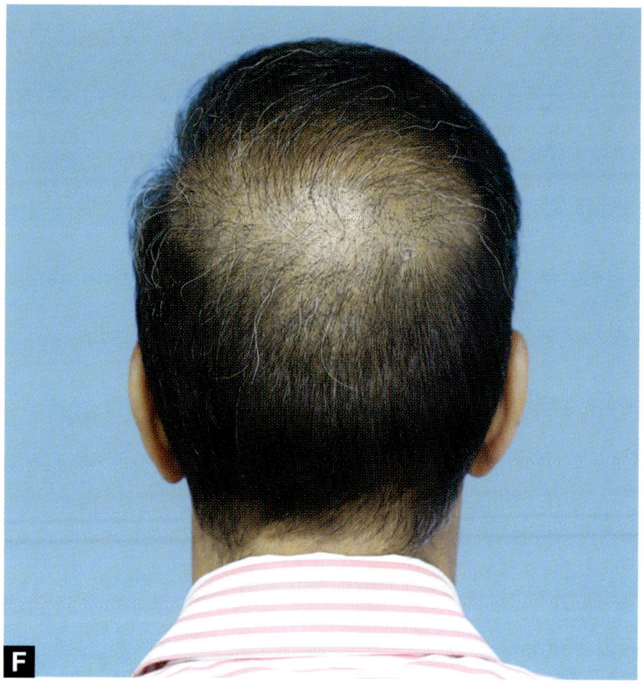

Back

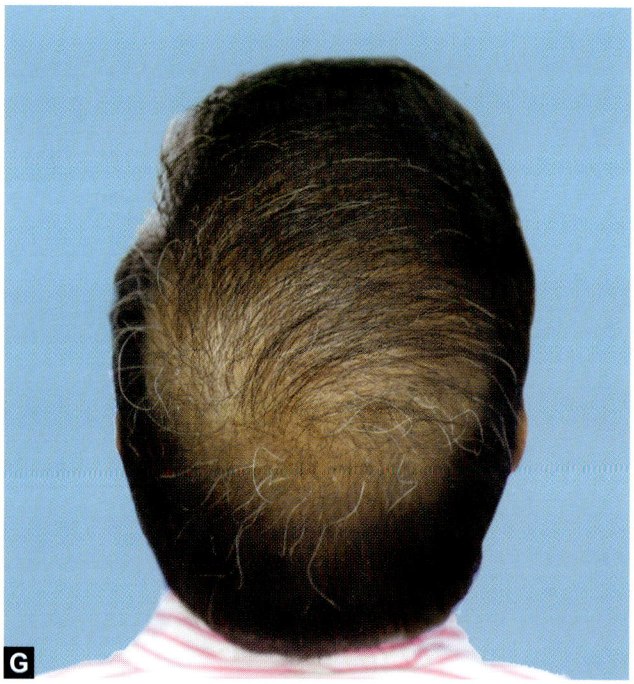

Roof view

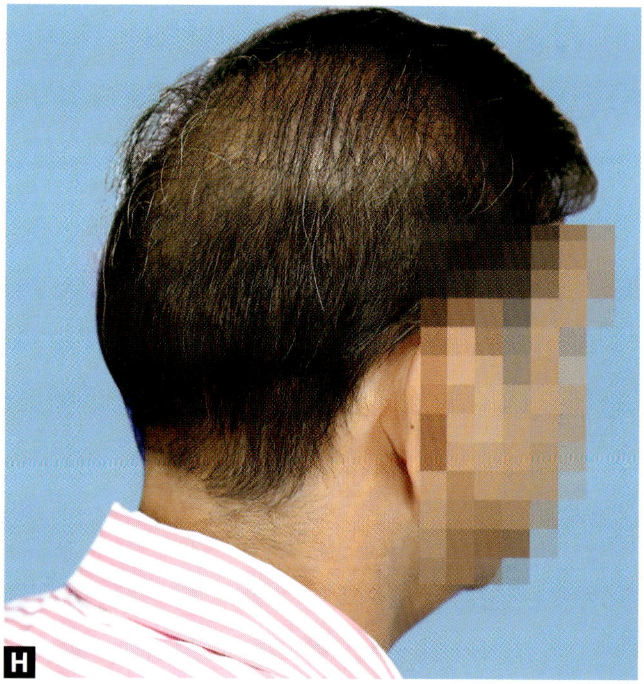

Right posterior oblique

Figures 17.5E to H

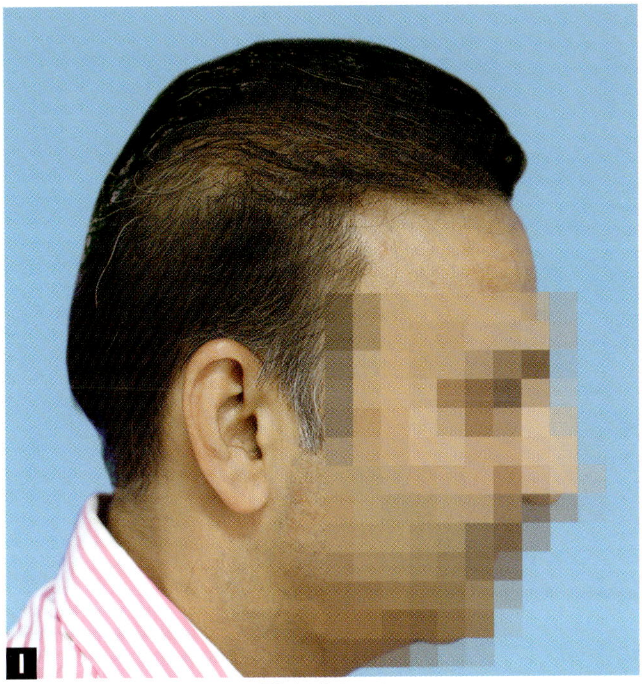

I

Right lateral

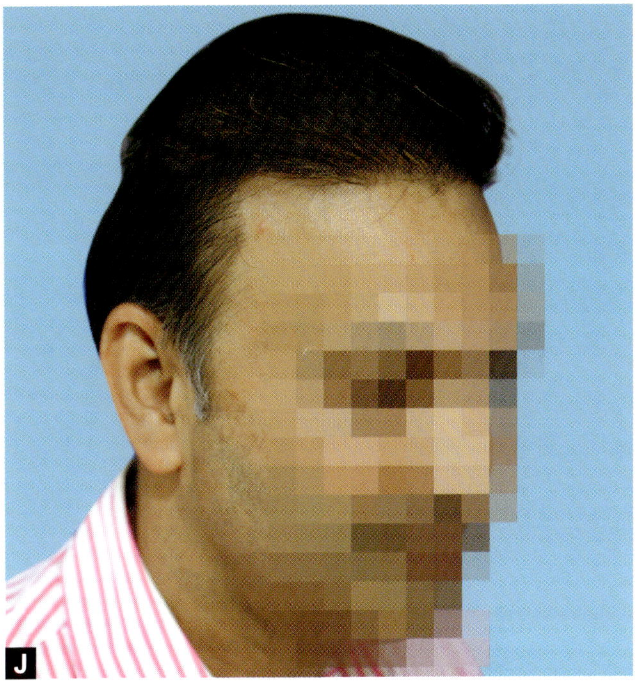

J

Right anterior oblique

Figures 17.5I and J

Figures 17.5A to J

The figures show the ten photographic angles of the patient which needs to be taken.

Photographic evidence of trimmed donor area, slits and beard (before and after extraction and even monthly to check it healing and presence and absence of redness) should also be kept for evaluation thereafter (Figs. 17.6A to C).

Various stages at which photograph should be taken are as follows:

1. Preoperative photograph in all above mentioned photographic angles.
2. Photograph after trimming and hairline designing.
3. Immediate postoperative photograph in all above mentioned photographic angles.
4. Photograph after head wash on day 7.
5. Monthly photographs till patient get his complete result, any visit thereafter.

How to take good quality photograph of smaller structures?[2]

Catching the details of smaller structure like grafts, cowlick, donor density, photographic image of slits, final hairline is an art which should be mastered by hair transplant surgeon. It is difficult to take good pictures without having a solid understanding of Shutter Speed, Aperture and ISO—the three Kings of Photography, also known as the *"Exposure Triangle"* (Figs. 17.7A and B). Surgeon should have complete understanding of manual mode of DSLR camera.

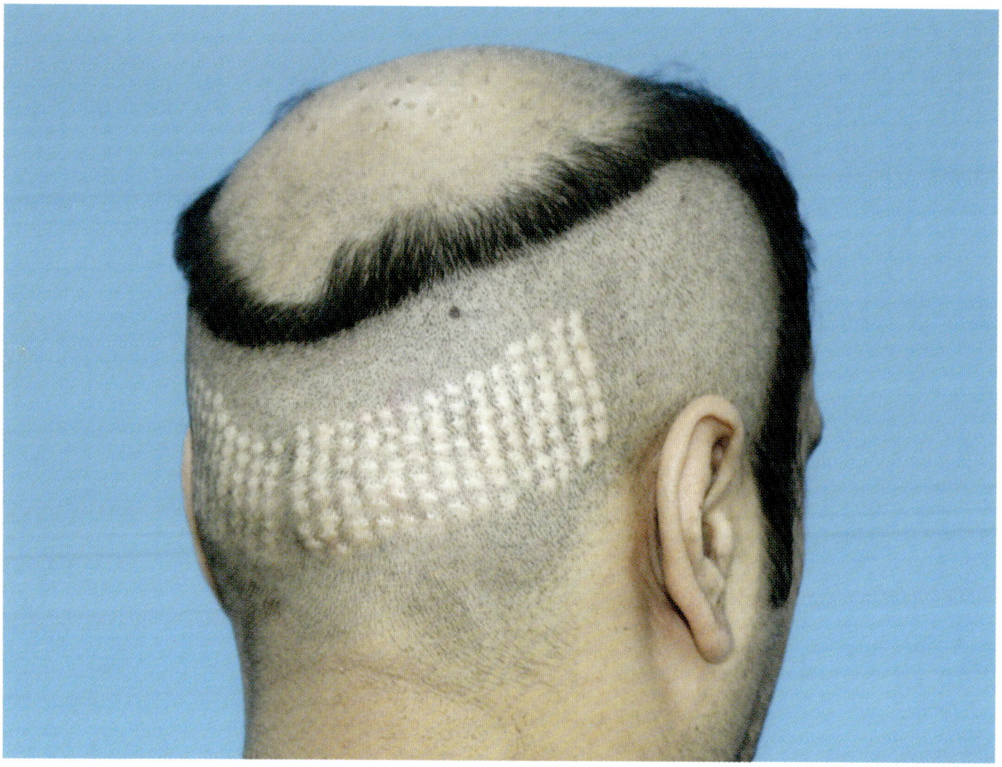

Figure 17.6A

Photographic evidence of trimmed donor.

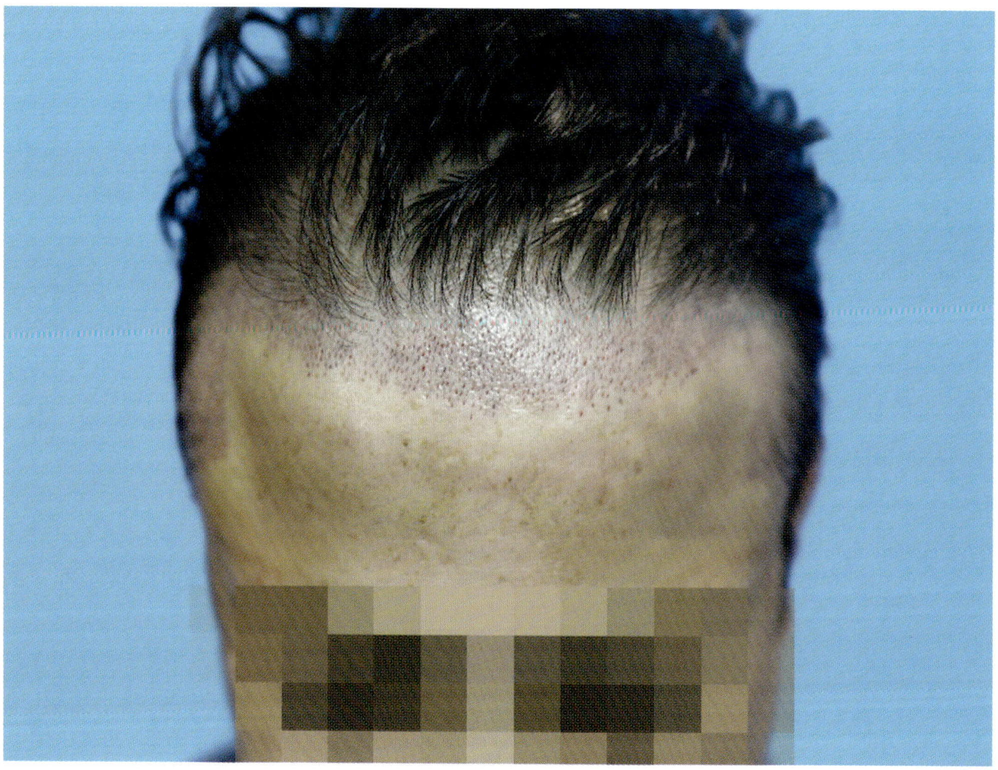

Figure 17.6B

Photographic evidence of slits.

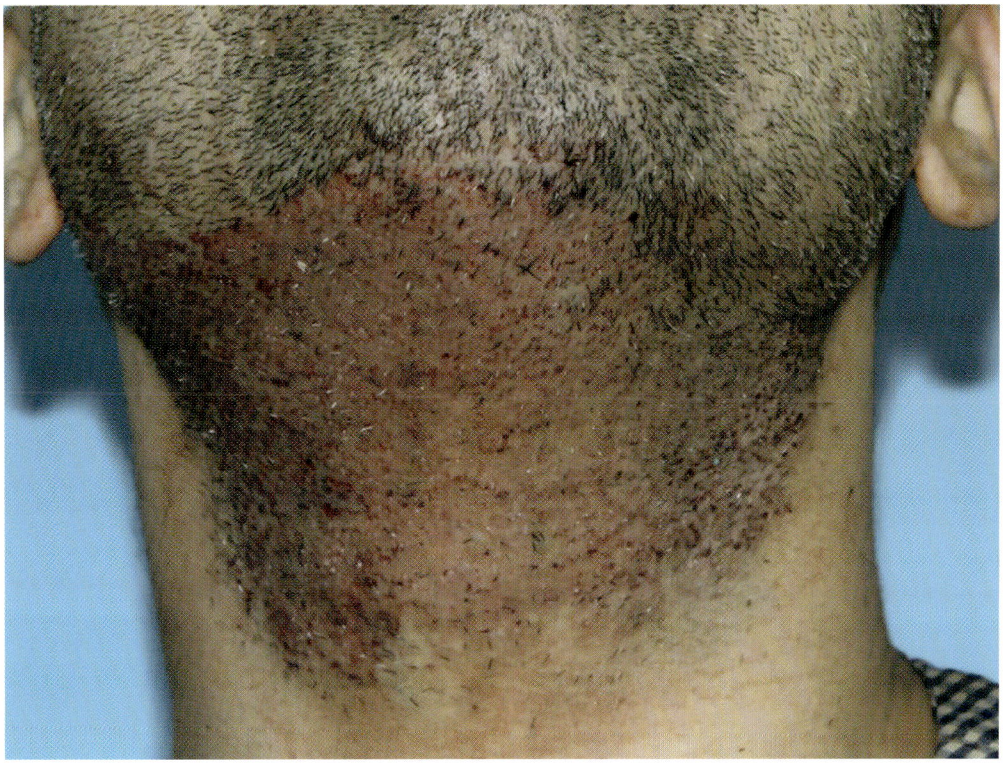

Figure 17.6C

Photograph of beard after extraction of beard grafts.

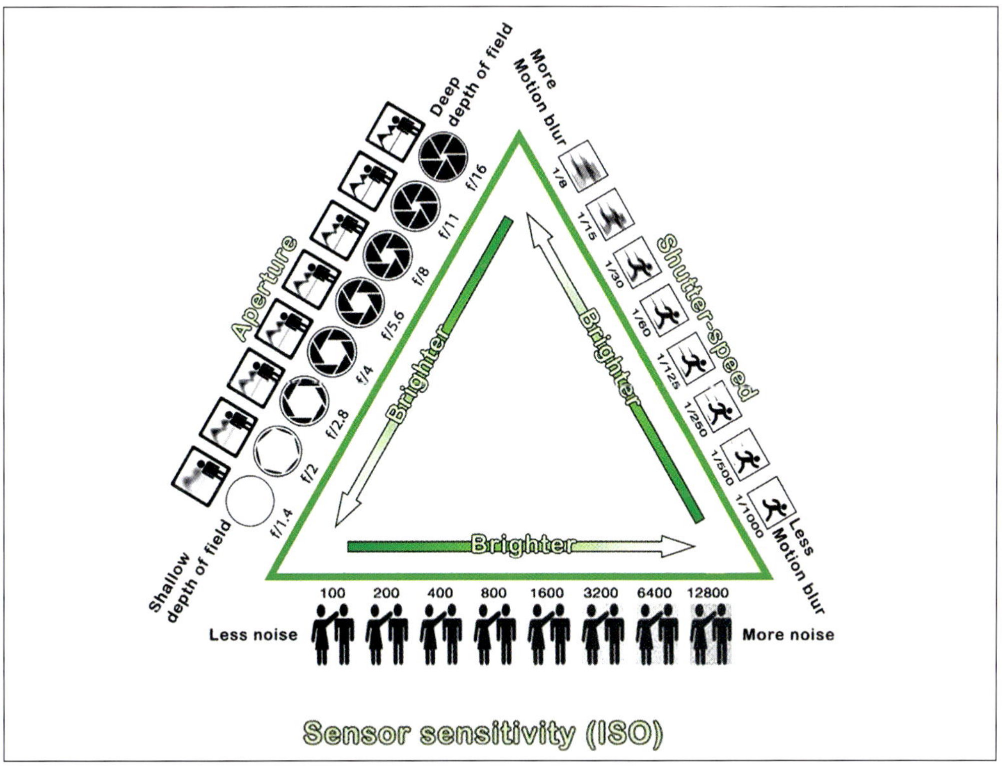

Figure 17.7A

The exposure triangle.[3] A basic understanding of these three setting can help you get best of images with even a basic DSLR camera.

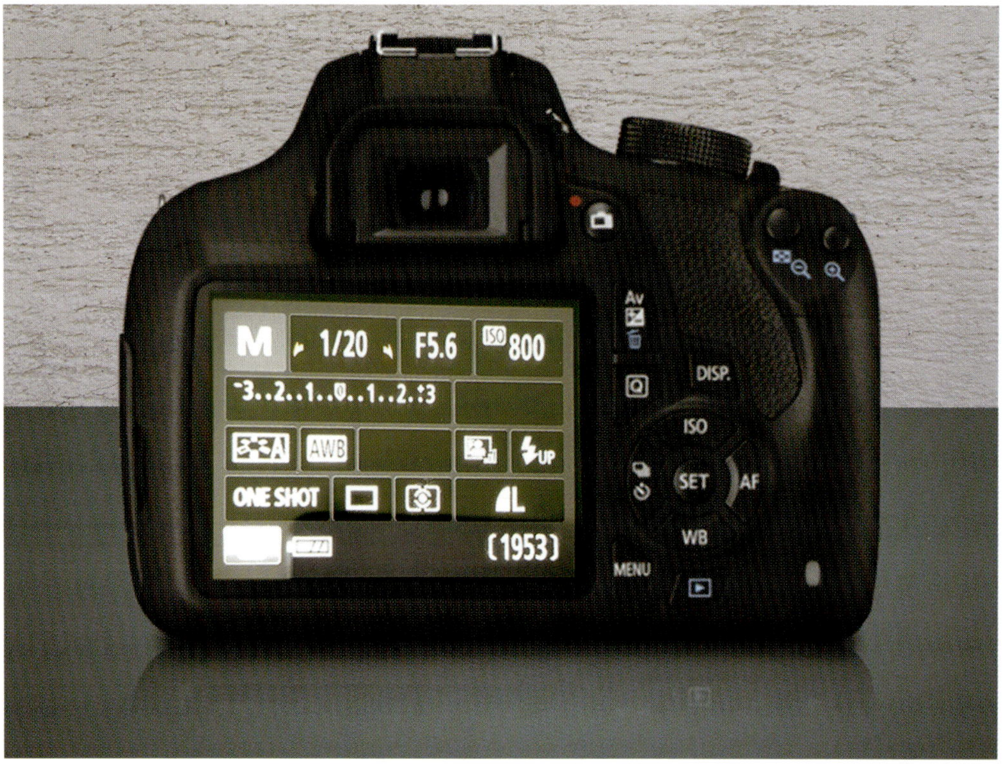

Figure 17.7B

Shows Shutter speed, F value, and ISO value on a DSLR camera (Manual Mode).

A good photographer uses manual mode to the maximum and minimizes the uses the auto mode for taking such photograph. One should have the basic understanding of the lens type and the use of flash. The following description about the basic functioning of camera should be known to a surgeon:

- *Shutter speed:* The length of time a camera shutter is open to expose light into the camera sensor. Shutter speeds are typically measured in fractions of a second, when they are under a second. Slow shutter speeds allow more light into the camera sensor and are used for low-light and night photography, while fast shutter speeds help to freeze motion. Examples of shutter speeds: 1/15 (1/15th of a second), 1/30, 1/60, and 1/125.
- *Aperture:* A hole within a lens, through which light travels into the camera body. The larger the hole, the more light passes to the camera sensor. Aperture also controls the depth of field, which is the portion of a scene that appears to be sharp. If the aperture is very small, the depth of field is large, while if the aperture is large, the depth of field is small. In photography, aperture is typically expressed in "f" numbers (also known as "focal ratio", since the f-number is the ratio of the diameter of the lens aperture to the length of the lens). Examples of f-numbers are: f/1.4, f/2.0, f/2.8, f/4.0, f/5.6, and f/8.0.
- *ISO:* A way to brighten your photos if you cannot use a longer shutter speed or a wider aperture. It is typically measured in numbers, a lower number representing a darker image, while higher numbers mean a brighter image.

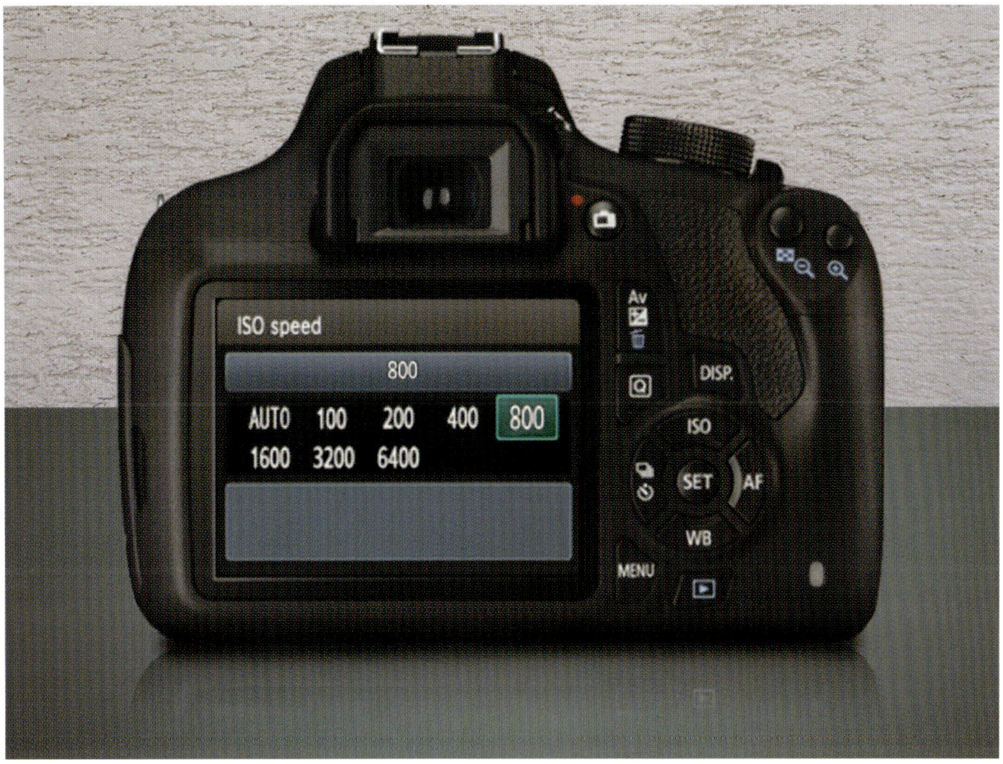

Figure 17.7C

ISO speed. Its way to brighten your image. However, as you increase the ISO, graininess of the image increases. Thus, image should be taken preferably in good light by playing with shutter speed and aperture.

However, raising your ISO comes at a cost. As the ISO rises, so does the visibility of graininess or noise in your images. Examples of ISO: 100, 200, 400, 800, and 1600 (Fig. 17.7C).

Example 1 (Figs. 17.8A to C)

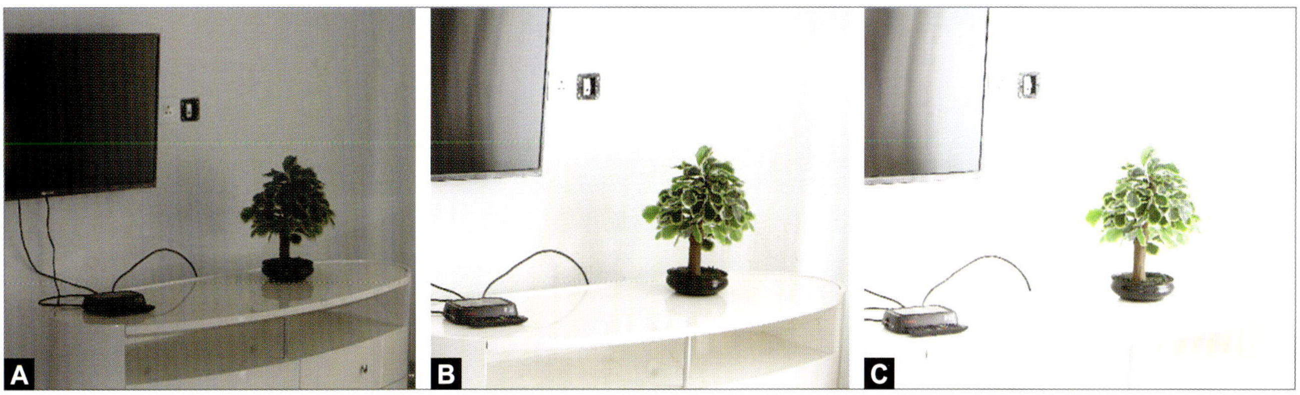

Figures 17.8A to C

Shows set of three images of the same object (plant). The central image is the best. We played with the shutter speed and gradually decreased the shutter speed from 1/80 to 1/40 to 1/20th of a second keeping the ISO and aperture value constant. This ensured increased exposure timing as we moved from first image to third. However, the third suffered from over exposure.

Example 2 (Figs. 17.9A to C)

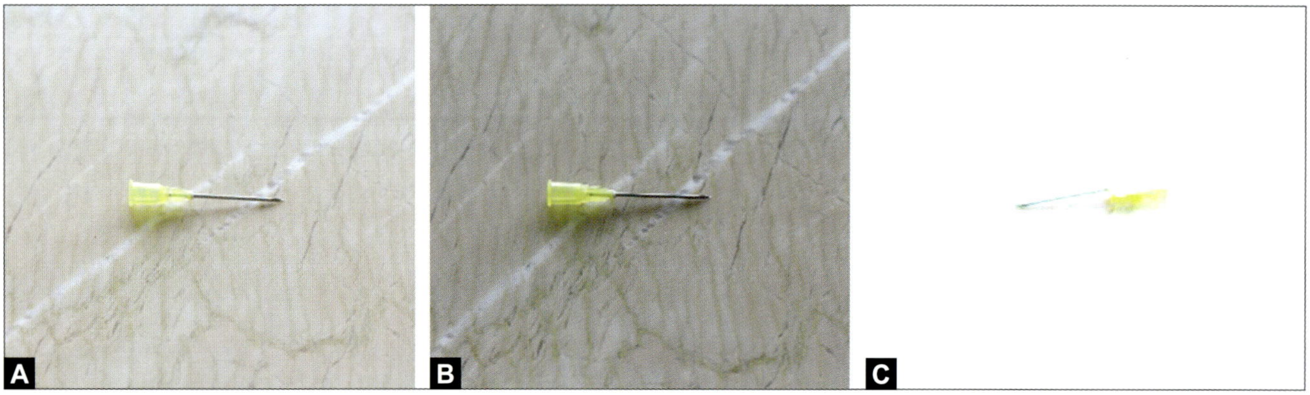

Figures 17.9A to C

Shows set of three images taken with a 50-mm lens taken in manual mode in good day light. The central image came out to be best. The ISO was kept at 100 due to daylight condition. The initial setting was shutter speed 1/10, ISO 100, and F/5.0, respectively. The first image suffers from excessive brightness; thus, shutter speed was increased from 1/10 to1/20th of a second with aperture value same as previous setting (F/5.0). The third image was taken with setting of shutter speed 1/20, with aperture value increased to F/2.0 with same value of ISO100. This increased the white balance of image and the needle is almost invisible in third image.

SUMMARY

- Photography room is the real workshop for designing the hairline and for planning the procedure.
- Scientific photograph should be taken before the procedure, immediately after the procedure and monthly after surgery.
- This may help the doctor and the patient understand the change in the look because of hair transplant and avoid legal hassles in future.

REFERENCES

1. Ashique K, Kaliyadan F. Clinical Photography for Trichology Practice: Tips and Tricks. Int J Trichol. 2011;3(1):7-13.
2. Photography Life. (2018). Understanding ISO, Shutter Speed and Aperture: A Beginner's Guide. [online] Available from https://photographylife.com/iso-shutter-speed-and-aperture-for-beginners [Accessed September 2018].
3. PhotoBlog. Exposure Triangle: How ISO, Shutter Speed, Aperture Affect Exposure. [online] Available from https://www.photoblog.com/learn/exposure-triangle-guide/ [Accessed September 2018].

Case Studies

- Case 1
- Case 2
- Case 3
- Case 4
- Case 5
- Case 6
- Case 7
- Case 8
- Case 9
- Case 10
- Case 11
- Case 12
- Case 13
- Case 14
- Case 15
- Case 16

CASE 1

1st Sitting	
Age	65 years
Donor area	Scalp and beard
Grafted area	Front and temple
Number of grafts planted	5455

FRONT

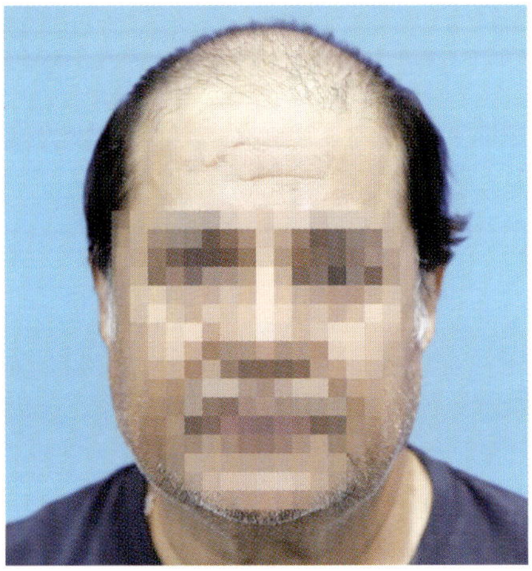

Before

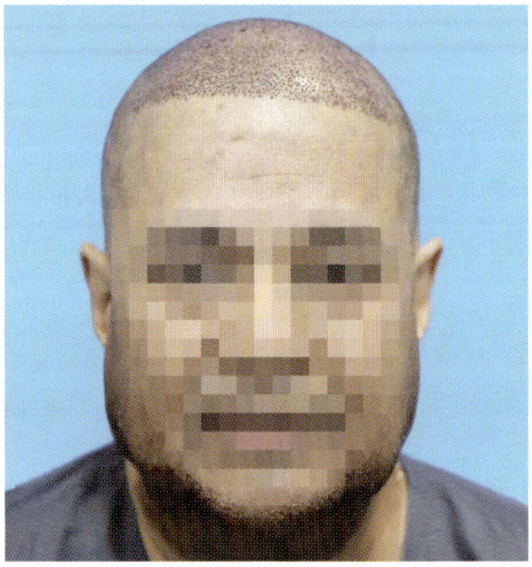

Immediate postoperative

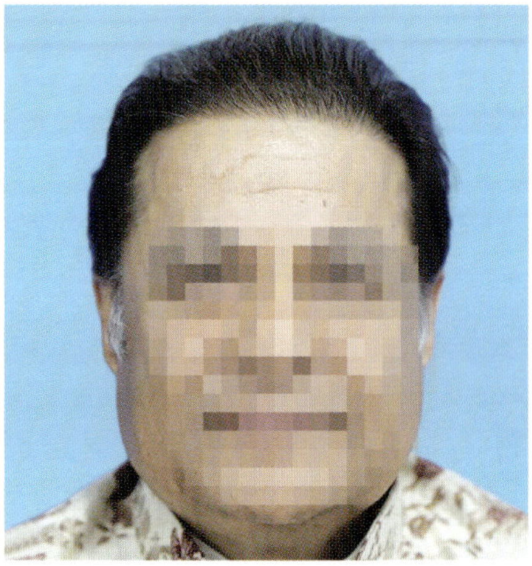

After 7 months

HEAD DOWN

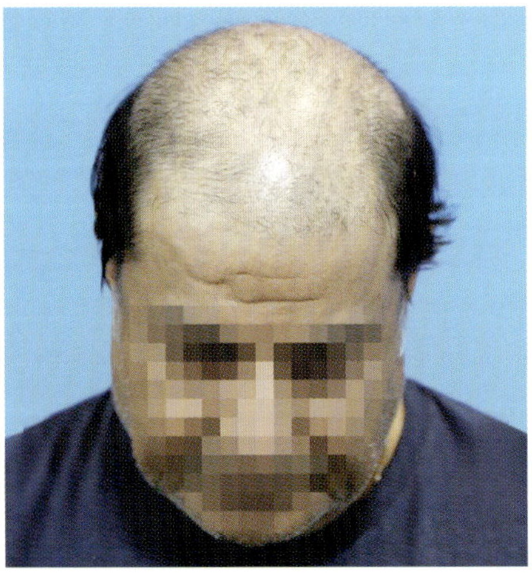

Before

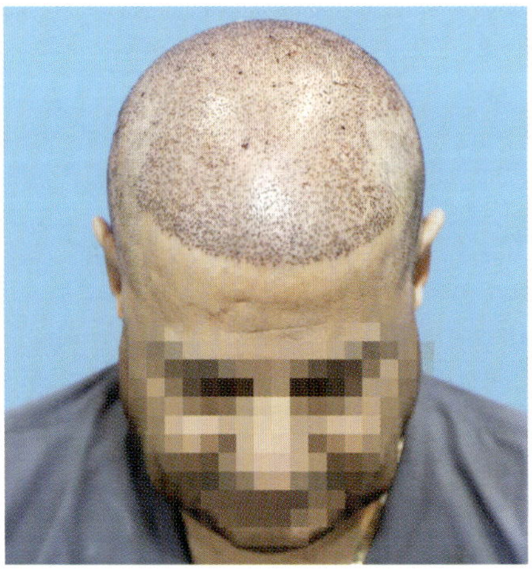

Immediate postoperative

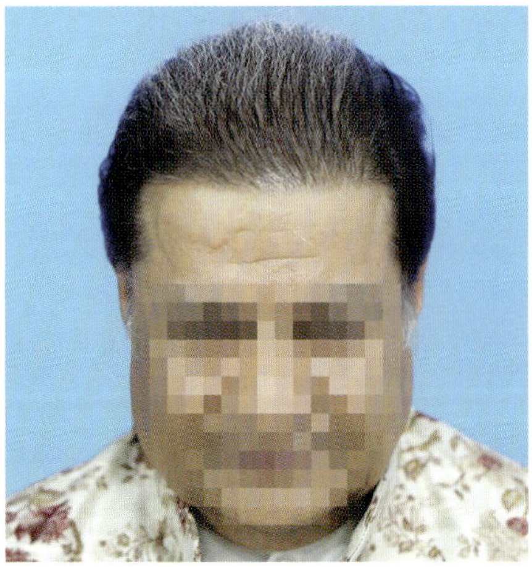

After 7 months

LEFT LATERAL

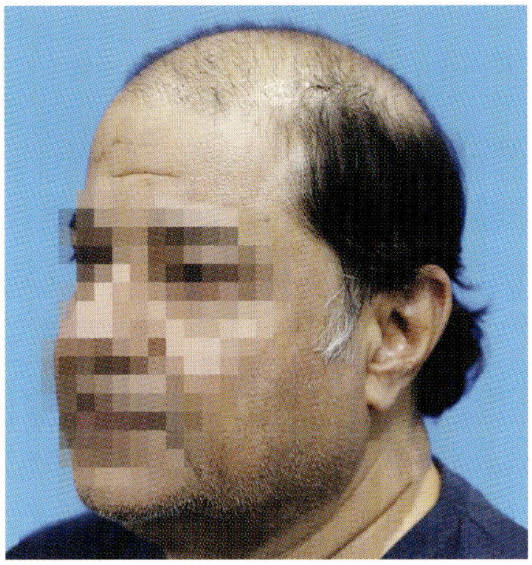

Before

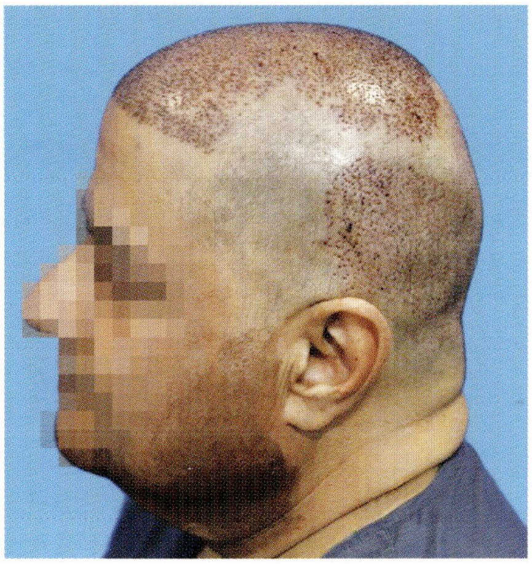

Immediate postoperative

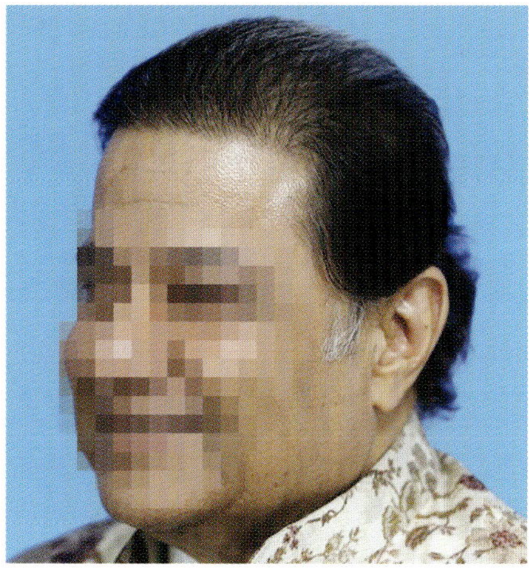

After 7 months

RIGHT LATERAL

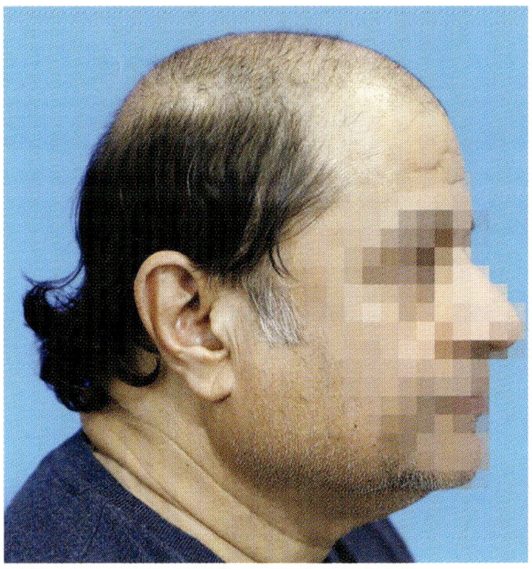

Before

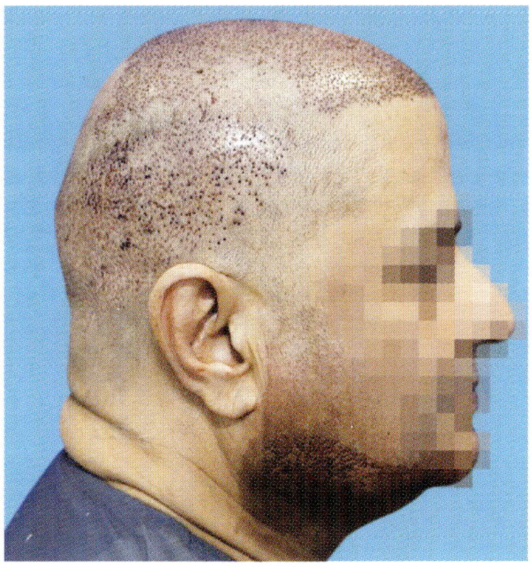

Immediate postoperative

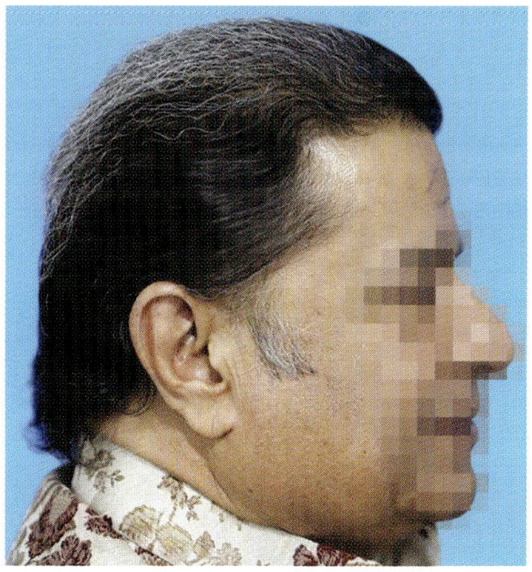

After 7 months

2nd Sitting

Donor area	**Scalp and beard**
Grafted area	**Crown**
Number of grafts planted	**2300**

BACK

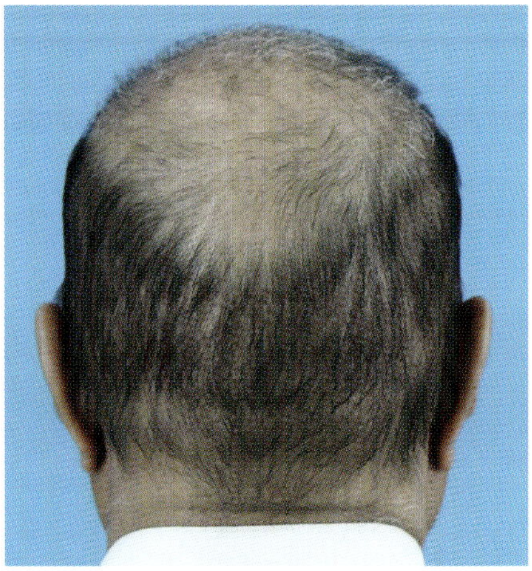

Before

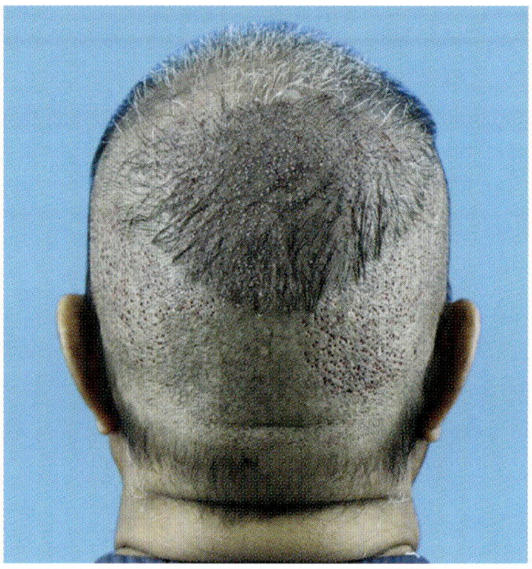

Immediate postoperative

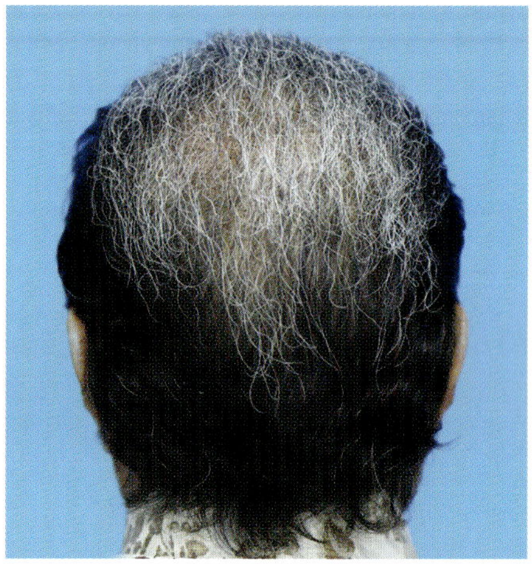

After 7 months

ROOF TOP VIEW

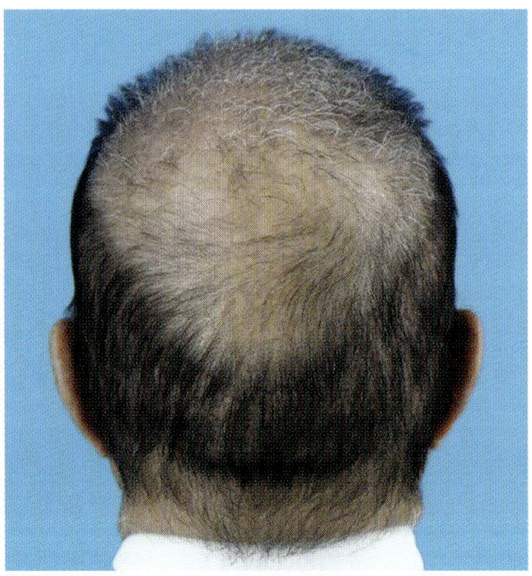

Before

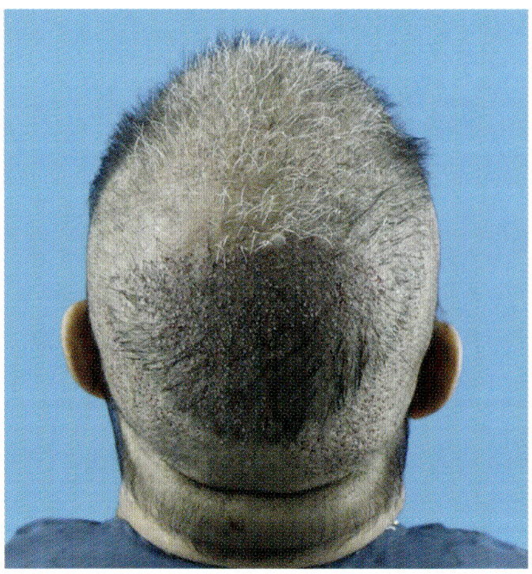

Immediate postoperative

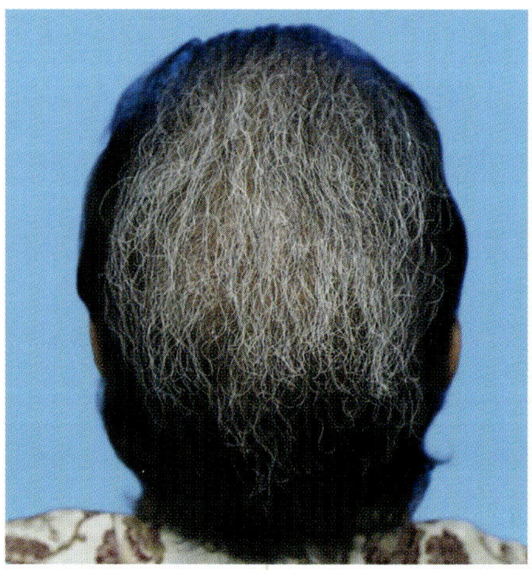

After 7 months

CASE 2

Surgery date	**21-06-2018**
Age	**41 years**
Donor area	**Scalp and beard**
Grafted area	**Front, mid-scalp**
Number of grafts planted	**5070**

FRONT

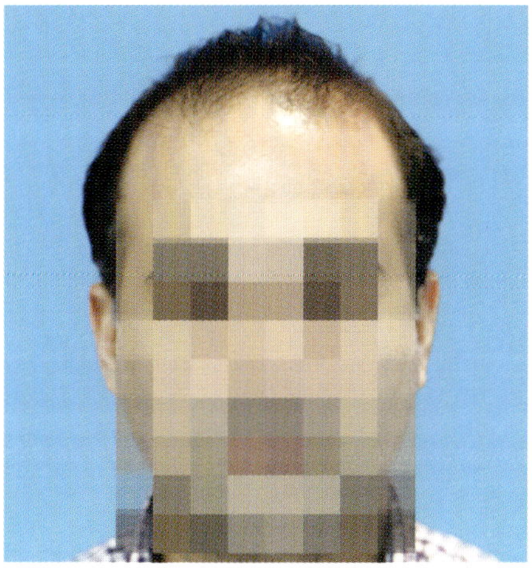
Before

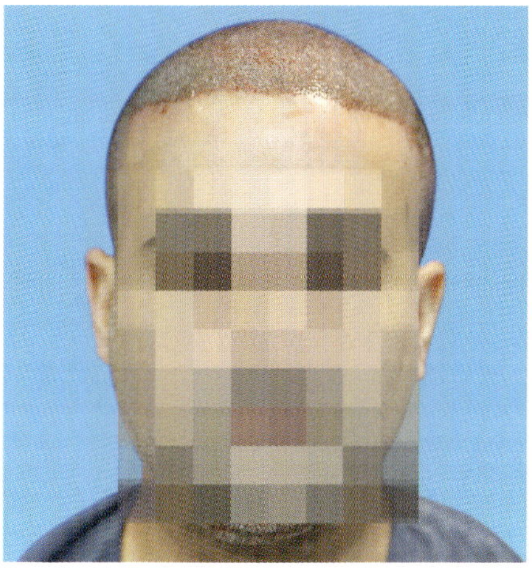
Immediate postoperative

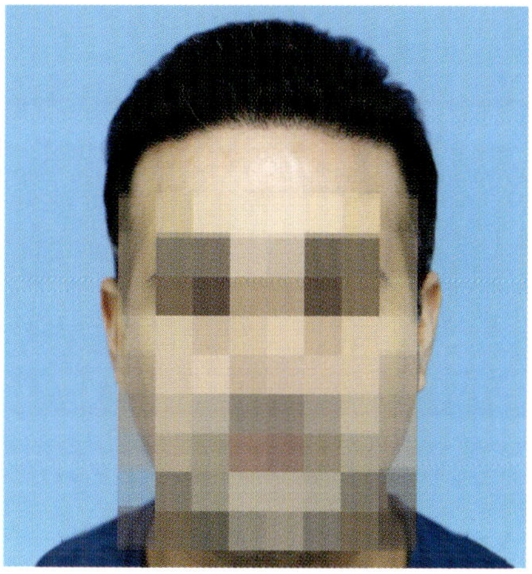
After 1 year

HEAD DOWN

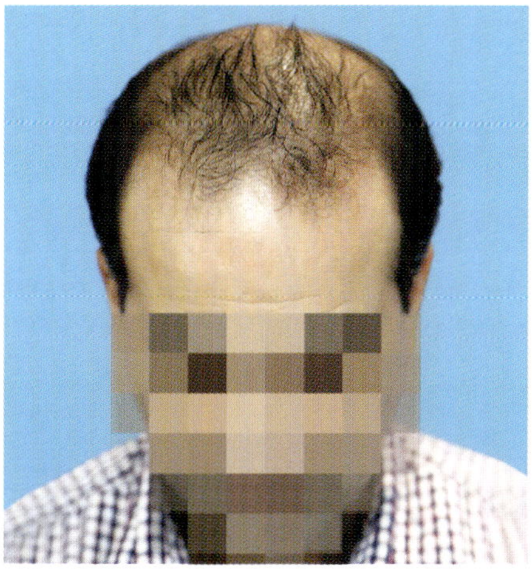
Before

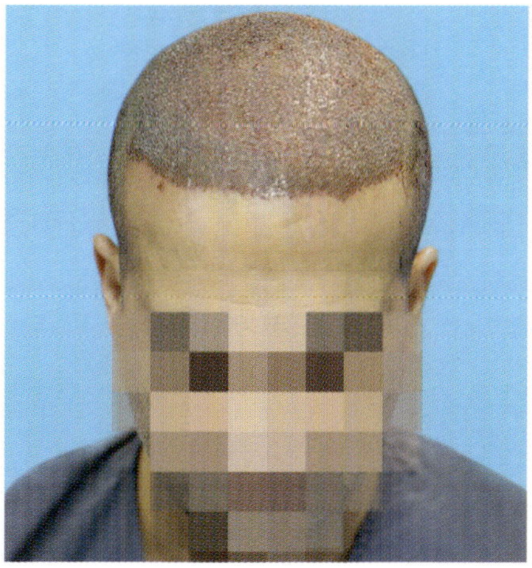
Immediate postoperative

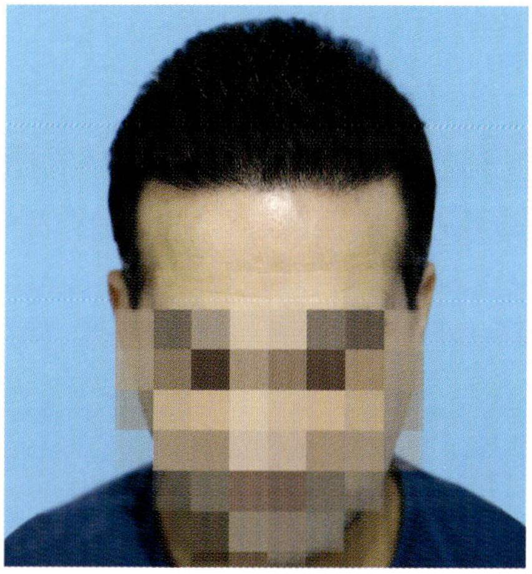
After 1 year

LEFT LATERAL

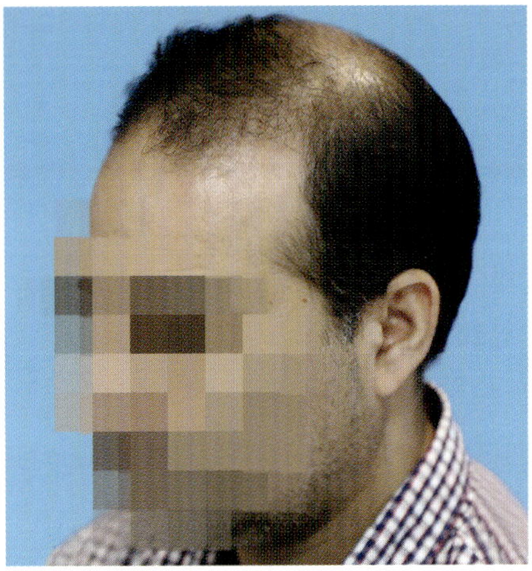

Before

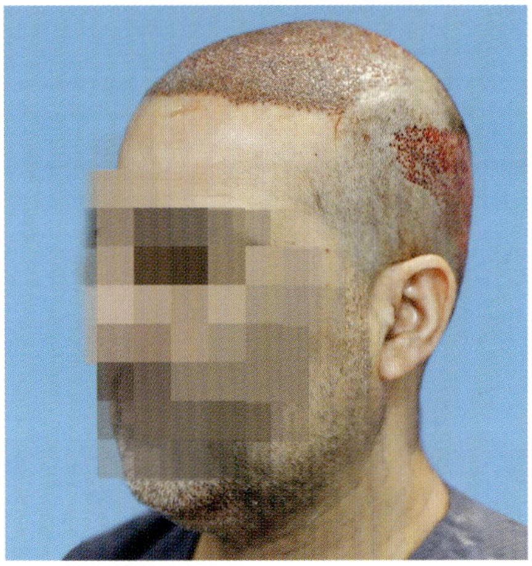

Immediate postoperative

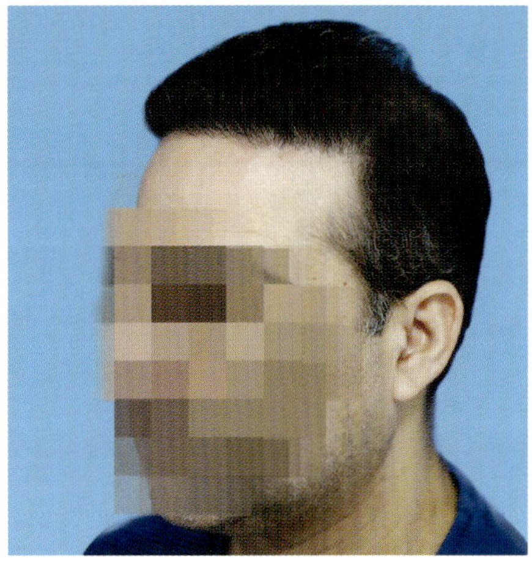

After 1 year

RIGHT LATERAL

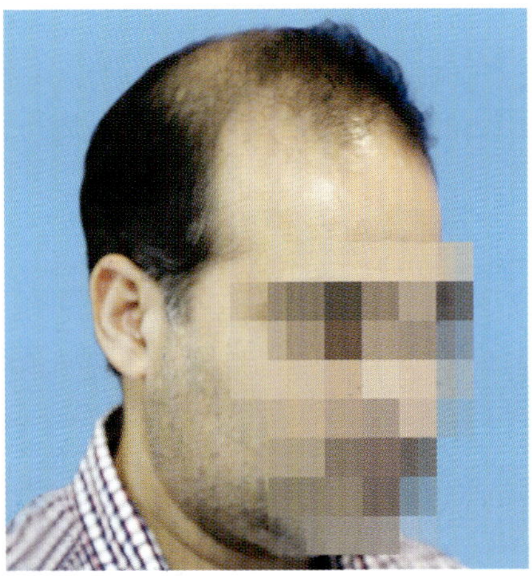

Before

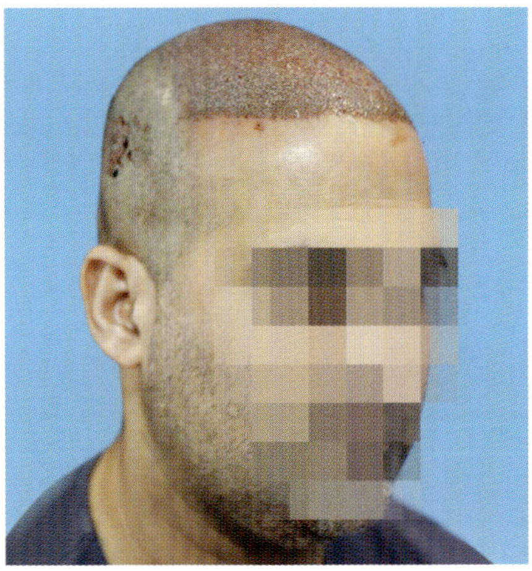

Immediate postoperative

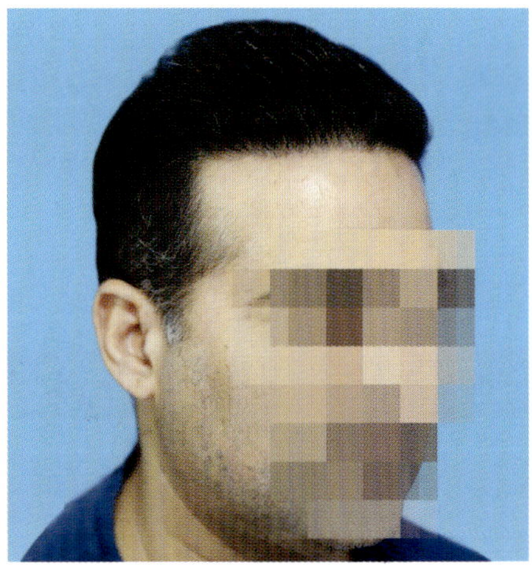

After 6 Months

BACK

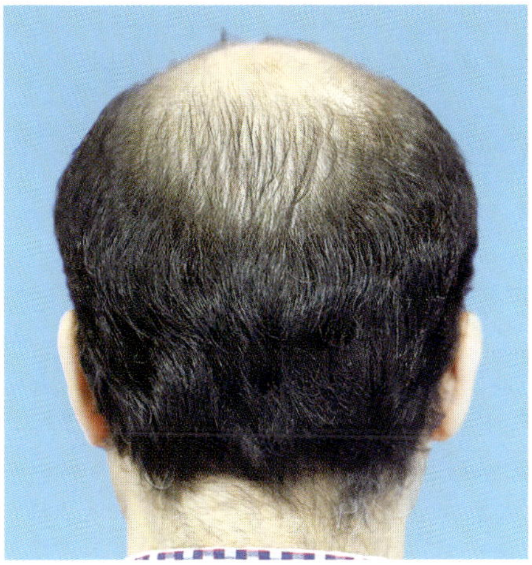
Before

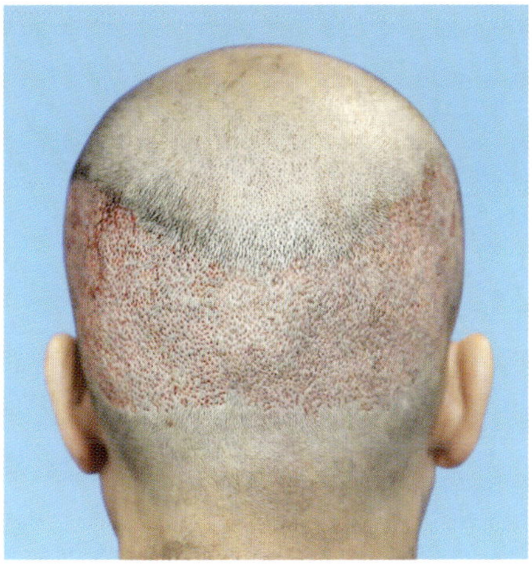
Immediate postoperative

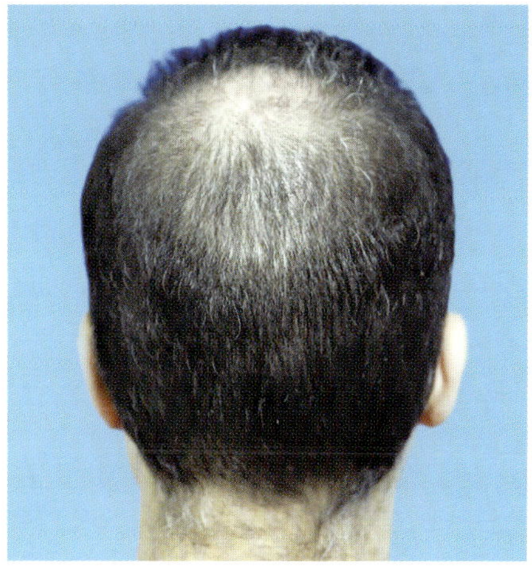
After 6 months

ROOF TOP VIEW

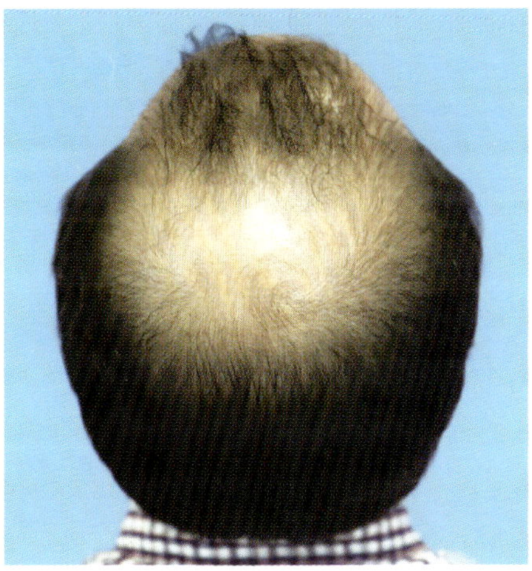
Before

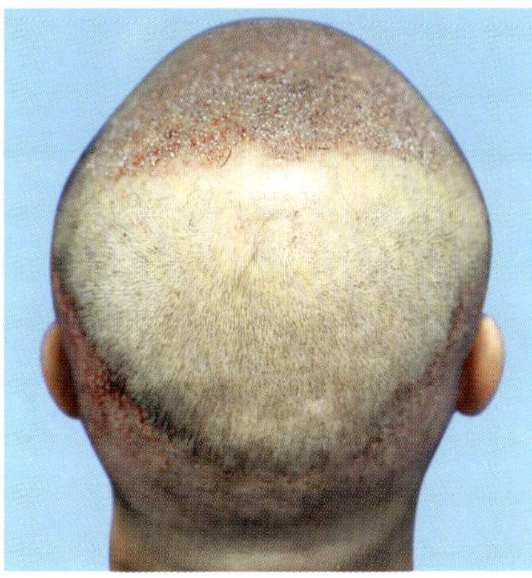
Immediate postoperative

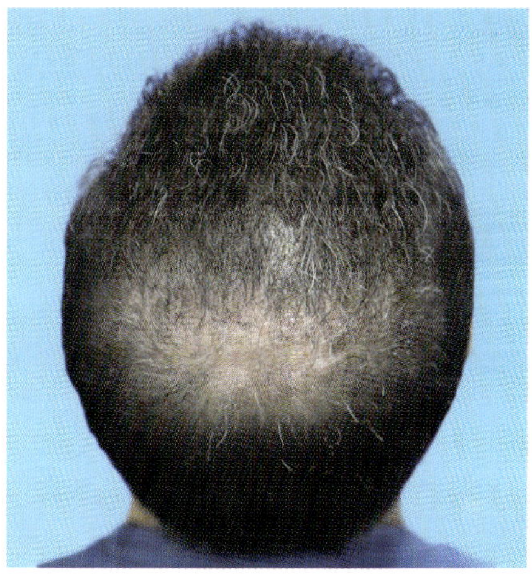
After 6 months

CASE 3

Surgery date	**23-01-2018**
Age	**32 years**
Donor area	**Scalp and beard**
Grafted area	**Front, mid-scalp, and crown**
Number of grafts planted	**5,060**
Single follicles	**1,230**

FRONT

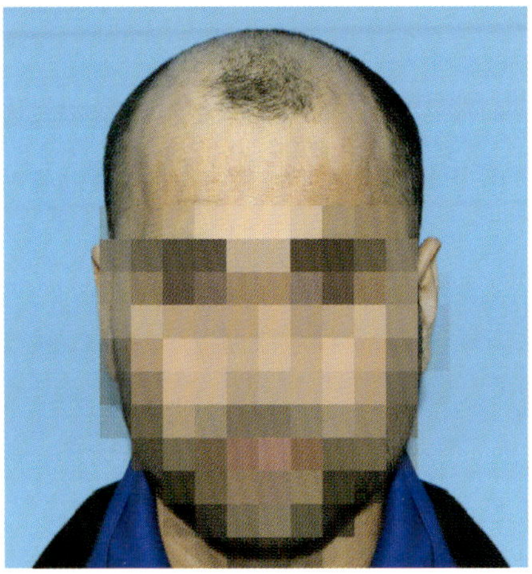
Before

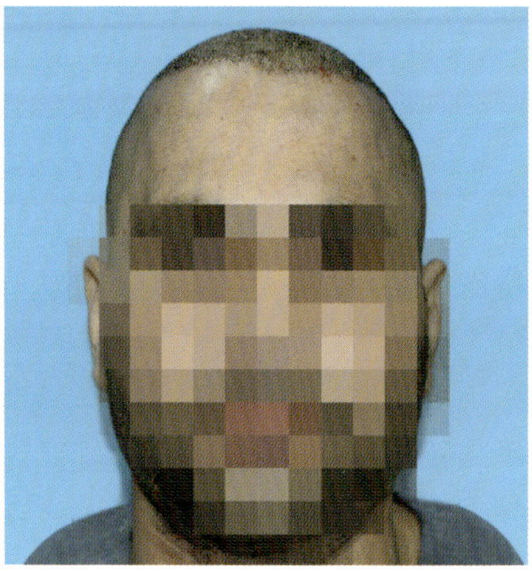
Immediate postoperative

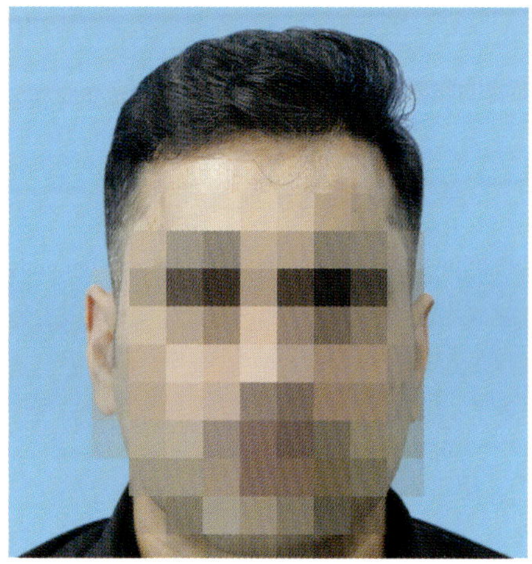
After 8 months

HEAD DOWN

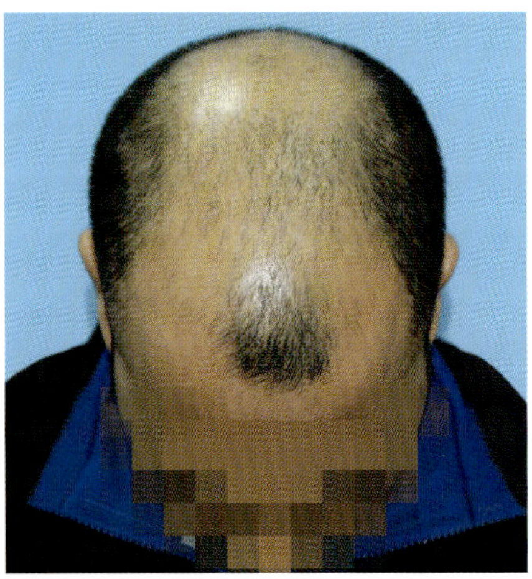
Before

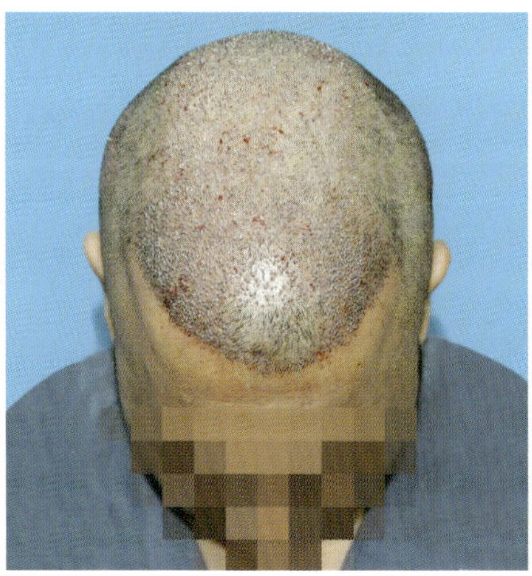
Immediate postoperative

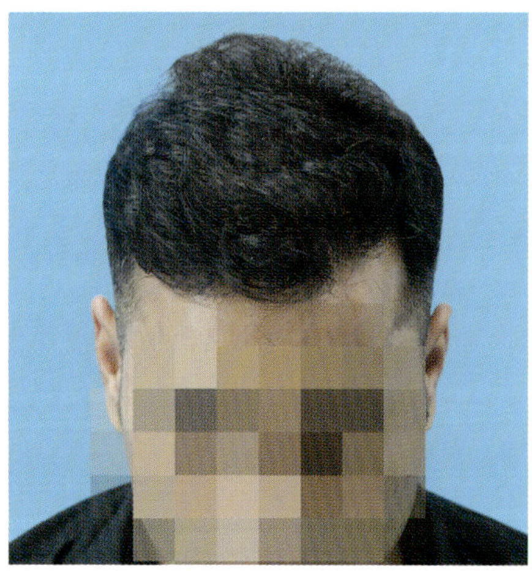
After 8 months

RIGHT LATERAL

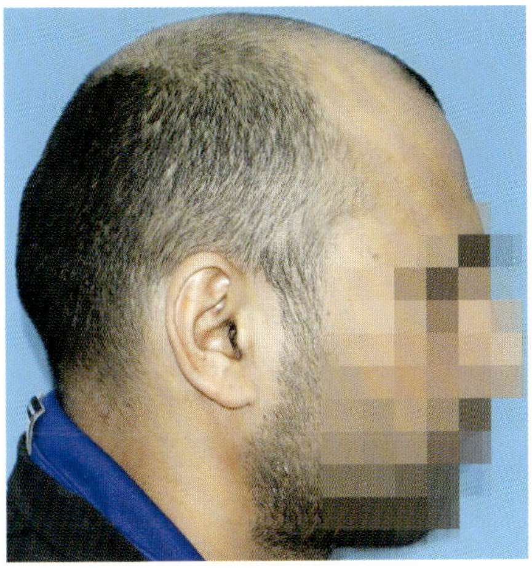

Before

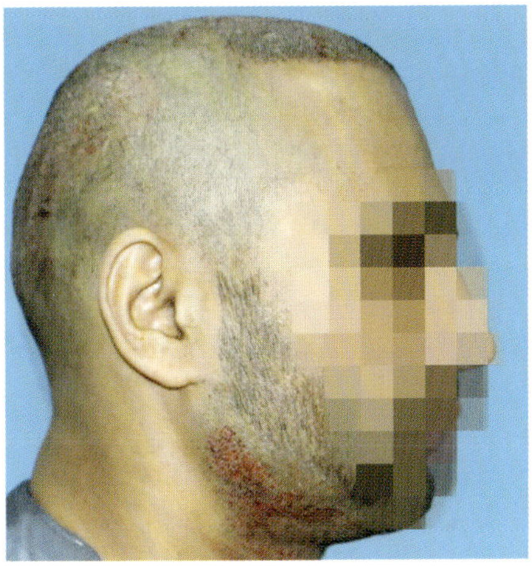

Immediate postoperative

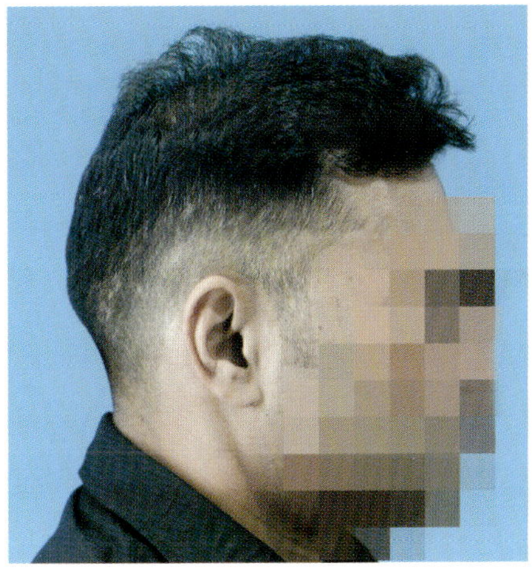

After 8 months

LEFT LATERAL

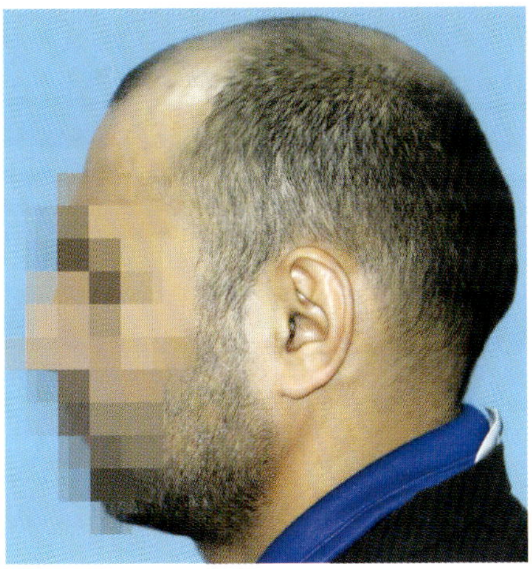

Before

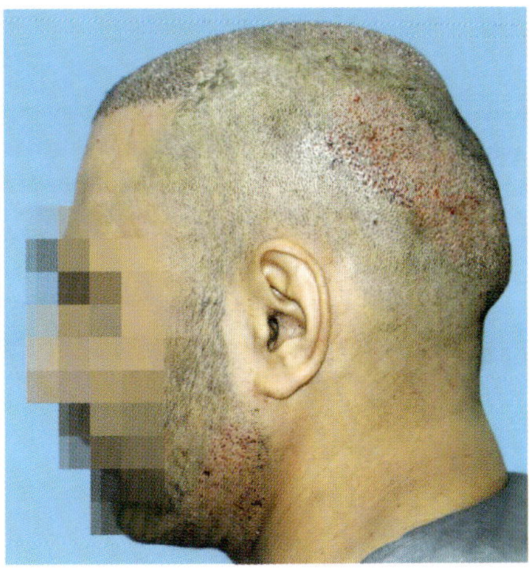

Immediate postoperative

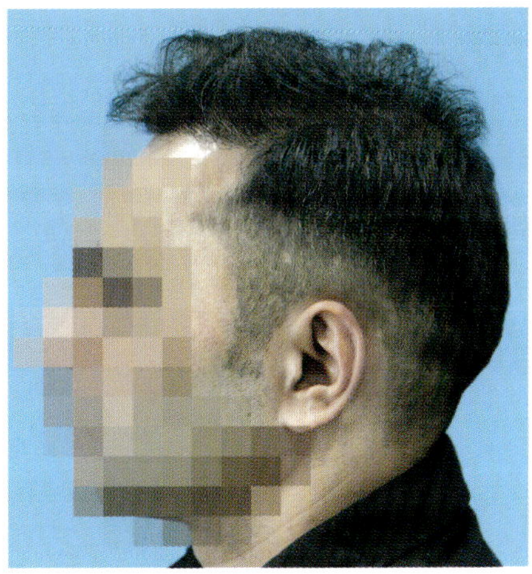

After 8 months

BACK

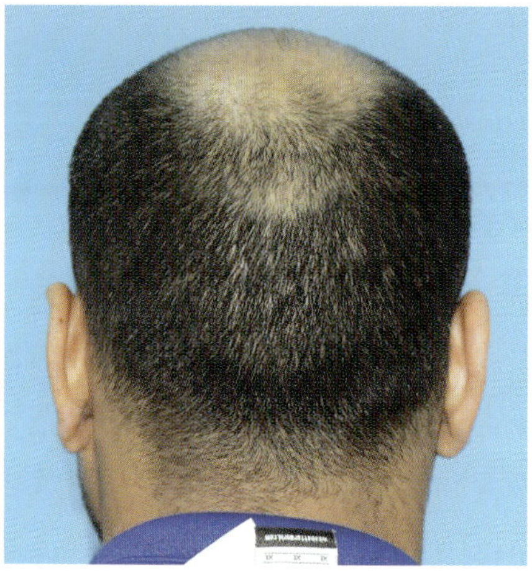

Before

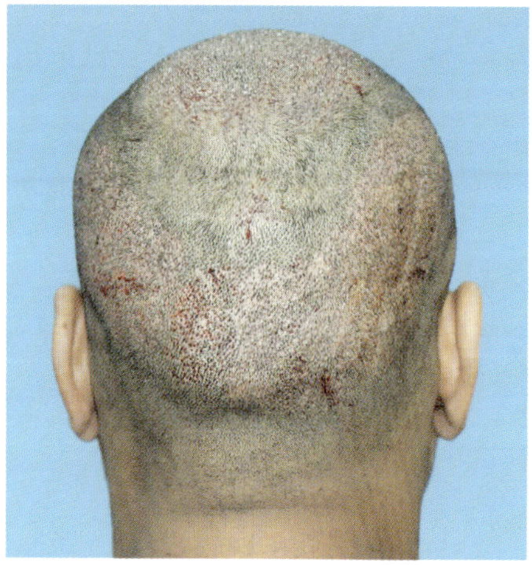

Immediate postoperative

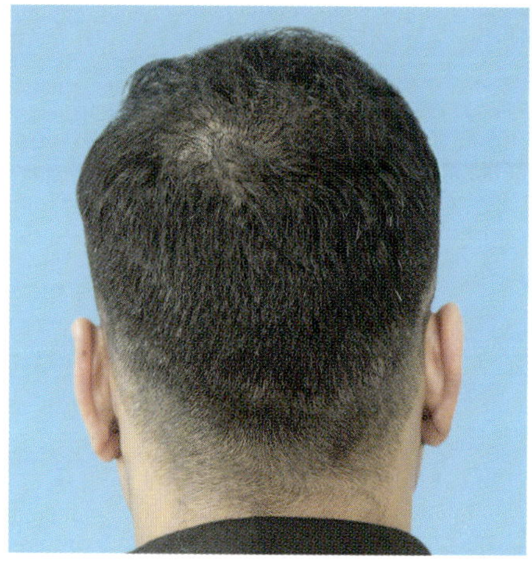

After 8 months

ROOF TOP VIEW

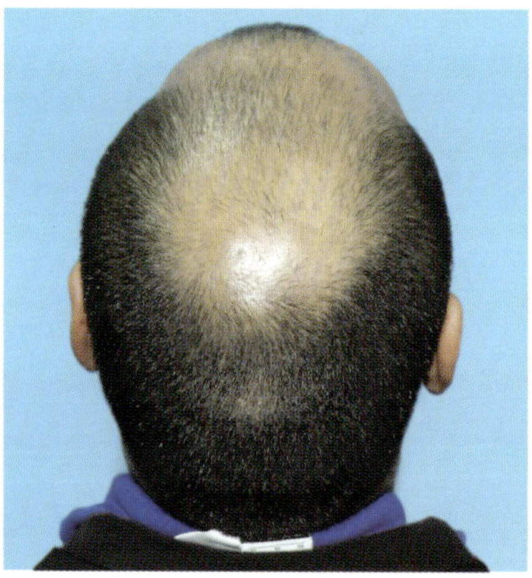

Before

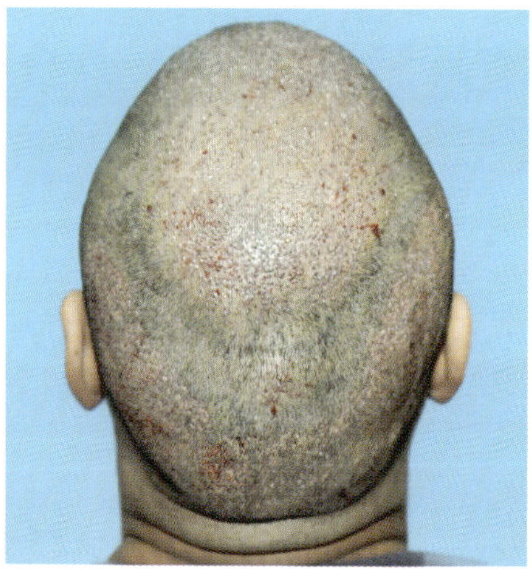

Immediate postoperative

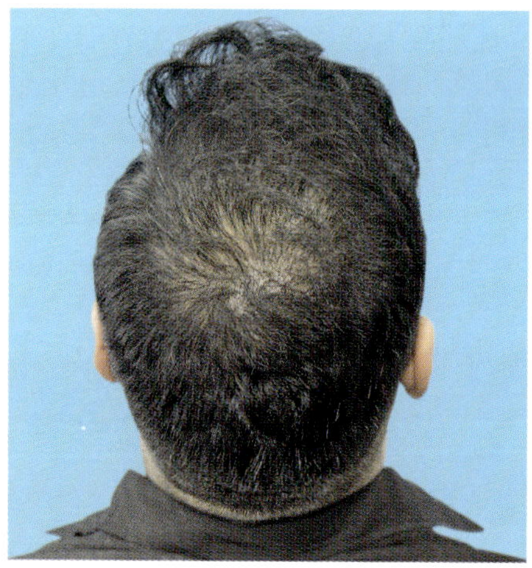

After 8 months

CASE 4

Surgery date	30-11-2016
Age	27 years
Donor area	Scalp and beard
Grafted area	Front and mid-scalp
Number of grafts planted	3,500
Single follicles	363

FRONT

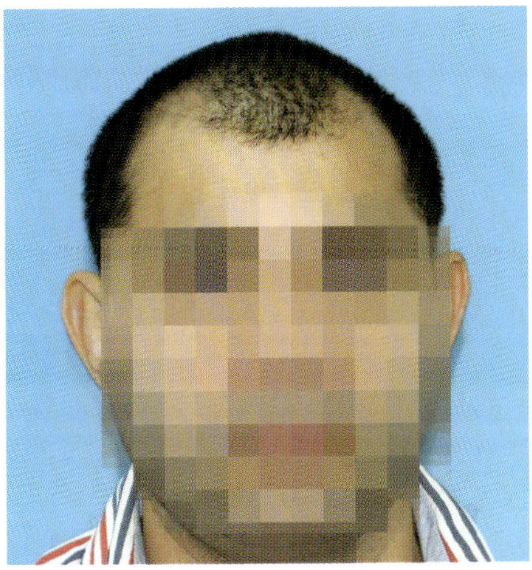
Before

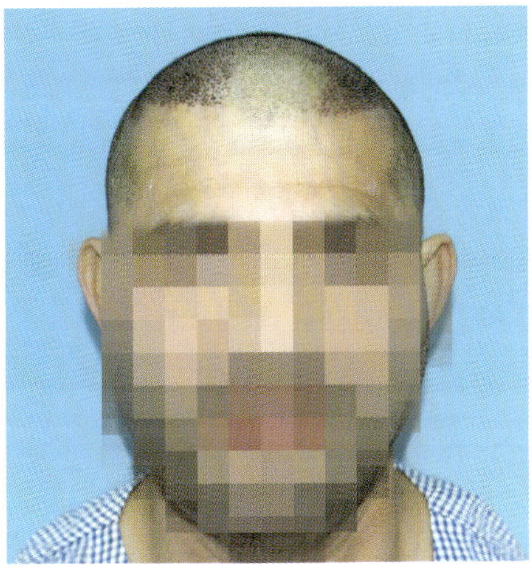
Immediate postoperative

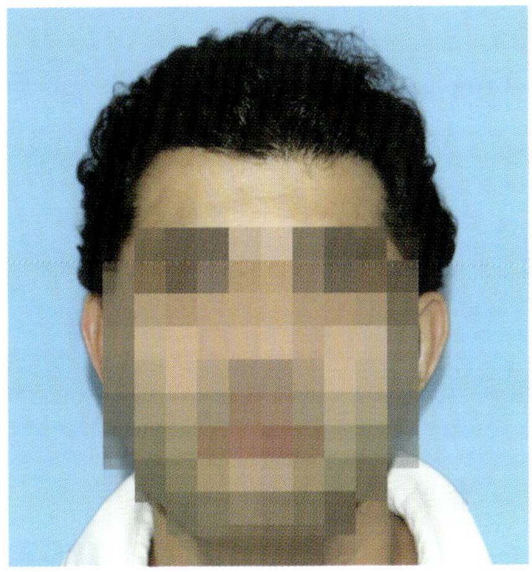
After 9 months

HEAD DOWN

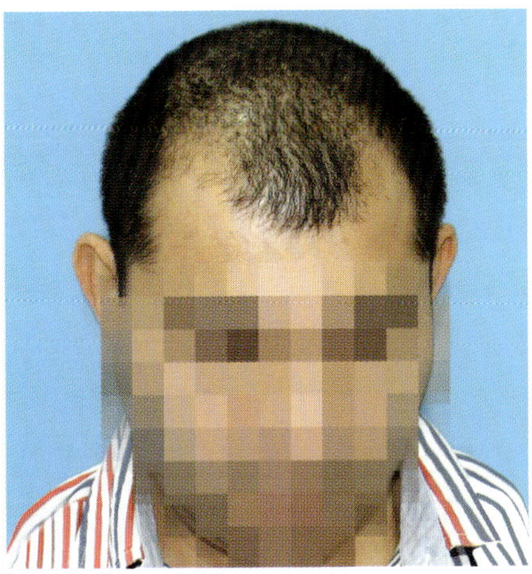
Before

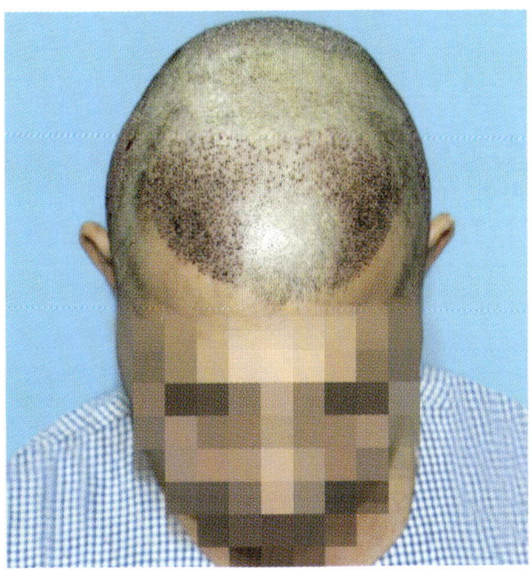
Immediate postoperative

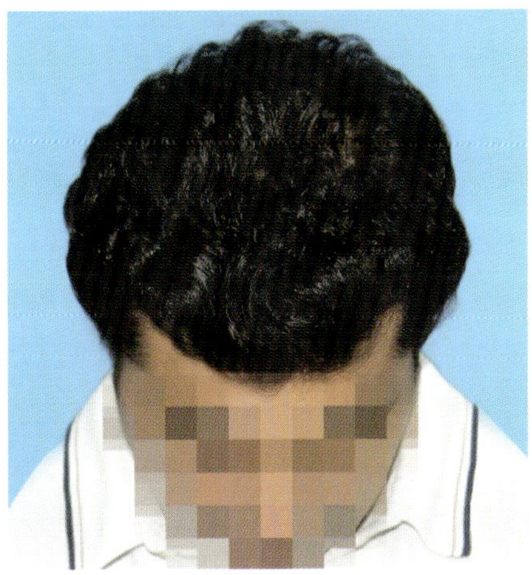
After 9 months

RIGHT LATERAL

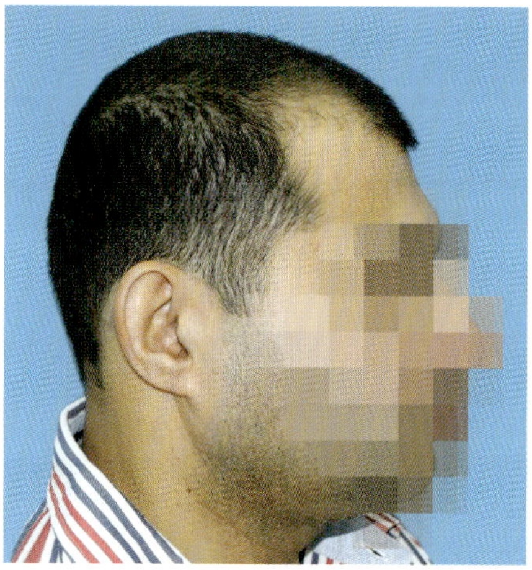

Before

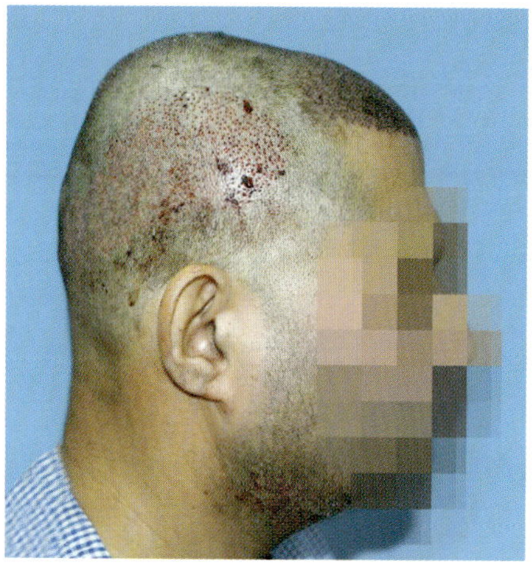

Immediate postoperative

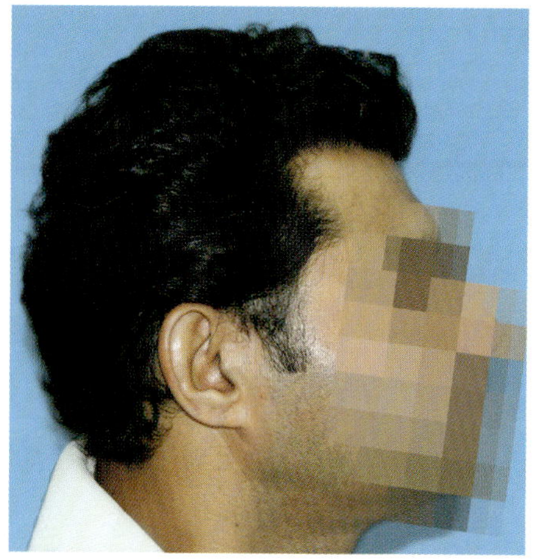

After 9 months

LEFT LATERAL

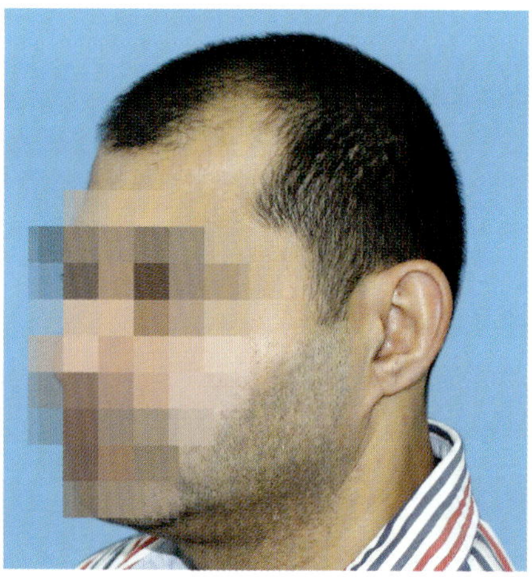

Before

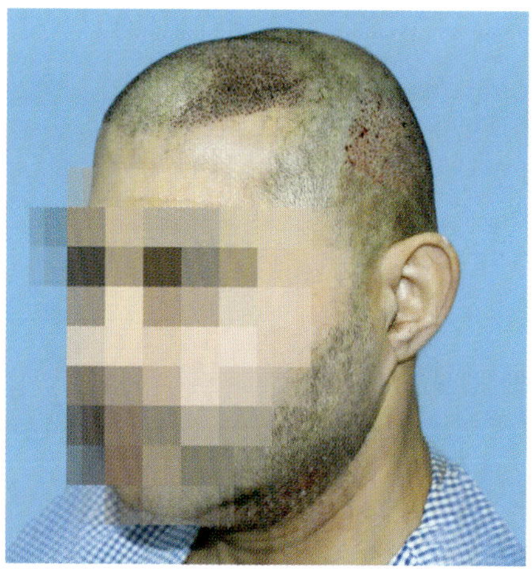

Immediate postoperative

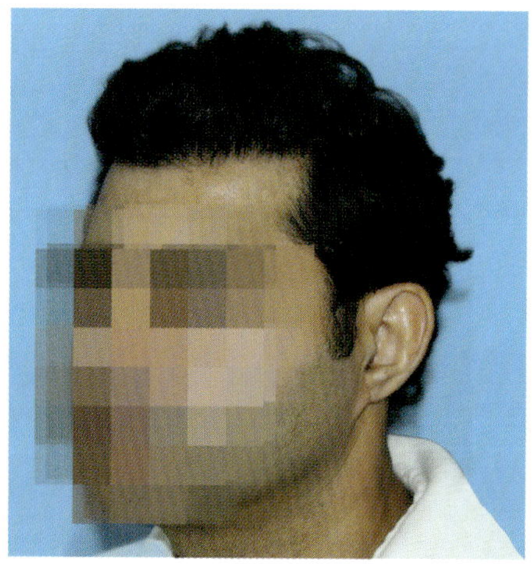

After 9 months

BACK

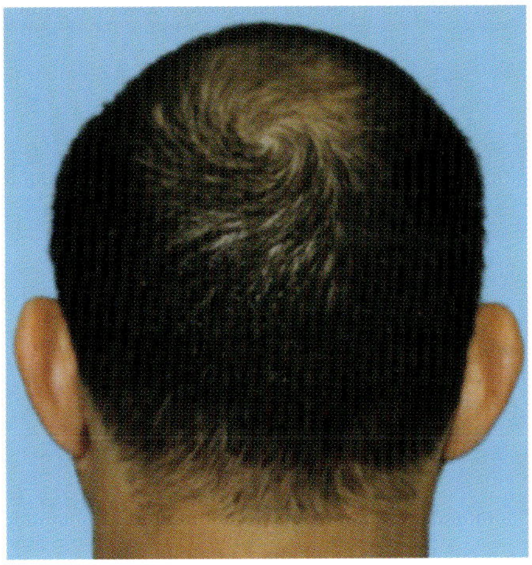
Before

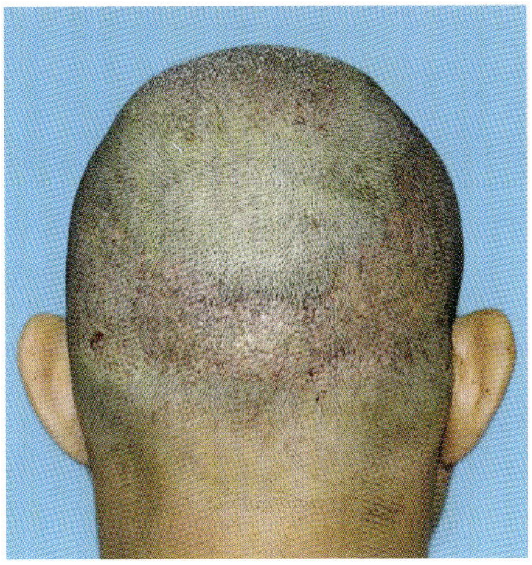
Immediate postoperative

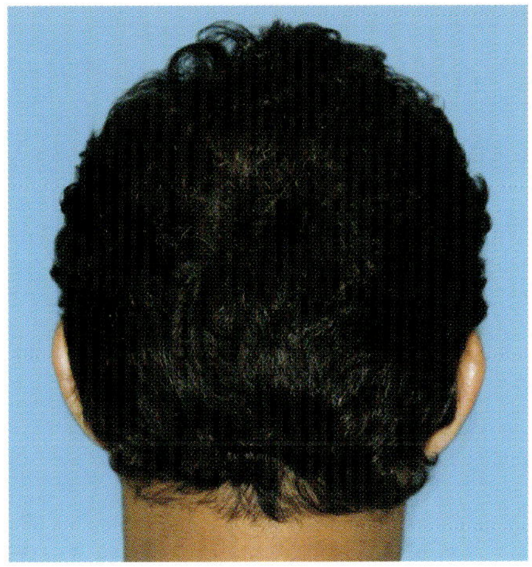
After 9 months

ROOF TOP VIEW

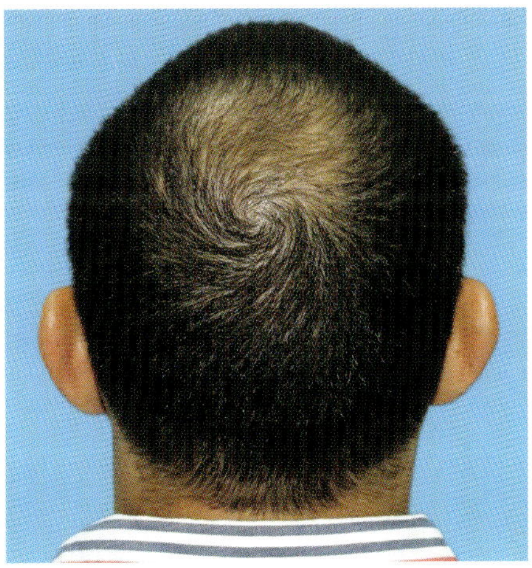
Before

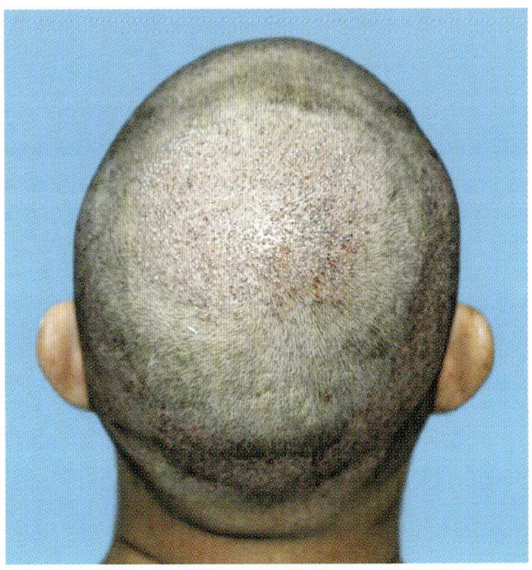
Immediate postoperative

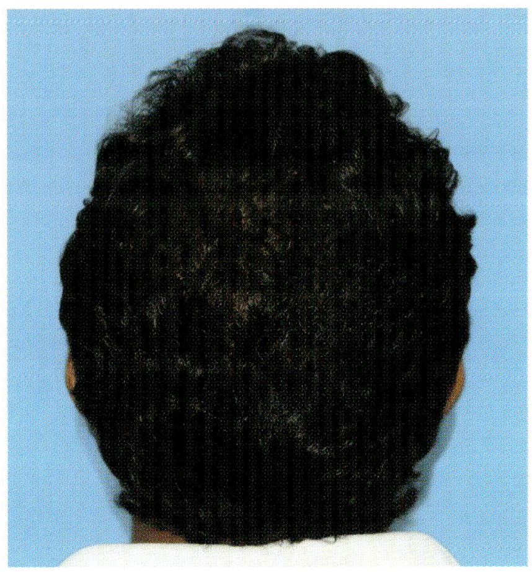
After 9 months

CASE 5

Surgery date	**26-08-2016**
Age	**58 years**
Donor area	**Scalp and beard**
Grafted area	**Front and temple**
Number of grafts planted	**7,390**
Single follicles	**432**

FRONT

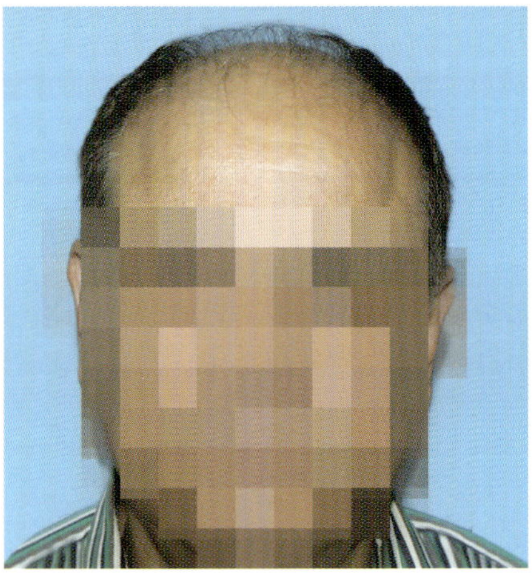

Before

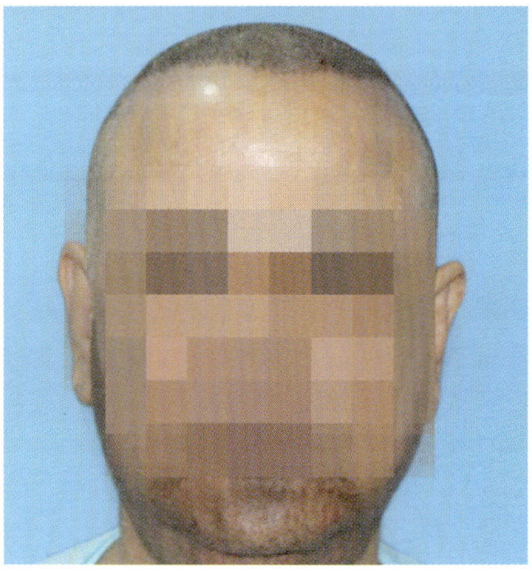

Immediate postoperative

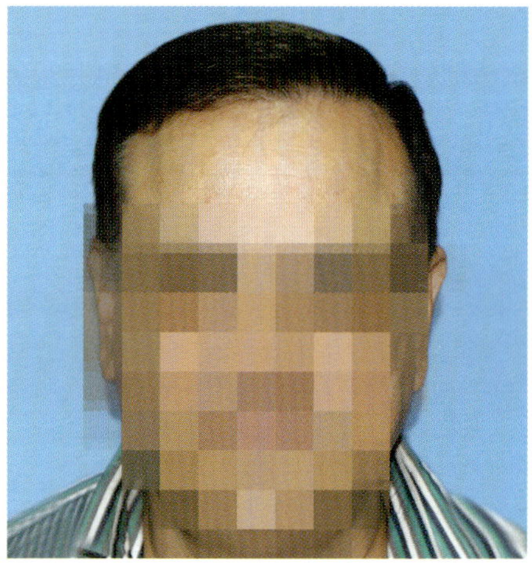

After 9 months

HEAD DOWN

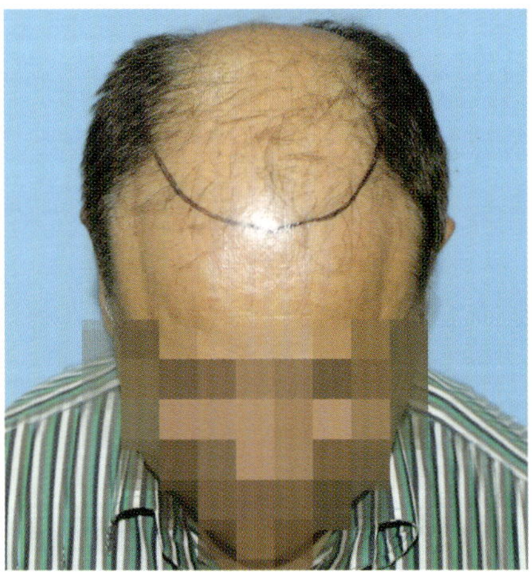

Before

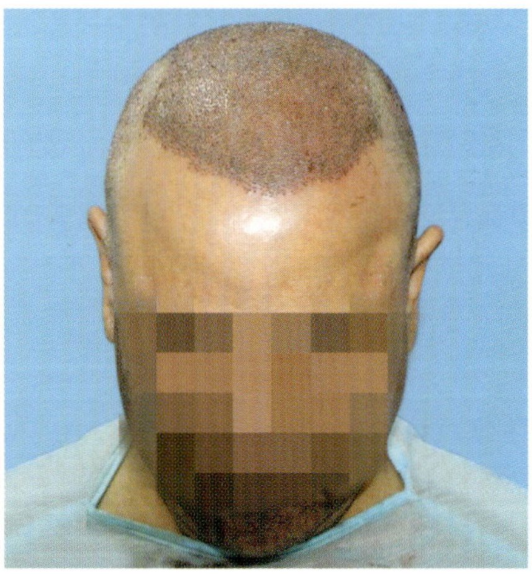

Immediate postoperative

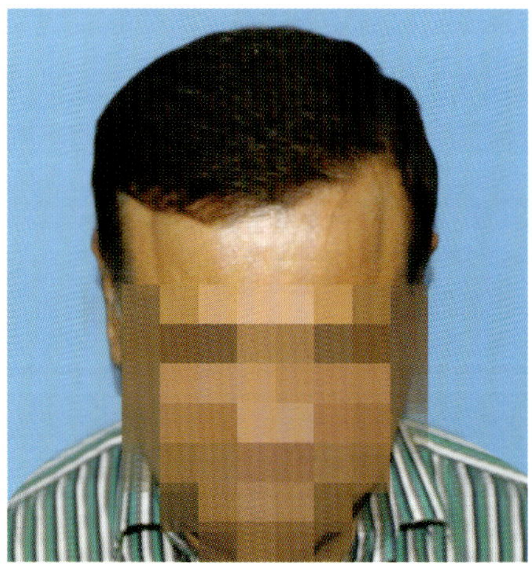

After 9 months

RIGHT LATERAL

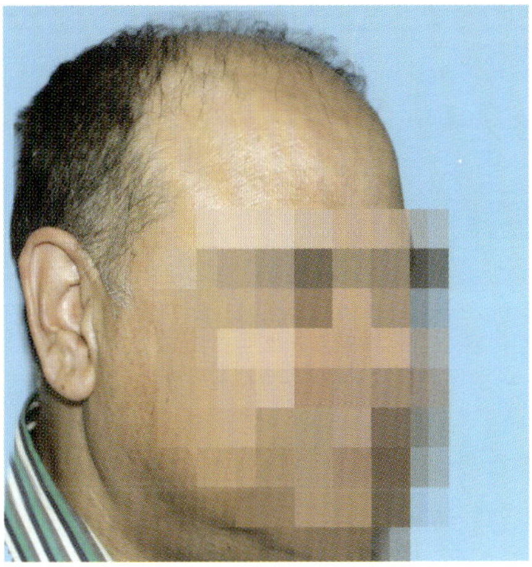
Before

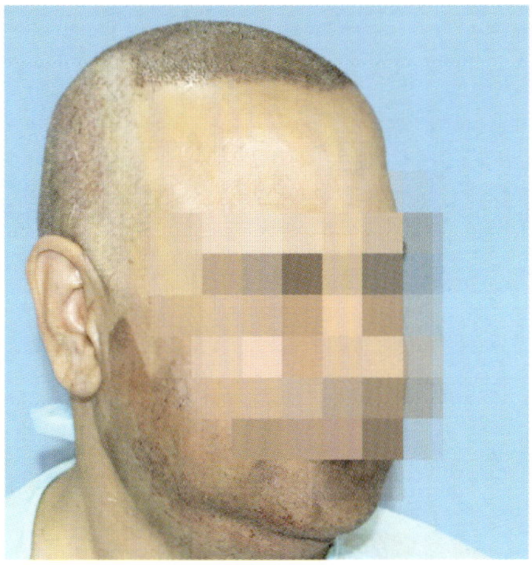
Immediate postoperative

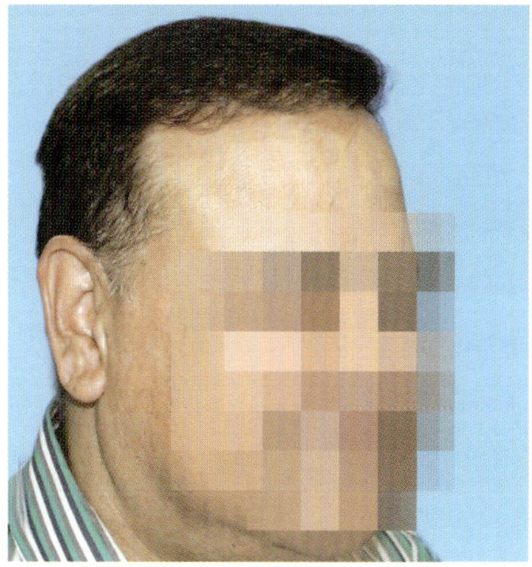
After 9 months

LEFT LATERAL

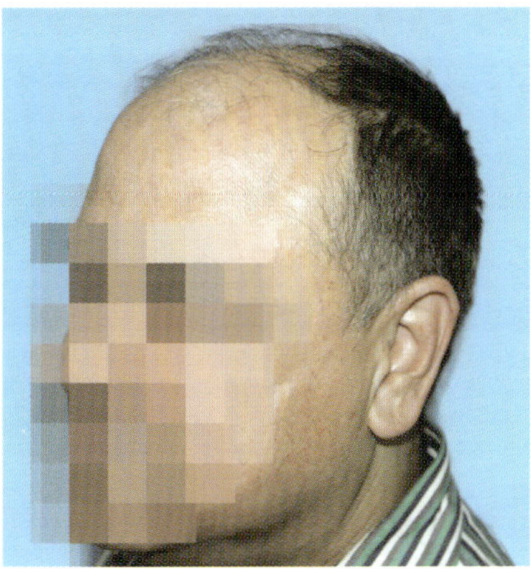
Before

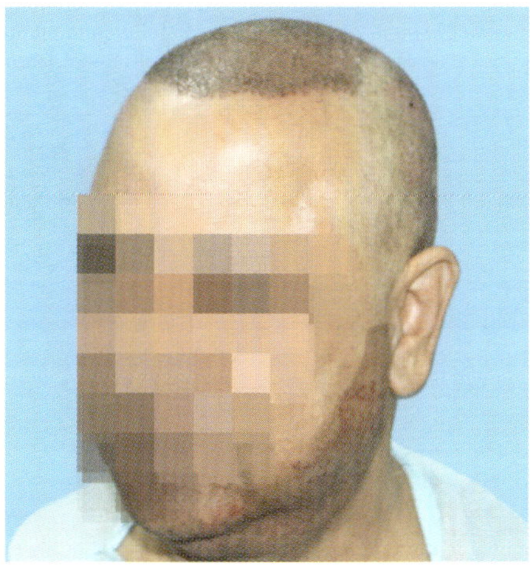
Immediate postoperative

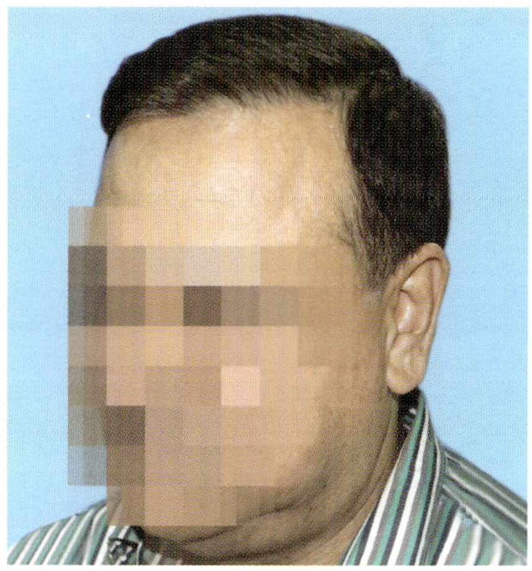
After 9 months

BACK

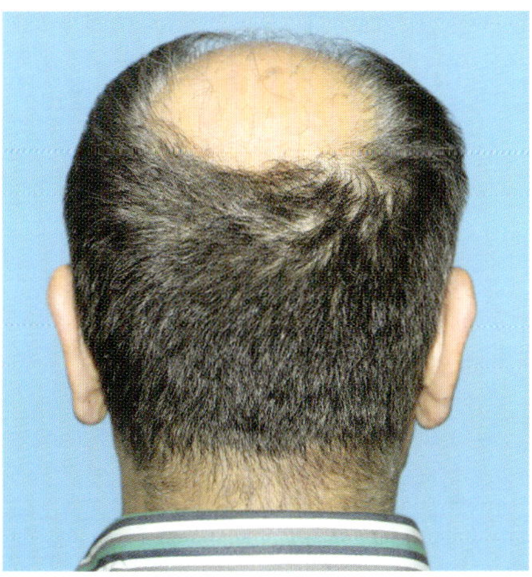
Before

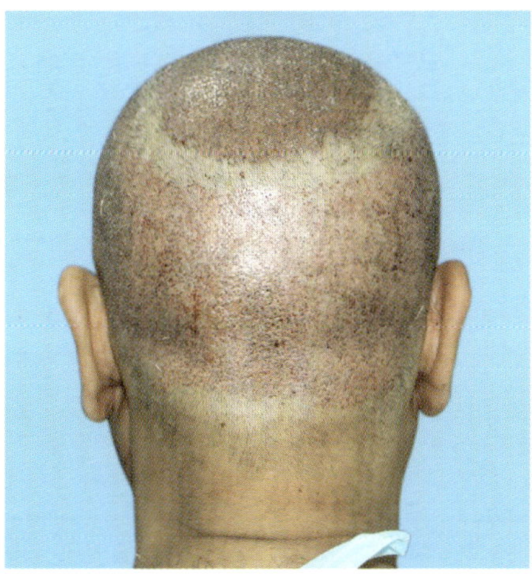
Immediate postoperative

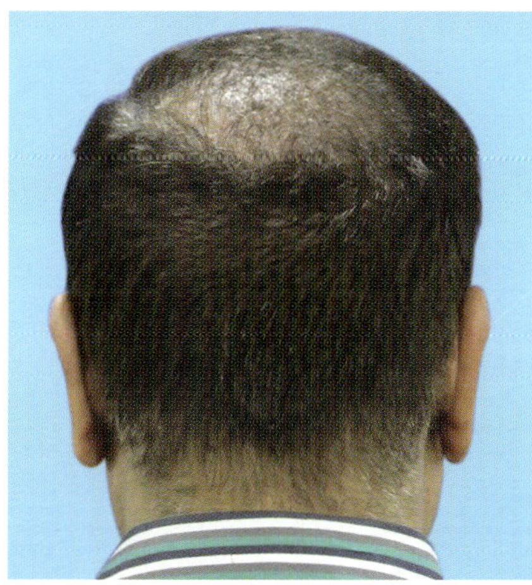
After 9 months

CASE 6

Surgery date	**26-01-2018**
Age	**33 years**
Donor area	**Scalp and beard**
Grafted area	**Front and middle**
Number of grafts planted	**6,386**
Single follicles	**578**

FRONT

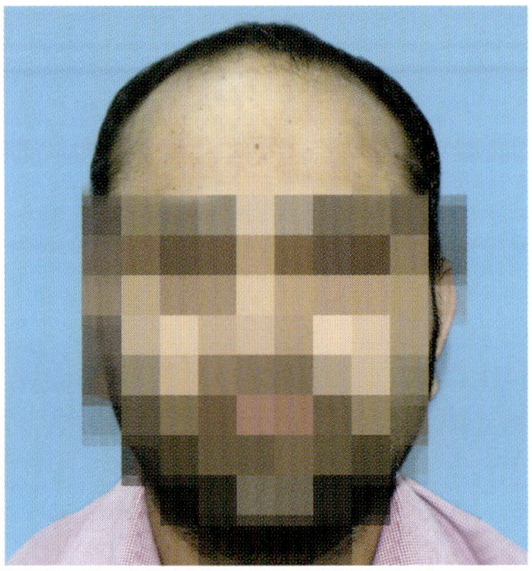
Before

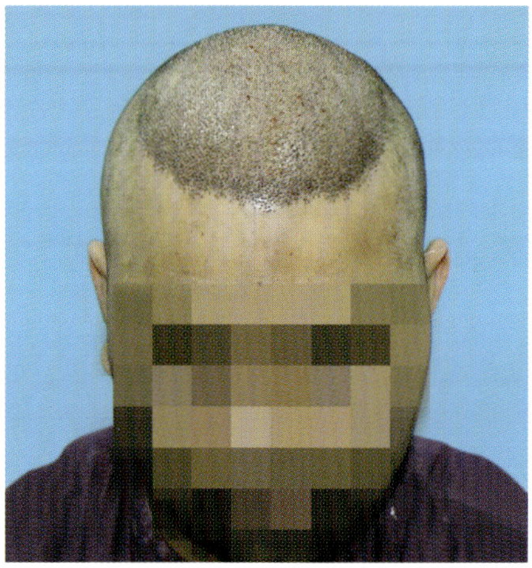
Immediate postoperative

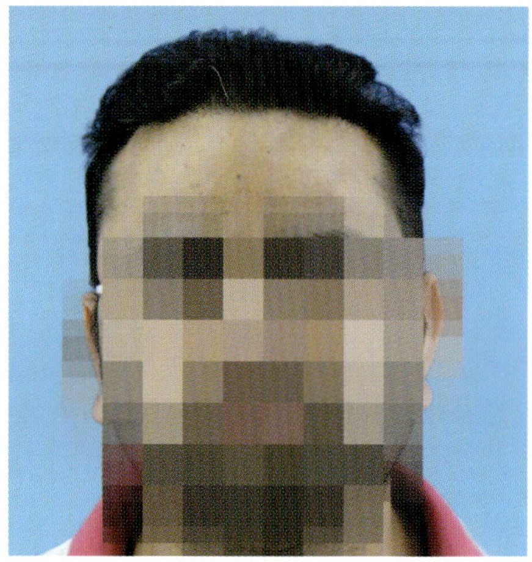
After 9 months

HEAD DOWN

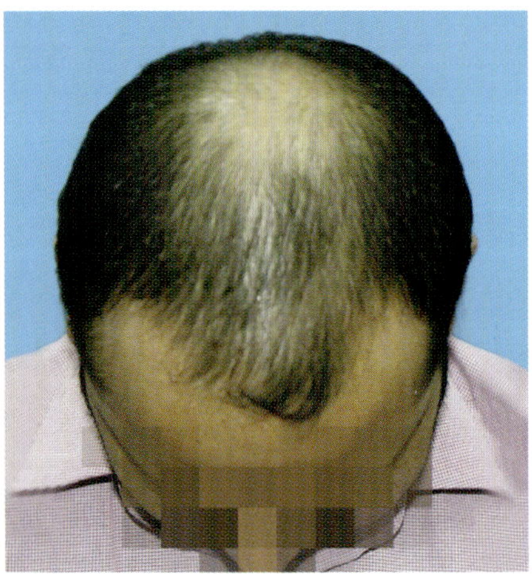
Before

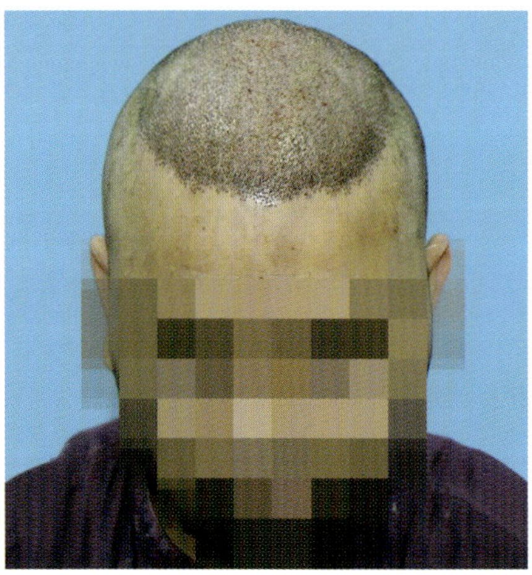
Immediate postoperative

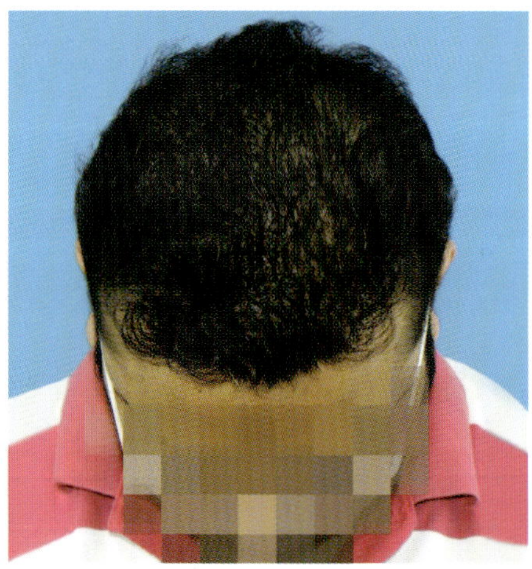
After 9 months

RIGHT LATERAL

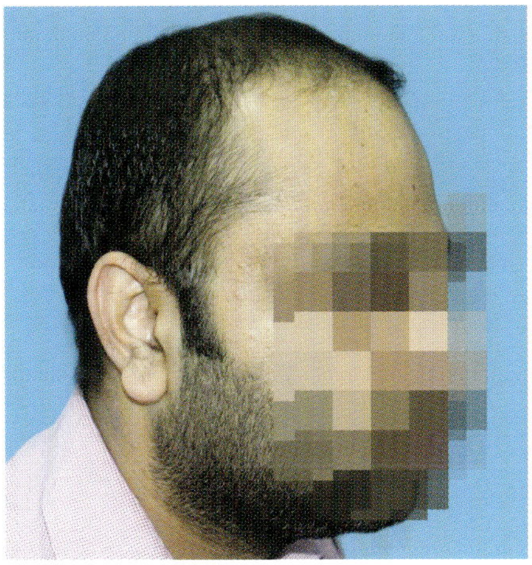
Before

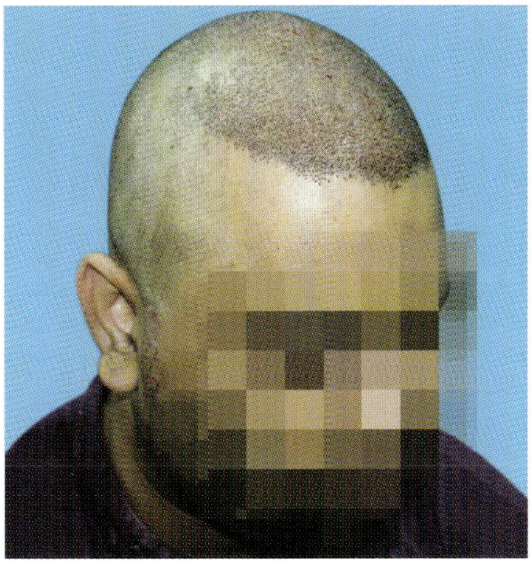
Immediate postoperative

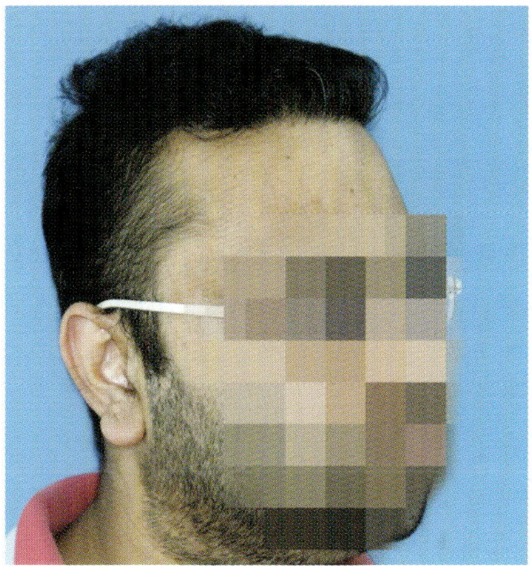
After 9 months

LEFT LATERAL

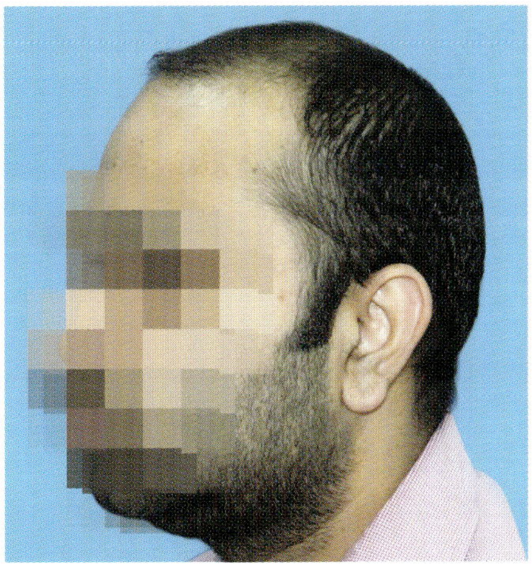
Before

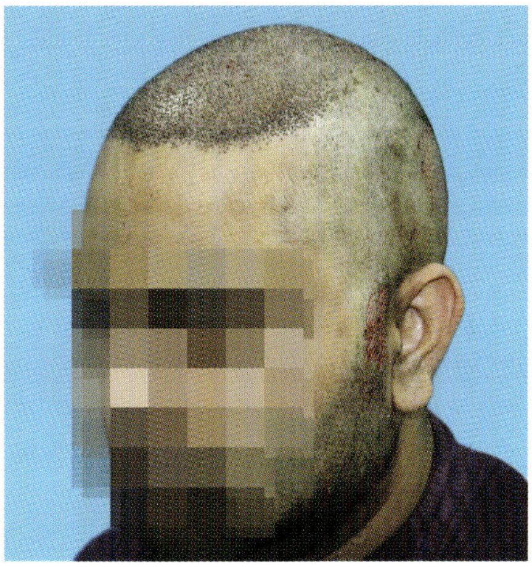
Immediate postoperative

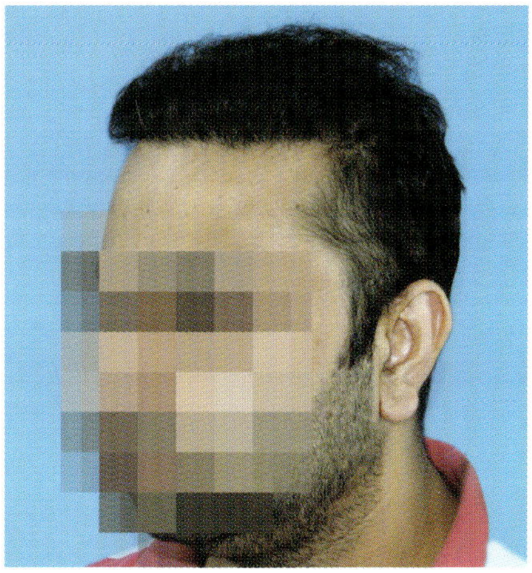
After 9 months

BACK

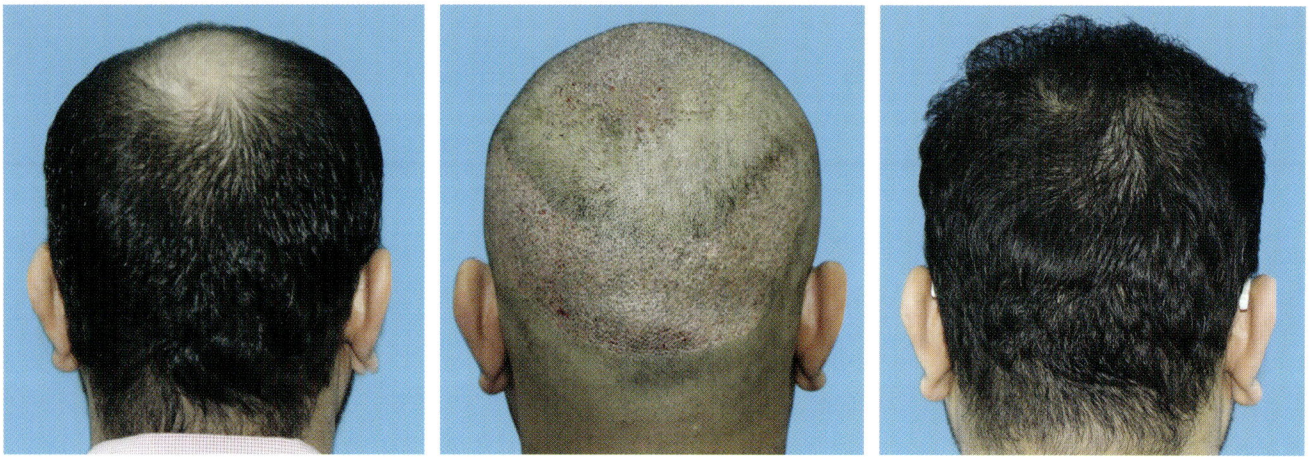

Before | Immediate postoperative | After 9 months

ROOF TOP VIEW

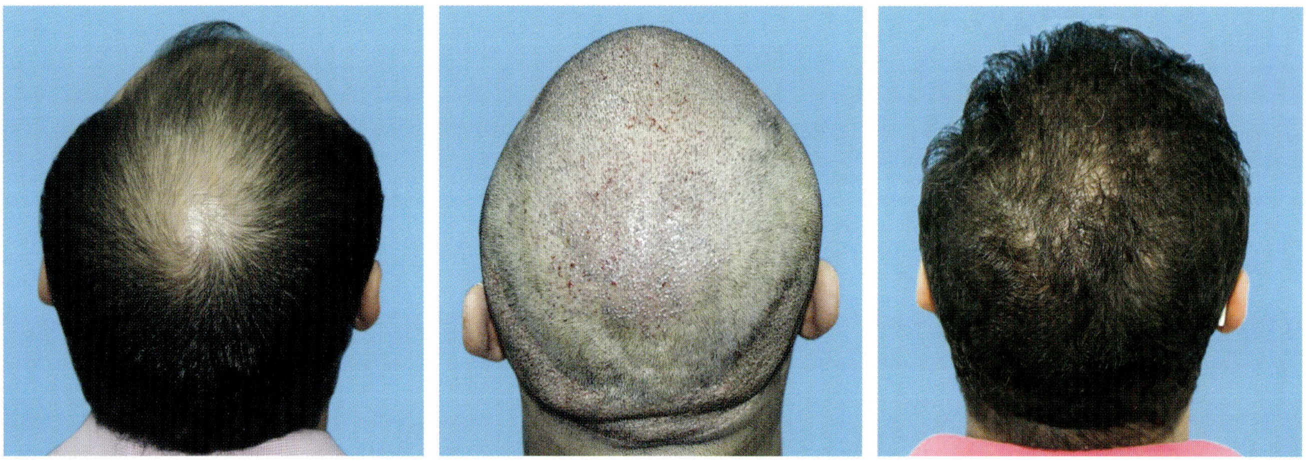

Before | Immediate postoperative | After 9 months

CASE 7

Surgery date	24-04-2017
Age	41 years
Donor area	Scalp and beard
Grafted area	Front, mid-scalp, and crown
Number of grafts planted	6,802
Single follicles	453

FRONT

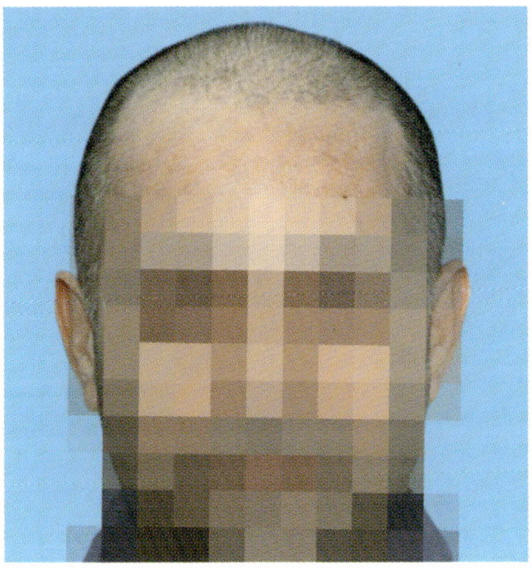
Before

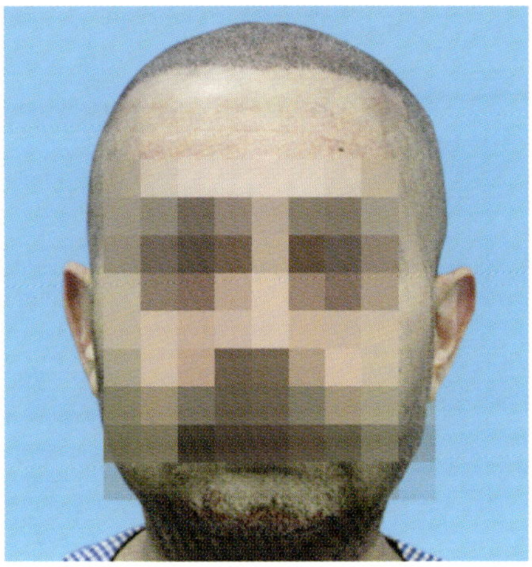
Immediate postoperative

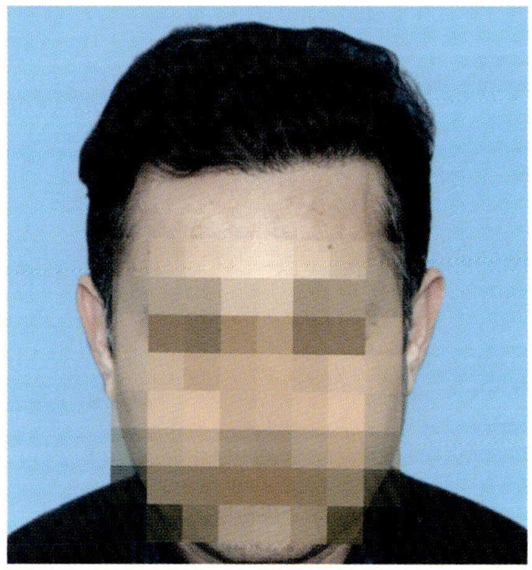
After 9 months

HEAD DOWN

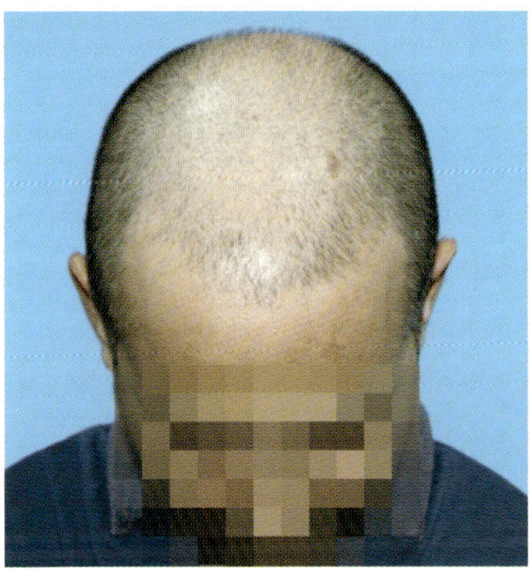
Before

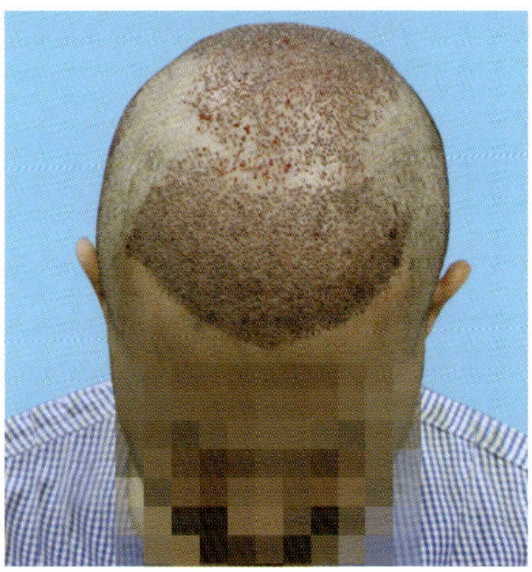
Immediate postoperative

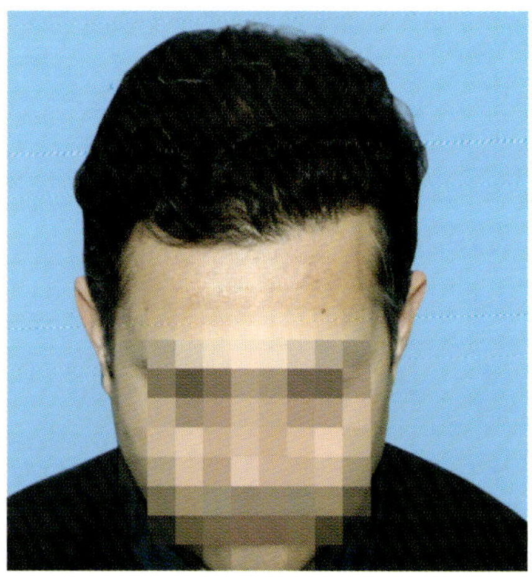
After 9 months

RIGHT LATERAL

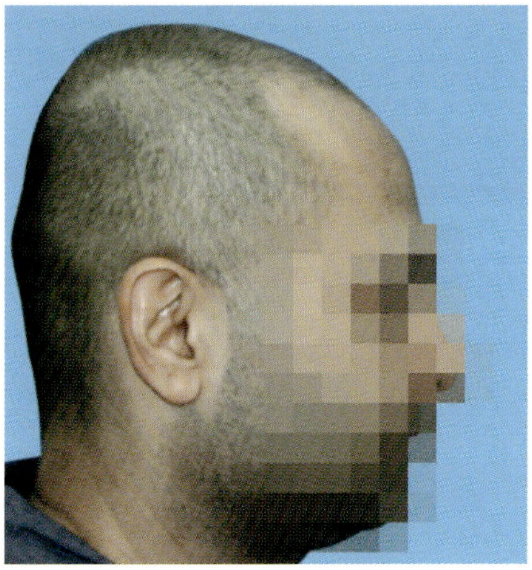

Before

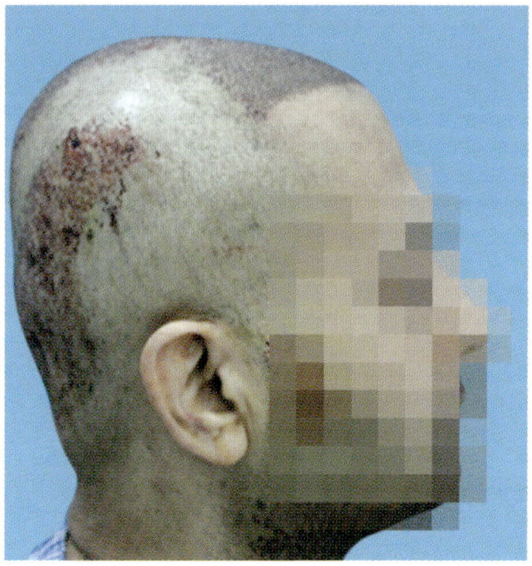

Immediate postoperative

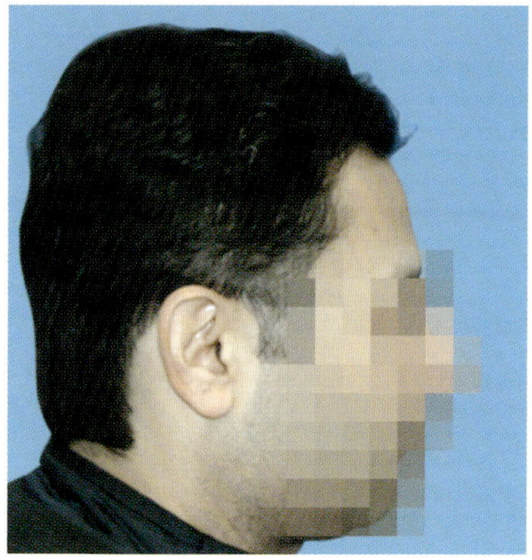

After 9 months

LEFT LATERAL

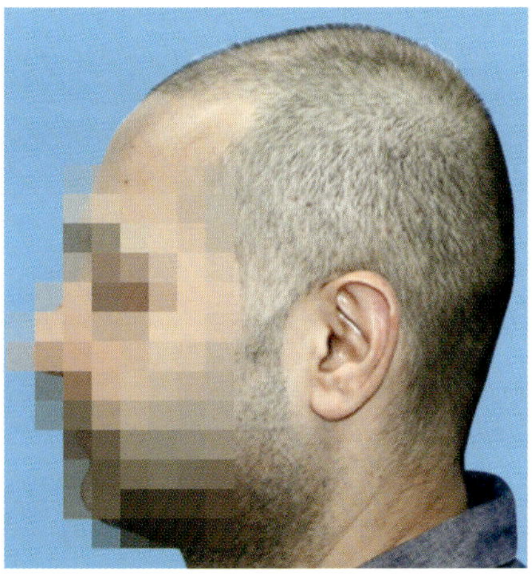

Before

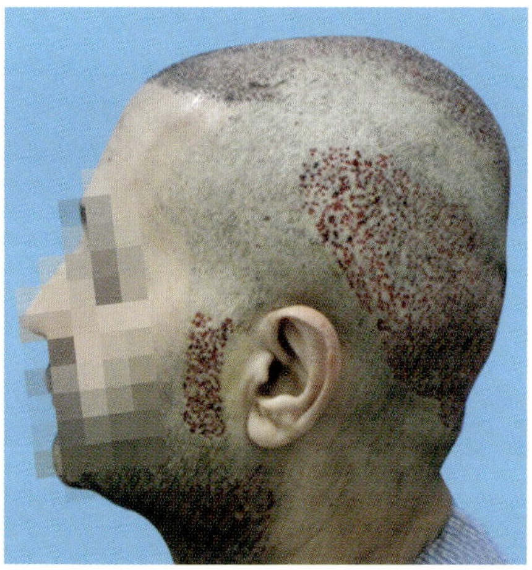

Immediate postoperative

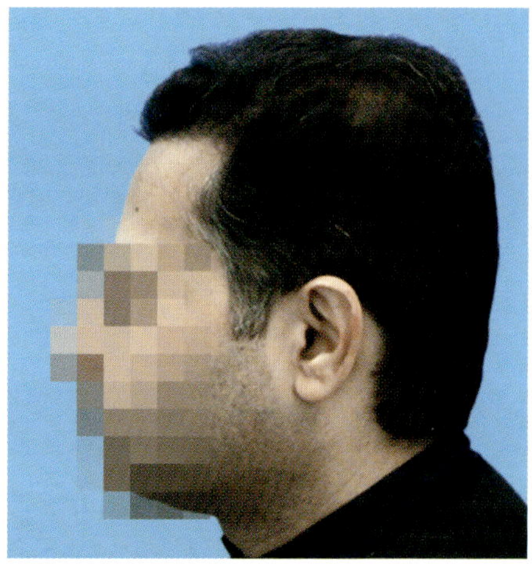

After 9 months

BACK

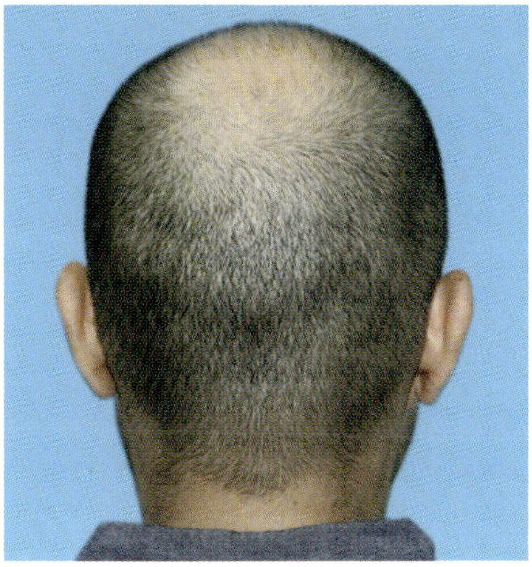

Before

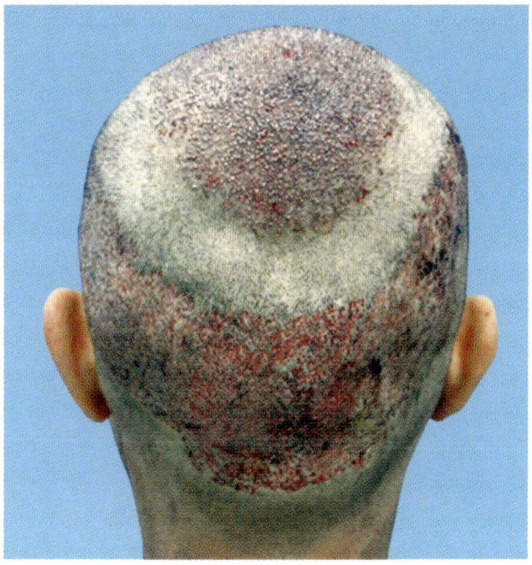

Immediate postoperative

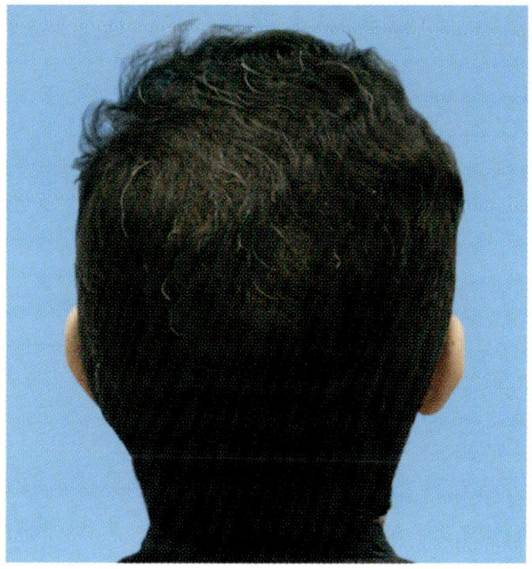

After 9 months

ROOF TOP VIEW

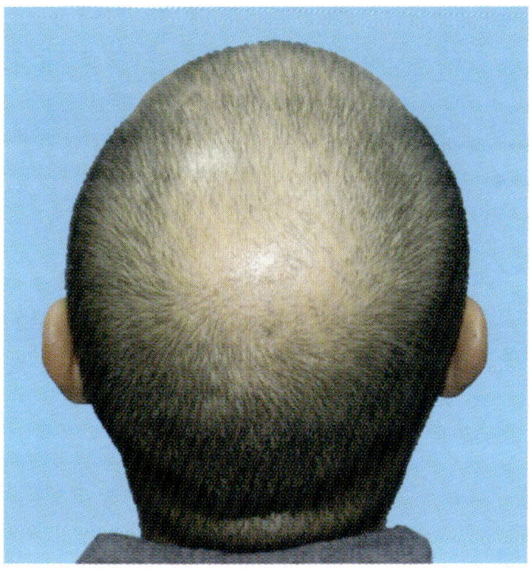

Before

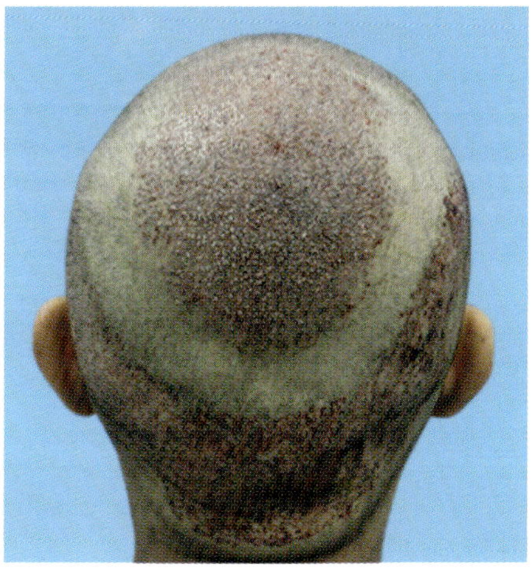

Immediate postoperative

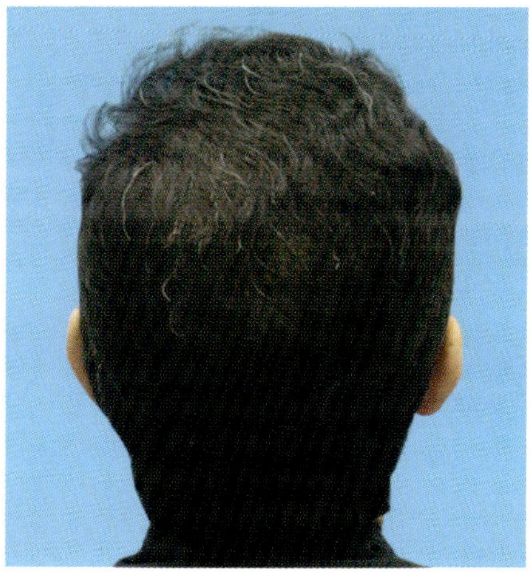

After 9 months

CASE 8

Surgery date	**24-12-2015**
Age	**38 years**
Donor area	**Scalp and beard**
Grafted area	**Front and mid-scalp, few on the crown (Focus: front and mid-scalp)**
Number of grafts planted	**6,518**
Single follicles	**626**

FRONT

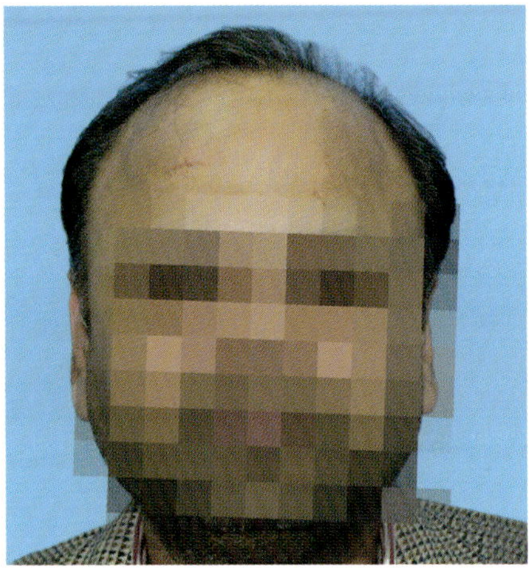

Before

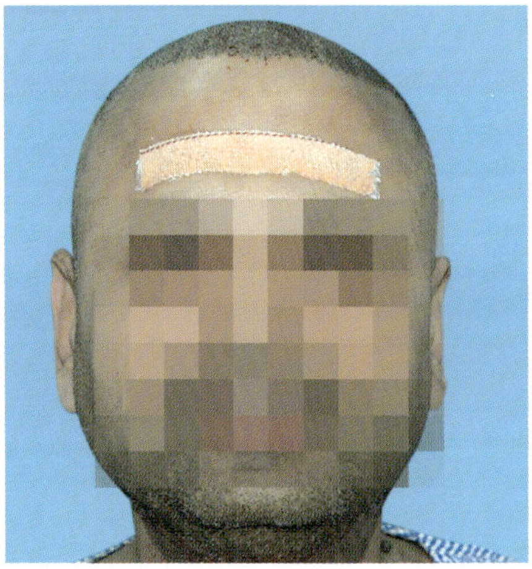

Immediate postoperative

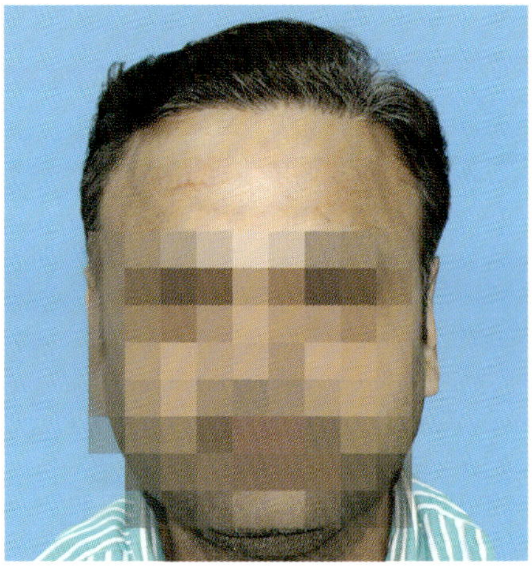

After 8 months

HEAD DOWN

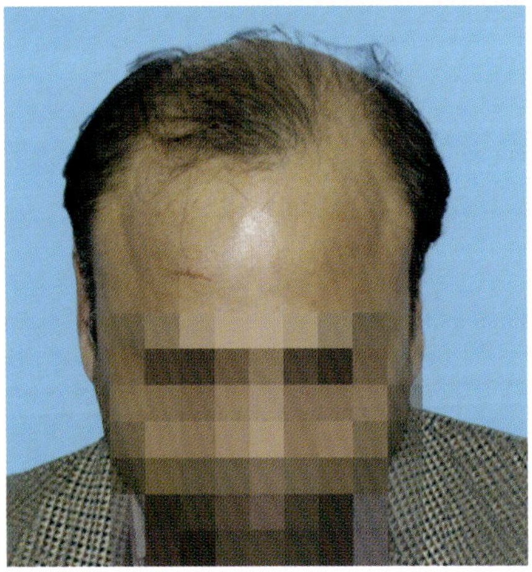

Before

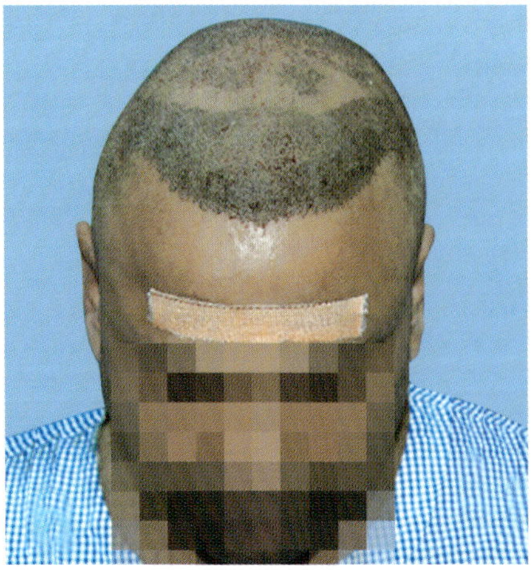

Immediate postoperative

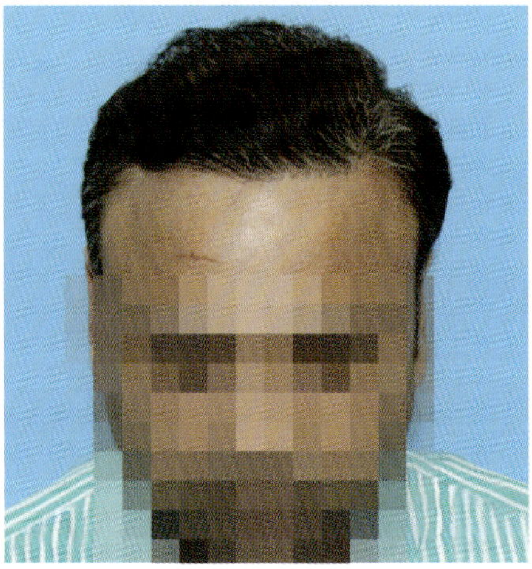

After 8 months

RIGHT LATERAL

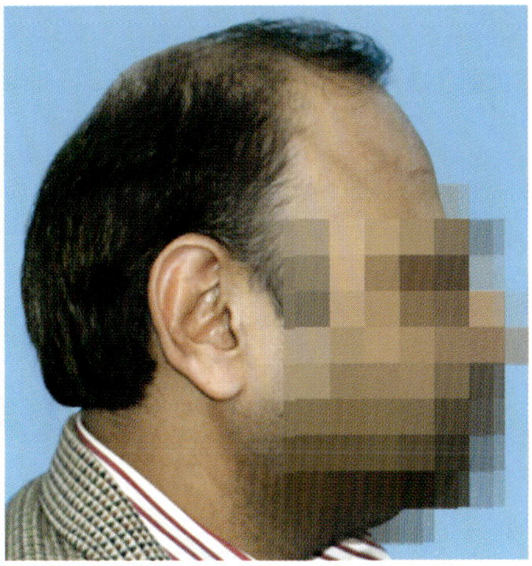

Before

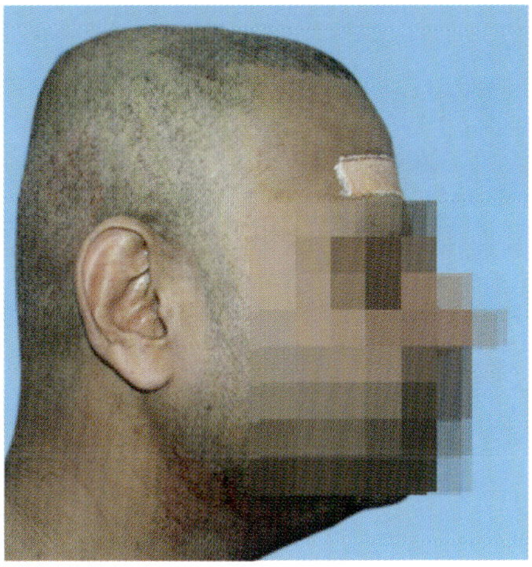

Immediate postoperative

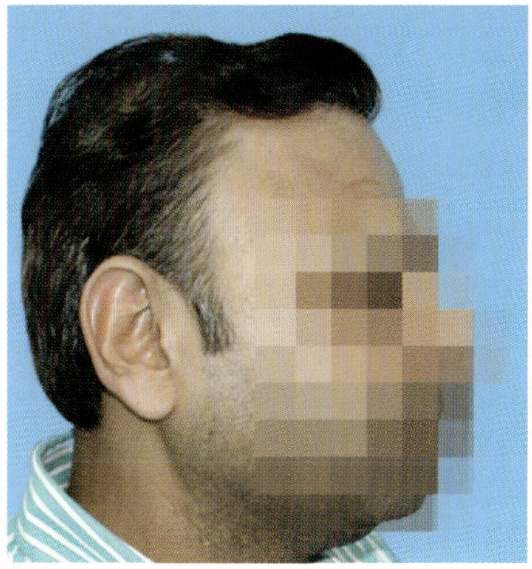

After 8 months

LEFT LATERAL

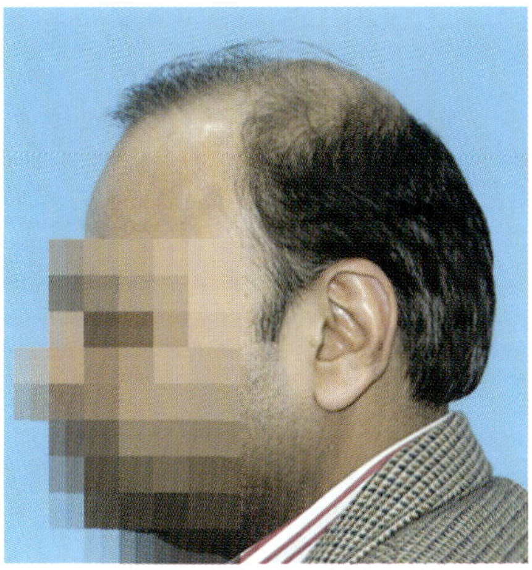

Before

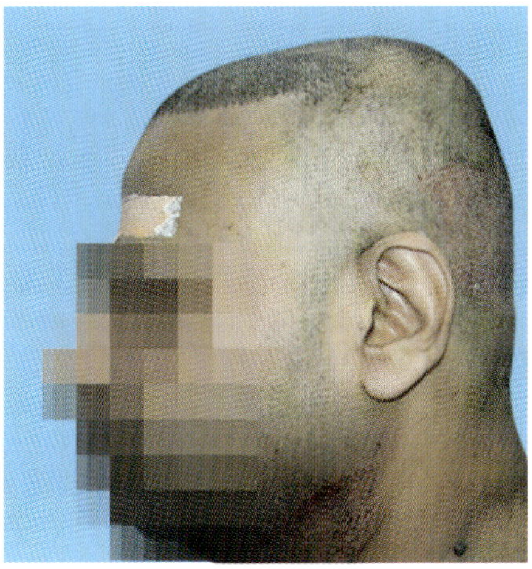

Immediate postoperative

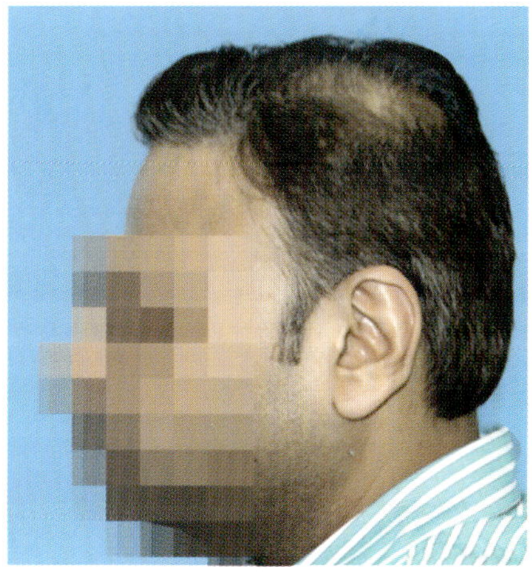

After 8 months

BACK

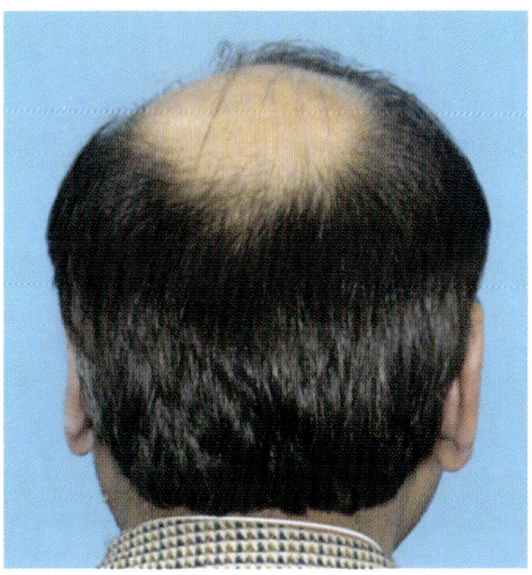

Before

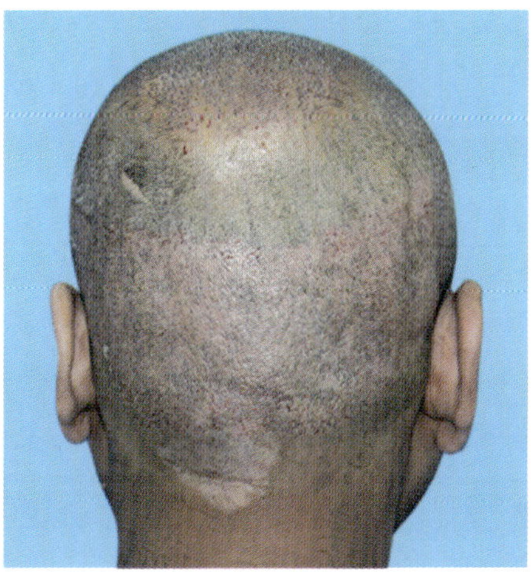

Immediate postoperative

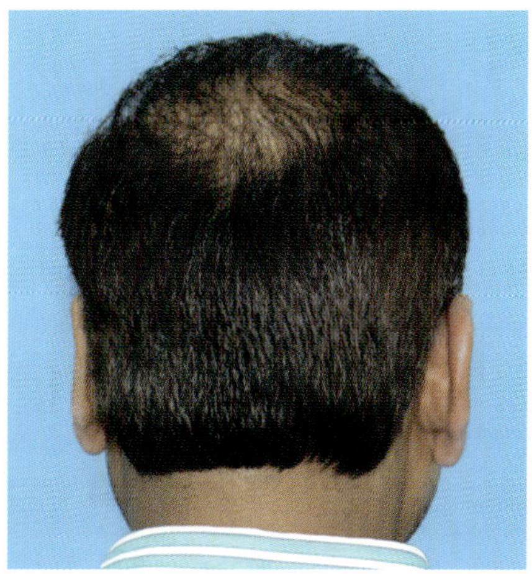

After 8 months

CASE 9

Surgery date	07-10-2016
Age	50 years
Donor area	Scalp and beard
Grafted area	Front, mid-scalp
Number of grafts planted	5,080
Single scalp follicles	431

FRONT

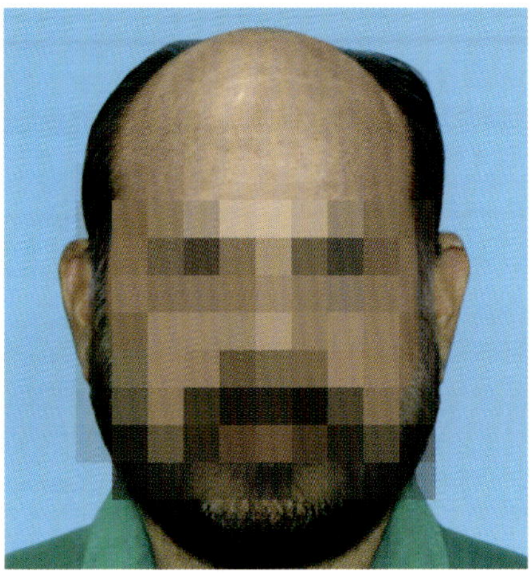

Before

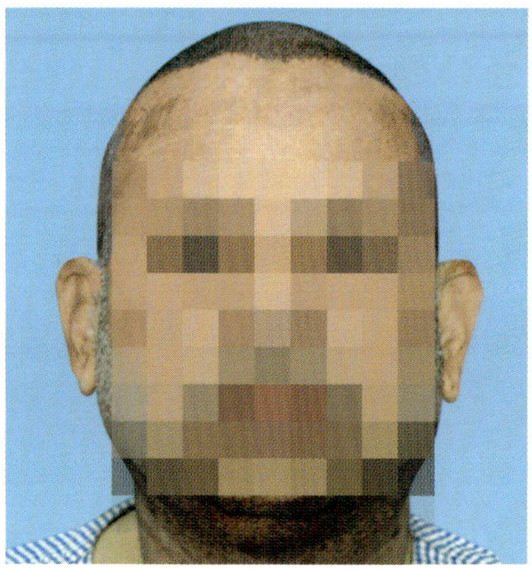

Immediate postoperative

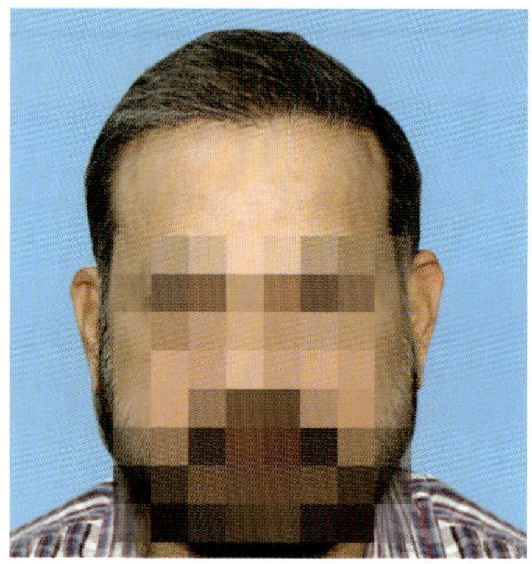

After 9 months

HEAD DOWN

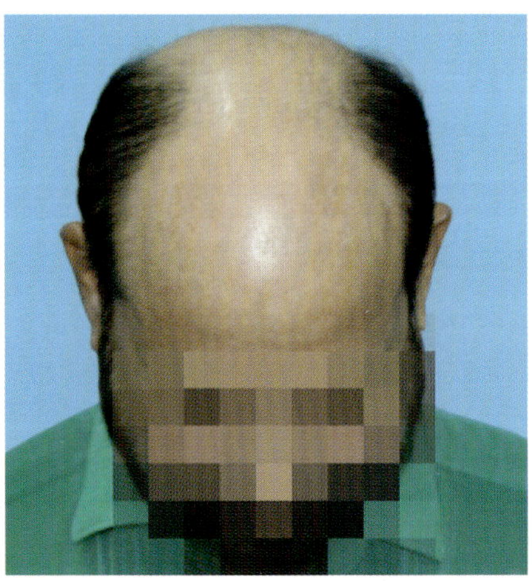

Before

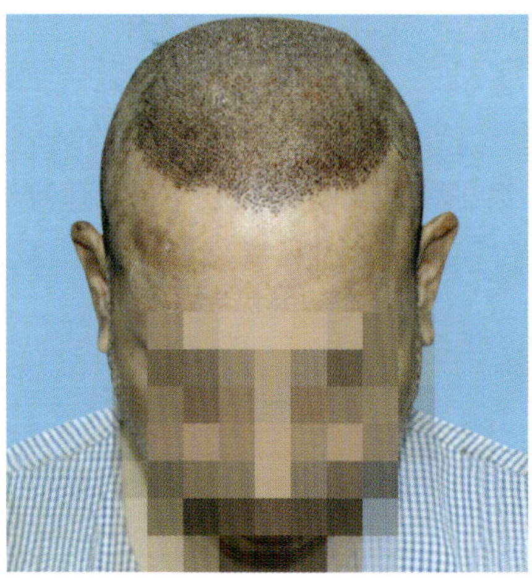

Immediate postoperative

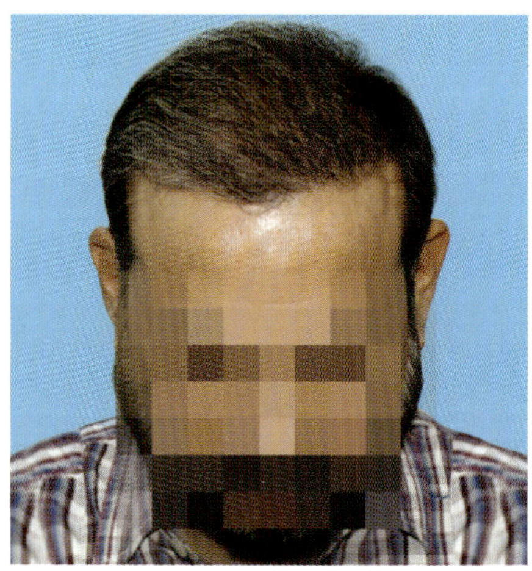

After 9 months

RIGHT LATERAL

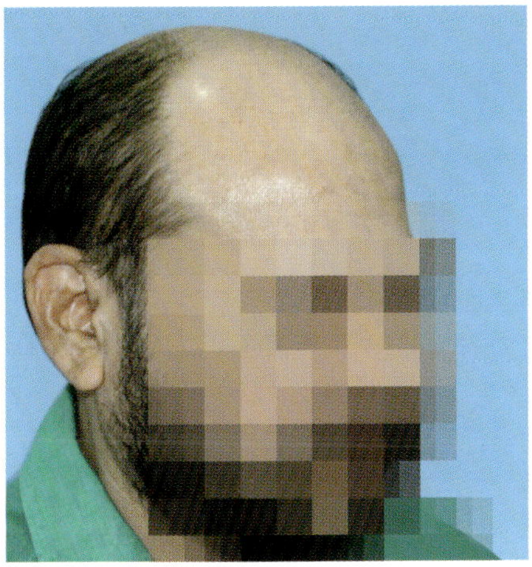

Before

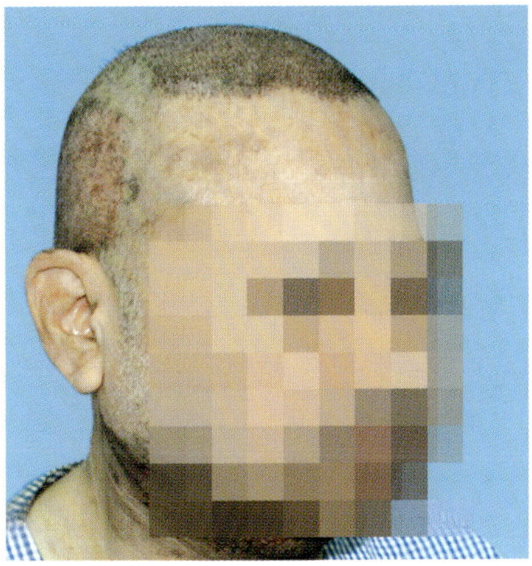

Immediate postoperative

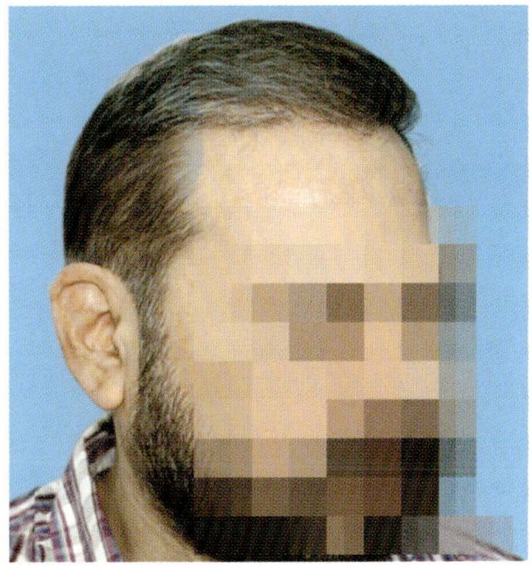

After 9 months

LEFT LATERAL

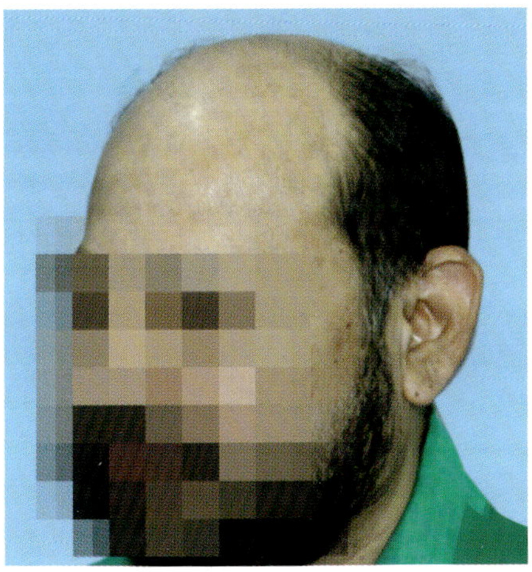

Before

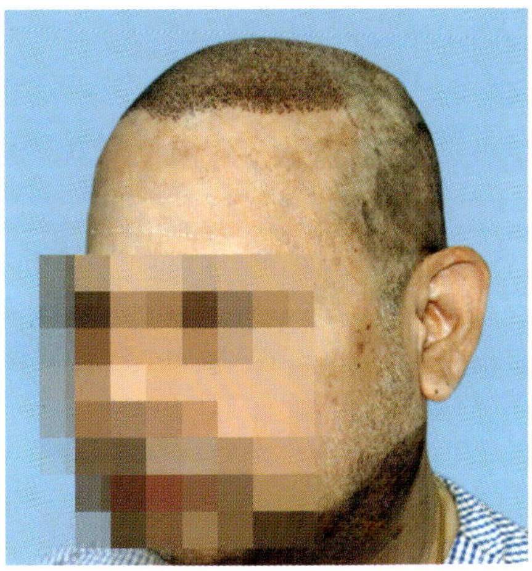

Immediate postoperative

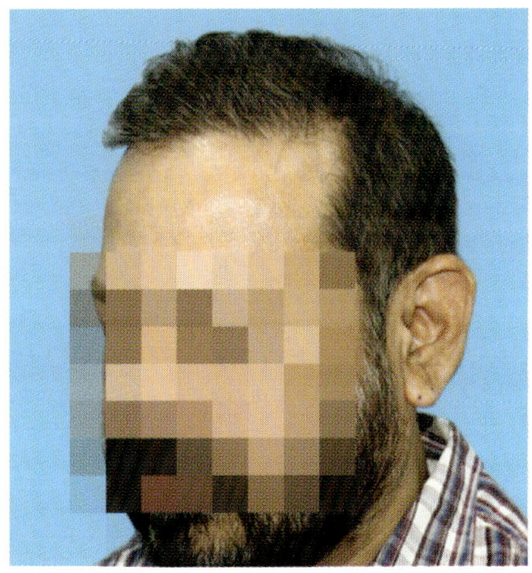

After 9 months

BACK

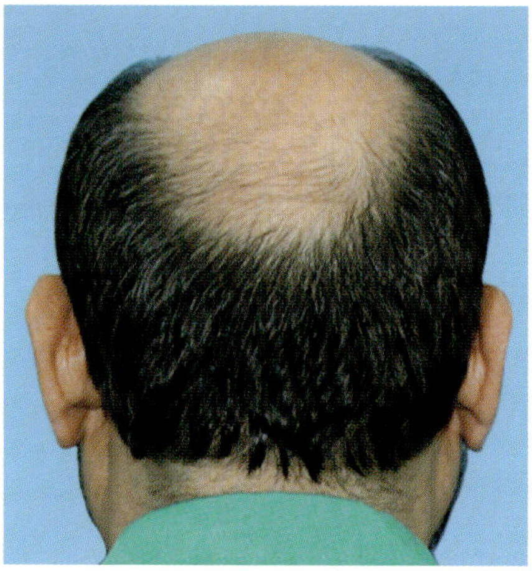

Before

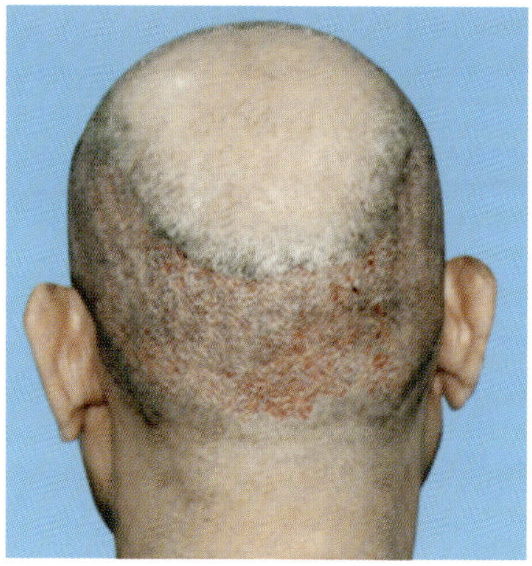

Immediate postoperative

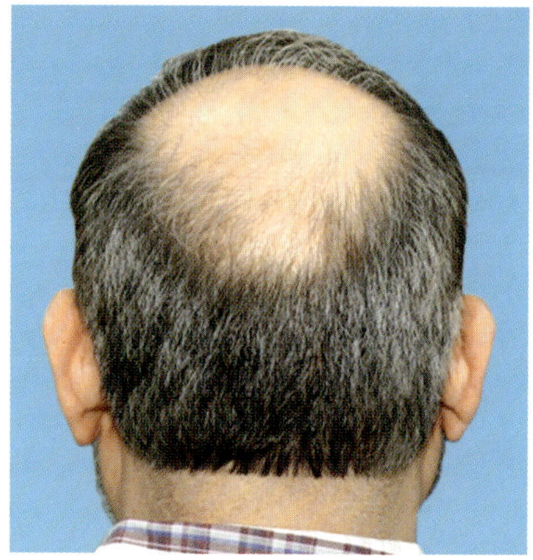

After 9 months

ROOF TOP VIEW

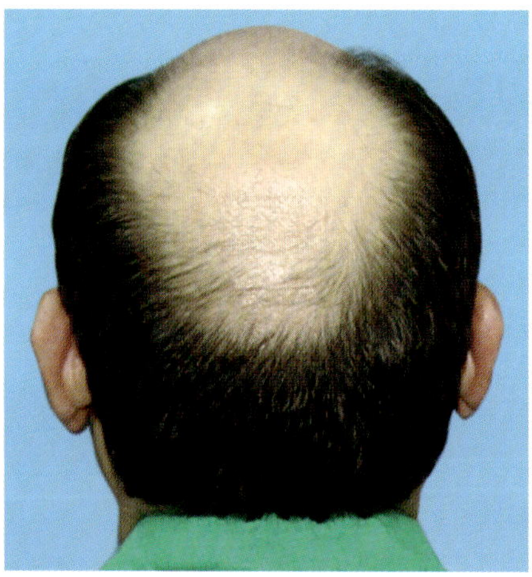

Before

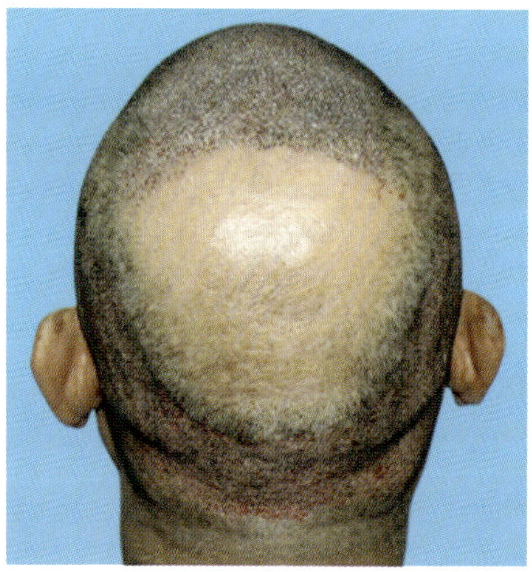

Immediate postoperative

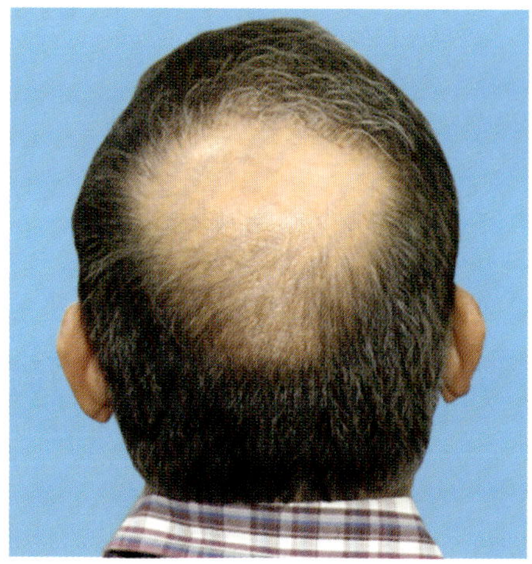

After 9 months

CASE 10

Surgery date	03-10-2016
Age	30 years
Donor area	Scalp and beard
Grafted area	Front and temple
Number of grafts planted	7,302
Single follicles	432

FRONT

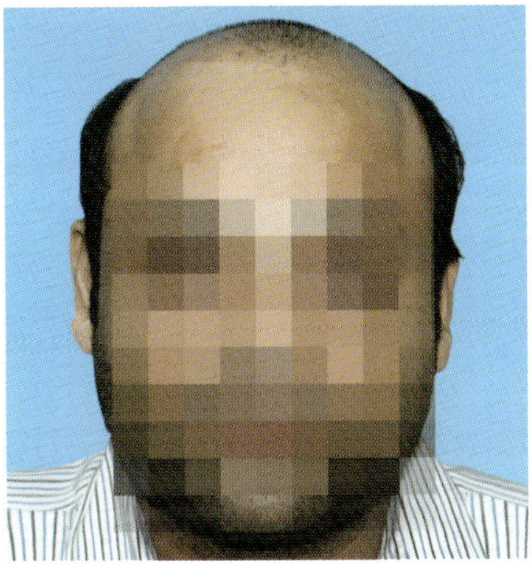
Before

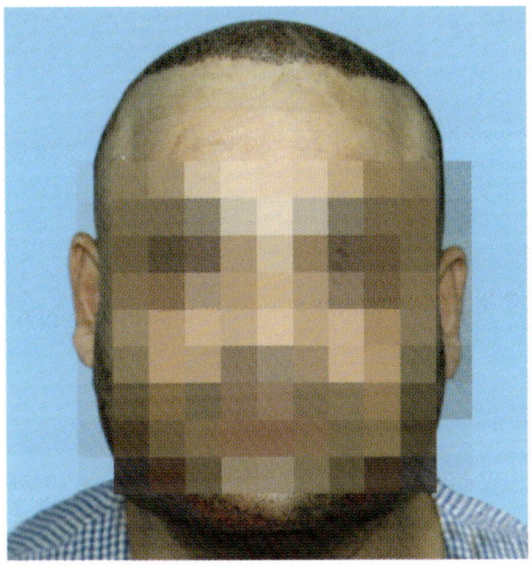
Immediate postoperative

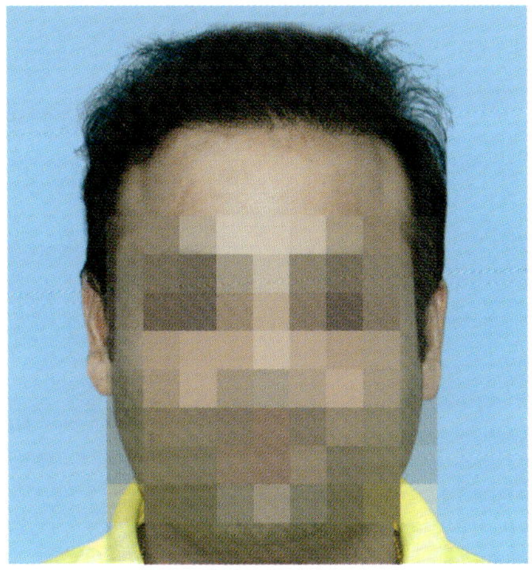
After 9 months

HEAD DOWN

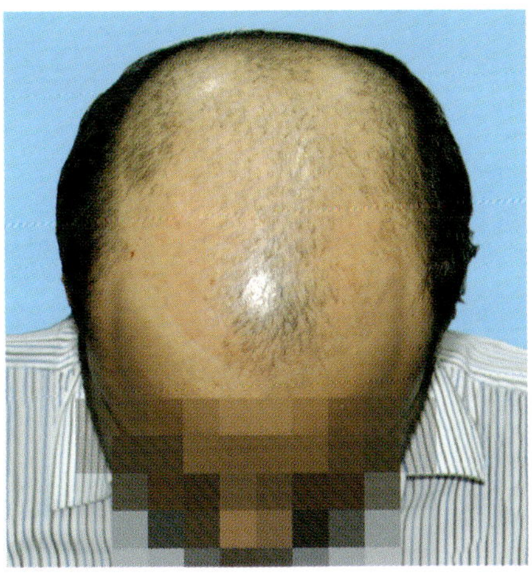
Before

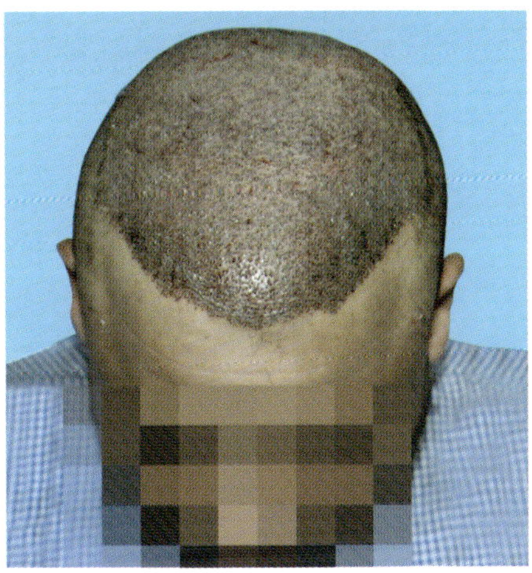
Immediate postoperative

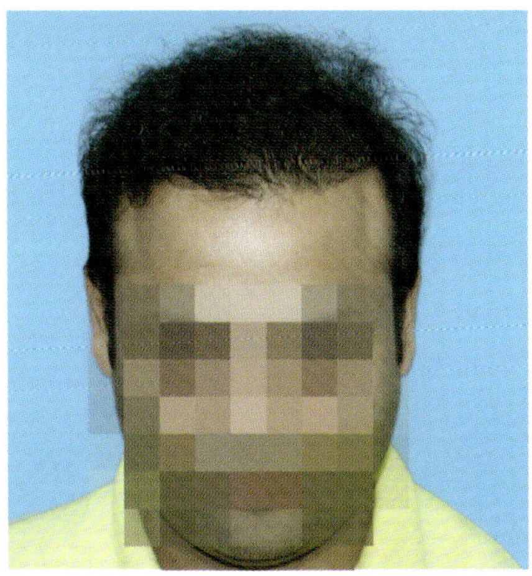
After 9 months

RIGHT LATERAL

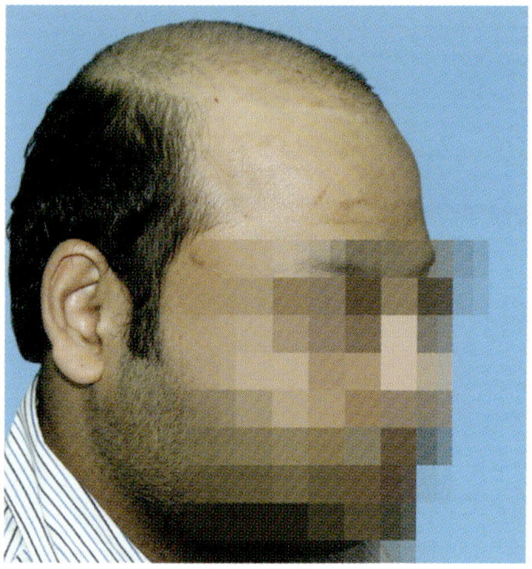
Before

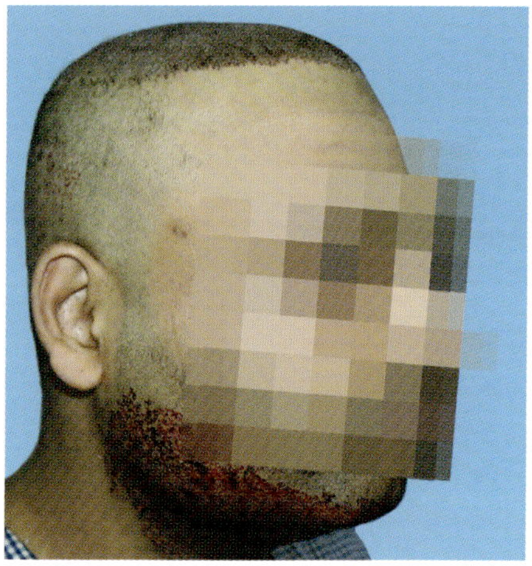
Immediate postoperative

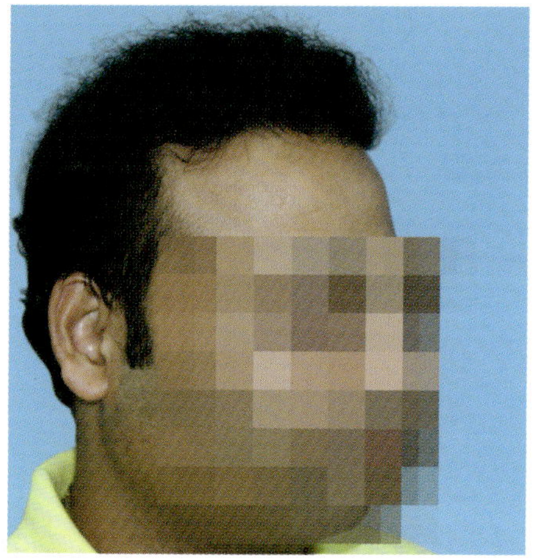
After 9 months

LEFT LATERAL

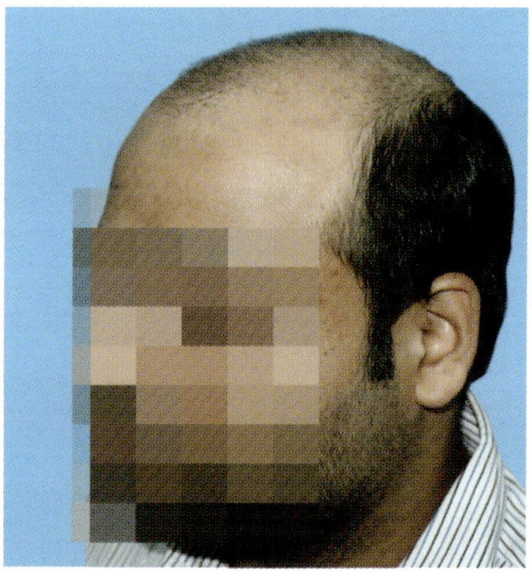
Before

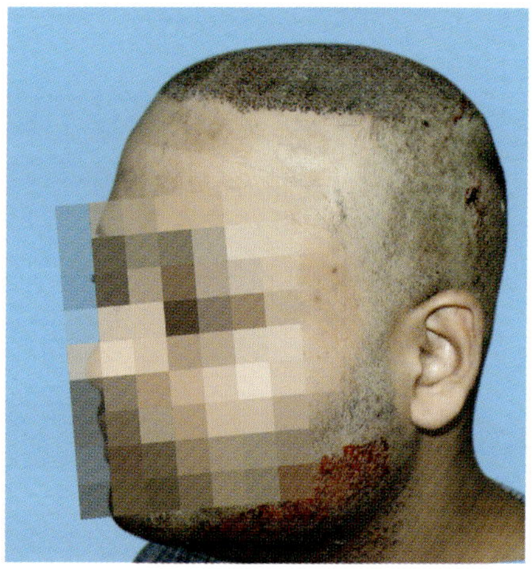
Immediate postoperative

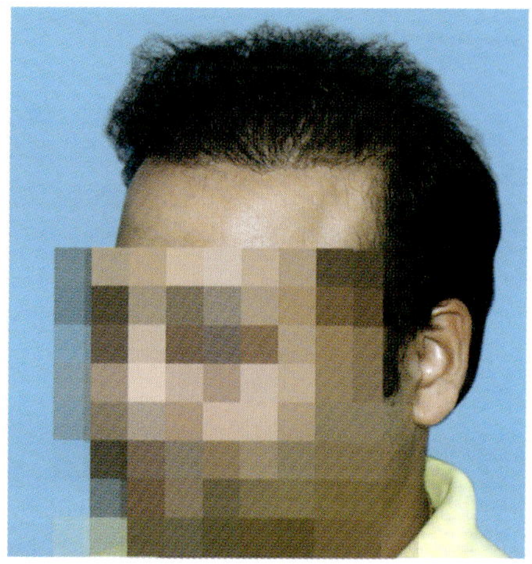
After 9 months

BACK

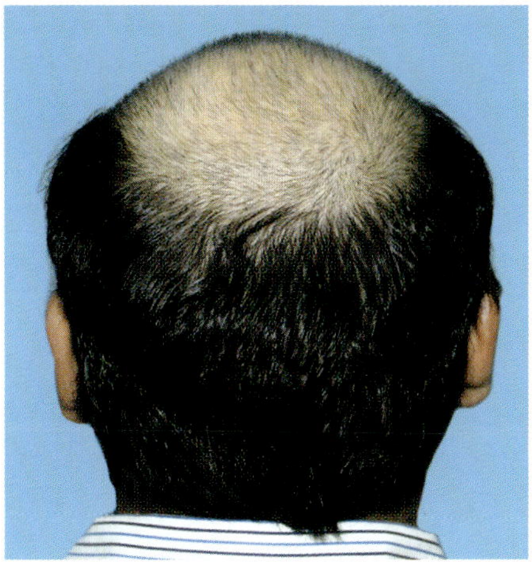

Before

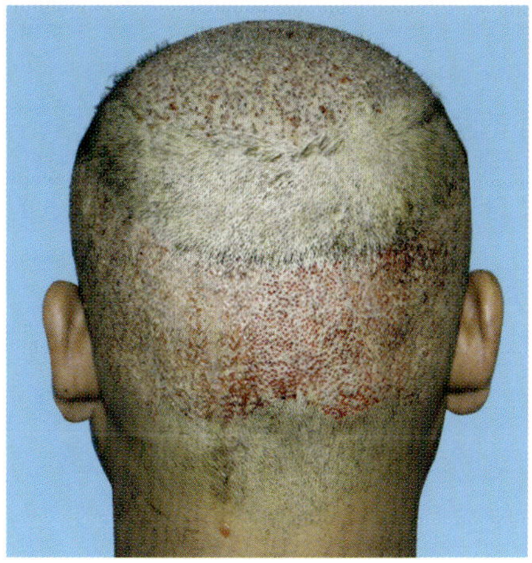

Immediate postoperative

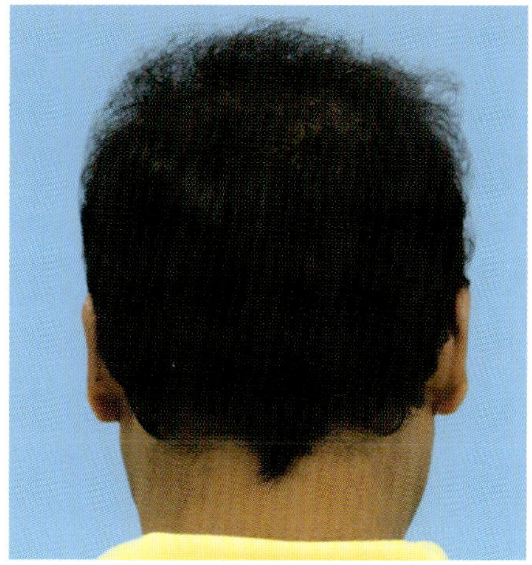

After 9 months

ROOF TOP VIEW

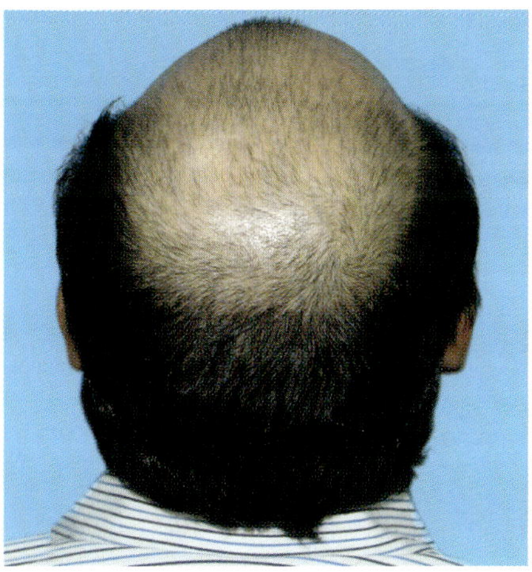

Before

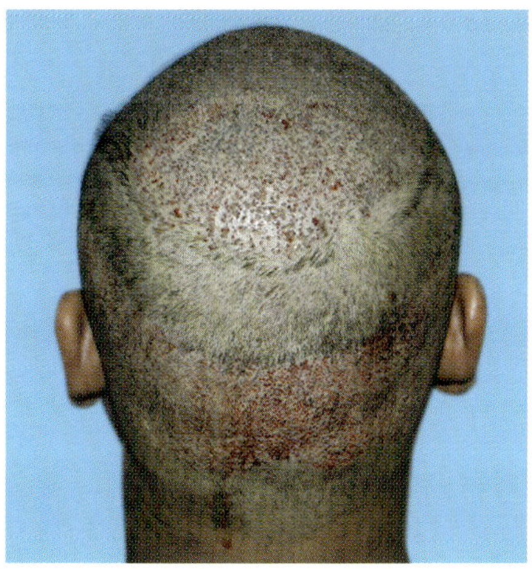

Immediate postoperative

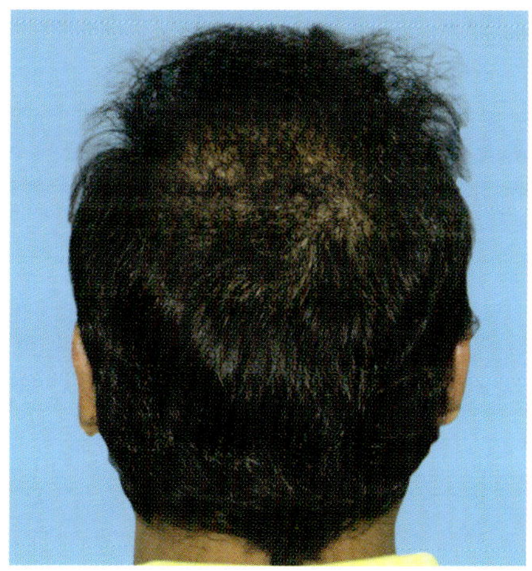

After 9 months

CASE 11

Surgery date	29-09-2017
Age	60 years
Donor area	Scalp
Grafted area	Front and mid-scalp
Number of grafts planted	3,491
Single follicles	430

FRONT

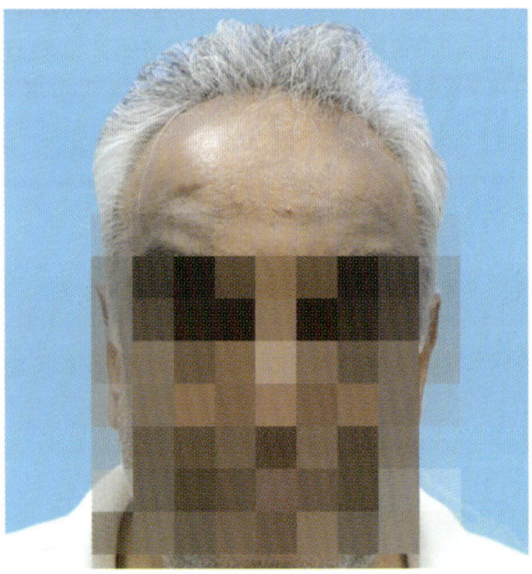

Before

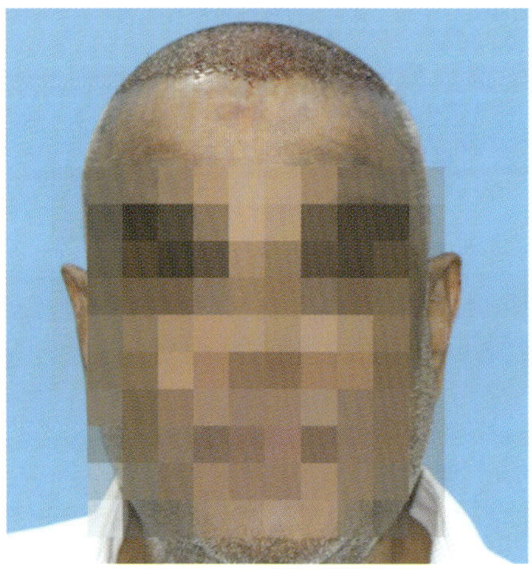

Immediate postoperative

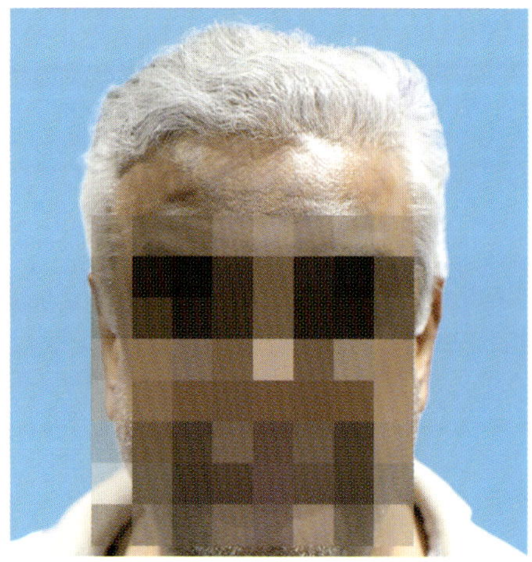

After 7 months

HEAD DOWN

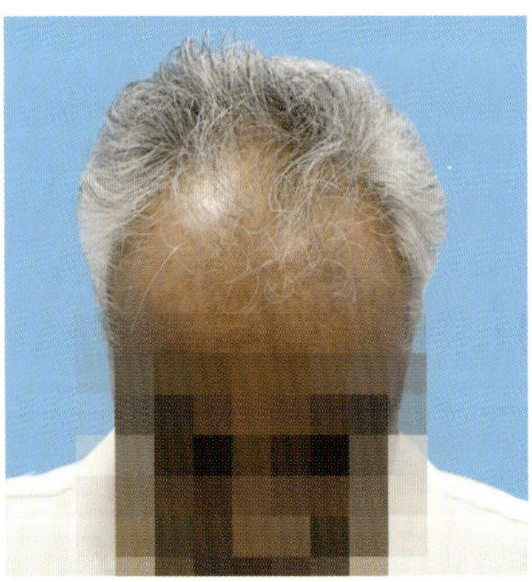

Before

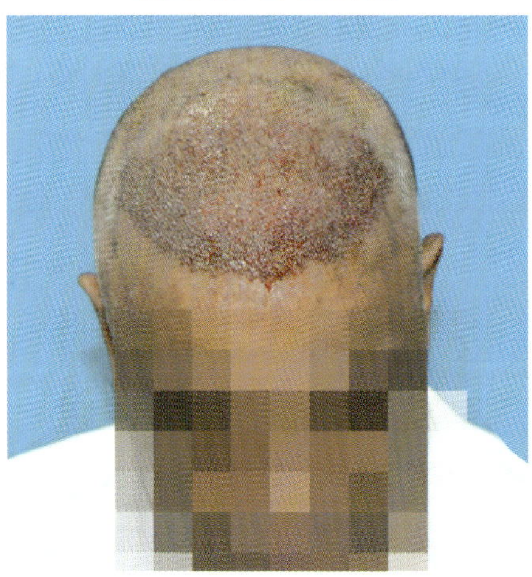

Immediate postoperative

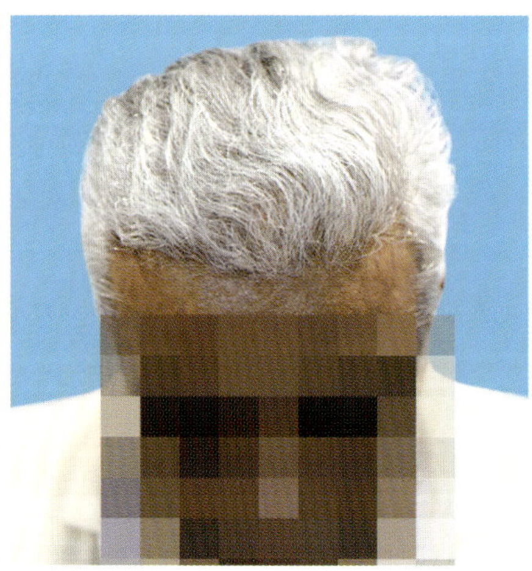

After 7 months

RIGHT LATERAL

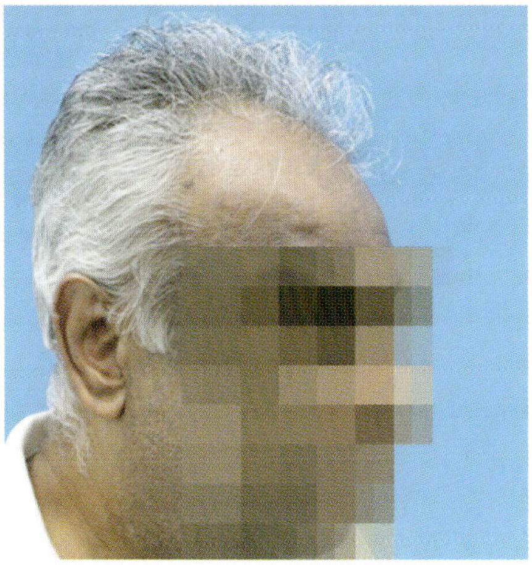

Before

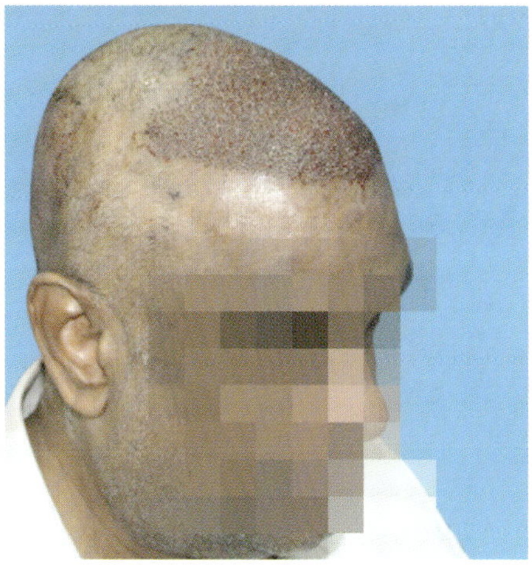

Immediate postoperative

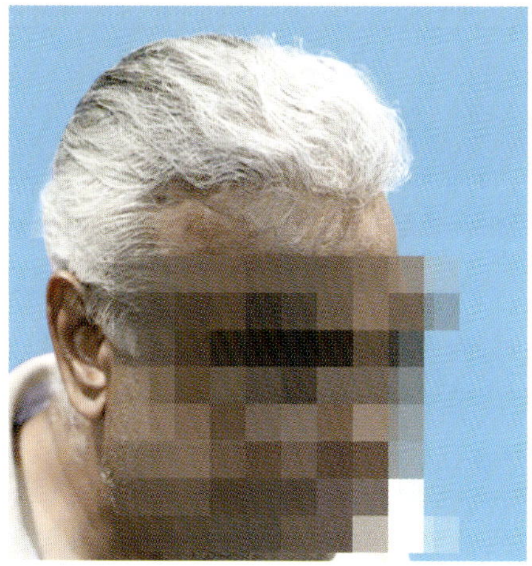

After 7 months

LEFT LATERAL

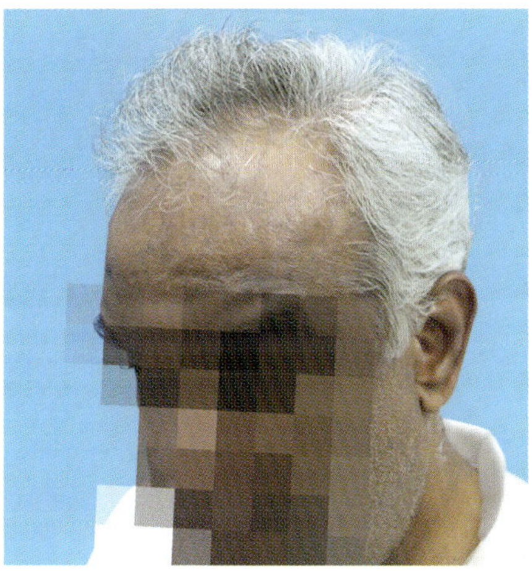

Before

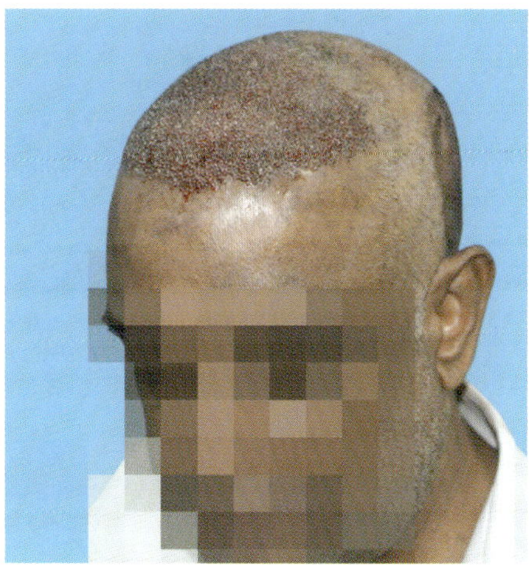

Immediate postoperative

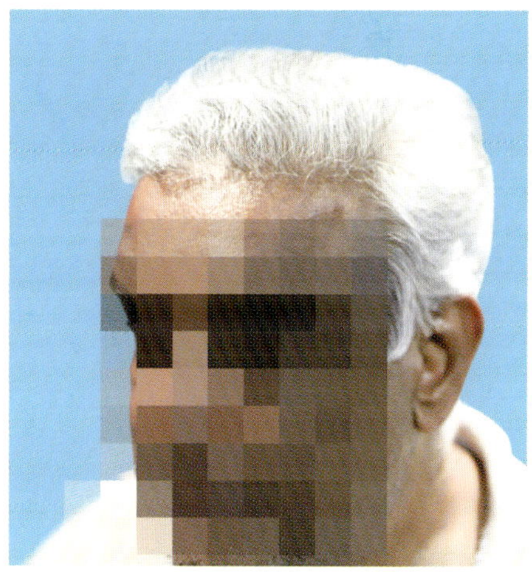

After 7 months

BACK

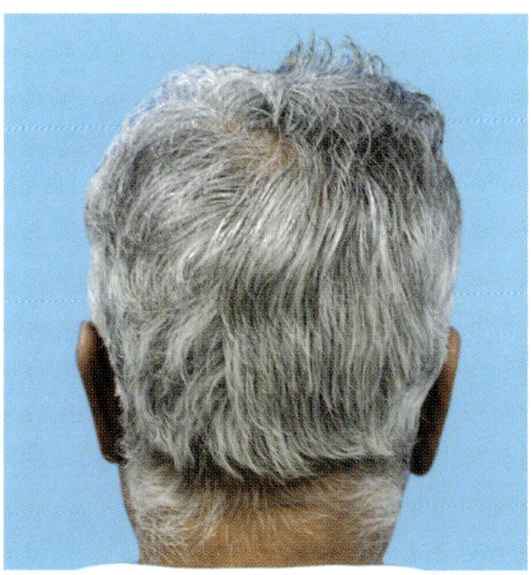

Before

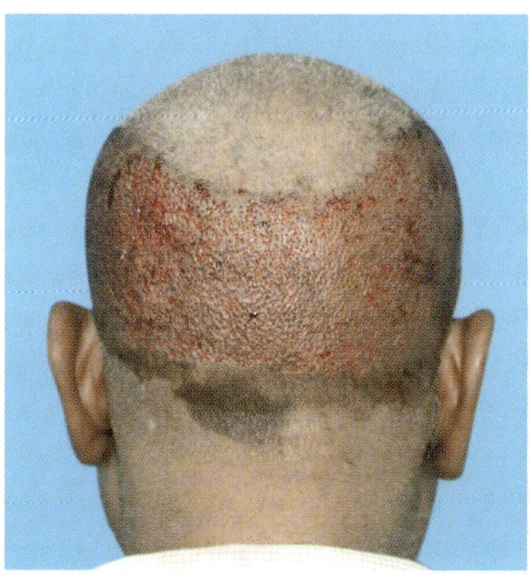

Immediate postoperative

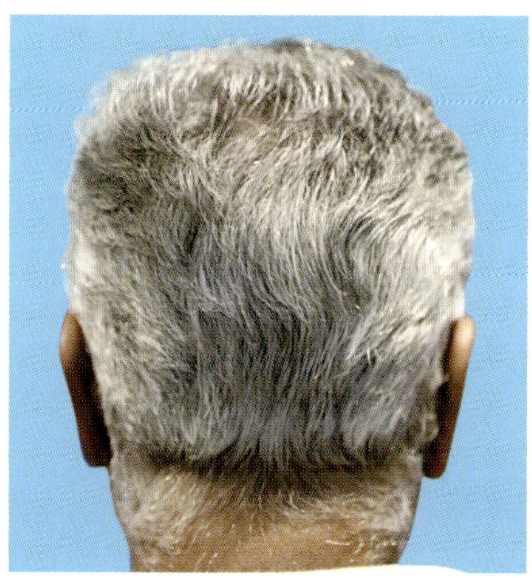

After 7 months

CASE 12

Surgery date	**04-02-2016**
Age	**31 years**
Donor area	**Scalp and beard**
Grafted area	**Front and mid-scalp**
Number of grafts planted	**5,500**
Single follicles	**418**

FRONT

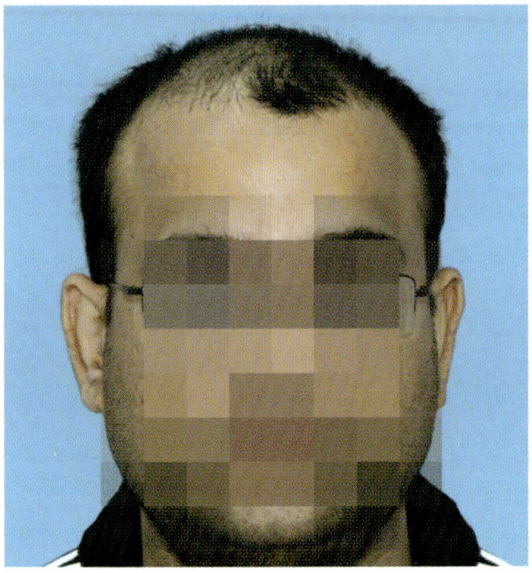
Before

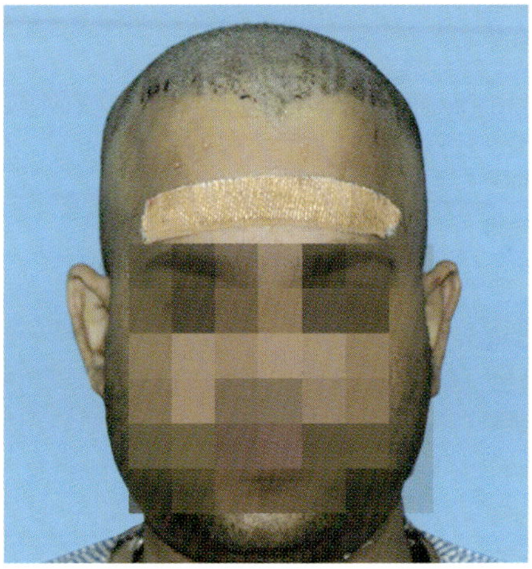
Immediate postoperative

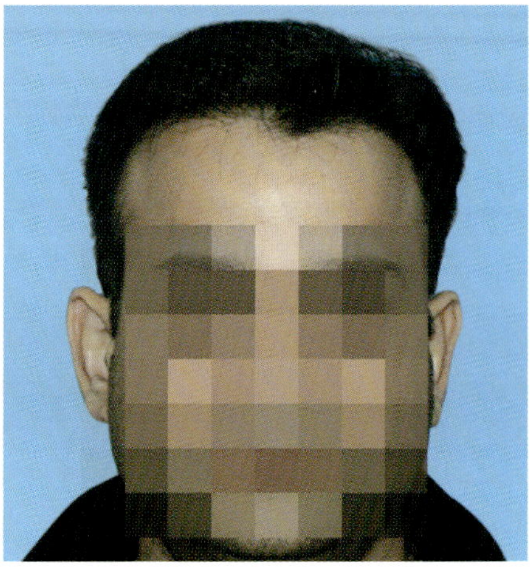
After 6 months

HEAD DOWN

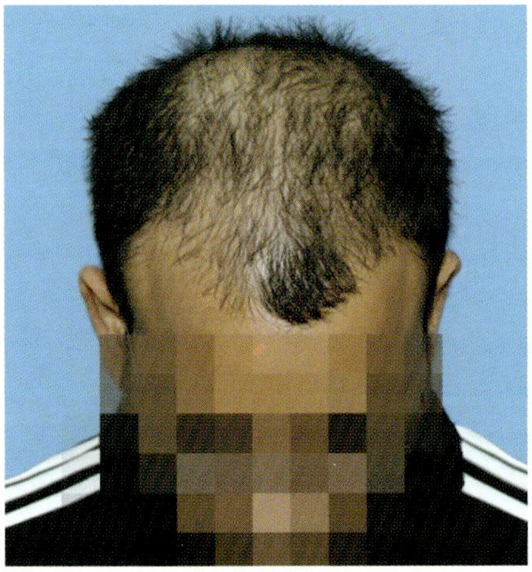
Before

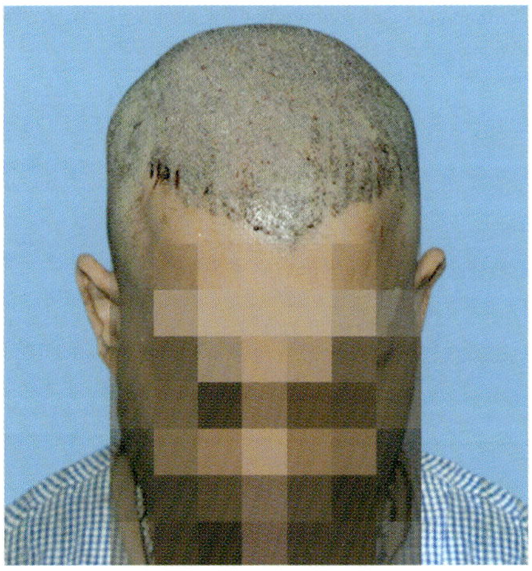
Immediate postoperative

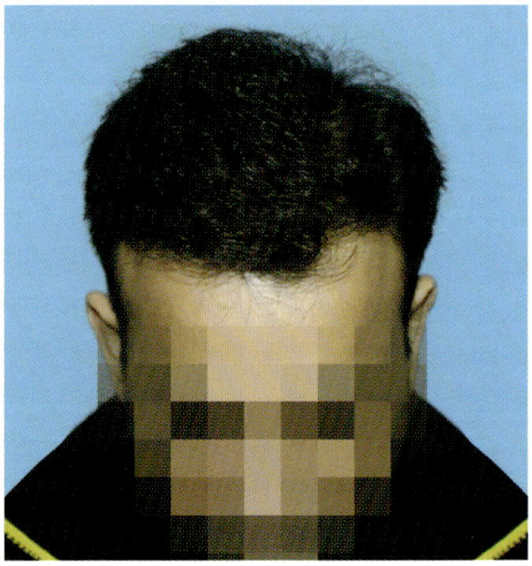
After 6 months

RIGHT LATERAL

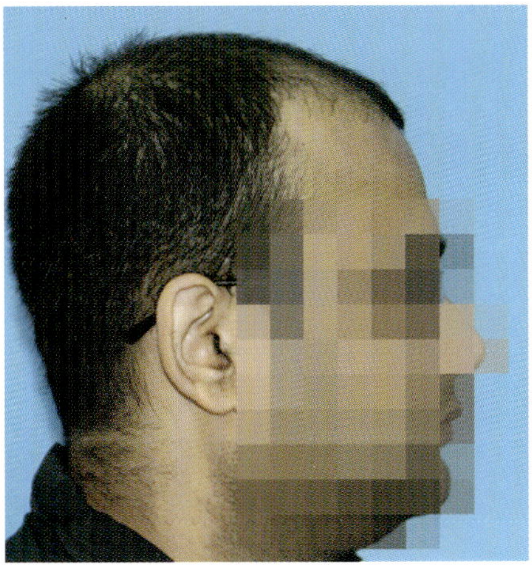

Before

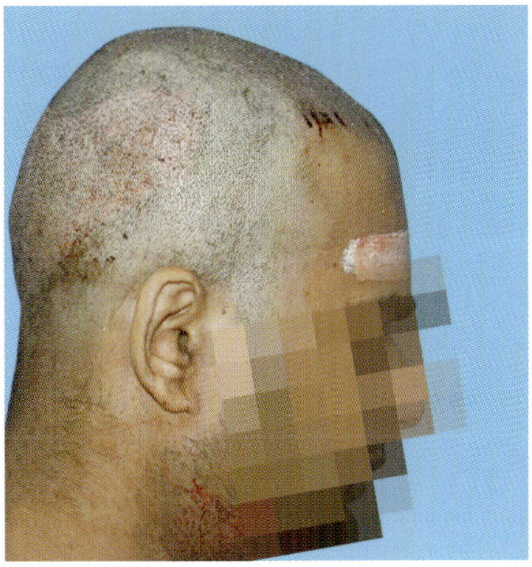

Immediate postoperative

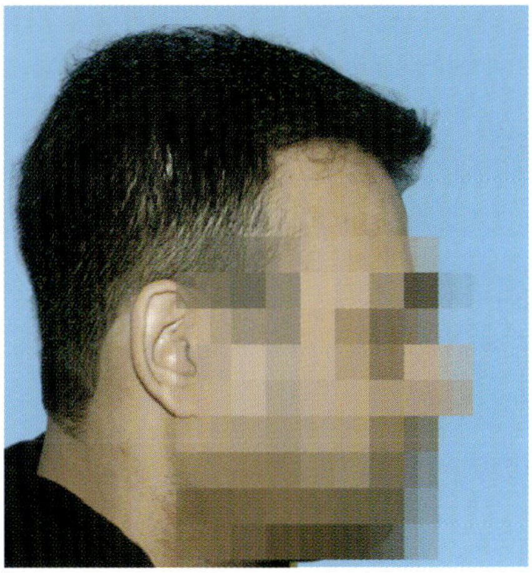

After 6 months

LEFT LATERAL

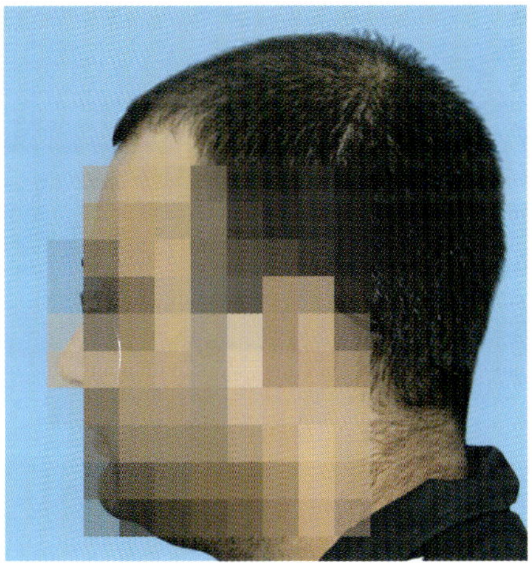

Before

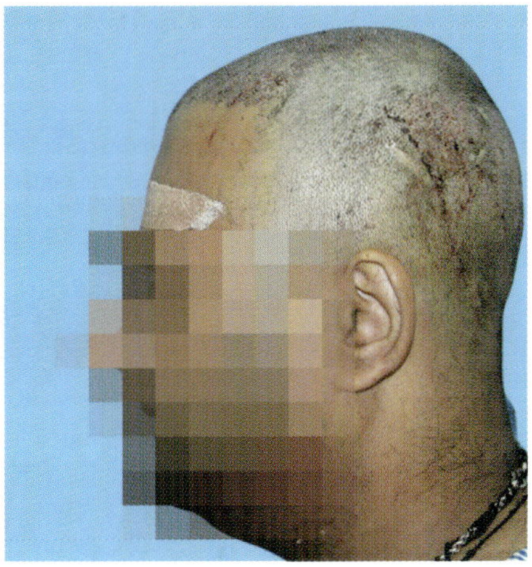

Immediate postoperative

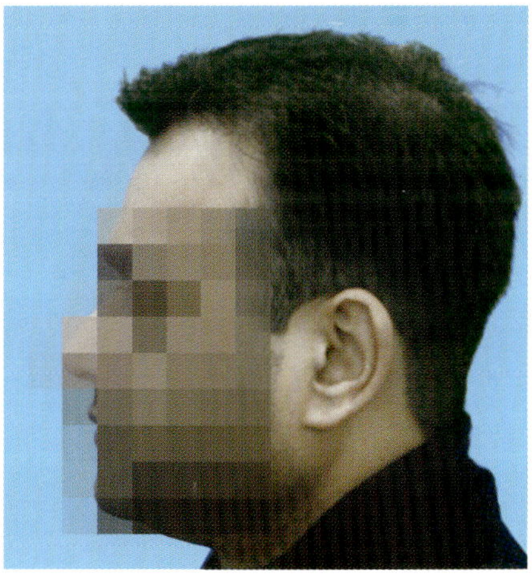

After 6 months

BACK

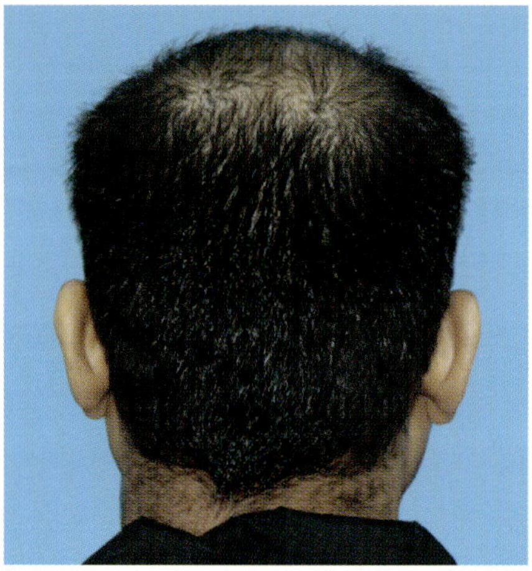

Before

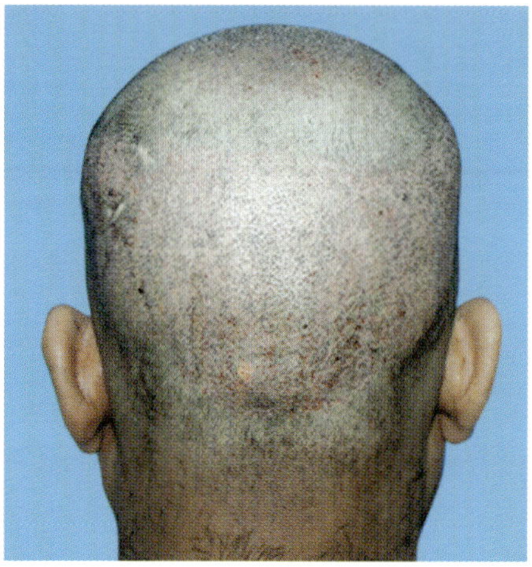

Immediate postoperative

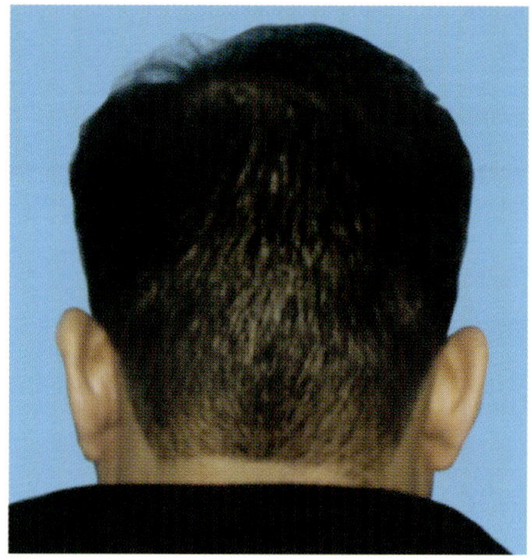

After 6 months

ROOF TOP VIEW

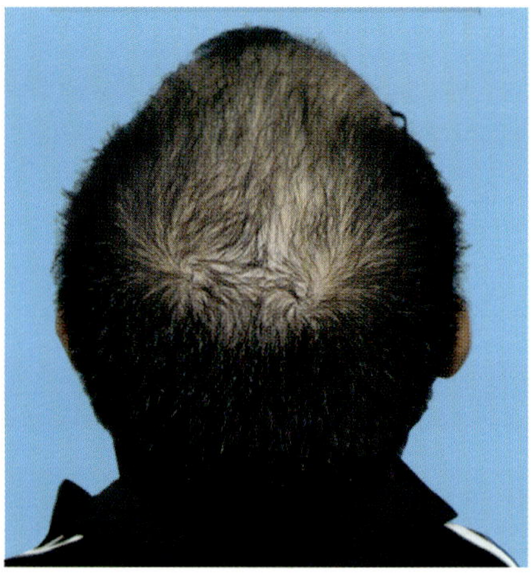

Before

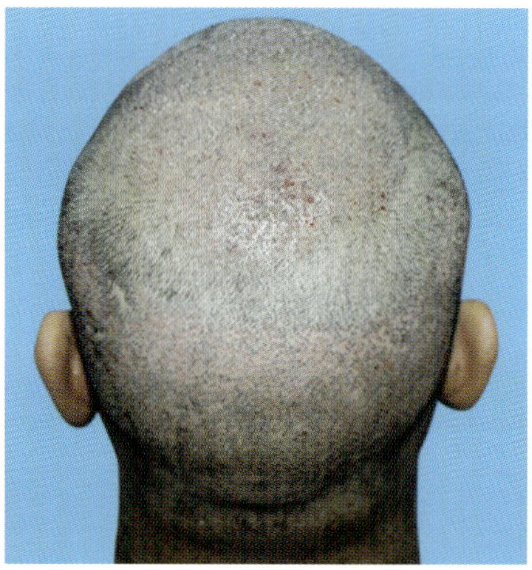

Immediate postoperative

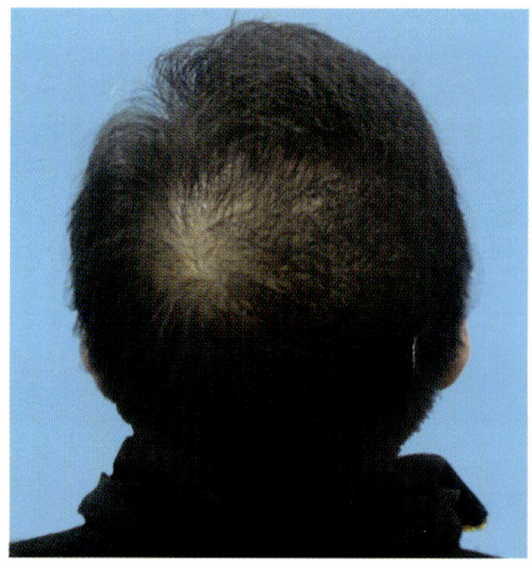

After 6 months

CASE 13

Age	**33 years**
Donor area	**Scalp**
Grafted area	**Front and temple**
Number of grafts planted	**1418**

FRONT

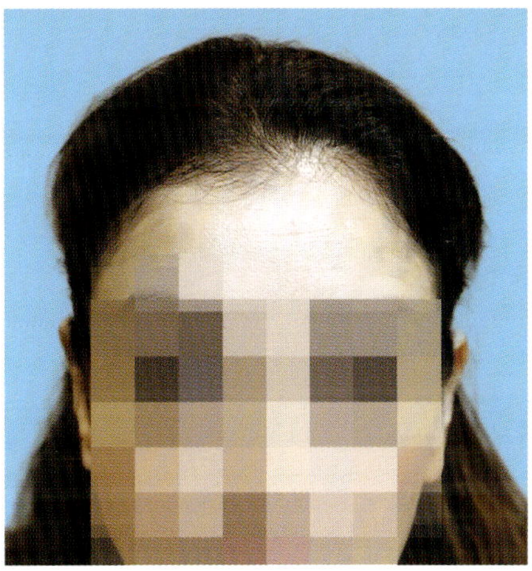

Before

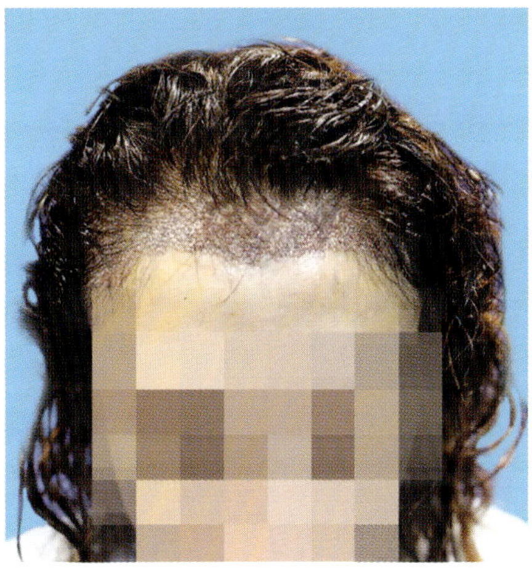

Immediate postoperative

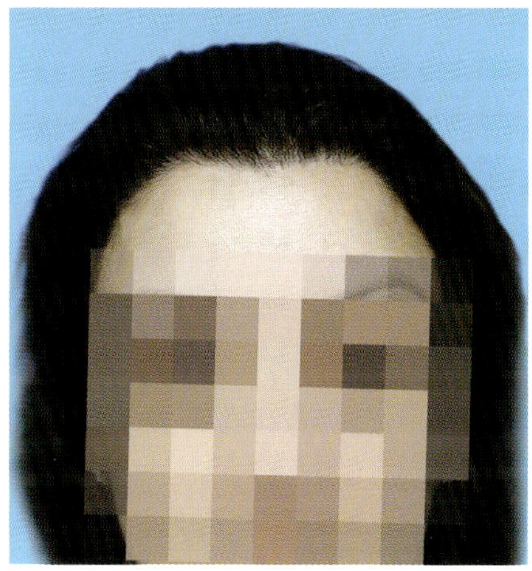

After 6 months

HEAD DOWN

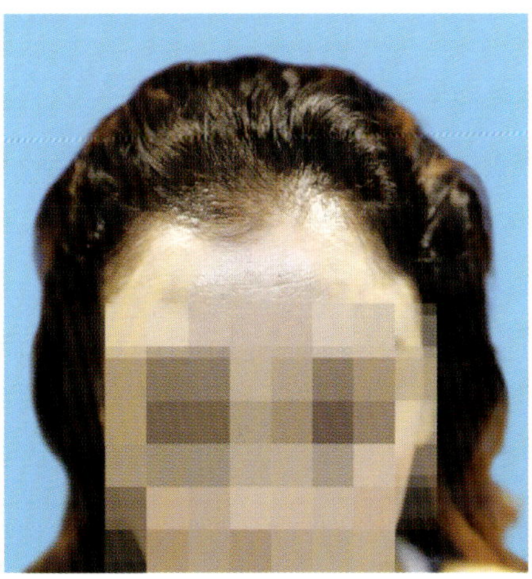

Before

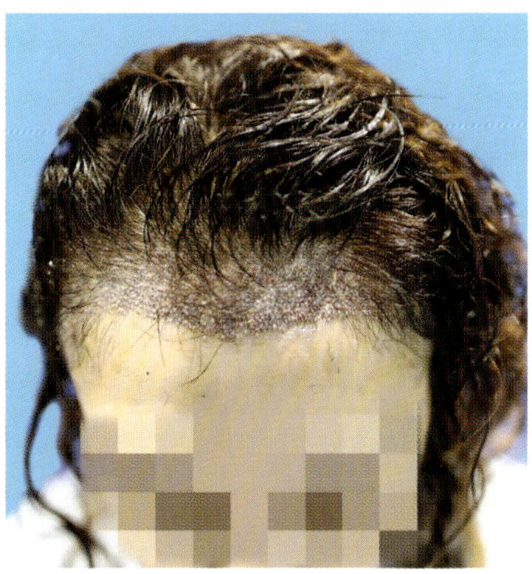

Immediate postoperative

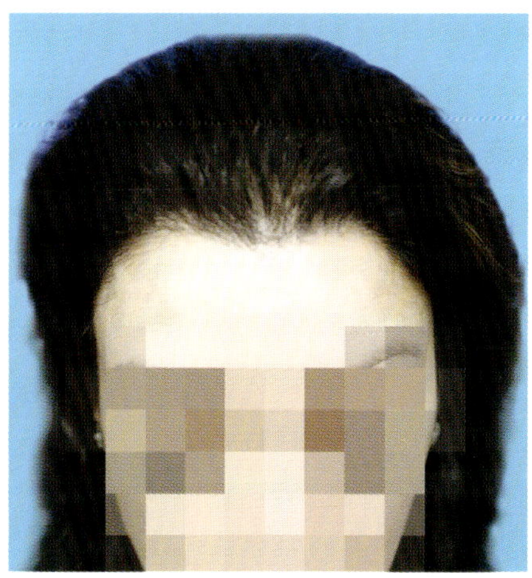

After 6 months

RIGHT LATERAL

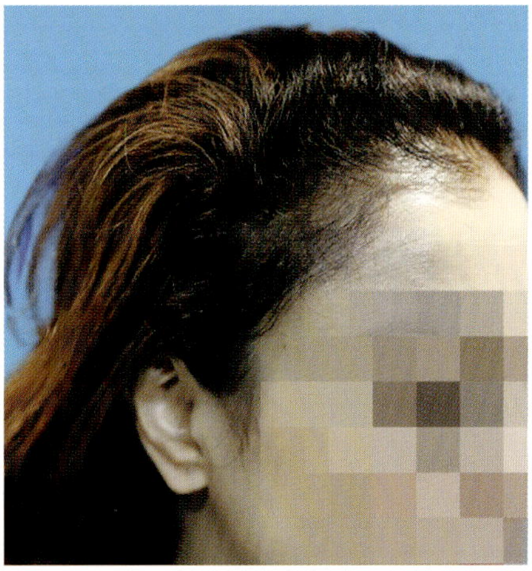

Before

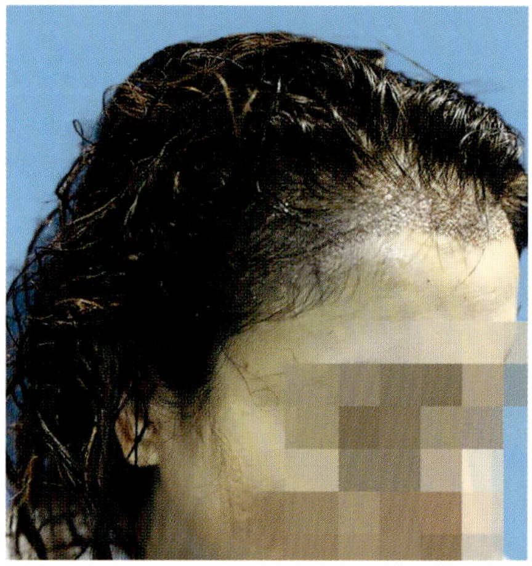

Immediate postoperative

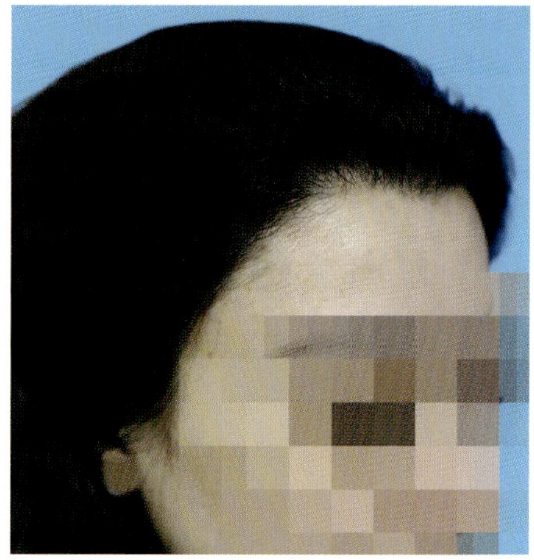

After 6 months

LEFT LATERAL

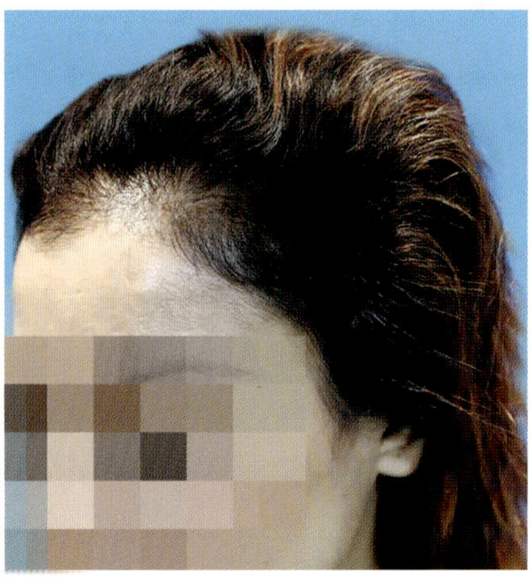

Before

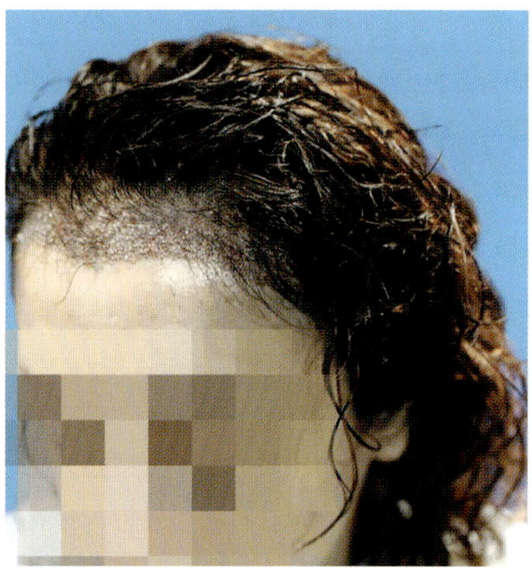

Immediate postoperative

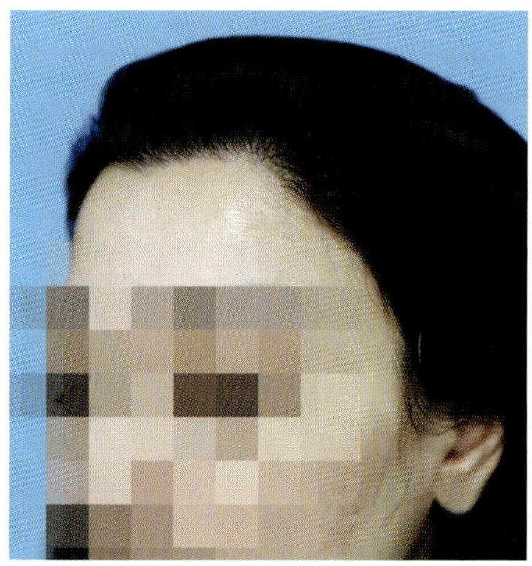

After 6 months

CASE 14

Age	**29 years**
Donor area	**Scalp**
Grafted area	**Front and mid-scalp**
Number of grafts planted	**2815**
Single follicles	**430**

FRONT

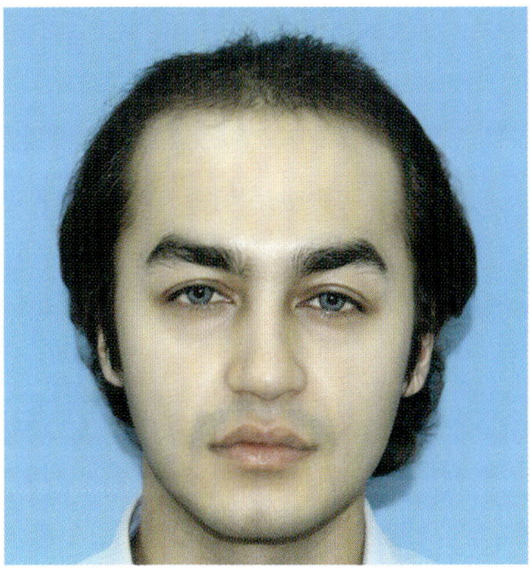

Before

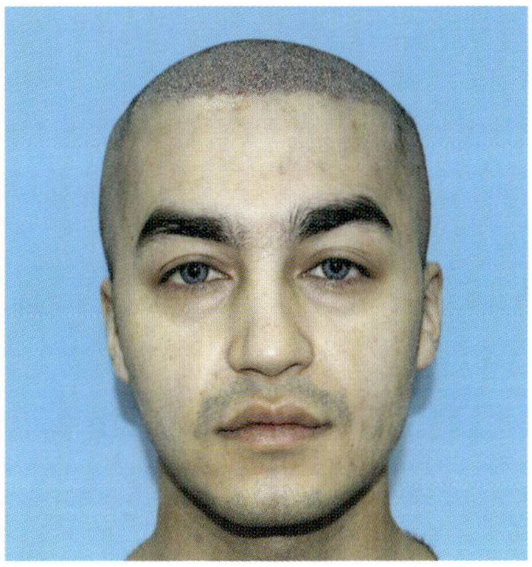

Immediate postoperative

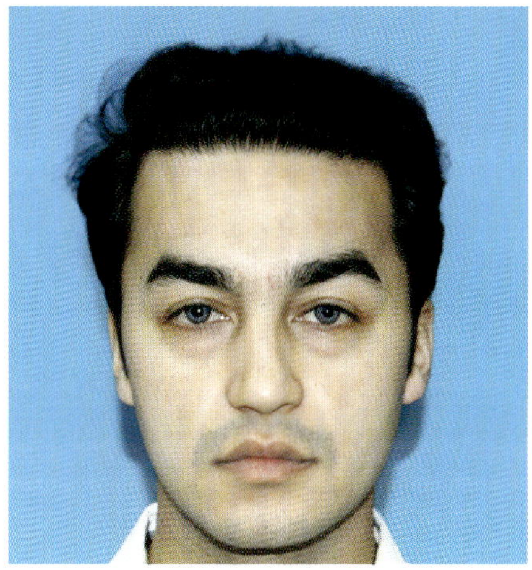

After 10 months

HEAD DOWN

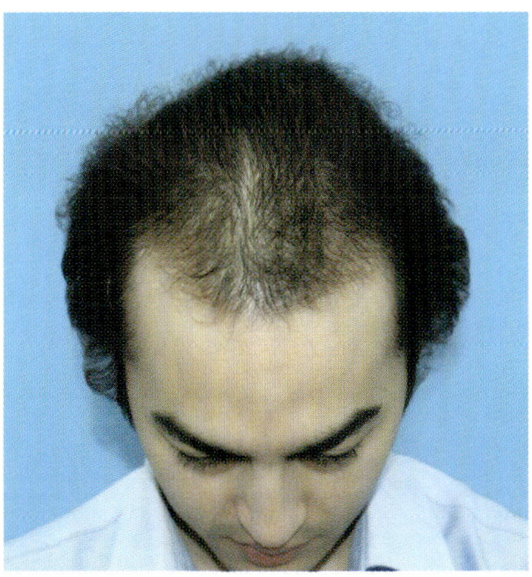

Before

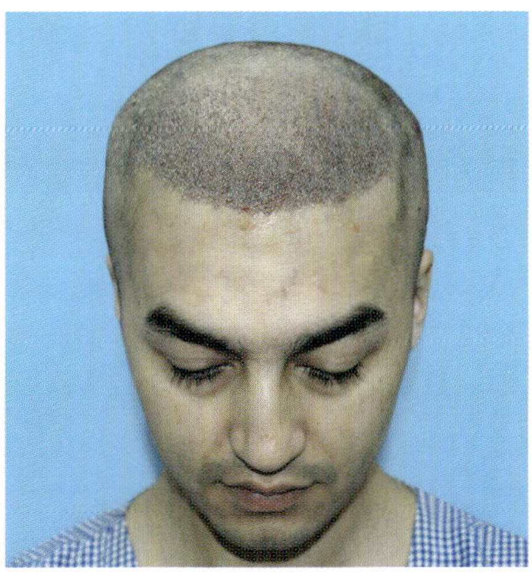

Immediate postoperative

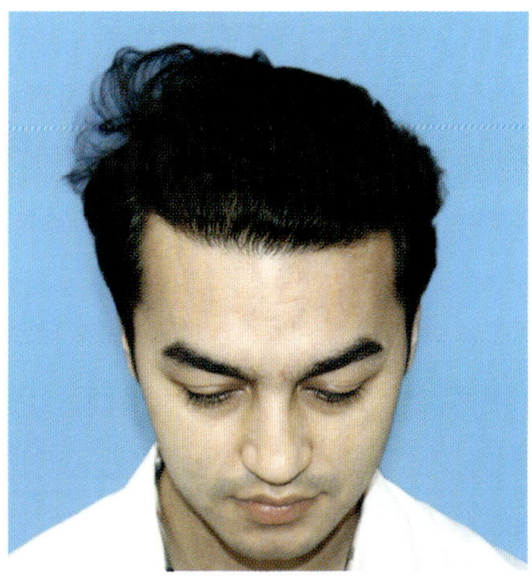

After 10 months

RIGHT LATERAL

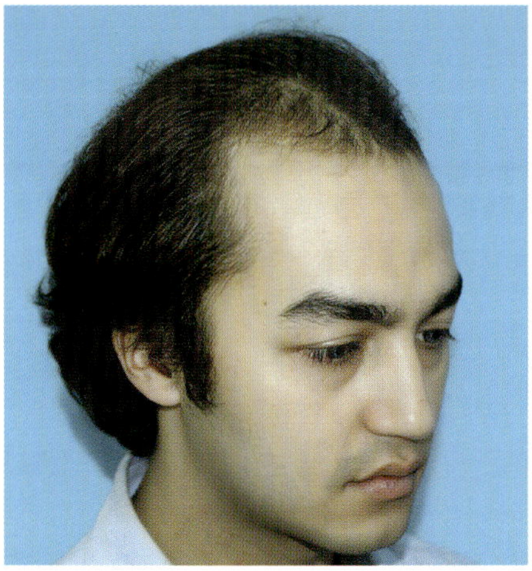

Before

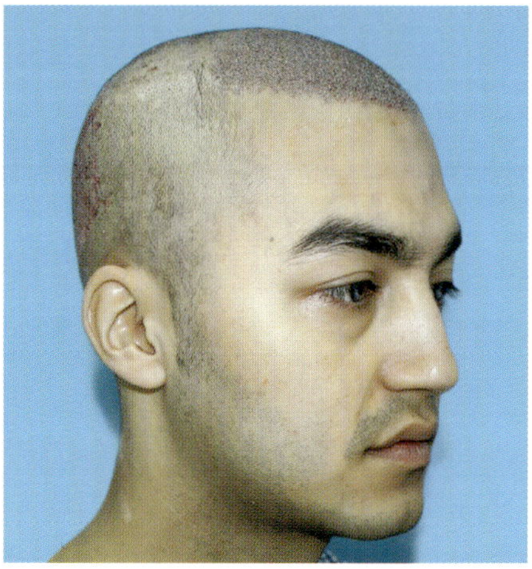

Immediate postoperative

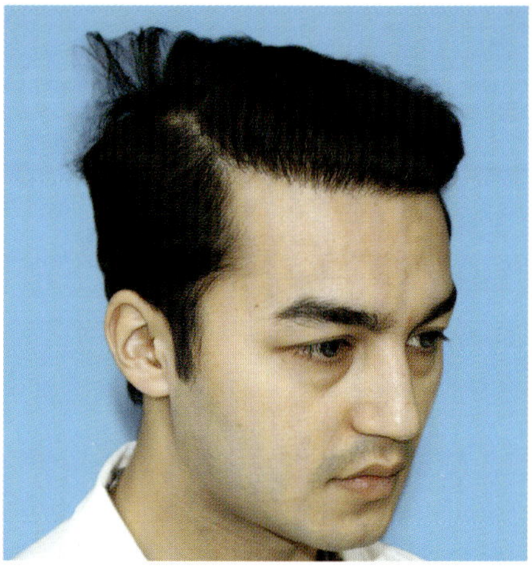

After 10 months

LEFT LATERAL

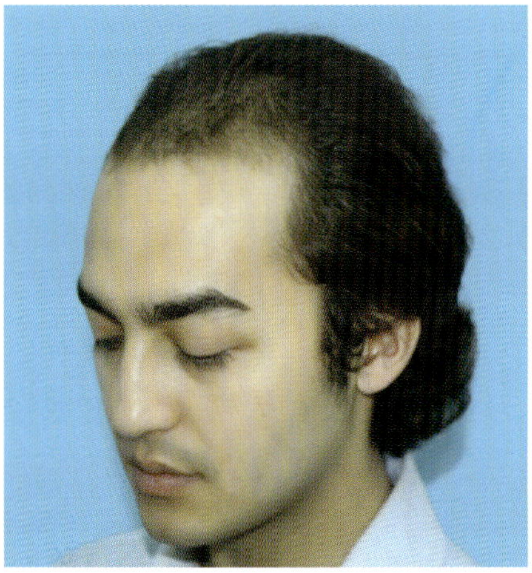

Before

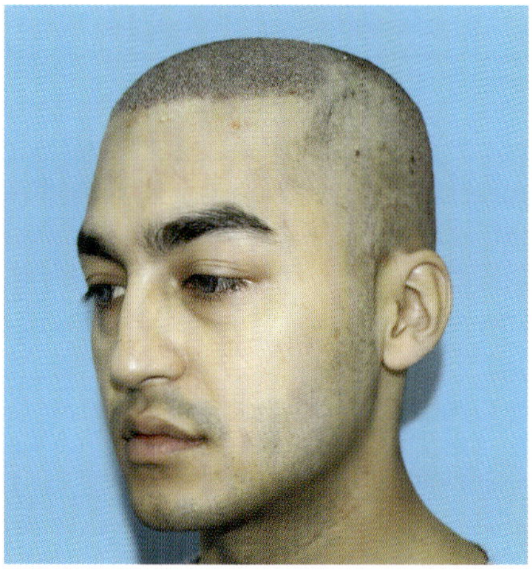

Immediate postoperative

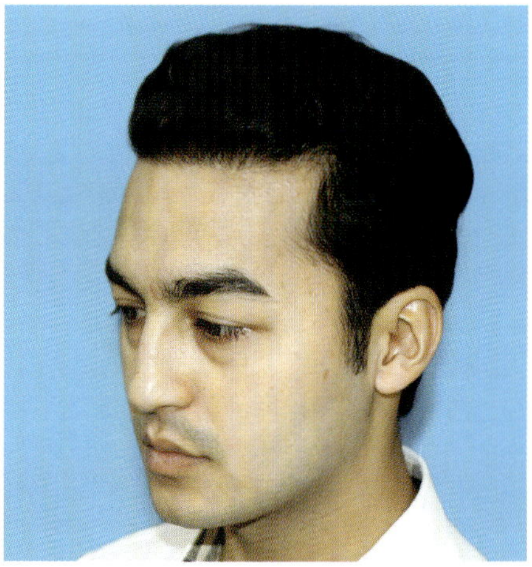

After 10 months

BACK

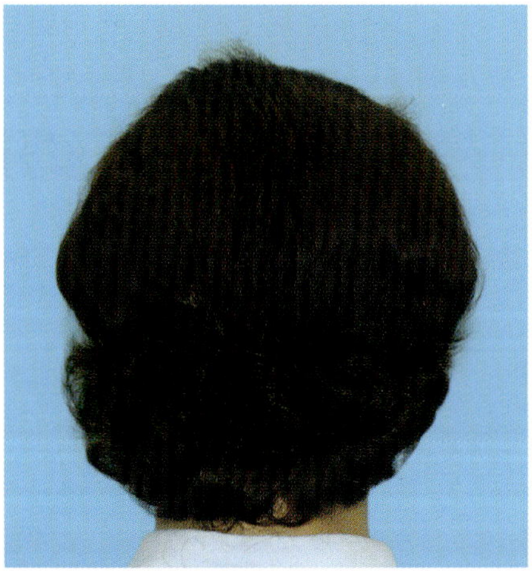

Before

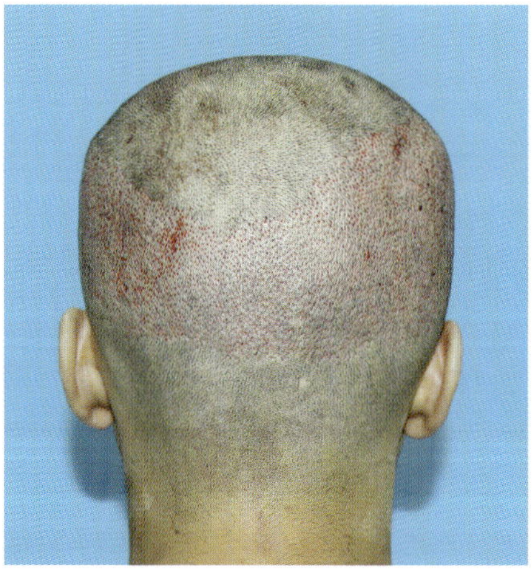

Immediate postoperative

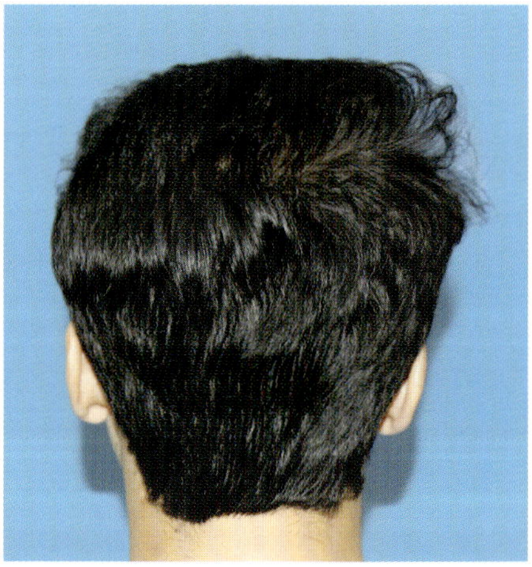

After 10 months

CASE 15

Surgery date	**12-04-2016**
Age	**47 years**
Donor area	**Scalp**
Grafted area	**Front**
Number of grafts planted	**1310**

FRONT

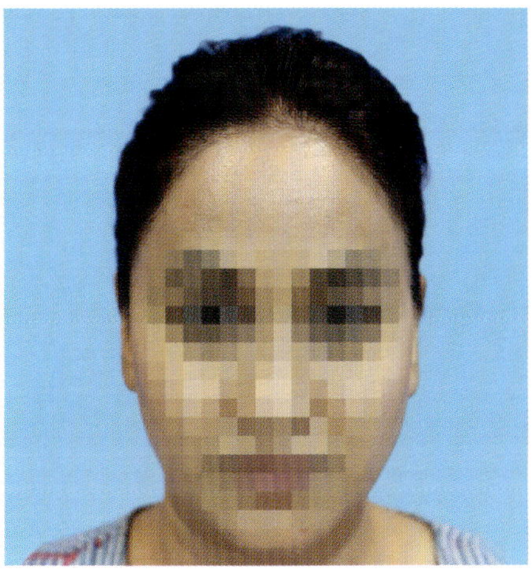

Before

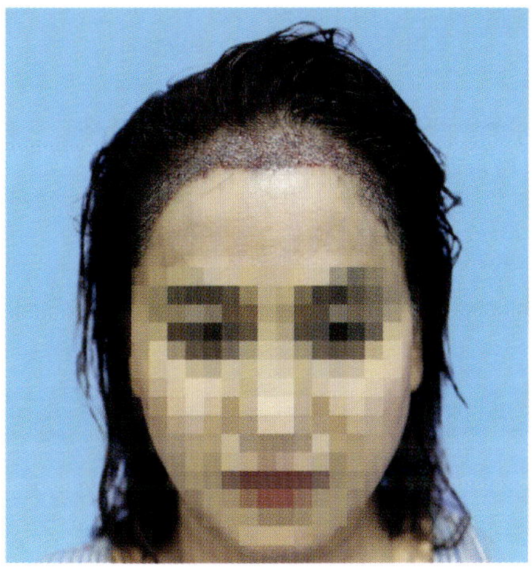

Immediate postoperative

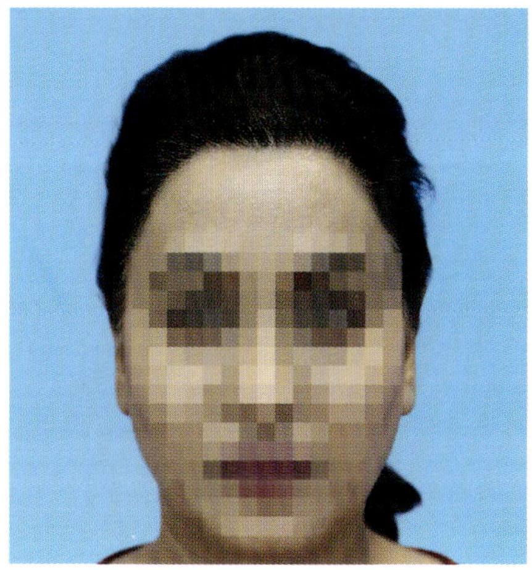

After 4 months

HEAD DOWN

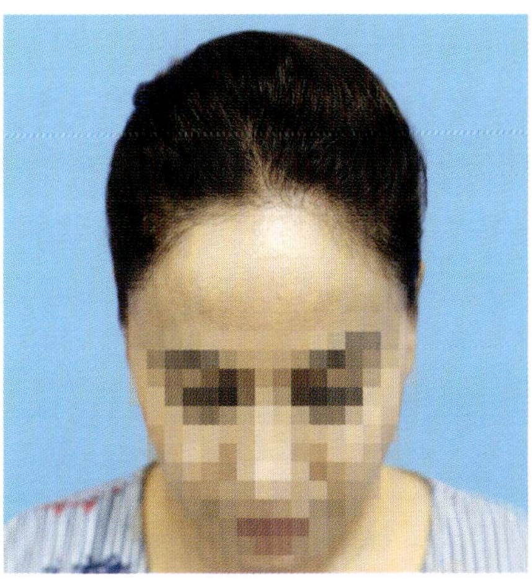

Before

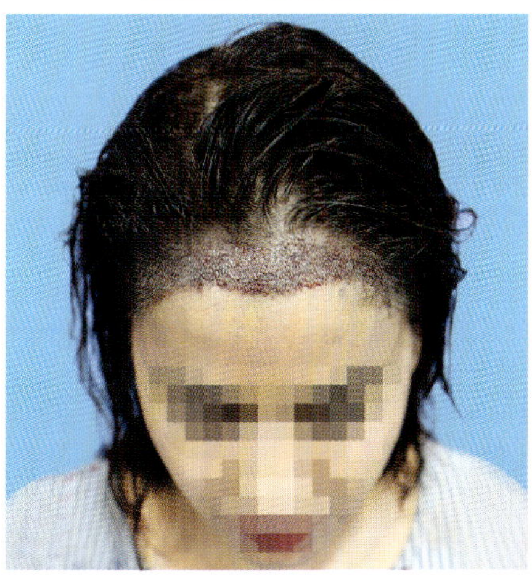

Immediate postoperative

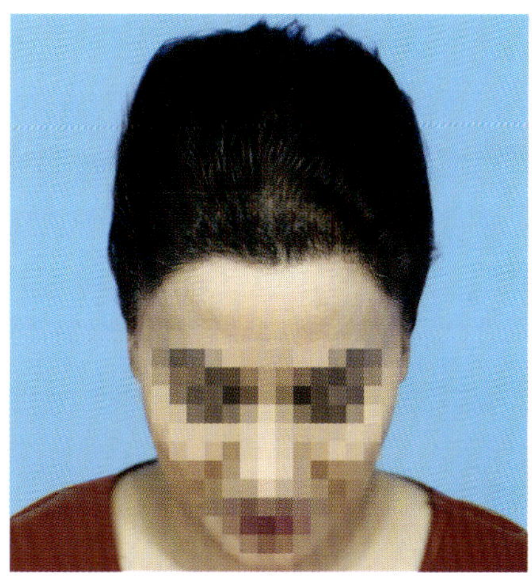

After 4 months

RIGHT LATERAL

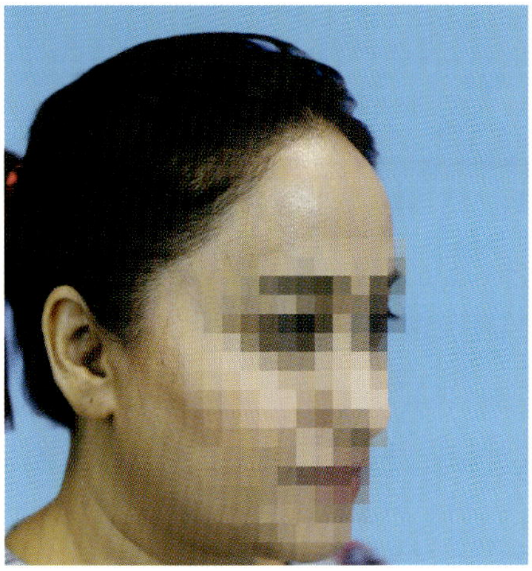

Before

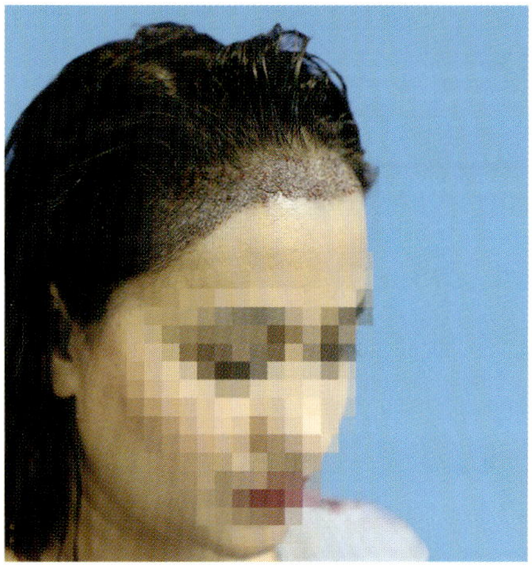

Immediate postoperative

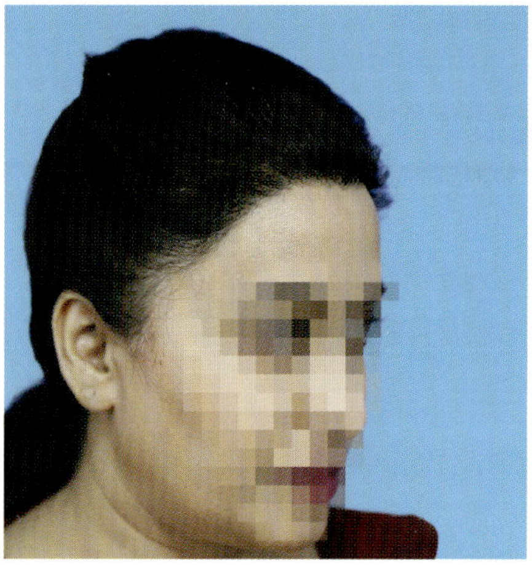

After 4 months

LEFT LATERAL

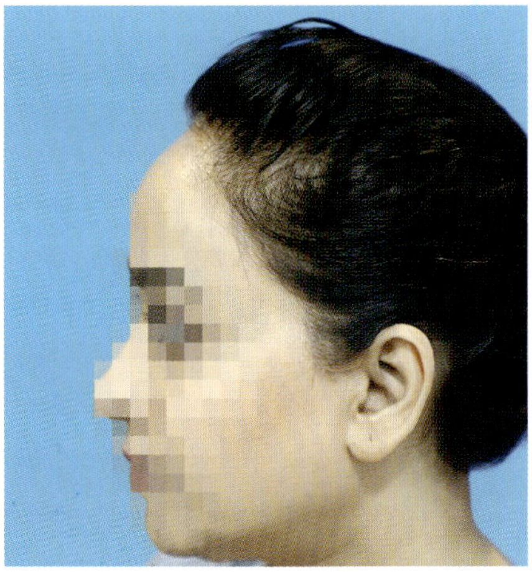

Before

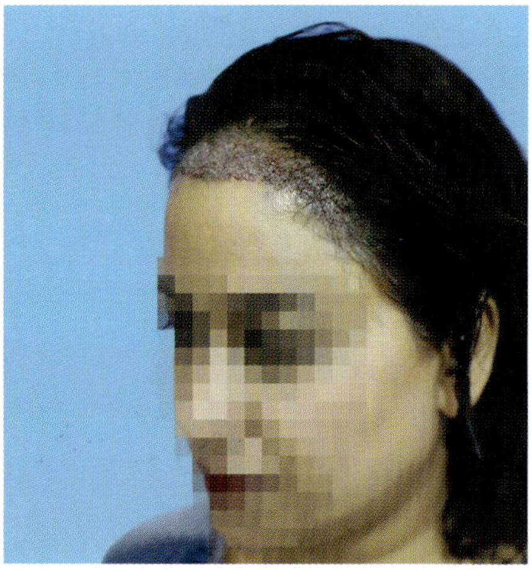

Immediate postoperative

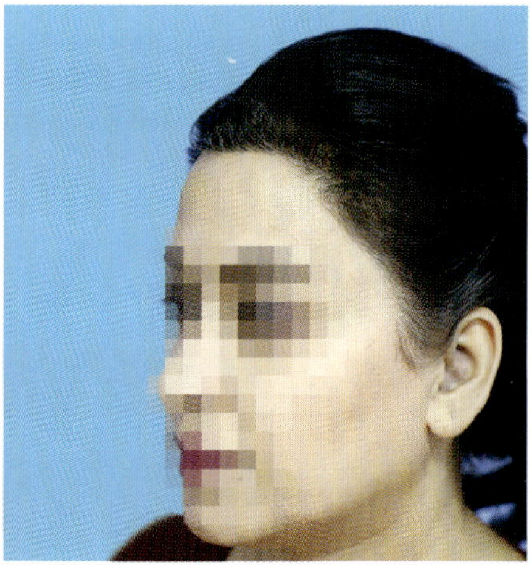

After 4 months

CASE 16

Surgery date	**12-04-2016**
Age	**28 years**
Donor area	**Scalp**
Grafted area	**Front and mid-scalp**
Number of grafts planted	**4000**

FRONT

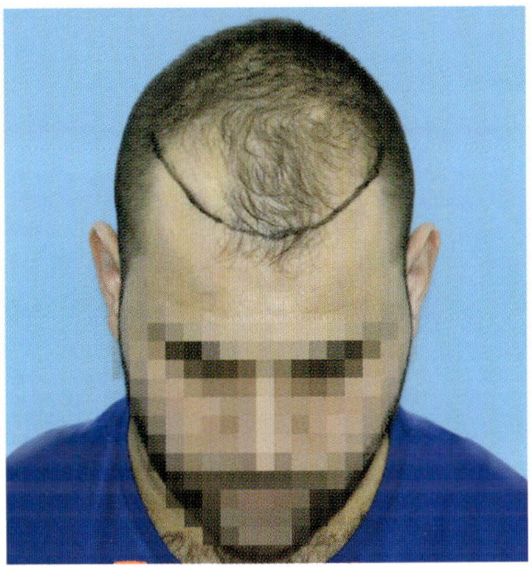

Before

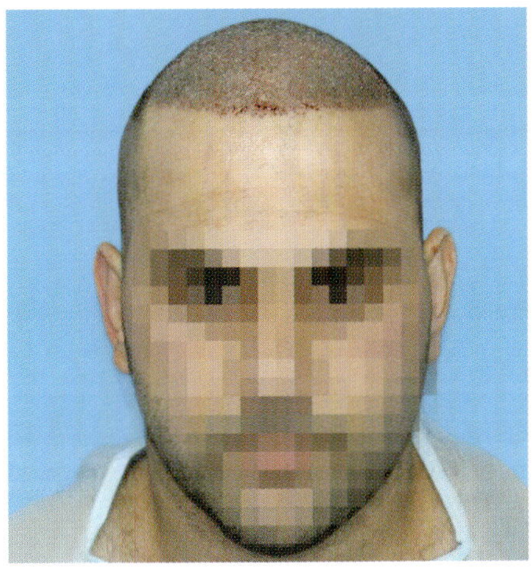

Immediate postoperative

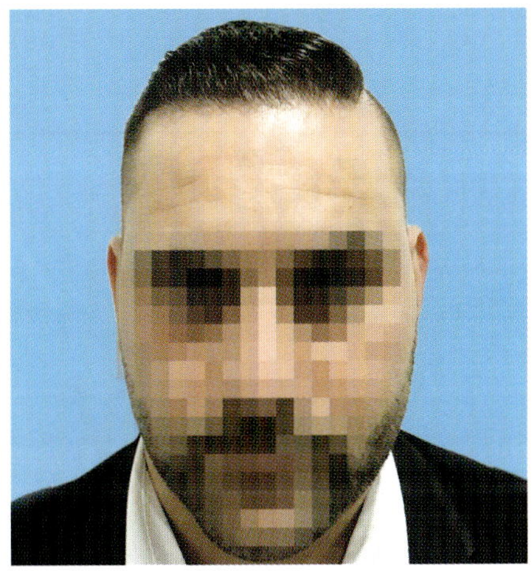

After 14 months

HEAD DOWN

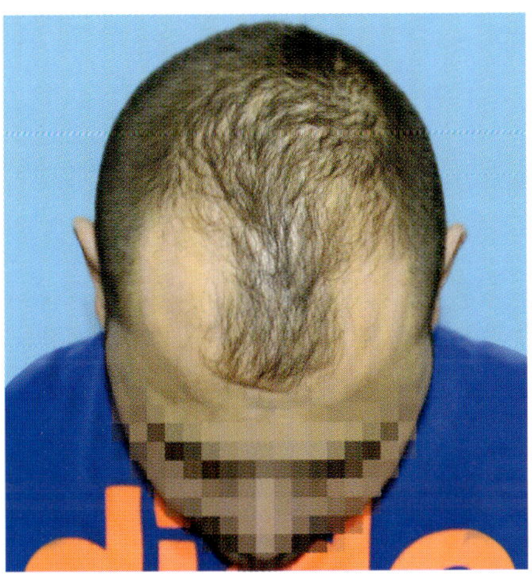

Before

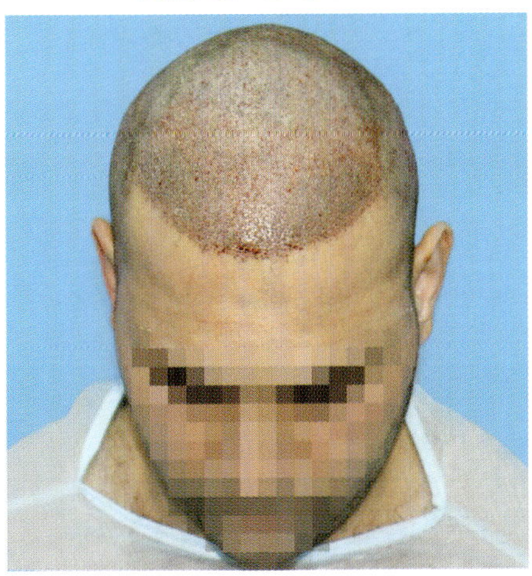

Immediate postoperative

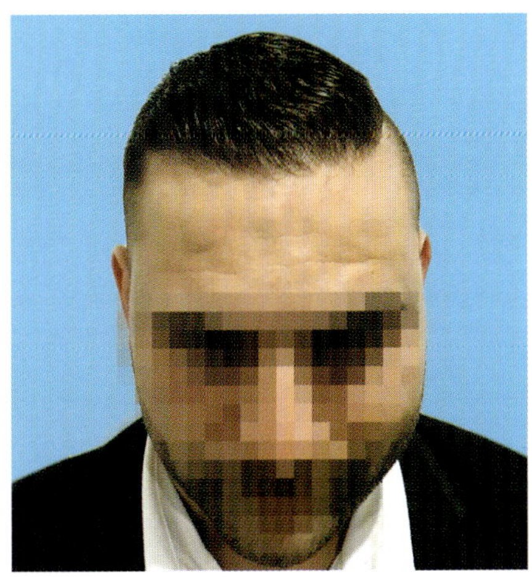

After 14 months

RIGHT LATERAL

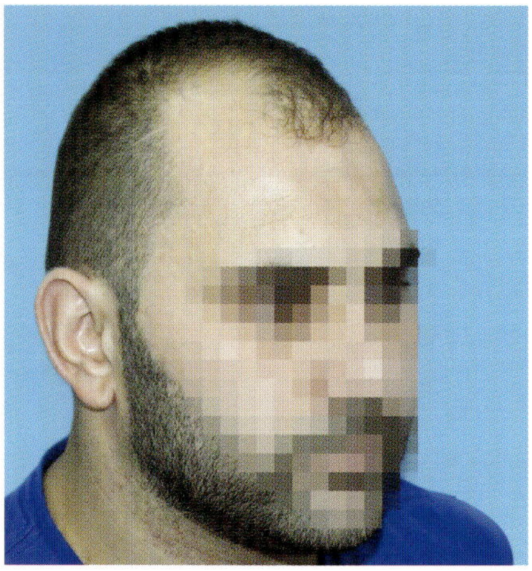
Before

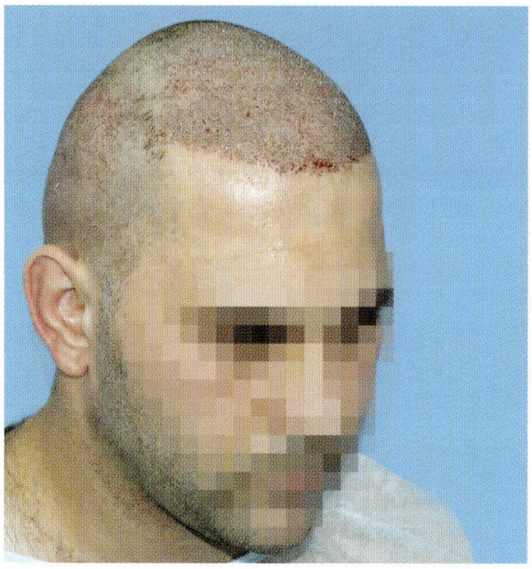
Immediate postoperative

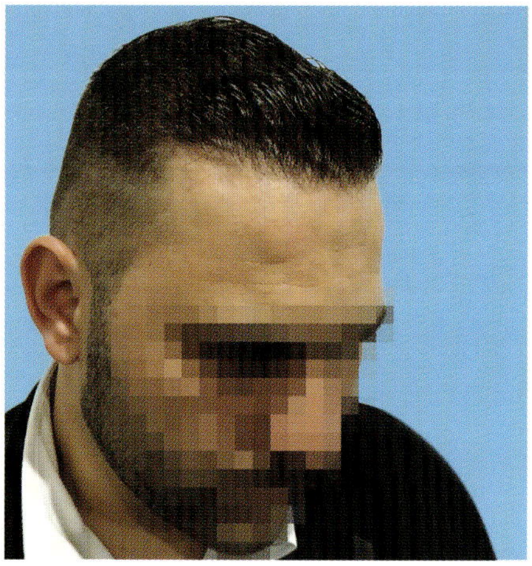
After 14 months

LEFT LATERAL

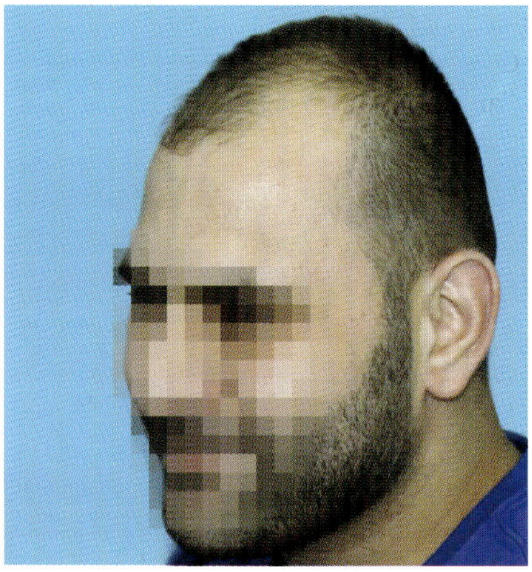
Before

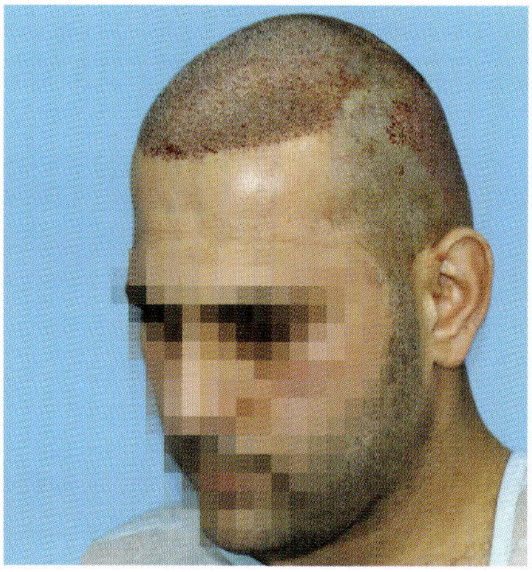
Immediate postoperative

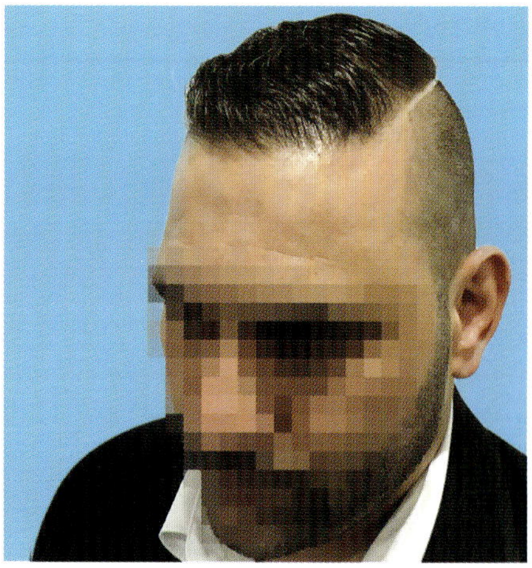
After 14 months

BACK

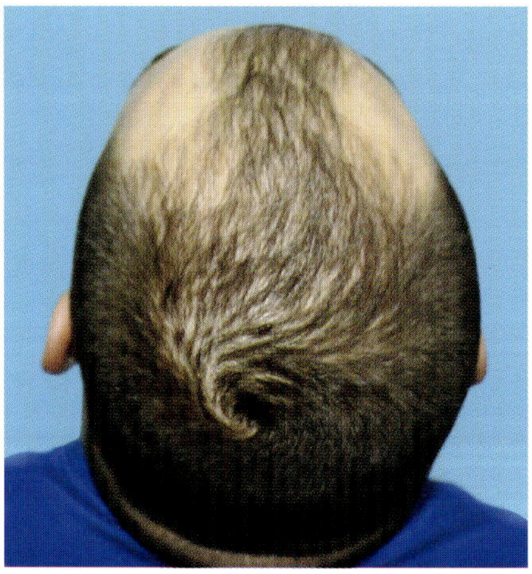
Before

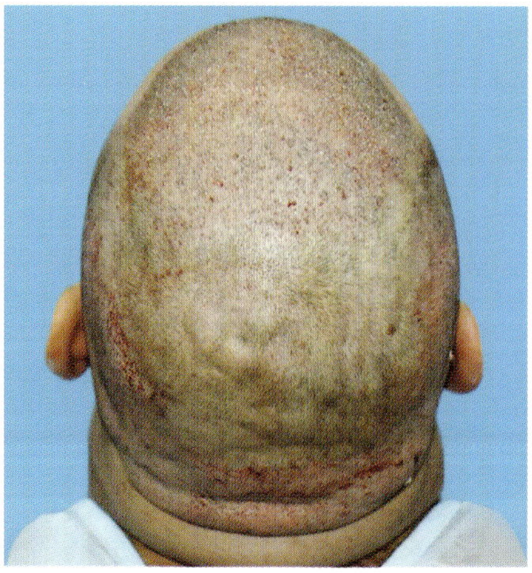
Immediate postoperative

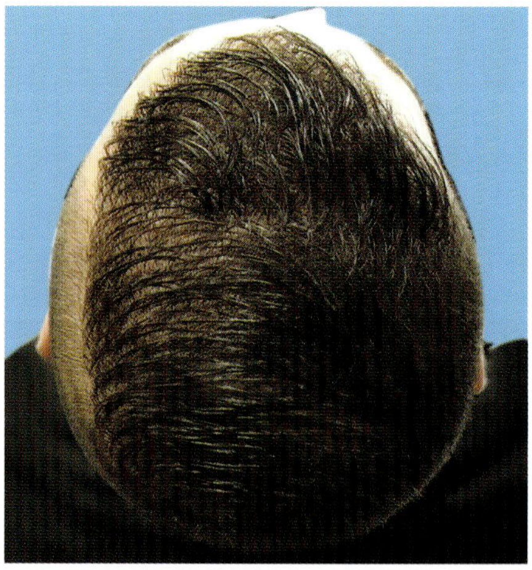
After 14 months

INDEX

Page numbers followed by *f* refer to figure and *t* refer to table.

S

T

V

W

Z